DUTTON'S INTRODUCTORY SKILLS AND PROCEDURES FOR THE PHYSICAL THERAPIST ASSISTANT

DUTTON'S INTRODUCTORY SKILLS AND PROCEDURES FOR THE PHYSICAL THERAPIST ASSISTANT

Mark Dutton, PT

New York   Chicago   San Francisco   Athens   London   Madrid   Mexico City
Milan   New Delhi   Singapore   Sydney   Toronto

Dutton's Introductory Skills and Procedures for the Physical Therapist Assistant

1 2 3 4 5 6 7 8 9   DSS   26 25 24 23 22 21

ISBN 978-1-264-26717-0
MHID 1-264-26717-7

The editors were Michael Weitz and Christina M. Thomas.
The production supervisor was Richard Ruzycka.
Project management was provided by Tasneem Kauser, KnowledgeWorks Global Ltd.
The cover designer was W2 Design.

Library of Congress Cataloging-in-Publication Data

Names: Dutton, Mark, author.
Title: Dutton's introductory skills and procedures for the physical
   therapist / Mark Dutton.
Other titles: Introductory skills and procedures for the physical therapist
Description: New York : McGraw Hill, [2022] | Includes bibliographical references and index. |
   Summary: "This book introduces a conceptual framework about the art of physical
   therapy to give the entry-level physical therapist assistant (PTA) student a broad
   foundation from which to support their journey through a typical curriculum. The
   purpose of this text is to cover the fundamental skills that most PTAs will use for the
   rest of their careers. This text provides a historical perspective on the physical therapy
   profession, an introduction to healthcare policy, and a definition of evidence-informed
   practice, and various chapters describing specific areas of clinical expertise, including how
   to enhance a patient's function in such tasks as bed mobility, transfers, and gait training.
   Chapter 1 provides a historical perspective on the physical therapy profession. Chapter 2
   introduces the reader to essential healthcare policies. Chapter 3 describes the importance
   of evidence-informed practice and clinical decision-making. Chapter 4 outlines clinical
   documentation. With every patient interaction, the clinician should always ensure patient
   and clinician safety. Throughout the remaining chapters, the emphasis is placed on patient
   and clinician safety through correct body mechanics, the application of assistive and safety
   devices, and the effective use of infection control procedures. Chapter 5 helps prepare the
   clinician for patient care. Chapter 6 describes the various methods by which a clinician can
   take a patient's vital signs and the significance of each of these vital signs. Chapter 7 covers
   the various methods to perform bed mobility skills, correctly drape and position a patient.
   Chapter 8 teaches the reader how to perform range of motion assessments and apply range
   of motion techniques as a treatment method. Chapter 9 describes the various methods
   to accurately test the strength of each of the patient's muscles. Chapter 10 describes
   wheelchair mobility skills and the various methods by which the clinician or clinical
   team can transfer a patient from and to various surfaces. Chapter 11 details the various
   components and parameters of gait and how to train a patient to ambulate with or without
   an assistive device. Finally, chapter 12 attempts to put all of the information together by
   providing a patient example"—Provided by publisher.
Identifiers: LCCN 2021019718 (print) | LCCN 2021019719 (ebook) | ISBN
   9781264267170 (paperback) | ISBN 9781264267187 (ebook)
Subjects: MESH: Physical Therapy Specialty | Physical Therapy Modalities |
   Physical Therapist Assistants | Patient Safety
Classification: LCC RM725 (print) | LCC RM725 (ebook) | NLM WB 460 | DDC
   615.8/2—dc23
LC record available at https://lccn.loc.gov/2021019718
LC ebook record available at https://lccn.loc.gov/2021019719

McGraw Hill books are available at special quantity discounts to use as premiums and sales promotions, or for use in corporate training programs. To contact a representative please visit the Contact Us pages at www.mhprofessional.com.

Contents

Acknowledgments

Any work, however enjoyable, takes time away from family members and friends. I would thus like to take this opportunity to thank the following:

▶ My family, especially my daughters Leah and Lauren.

▶ My parents.

▶ The exceptional team at McGraw Hill—Michael Weitz and Christina Thomas.

▶ To the production crew of KnowledgeWorks Global Ltd., especially the Project Coordinator, Tasneem Kauser.

Introduction

This book introduces a conceptual framework about the art of physical therapy to give the entry-level physical therapist assistant (PTA) student a broad foundation from which to support their journey through a typical curriculum. The purpose of this text is to cover the fundamental skills that most PTAs will use for the rest of their careers.

This text provides a historical perspective on the physical therapy profession, an introduction to healthcare policy, and a definition of evidence-informed practice, and various chapters describing specific areas of clinical expertise, including how to enhance a patient's function in such tasks as bed mobility, transfers, and gait training.

Chapter 1 provides a historical perspective on the physical therapy profession.

Chapter 2 introduces the reader to essential healthcare policies.

Chapter 3 describes the importance of evidence-informed practice and clinical decision-making.

Chapter 4 outlines clinical documentation.

With every patient interaction, the clinician should always ensure patient and clinician safety. Throughout the remaining chapters, the emphasis is placed on patient and clinician safety through correct body mechanics, the application of assistive and safety devices, and the effective use of infection control procedures.

Chapter 5 helps prepare the clinician for patient care.

Chapter 6 describes the various methods by which a clinician can take a patient's vital signs and the significance of each of these vital signs.

Chapter 7 covers the various methods to perform bed mobility skills, and correctly drape and position a patient.

Chapter 8 teaches the reader how to perform range of motion assessments and apply range of motion techniques as a treatment method.

Chapter 9 describes the various methods to accurately test the strength of each of the patient's muscles.

Chapter 10 describes wheelchair mobility skills and the various methods by which the clinician or clinical team can transfer a patient to and from various surfaces.

Chapter 11 details the various components and parameters of gait and how to train a patient to ambulate with or without an assistive device.

Finally, Chapter 12 attempts to put all of the information together by providing a patient example.

CHAPTER 1

The Physical Therapy Profession

After this chapter, the reader will be able to:

1. Define physical therapy
2. Give a historical perspective of how the role of a physical therapist assistant (PTA) has changed over the years
3. Name some of the pioneers who played a significant role in the development of today's physical therapy profession
4. Describe how the name of the American Physical Therapy Association (APTA) was derived
5. Describe how social change affected the growth of physical therapy in the United States
6. Discuss the purposes of having a code of ethics for a profession
7. Describe the differences between morals and ethics
8. Have a good understanding of the APTA policies that address practice standards, ethical conduct, and professionalism
9. Describe the various members of the healthcare team
10. Describe the different physical therapy practice settings
11. Describe some of the challenges faced by healthcare workers

OVERVIEW

The American Physical Therapy Association (APTA) is the national organization that represents the physical therapist (PT) and the physical therapist assistant (PTA). It currently has a national office in Alexandria, Virginia, and a chapter office in almost every state. APTA membership for PTs, PTAs, and their respective student categories is voluntary and not mandatory for licensure. Several APTA publications, including *The Guide to Physical Therapist Practice 3.0* ("the Guide")[1] and a monthly journal aptly named *Physical Therapy*, guide the physical therapy profession.

The House of Delegates (HOD), composed of voting delegates from all chapters and nonvoting delegates from each section, is the APTA's policymaking body. The HOD works closely with the Board of Directors (BOD), the latter of which consists of six APTA officers and nine directors, to establish the APTA's policies and directives.

CLINICAL PEARL

The organizational structure of the APTA consists of four main levels:

▶ *District*: Although not located in all jurisdictions, a district represents the APTA at the local level.
▶ *Chapter*: There is a chapter in each state and the District of Columbia, and each has proportional representation at the national level. Each chapter requires dues from PT and PTA members.
▶ *Section*: Each of the 18 sections provides members with similar areas of interest to interact with each other. The various sections meet annually at the Combined Sections Meeting (CSM) in early February.
▶ *Assembly*: Members of an assembly belong to the same class (category) and can exist at the state and national levels.

PTAs are healthcare professionals who help maintain, restore, and improve movement, activity, and health, enabling an individual to have optimal functioning and quality of life while ensuring patient safety and applying evidence to provide efficient and effective care. PTAs are involved in promoting health, wellness, and fitness by implementing services to reduce risk, slow the progression of or prevent functional decline and disability, and enhance participation in chosen life situations.[1] The Guide, which outlines the roles of PTs and PTAs across a broad range of settings and practice opportunities, has defined physical therapy as follows[1]:

> Physical therapy is a dynamic profession with an established theoretical and scientific base and widespread clinical applications in the restoration, maintenance, and promotion of optimal physical function. Physical therapy services prevent, minimize, or eliminate impairments of body functions and structures, activity limitations, and participation restrictions.

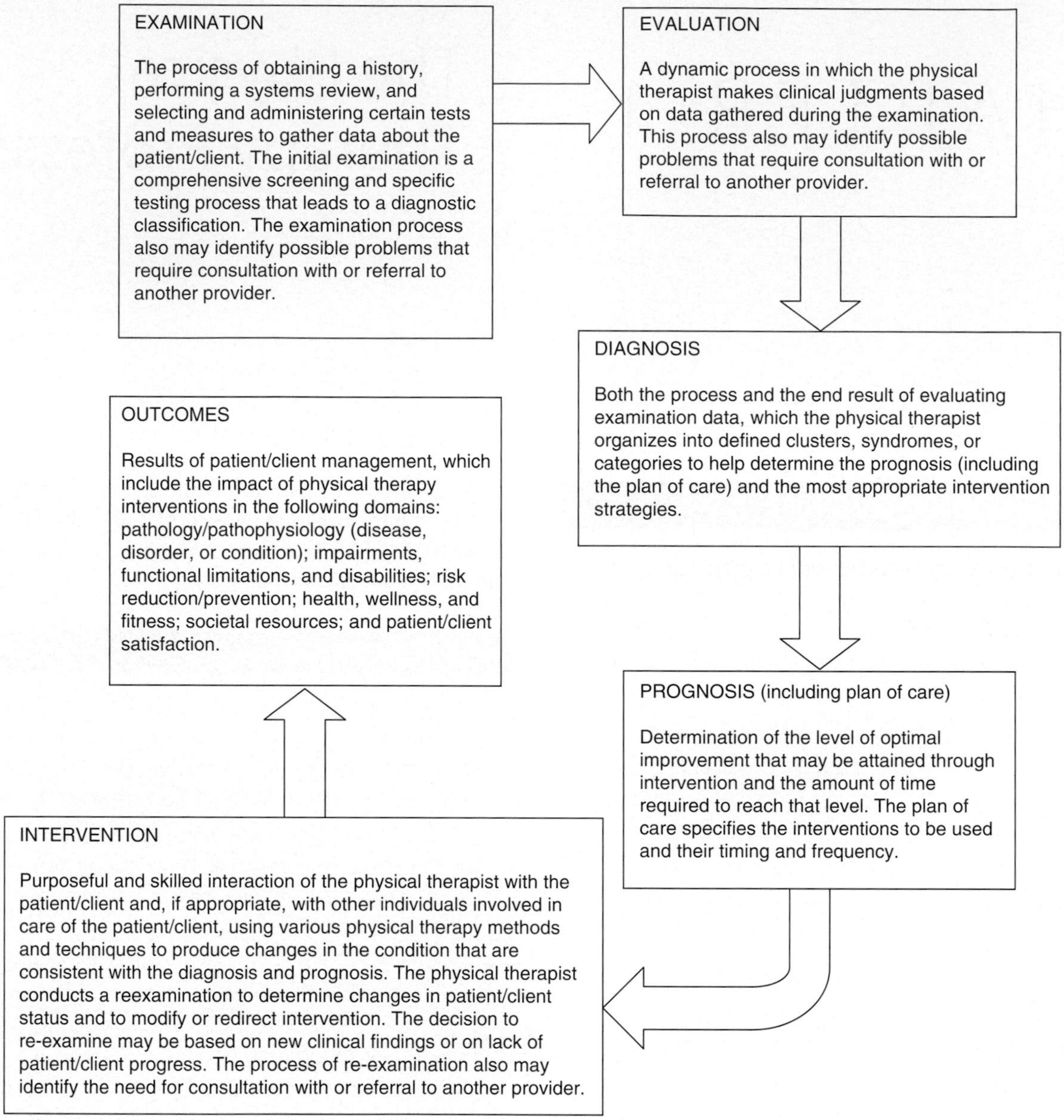

EXAMINATION

The process of obtaining a history, performing a systems review, and selecting and administering certain tests and measures to gather data about the patient/client. The initial examination is a comprehensive screening and specific testing process that leads to a diagnostic classification. The examination process also may identify possible problems that require consultation with or referral to another provider.

EVALUATION

A dynamic process in which the physical therapist makes clinical judgments based on data gathered during the examination. This process also may identify possible problems that require consultation with or referral to another provider.

OUTCOMES

Results of patient/client management, which include the impact of physical therapy interventions in the following domains: pathology/pathophysiology (disease, disorder, or condition); impairments, functional limitations, and disabilities; risk reduction/prevention; health, wellness, and fitness; societal resources; and patient/client satisfaction.

DIAGNOSIS

Both the process and the end result of evaluating examination data, which the physical therapist organizes into defined clusters, syndromes, or categories to help determine the prognosis (including the plan of care) and the most appropriate intervention strategies.

PROGNOSIS (including plan of care)

Determination of the level of optimal improvement that may be attained through intervention and the amount of time required to reach that level. The plan of care specifies the interventions to be used and their timing and frequency.

INTERVENTION

Purposeful and skilled interaction of the physical therapist with the patient/client and, if appropriate, with other individuals involved in care of the patient/client, using various physical therapy methods and techniques to produce changes in the condition that are consistent with the diagnosis and prognosis. The physical therapist conducts a reexamination to determine changes in patient/client status and to modify or redirect intervention. The decision to re-examine may be based on new clinical findings or on lack of patient/client progress. The process of re-examination also may identify the need for consultation with or referral to another provider.

FIGURE 1-1 The six elements of physical therapy patient/client management. (Reproduced with permission from Dutton M: Introduction to Physical Therapy and Patient Skills, 2nd ed. New York, NY: McGraw Hill; 2014.)

The Guide, together with the Standards of Ethical Conduct of the Physical Therapist Assistant, another document provided by the APTA, outlines the PTA's role (Appendix A). The Guide[1] describes six elements of the physical therapy patient/client management (Figure 1-1). The only one of the six elements that may be delegated to a qualified PTA is the intervention—the purposeful and skilled interaction of the PTA using various physical therapy methods and techniques to produce changes in the condition consistent with the diagnosis and prognosis.[1] The PTA cannot evaluate, reevaluate, or discharge a patient. However, the PTA can perform most tests and measures related to the intervention in a continuous data collection process. Thus, the PTA reviews the initial documentation, including the plan of care (POC), notes which interventions to use during the first and ensuing treatment sessions, and effectively arranges those interventions within each session while using suitable tests and measures to measure the patient's progress toward the goals while monitoring any patient response to the interventions used. Some of this data is then documented according to facility policy and/or provided orally to the supervising PT.

In addition to providing habilation and rehabilitation services and prevention and risk reduction services, PTAs also collaborate with other healthcare professionals to address patient needs, increase communication, and provide efficient and effective care. PTAs also provide education, research, and administration services across healthcare settings.

As we move forward in the twenty-first century, the practice of physical therapy continues to evolve. Many of the challenges facing today's PTA are due to an increased prevalence of certain contemporary lifestyle conditions. These include hypertension, obesity, diabetes, ischemic heart disease, cerebrovascular accidents, and smoking-related diseases. In addition to having a primary focus on rehabilitating those individuals with impairments and dysfunction, today's PTAs are becoming more involved in multipronged strategies to help reduce or prevent poor lifestyle choices. The evolution of the PTA can best be appreciated from a historical perspective.

HISTORICAL PERSPECTIVE

Descriptions of the early years of the United States' physical therapy profession began at the beginning of the twentieth century. Much of the impetus behind the profession during these times resulted from the high incidence of acute anterior poliomyelitis, referred to as infantile paralysis, which occurred in 1916 (Figure 1-2) in areas of Louisiana, Boston, and New York.[2] Rehabilitation medicine became involved with polio first when orthopedic surgeons adopted what they referred to as aftercare rehabilitation programs for the children and adults affected. The best known of these programs, led by Robert Lovett, a professor of orthopedic surgery at Harvard, and Wilhelmine Wright, a PT, was a statewide program that came to be known as the Vermont Plan. Wilhelmine Wright developed the training technique of ambulation with crutches for patients with paraplegia or paralysis caused by polio. She also introduced manual muscle testing concepts in physical therapy, which appeared in a book called *Muscle Function*.

Dr. Lovett discovered that muscle training exercises were the most important early therapeutic measures for polio treatment and organized teams of workers, including physicians, nurses, and other nonphysician personnel, to provide interventions. The nonphysician personnel included three individuals—Wilhelmine Wright, Janet Merrill, and Alice Lou Plastridge—who received special training in massage, muscle training, and corrective exercises from Dr. Lovett.

The United States entered World War I by declaring war on Germany in 1917, and the Army recognized the need to rehabilitate soldiers injured in the war.[3] This caused a change in focus on using multiple and combined methods to restore physical function in the military forces and the civilian workforce under the umbrella term *physical reconstruction*. Physical reconstruction was defined as the "maximum mental and physical restoration of the individuals achieved by the use of medicine and surgery, supplemented by physical therapy, occupational therapy or curative workshop activities, education, recreation, and vocational training." Many of the exercises used were based on Pehr Henrik Ling's Swedish exercise/gymnastics

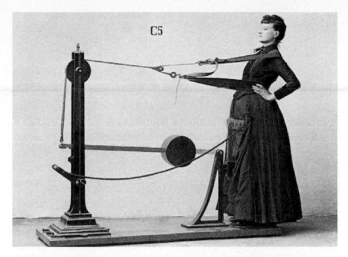

FIGURE 1-3 Exercises using machines.

and Dr. Jonas Gustaf Wilhelm Zander's exercise machines (Figure 1-3) (see Box 1-1). These exercise-based approaches and their subsequent outcomes began to change the belief that disability was irreversible.

CLINICAL PEARL

► Physical therapy practice in the United States evolved around two major historical events: the poliomyelitis epidemics of the 1800s through the 1950s and the effects of several wars, including World War I, World War II, and the Korean conflict.

► Historically, physical therapy emerged as a profession within the medical model, not as an alternative to medical care.[4]

A report from the Division of Orthopedic Surgery of the Army Medical Department suggested that the US medical schools develop the standards, and in 1917, a special unit of the Army Medical Department, the Division of Special Hospitals and Physical Reconstruction, developed 15 "reconstruction aide" training programs to respond to the need for medical workers with expertise in rehabilitation to treat the more than 200,000 US troops wounded in battle (Figure 1-4). Individuals who completed the courses and who worked in the Division of Special Hospitals and Physical Reconstruction in the Office of the Surgeon General, US Army, were given the title Reconstruction Aide (those practitioners rendering similar service in civilian facilities were referred to as physical therapy technicians, physiotherapy aides, and physiotherapy technicians).

By 1918, outlines for a 3-month course to be used in training programs had been developed to prepare practitioners who would serve, in a civilian capacity, as reconstruction aides in the recently established Division of Special Hospitals and Physical Reconstruction.

As World War I drew to a close, physical reconstruction practices, which had previously been directed toward preserving, restoring, and maintaining a fighting force, were directed toward preserving and maintaining a working force.

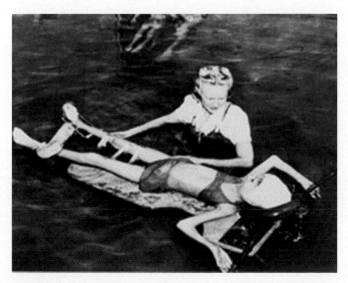

FIGURE 1-2 Early treatment approach to poliomyelitis.

Box 1-1

- ▶ Approximately 1000 CE: Taoist priests in China describe a type of exercise, which involves body positioning and breathing routines to relieve pain and other symptoms.

- ▶ Approximately 500 CE: A Greek physician called Herodicas gives written descriptions about an elaborate exercise system called Ars Gymnastica, which consisted of various gymnastic exercises.

- ▶ Approximately 400 CE: Hippocrates, considered the father of medicine, recommends using muscle strengthening exercises, an early form of transverse friction massage, and therapeutic massage. Hippocrates was also the first to use electrical stimulation.

- ▶ Approximately 180 CE: The ancient Romans introduce a series of therapeutic exercises that they call gymnastics.

- ▶ Approximately 200 BCE: Galen, a renowned physician of ancient Rome, emphasizes the importance of moderate exercise to strengthen the body, increase body temperature, allow the pores of the skin to open, and improve a person's spiritual well-being.

- ▶ Approximately 1400 BCE: Therapeutic exercises are introduced into schools as physical education courses.

- ▶ Approximately 1500 BCE: The first printed book on exercise is published in Spain.

- ▶ Approximately 1700 BCE: Mass hydrotherapy and exercises are first introduced in the United States.

- ▶ 1723 BCE: Nicholas Andry, considered the grandfather of orthopedics, emphasizes the importance of exercise to cure many infirmities of the body.

- ▶ Mid-1700s BCE: Exercise equipment appears on the market.

- ▶ 1800s BCE: Introduction of Swedish exercise/gymnastics by Pehr Henrik Ling. Dr. Johann Georg Mezger adapts these exercises and introduces the terms *effleurage*, *petrissage*, and *tapotement*, known as Swedish massage. In 1864, Gustav Zander introduces 71 different types of apparatus to assist in the performance of Swedish exercise/gymnastics and opens numerous Zander institutes throughout Europe and the United States. At the end of the 1800s, H.S. Frenkel introduces a series of neurological exercises and rehabilitation techniques to enhance coordination and gait in those patients with ataxia resulting from nerve cell destruction. Frenkel's exercises continue to be used today.

CLINICAL PEARL

The American Women's Physical Therapeutics Association (AWPTA) was founded in 1921.[5] Mary McMillan, trained in England and credited as the first PT in the United States, was elected the first president of the AWPTA by a mail-in vote. The first issue of the association's official publication, *The PT Review,* appeared on March 1, 1921. Today, the *PT Review* is called *Physical Therapy* and is the official publication of the APTA. From 1929 until 1933, an American Physical Therapy Association existed as an organization formed through two physician organizations, the Western Association of Physical Therapy and the American Electrotherapeutic Association. In 1922, at its first conference, the name of the AWPTA was changed to the American Physiotherapy Association (APA)[5] in recognition of the fact that men also practiced physiotherapy, and subsequently, in 1947, to its current name, the American Physical Therapy Association (APTA).[6]

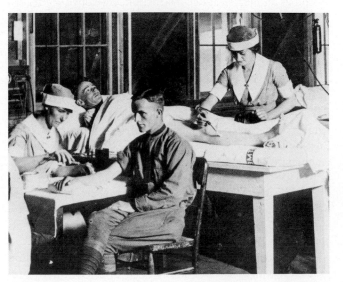

FIGURE 1-4 Rehabilitation of US troops wounded in battle. (U.S. Army Photo. Courtesy of the American Physical Therapy Association)

In 1921, Mary McMillan (Figure 1-5) published *Massage and Therapeutic Exercise* (Figure 1-6), the first textbook written by a physiotherapist.[7] McMillan referred to four distinct branches in physical therapeutics: hydrotherapy (Figure 1-7), massage, therapeutic exercise, and electrotherapy.

CLINICAL PEARL

Today, the APTA is the one national organization recognized as speaking for the profession of physical therapy. The association's members are PTs, PTAs, and students who voluntarily join. To join the APTA, an individual must be accepted, currently enrolled, or a graduate of an accredited PT or PTA program.

In 1925, a group of physical therapy physicians founded the American College of Physical Therapy (ACPT) and then established the American Registry of Physical Therapy Technicians to bestow a registered title on physiotherapists who

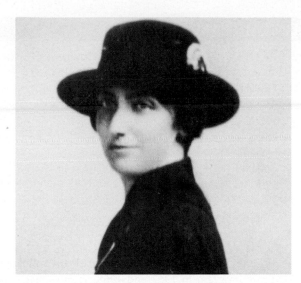

FIGURE 1-5 Mary McMillan. (Courtesy of the American Physical Therapy Association)

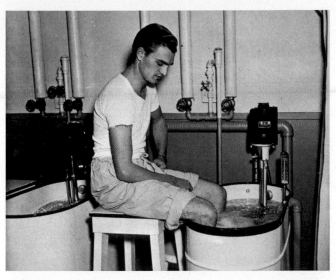

FIGURE 1-7 Hydrotherapy. (Reproduced with permission from Dutton M: Introduction to Physical Therapy and Patient Skills, 2nd ed. New York, NY: McGraw Hill; 2014.)

passed the test.[7] Under this plan, registered physiotherapists remained technicians under the supervision of physicians.[7] Later that year, the ACPT joined the American Medical Association (AMA) and changed its name to the American Congress of Physical Therapy. By 1937, physical therapy physicians had achieved recognition as a medical specialty. At that time, to further distinguish themselves from physiotherapists and gain respect within the medical profession, the physical therapy physicians began to call themselves "physiatrists."[7] The AMA became concerned that the public might consider physiotherapists to be physicians. This concern led to a name change from *physiotherapists* to *physical therapists* in the early 1940s.

The advent of World War II resulted in an ever-increasing demand for physical therapy specialists. During this time, drastic improvements in medical management and surgical techniques led to growing numbers of survivors, albeit with disabling war wounds.[8] Wounded veterans who returned home with amputations, burns, cold injuries, wounds, fractures, and nerve and spinal cord injuries required the attention of physical therapists in the first half of the 1940s, with World War II at its peak.[9] The subsequent demand for specialized techniques propelled physical therapy practice through a major growth period as the attention switched to a focus on applying neurophysiologic principles, which prompted the advent of some techniques still used today, including progressive resistive exercise (PRE).

In 1945, Thomas DeLorme, a physician, first introduced the concept of PREs after using increasing resistance on himself following knee surgery.

The passage of the Hospital Survey and Construction Act of 1946, also known as the Hill-Burton Act, initiated a nationwide hospital-building program and increased public access to hospitals and healthcare facilities, which in turn led to an increase in hospital-based practice for physical therapists.

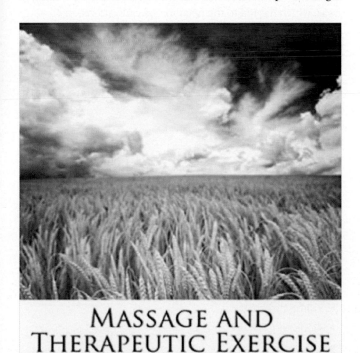

FIGURE 1-6 *Massage and Therapeutic Exercise*, the first textbook written by a physiotherapist (*Massage and Therapeutic Exercise*).

CLINICAL PEARL

After World War II, many patients who had sustained brain injuries sought the services of physical therapists. Signe Brunnström, a Swedish physical therapist, documented new approaches for assessing and treating individuals with cerebrovascular accidents (CVAs) and, after observing thousands of patients, delineated stroke recovery stages.[10] Also, during this time, Berta Bobath and Dr. Karl Bobath began to develop their reflex-inhibiting postures for the management of children with cerebral palsy, which utilized specialized handling techniques to decrease tone and stiffness, increase muscle control against gravity, and help stabilize muscle activity.[11]

The physical therapist's role progressed further in the 1950s from that of a technician to a professional practitioner.[7]

The outbreak of the Korean War in 1950 involved the United States in yet another war effort.[7] It is during this period that Margaret Rood, a physical and occupational therapist, broke new ground in the treatment of individuals with central nervous system (CNS) disorders.[12]

The 1950s were a pivotal time for the physical therapy profession to gain independence, autonomy, and professionalism. For example, during the late 1950s and into the 1960s, increasing numbers of states enacted state licensure laws for physical therapists, and in 1954, a seven-hour professional competency exam was developed by the APTA in conjunction with the Professional Examination Service of the American Public Health Association.[7] By 1959, 45 states and the territory of Hawaii had physical therapy practice acts in place.[5]

CLINICAL PEARL

► At the beginning of the 1950s, a neurophysiologist named Herman Kabat introduced the neurological concepts of tonic neck reflex, flexion reflex, and stretch reflex and applied these concepts to develop neurological exercises called proprioceptive facilitation. In 1956, Margaret Knott and Dorothy Voss[13] expanded on this work, and similar work by Arnold Gesell, René Cailliet, Myrtle McGraw, and Charles Sherrington and established the concepts of proprioceptive neuromuscular facilitation (PNF) as a treatment for patients with paralysis.

► In 1953, Paul C. Williams introduced a series of postural exercises, known today as the Williams exercises, which were designed to strengthen the spine flexors and extensors and relieve back pain.

► In the 1950s and 1960s, Robin McKenzie pioneered a series of back extension exercises that complemented the Williams exercises.

The 1960s brought profound changes in the US healthcare system as increasing numbers of states began to enact some practice acts.[5] Also, the polio vaccine had virtually eradicated poliomyelitis in the United States by 1961. By the 1960s, due to a shortage of physical therapists to fill the growing demand, the physical therapy profession began to look at ways to introduce personnel beyond rehabilitation aides. In 1964 an ad hoc committee was formed to study the utilization and training of nonprofessional assistants and, in 1967, the committee submitted a report to the HOD with a policy statement entitled "Training and Utilization of the Physical Therapy Assistant," which outlined a policy on the function, supervision, education, and regulation for the physical therapy assistant. In 1969, 15 students graduated with 2-year associate's degrees from the first PTA programs at Miami Dade College in Florida and St. Mary's Campus of the College of St. Catherine in Minnesota. As more community and technical colleges began offering PTA programs, the program directors formed the Physical Therapist Assistant Education Group (PTAEG), which eventually became the PTA Educators Special Interest Group of the Education Section.

CLINICAL PEARL

The PTA education program's focus is to prepare PTA students to assist the PT in delivering physical therapy interventions and the associated data collection. Although the PT's education requirements have changed over the years from an entry-level degree toward the Doctor of Physical Therapy (DPT), the educational program for the PTA has essentially remained unchanged despite the increased autonomy of the profession in healthcare. The change in the PT's education is mainly because, despite the increase in physical therapy autonomy, the PTA's role in the clinic did not undergo a similar evolution.

The earlier efforts to gain state licensure clearly influenced the Medicare program in 1967 and 1968, as most states had licensure laws by this time, which regulated the practice of physical therapy. Amendments to the Social Security Act (SSA) in 1967 added a definition of "outpatient physical therapy services," resulting in the Social Security organization recognizing physical therapy services as a healthcare provider for reimbursement. This amendment also resulted in dramatic changes to the practice of physical therapy for patients with neuromuscular disorders. Influenced by the earlier work of Margaret Rood, Margaret Knott, Dorothy Voss, and Signe Brunnström, Berta and Karl Bobath developed techniques for adults with a cerebrovascular accident (stroke), cerebral palsy, and other disorders of the central nervous system.[9] Since that time, the physical therapy profession has continued to expand its treatment areas, which has led to the need for specializations.

CLINICAL PEARL

The APTA currently recognizes the following 18 specialty sections as part of the professional organization of physical therapy:

► Acute care
► Aquatic physical therapy
► Cardiovascular and pulmonary
► Clinical electrophysiology and wound management
► Education
► Federal physical therapy
► Geriatrics
► Hand rehabilitation
► Health policy and administration
► Home health
► Neurology
► Oncology
► Orthopedics
► Pediatrics
► Private practice
► Research
► Sports physical therapy
► Women's health

In the late 1960s and early 1970s, open-heart surgery became possible, and the physical therapy profession expanded the cardiovascular/pulmonary area of its practice with increasing chest physical therapy programs for pre- and postoperative patients. There was an expansion of joint replacements in the orthopedic practice arena, resulting in the emergence of new avenues for orthopedic physical therapy practice by introducing new options for patients with severe joint restrictions to live more independent and pain-free lives. During this time, technological advances provided new testing methodologies and options to improve patient function, which allowed the profession opportunities to develop more objective outcome measures, new intervention strategies, and an increase in the types of diseases and conditions that physical therapy could positively influence. In 1970, PTAs were granted temporary membership into the APTA. PTAs were admitted as affiliate members in 1973, and, since 1992, PTAs have been able to hold offices (except for president) on the state and national levels of the APTA.

CLINICAL PEARL

▶ The APTA HOD adopted the Physical Therapist Assistant (PTA) Policy, and affiliate membership was granted to PTAs in 1973.

▶ The APTA HOD adopted its first Standards for Services and Practice in 1975.

▶ The first Combined Sections Meeting was held in Washington, DC, in 1976.

▶ The PT Fund became the Foundation for Physical Therapy in 1979. The Foundation promotes and provides financial support for clinically focused research to improve physical therapy's practice and cost effectiveness.

The 1970s and 1980s saw an increase in opportunities for practice with the implementation of Occupational Safety and Health Administration (OSHA) rules and regulations, the passage of the Education for All Handicapped Children Act (PL 94-142), and the epidemic spread of acquired immunodeficiency syndrome (AIDS). OSHA was formed for the prevention, management, and compensation of on-the-job injuries. The AIDS epidemic again highlighted the need for physical therapy to provide services to patients with multisystem involvement. Also, physical therapy services evolved into women's health, oncology, and hand rehabilitation.

In the early 1980s, the APTA adopted a policy indicating that "physical therapy practice independent of practitioner referral was ethical as long as it was legal in the state."[9]

Also significant during this time was the formation of the Federation of State Boards of Physical Therapy (FSBPT) in 1986, providing an independent organization through which member licensing authorities could coordinate to promote and protect the health, welfare, and safety of American communities.[4] The FSBPT also develops, maintains, and administers the national licensing examination for PTs and PTAs and creates a model state practice act for physical therapy.

Substantial changes in the healthcare delivery system in the United States required a major association focus in the 1990s, influencing physical therapy practice in ways that continue today.[4] The Americans with Disabilities Act (ADA) and the National Center for Medical Rehabilitation Research (NCMRR) led to new practice opportunities. The physical therapy profession was faced with the challenges of increasing governmental cost savings, decreasing reimbursement, increasing governmental regulations, the influences of the insurance industry and corporate America, and the rapid personnel supply exceeding demand for services.[7]

In August 1997, President Clinton signed the Balanced Budget Act (BBA) to eliminate the Medicare deficit. The BBA, which took effect in January 1999, applied an annual cap of $1500 (for physical therapy and speech therapy services) per beneficiary for all outpatient rehabilitation services. These changes had a dramatic effect, reducing rehabilitation services to Medicare patients. In November 1999, because of increasing pressure from the public, President Clinton signed the Refinement Act, which suspended the $1500 cap for two years in all rehabilitation settings starting on January 3, 2000.

CLINICAL PEARL

The 1990s introduced some major changes in the healthcare delivery system, including managed care, point-of-service plans, and other alternative organizational structures (see Chapter 2). Also, skilled nursing facilities (SNFs) were affected by the following regulations[7]:

▶ *PPS:* Medicare Prospective Payment System. PPS is a Medicare reimbursement method intended to motivate providers to deliver patient care effectively, efficiently, and without overutilization of services in hospitals, SNFs, and home health agencies. The payment is based on a unique assessment classification of each patient, and the payment amount for a particular service is derived based on a classification system (eg, per diem or per stay).

▶ *MDS:* Minimum Data Set. MDS is part of a federally mandated process for all residents in Medicare- or Medicaid-certified nursing facilities regardless of the individual resident's source of payment. The MDS is a comprehensive resident assessment instrument (RAI) that measures functional, mental health, and behavioral status to identify chronic-care patient needs and formalize a care plan in response to 18 resident assessment protocols (RAPs). Under federal regulation, assessments are conducted at the time of admission into a nursing facility, on return from a 72-hour hospital admission, whenever there is a significant change in status, quarterly and annually. In most cases, participants in the assessment process are licensed healthcare professionals employed by the facility. Data collected from the MDS assessments are used for the Medicare reimbursement system, many state Medicaid reimbursement systems, and to monitor the quality of care provided to nursing facility residents.

▶ *RUGs:* Resources Utilization Groups. A RUG is a mutually exclusive category that reflects various levels of resources needed in long-term care (LTC). These categories, which are assigned to individuals based on data elements derived from the LTC Minimum Data Set (MDS), are primarily used to facilitate Medicare and Medicaid payment. Each RUG, which is organized hierarchically, is associated with relative weighting factors. Several RUGs have evolved over the years:

- *RUG 34:* An initial set of RUGs developed primarily to support resource risk adjustment for Medicaid payment.

- *RUG 44:* An expanded version of RUG 34 that included 14 Rehab RUGs and a new hierarchical order to support Medicare PPS starting in 1998.

- *RUG 53:* An expanded version of RUG 44 that included nine mixed Rehab and Extensive Service RUGs, which were used to support Medicare PPS since January 2006.

► *OBRA:* Omnibus Budget Reconciliation Act of 1987. OBRA requires a comprehensive assessment of all nursing facility residents within 14 days of admission, a quarterly assessment (within 92 days) after that, and a full annual assessment (within 366 days of prior full assessment).

Prompted by a need to formally define the practice of physical therapy, the Guide was created. This model for PT practice was adopted in 1997, and the *Guide to Physical Therapist Practice,* published in 1999, introduced the terminology of examination, evaluation, diagnosis, prognosis, intervention, reexamination, and the assessment of outcomes.[1,7]

In 2000, the position statement "Procedural Interventions Exclusively Performed by Physical Therapists"[14] defined interventions beyond the scope of work of the PTA. Then, in 2008, the APTA BOD adopted the document "Minimum Required Skills of Physical Therapist Assistants at Entry-Level."[15]

CLINICAL PEARL

In 2009, the APTA BOD issued a resolution reaffirming that the PTA is the sole extender of the physical therapist, which highlighted the fact that the PTA is the "only individual permitted to assist a PT in selected interventions under the direction and supervision of a physical therapist."[16]

Currently, PTAs, licensed or otherwise regulated in all 50 states and the District of Columbia, work under the physical therapist's direction and supervision, who directs appropriate physical therapy interventions to the PTA. A PTA may implement selected components of patient/client interventions; obtain outcomes data related to the interventions provided; modify interventions either to progress the patient/client as directed by the PT or to ensure patient/client safety and comfort; educate and interact with other healthcare providers, students, aides/technicians, volunteers, and patients/clients and their families and caregivers; and respond to patient/client and environmental emergencies (see Figure 1-8). The

PTA can adjust, modify, or discontinue an intervention within the POC established by the PT based on clinical indications.[15] Thus, the PTA must determine the effectiveness of the intervention so that adjustments can be made to improve the patient/client response or patient/client safety or comfort.

CLINICAL PEARL

The PTA operates within the scope of work and supervision requirements defined by the physical therapy practice act in each state.

The PTA's main clinical role occurs within implementing the POC (intervention) component of the patient/client management model (Figure 1-1). A PTA may modify an intervention only following patient status changes within the established POC developed by the PT.

It is important to remember that, based on the APTA statement regarding the direction and supervision of the PTA,[16] the delegation of selected interventions by the PT to the PTA requires the education, expertise, and professional judgment of the PT (Figure 1-9) (see Appendix B).

CLINICAL PEARL

The PT directs and supervises the PTA consistent with APTA HOD positions, including direction and supervision of the PTA; APTA core documents, including standards of ethical conduct; federal and state legal practice standards; and institutional regulations.

The PTA may supervise or direct individuals, including physical therapy aides, transport staff, cleaning staff, and administration members.

CLINICAL PEARL

A PTA must practice within the scope of physical therapy practice defined by the state licensure laws (physical therapy practice acts) in the state in which he or she practices. The entire practice act, including accompanying rules, constitutes the law governing physical therapy practice within a state. Included within these practice acts are definitions as to what constitutes the requirements to practice as a PTA, what defines physical therapy, and directions on such topics as:

► The required level of direct on-premises supervision (this can vary widely based on the state from the PT being in the facility, to the PTA being directly supervised by a PT for 50% of the hours worked by the PTA, to the PT being within a 100-mile radius of the treatment location but available by telecommunication).

► Definitions on what constitutes mobilization/manual therapy (normally defined as a group of techniques comprising a continuum of skilled passive movements to the joints and/or related soft tissues throughout the normal physiological range of motion).

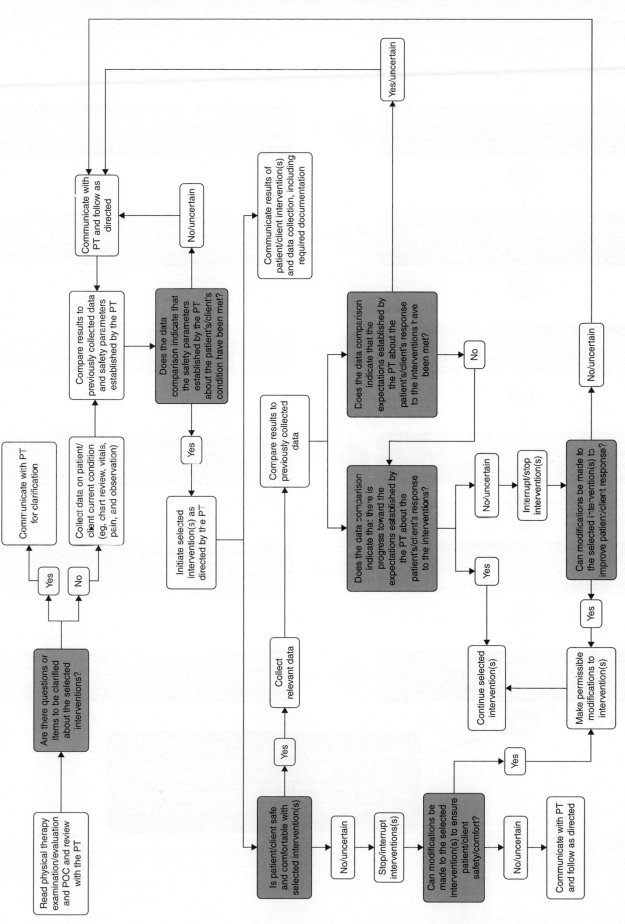

FIGURE 1-8 A one-page summary of the thought processes of a physical therapist assistant. Red font represents decisions to be made. (Reprinted from [http://www.apta.org], with permission of the American Physical Therapy Association. © 2021 American Physical Therapy Association. All rights reserved.)

PTA Direction Algorithm

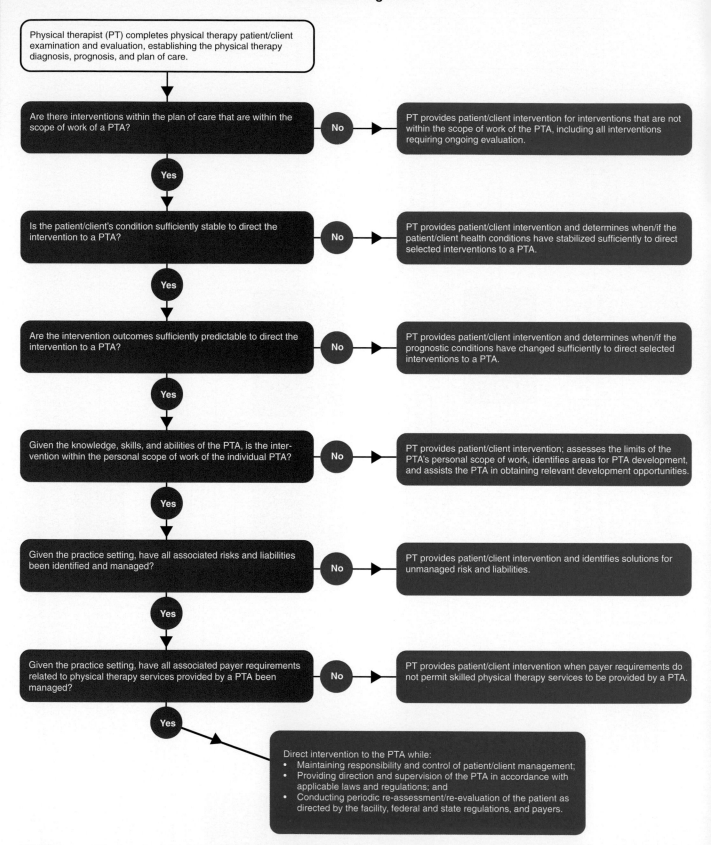

Physical therapist (PT) completes physical therapy patient/client examination and evaluation, establishing the physical therapy diagnosis, prognosis, and plan of care.

Are there interventions within the plan of care that are within the scope of work of a PTA?

No → PT provides patient/client intervention for interventions that are not within the scope of work of the PTA, including all interventions requiring ongoing evaluation.

Yes

Is the patient/client's condition sufficiently stable to direct the intervention to a PTA?

No → PT provides patient/client intervention and determines when/if the patient/client health conditions have stabilized sufficiently to direct selected interventions to a PTA.

Yes

Are the intervention outcomes sufficiently predictable to direct the intervention to a PTA?

No → PT provides patient/client intervention and determines when/if the prognostic conditions have changed sufficiently to direct selected interventions to a PTA.

Yes

Given the knowledge, skills, and abilities of the PTA, is the intervention within the personal scope of work of the individual PTA?

No → PT provides patient/client intervention; assesses the limits of the PTA's personal scope of work, identifies areas for PTA development, and assists the PTA in obtaining relevant development opportunities.

Yes

Given the practice setting, have all associated risks and liabilities been identified and managed?

No → PT provides patient/client intervention and identifies solutions for unmanaged risk and liabilities.

Yes

Given the practice setting, have all associated payer requirements related to physical therapy services provided by a PTA been managed?

No → PT provides patient/client intervention when payer requirements do not permit skilled physical therapy services to be provided by a PTA.

Yes

Direct intervention to the PTA while:
- Maintaining responsibility and control of patient/client management;
- Providing direction and supervision of the PTA in accordance with applicable laws and regulations; and
- Conducting periodic re-assessment/re-evaluation of the patient as directed by the facility, federal and state regulations, and payers.

FIGURE 1-9 PTA direction algorithm. (Reprinted from [http://www.apta.org], with permission of the American Physical Therapy Association. © 2021 American Physical Therapy Association. All rights reserved.)

- The maximum PT: PTA ratio (eg, in Pennsylvania, a licensed PT cannot supervise more than three PTAs at any time.
- Definitions concerning entry-level education and continuing education requirements, examination and licensure standards, and professional misconduct disciplinary procedures. (State licensure is required in each state in which a PTA practices and must be renewed regularly [typically every two years], with a majority of states requiring continuing education units [CEUs] or other continuing competency requirements for renewal.)

Typically, a PT works with one or more PTAs within a group of other clinicians and health team members. Each clinician brings a unique set of experiences and backgrounds, so communicating through effective written and verbal means is paramount. The supervising PT must understand the PTA's competency and skill level when making delegation decisions (Figure 1-10). Similarly, if the PTA does not understand something or is being asked to do something that he or she is not trained in, the PTA must feel comfortable raising these issues with the supervising PT. Regardless of the PTA's competency and skill level, it is the PTA's responsibility to request a consultation with the supervising PT in the event of any of the following:

- If there is any need for clarification regarding the POC
- Any change in the status of the patient/client
- Any adverse response by the patient/client to an intervention
- If the patient/client is demonstrating a lack of expected progress
- Before making any change to the established POC

CLINICAL PEARL

Aside from the practice act of the state and the level of confidence by the PT in the PTA's skills and abilities, delegation by a PT is also governed by two other factors:

1. Payer reimbursement policies. For example, under Medicare, PTAs can provide therapy services in an outpatient private practice setting—provided that those services are performed under the direct supervision (physically present in the office—but not necessarily in the same room) of a licensed PT. However, in other settings such as home health agencies, a PT presence is not required on the premises but the PT must be available by phone.

2. Acuity of the caseload. The delegation to a PTA by a PT depends on the patient's skill level. A more compromised patient with additional comorbidities typically requires a higher level of intervention or an increased need for and frequency of PT reassessment.

THE FUTURE

Thus, throughout the twentieth century, biomedicine was the dominant medical care model focusing on an impairment model. During this time, healthcare priorities shifted from the prevention, cure, and management of acute infectious conditions to the present-day focus on the prevention, cure, and management of lifestyle conditions such as hypertension, obesity, and metabolic syndrome (a group of risk factors that occur together and increase the risk for coronary artery disease, cerebrovascular accident, and type 2 diabetes).[17]

With the twenty-first century's arrival, a vastly revised version of the Guide was published in 2001. Continued development of the Guide led to the development of an interactive CD-ROM version that included the specifics of all the tests and measures used in the PT examination process.[7]

That same year, the Hooked on Evidence project was developed to facilitate increasing practice based on evidence, when available. Legislation was introduced in 2001 in the House of Representatives to allow Medicare patients direct access to PT services.[7]

The momentum behind these publications and legislations was driven by a combination of increased life expectancy, end-of-life morbidity, and, thus, prolonged disability. Unfortunately, it had also become apparent that many of the lifestyle conditions that had only affected adults, such as heart disease, type 2 diabetes, and obesity, now impact the pediatric population. Thus, it became necessary to shift the focus from symptom reduction with drugs and surgery to one that addressed their causes through prevention at both the individual and societal levels. It became clear that many of the most common lifestyle conditions were preventable, and in some cases, reversible, with the removal of their associated risk factors.

The physical therapy environment continues to be subjected to multiple forces. These forces include[18]:

- Ethical considerations, including patient confidentiality and informed consent
- Societal and cultural beliefs and values
- Population demographics
- The economy
- Governmental legislation, rules, and regulations
- Public and private organizations and agencies
- Scientific and technological advances

Given that most people have one or more risk factors or adverse manifestations of lifestyle conditions, strategies to address these conditions in the twenty-first century have included multiple health behavior change strategies and evidence-informed interventions. These strategies are targeted at the individual based on an assessment of health and risk factors.[19] To be equipped to address present-day health issues, the physical therapy profession needs sufficient clinical competencies, knowledge, and expertise to serve as the primary caregiver concerning smoking cessation, basic nutritional recommendations, weight control, regular physical activity guidelines, exercise prescription, stress, sleep management, and recommendations for moderate rather than

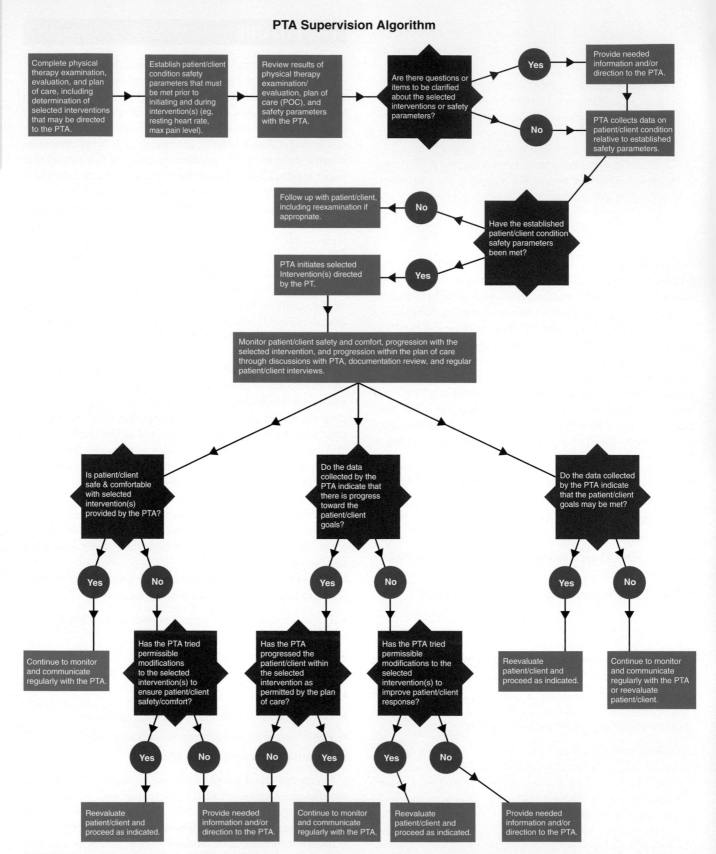

PTA Supervision Algorithm

FIGURE 1-10 PTA supervision algorithm. (Reprinted from [http://www.apta.org], with permission of the American Physical Therapy Association. © 2021 American Physical Therapy Association. All rights reserved.)

excessive alcohol consumption.[17] These noninvasive interventions will play an increasingly important role as the profession progresses through the twenty-first century.

The growing responsibility for physical therapists in patient care has led the APTA to develop a vision statement known as Vision 2020. The Vision 2020 states, "By 2020, physical therapy will be provided by physical therapists who are doctors of physical therapy, recognized by consumers and other healthcare professionals as practitioners of choice to whom consumers have direct access for the diagnosis of, interventions for, and prevention of impairments, functional limitations, and disabilities related to movement, function, and health." For Vision 2020 to be realized, there are six key elements:

1. *Autonomous practice.* The PT is solely responsible for the patient's physical therapy diagnosis, evaluation, intervention, and treatment outcomes. It is important to note that with this autonomy comes accountability and increased liability exposure.

2. *Direct access.* Direct access is a situation in which a state's licensure laws allow a PT to evaluate and treat a patient without the physician's referral or prescription requirement. At the time of writing, 43 states now have some form of direct access. For this to be effective, physical therapists must recognize the parameters associated within the scope of practice.

CLINICAL PEARL

An individual physical therapist's scope of practice is influenced by professional, jurisdictional, and scopes of practice.*

3. *Doctor of physical therapy.* By the year 2020, practicing physical therapists will have obtained a doctorate in physical therapy. This doctoral degree can take two forms:
   - An academic doctoral degree (PhD) in physical therapy
   - A transitional doctoral degree (DPT or tDPT) in physical therapy

4. *Evidence-based practice.* The goal is to provide the most cost-effective and beneficial treatment based on research (see Chapter 3). The APTA's Hooked on Evidence program now provides a platform called "Open Door: APTA's Portal to Evidence-based Practice" to help members obtain this goal.

5. *Practitioner of choice.* The goal for this is that PTs and PTAs will be the consumer's first choice for treating movement dysfunction, dysfunction related to pain, and restoration of function lost to diseases and disabilities. As with autonomy of practice, this describes a situation in which there is no one overseeing the evaluation of services the PT provides, which increases therapist liability.

6. *Professionalism.* The APTA has identified seven core values of professionalism in physical therapy:
   - Accountability
   - Altruism
   - Compassion/caring
   - Excellence
   - Integrity
   - Professional duty
   - Social responsibility

These are all broad terms describing professionalism. Specific examples include timeliness, appearance, and personality, all of which can impact one's reputation. The Normative Model of Physical Therapist Professional Education: Version 2004 (NMV2004) introduced several expectations, including professional practice, patient/client management, and practice management expectations[3]:

▶ Professional practice expectations include accountability, altruism, compassion/caring, integrity, professional duty, communication, cultural competence, clinical reasoning, evidence-based practice, and education.

▶ Patient/client management expectations include screening, examination, evaluation, diagnosis, prognosis, plan of care, intervention, and outcomes assessment.

▶ Practice management expectations include: 1) Prevention, health promotion, fitness, and wellness; 2) Management of care delivery; 3) Practice management; 4) Consultation; 5) Social responsibility and advocacy.

Perhaps the most contentious issue concerning PTAs these days is with the legal application of manual therapy techniques. At the time of writing, the delegation of many manual techniques is based on the supervising PT's discretion. There is also the issue of legality, which involves the licensing practice act of the state in which the PTA practices. In the United States, some states still do not have legal rules and regulations covering the service delivery of PTAs in general; other states have laws that limit the performance of specific PTA-related skills.

The APTA's practice/education unit and PTA services department have developed two algorithmic guides that are designed to (1) help the PT determine when to direct interventions to the PTA, (2) assist the PT in deciding which interventions may be appropriate to direct to the PTA, and (3) offer the PT guidance in the appropriate supervision the PTA, once selected interventions have been directed (Figure 1-9 and Figure 1-10).

STANDARDS OF PRACTICE

It is the role of the primary representative body for the physical therapy profession, the APTA, to outline and promote the expected level of quality of care for that profession. The APTA's commitment to society promotes optimal health and functioning in individuals by pursuing excellence in care.[4] To that end, the APTA has established the Standards of Practice for Physical Therapy (see Appendix C) and the corresponding Criteria for Standards of Practice in Physical

---

*APTA Guidelines: Scope of Practice (http://www.apta.org/uploadedFiles/APTAorg/About_Us/Policies/Practice/PTScopeOfPracticeCombined.pdf).

Therapy (see Appendix D). These are the profession's statements of conditions and performances essential for high-quality professional service to individuals in society and the necessary foundation for the assessment of physical therapy.

CODE OF ETHICS

It is generally recognized that a code of ethics is important to professions, professionals, and the public, such that every clinician-patient interaction should be performed with a high degree of professionalism. Some authors have elaborated on the purposes of a professional code of ethics, putting forth such descriptions as "providing a vocabulary for intraprofessional argument, self-criticism, and reform,"[20] and "a profession's code of ethics is perhaps its most visible and explicit enunciation of its professional norms."[21] A code not only embodies the profession's collective conscience and is a testimony to the group's recognition of its moral dimension[22] but also serves as a set of broad moral guidelines and a public document stating the moral commitments of a group at a period in time.

CLINICAL PEARL

A profession is an occupation that regulates itself through systematic, required training and collegial discipline; that has a base in technical, specialized knowledge; and that has a service rather than a profit orientation, enshrined in its code of ethics.[1]

Professionalism enhances trust. Throughout the history of physical therapy, PTAs have always been concerned about their profession's ethics. Members of the APA first adopted a formal set of ethical principles in 1935. The four principles listed covered professional practice, advertising, behavior, and discipline. In effect, the 1935 Code of Ethics sacrificed professional autonomy for stability in their relations with the medical profession.[22] Since then, the Code of Ethics has undergone some revisions and expansions. The Guide for Professional Conduct was issued by the Ethics and Judicial Committee of the APTA in 1981 (last amended in June 2009) and published as the *APTA Guide to Professional Conduct*. In July 2010, the HOD of the APTA implemented a major revision of the APTA Code of Ethics for physical therapists (see Appendix E) and the Standards of Ethical Conduct for the Physical Therapist Assistant (see Appendix A). It may be that the 2009 revision of the core ethics documents represents the culmination of increasing awareness within the profession and the professional organization of the ethical implications of the maturation of the profession.[21]

CLINICAL PEARL

Some professions and institutions distinguish between "codes of ethics" and "codes of conduct." When this distinction is made, the code of ethics typically outlines the general ethical principles or ideals, and the code of conduct provides specific rules for behavior.[22,23]

Two words that are commonly used when describing an individual's attitude and behavior are *morals* and *ethics*. Historically, the roots of the words *ethics* (from the ancient Greek word *ethikos*, derived from *ethos*, meaning character) and *morality* (from the Latin word *moralis*, meaning custom) meant the same thing, in that one was a translation of the other. Nowadays, however, while they are still sometimes used interchangeably, they are considered to have different meanings:

► *Morals.* Morals are the attitudes and behaviors that an individual feels are desirable and necessary for maximizing the realization of things they cherish the most.[24] Moral judgments are merely statements of a person's feelings or attitudes about what is right and wrong. Examples include honesty, a patient's rights to their life and autonomy, and character traits such as compassion, empathy, and conscientiousness.

► *Ethics.* Ethics is the study of morals and moral judgments that can be influenced by external sources such as religion and societal norms. An ethical dilemma is a situation in which there is no right answer. However, when individuals think ethically, they are at least giving some thought to something beyond themselves.

CLINICAL PEARL

Put simply, morals lean toward decisions based upon individual character through an individual's subjective understanding of right and wrong, whereas ethics emphasize a widely shared communal or societal norm about right and wrong. Thus, it is possible to act morally but still be confronted with ethical dilemmas. For example, a PTA treats a patient whose Living Will indicates that the patient does not want to be resuscitated (a DNR order) if their health status rapidly deteriorates. When the PTA is alone with this patient during a treatment session, the patient suffers a cardiac arrest while exercising. In this situation, the ethical decision is determined by the general principles set by the DNR, but the moral dilemma is the decision the PTA has to make—whether to adhere to the DNR order or make attempts to save the patient's life.

OTHER MEMBERS OF THE HEALTHCARE TEAM

As a PTA begins a healthcare career, they become part of the healthcare team, which depends on the facility type. For example, in an inpatient setting, interdisciplinary team meetings frequently occur so that information about a patient/client can be shared with the team members. The student PTA must understand the healthcare team's various members in terms of their roles and capabilities.

Primary Care Physician (PCP)

A practitioner, usually an internist, general practitioner, or family medicine physician, providing primary care services and managing routine healthcare needs. Most PCPs serve as gatekeepers for the managed-care health organizations—they provide authorization for referrals to other specialty physicians or services, including physical therapy. State medical boards require that physicians applying for a license should document a passing grade on national licensing examinations, certification of graduation from medical school, and, in most cases, completion of at least one year of residency training after medical school.

Physician Assistant (PA)

As the name suggests, a physician assistant (PA) works closely with physicians, especially in primary care and underserved communities. A PA can perform physical examinations, diagnose, prescribe medications, and administer therapies under a physician's supervision (see also Registered Nurse). Studies of PAs in primary care settings have found that the scope overlaps with approximately 80% of primary care physicians' work scope. A PA is usually licensed by the same state boards that license physicians. To be eligible for licensure in most states, a PA must have graduated from an accredited training program and pass the Physician Assistant National Certifying Examination.

Dentist and Oral Surgeon

The amount of involvement that physical therapy has with a dental practice is limited because the number of referrals for temporomandibular joint dysfunctions (TMDs) varies from practice to practice. However, they are included here for completeness. All dentists spend 7 or 8 years in college and dental school earning a DDS (Doctor of Dental Surgery) or DMD (Doctor of Dental Medicine). After earning the DDS or DMD degree, a general dentist must complete a licensure exam to practice in a particular area. In contrast, oral surgeons complete a 4- to 6-year surgical residency. Whereas a general dentist provides such services as teeth cleaning, routine X-rays, dental fillings, root canals, veneers, bridges, and crowns, an oral surgeon is a dental specialist that provides such services as teeth extractions, dental implant placement, repair of broken bones in the jaws and face, removal of cysts and tumors of the jaws, and jaw realignment surgery to correct bite discrepancies.

Physiatrist

A physiatrist specializes in physical medicine and rehabilitation and has been certified by the American Board of Physical Medicine and Rehabilitation. The physiatrist's primary role is to diagnose and treat patients with disabilities involving musculoskeletal, neurological, cardiovascular, or other body systems.

Nurse Practitioner

A nurse practitioner (NP) is an advanced-practice registered nurse who has completed graduate-level education at either a Master of Nursing or Doctor of Nursing Practice level in addition to the basic nurse training. NPs diagnose a wide range of acute and chronic diseases, provided that they are within their scope of practice and can provide appropriate treatment for patients, including prescribing medications. Licensing and related regulations for NPs are less uniform across states than those for physicians, PAs, and RNs. Instead of a single national licensing examination for all NPs, different organizations administer certification examinations that are specialty-specific, similar to medical specialty board certification. State boards of nursing vary in the scope of practice, with most states requiring NPs to collaborate with the physician.

Physical Therapy Director

The physical therapy director is responsible for the day-to-day running of the physical therapy department. The director is either promoted or hired because they have demonstrated the necessary education and experience in physical therapy and are willing to accept the role's inherent responsibilities.[1] The director of a physical therapy service must:

- Establish guidelines and procedures that will delineate the functions and responsibilities of all levels of physical therapy personnel in the service and the supervisory relationships inherent in the functions of the service and the organization.[1]
- Ensure that the service's objectives are efficiently and effectively achieved within the framework of the organization's stated purpose and per safe physical therapy practice through the design of policies and procedures.
- Interpret administrative policies.
- Act as a liaison between line staff and administration.
- Foster the professional growth of the staff.
- Be responsible for the departmental budget.

Physical Therapy Aide

A physical therapy aide is an individual who may be involved in support services under the direction and supervision of a PT or PTA. A physical therapy aide receives on-the-job training and is permitted to function only with continuous on-site supervision. A physical therapy aide's duties are limited to those methods and techniques that do not require clinical decision-making or problem-solving by a PT or a PTA.

Physical Therapist and Physical Therapist Assistant Student

The PT or PTA student can perform duties commensurate with their level of education.

CLINICAL PEARL

Patients, parents, or legal guardians can refuse treatment by a student practitioner.

Physical Therapy Volunteer

A volunteer is usually a member of the community who has an interest in assisting with departmental activities. Responsibilities of a volunteer include:

▶ Taking phone messages

▶ Basic nonclinical/secretarial duties

Home Health Aide

A home health aide provides health-related services to the elderly, disabled, and unwell in their homes. Their duties include performing housekeeping tasks, assisting with ambulation or transfers, and promoting personal hygiene. The registered nurse, PT/PTA, or social worker caring for the patient may assign specific duties to, and supervise, the home health aide.

Occupational Therapist

An occupational therapist (OT) assesses a patient's function in activities of daily living (ADLs), including dressing, bathing, grooming, meal preparation, writing, and driving, which are essential for independent living. In making treatment recommendations, the OT addresses many factors including, but not limited to, (1) fatigue management; (2) upper body strength, movement, and coordination; (3) adaptations to the home and work environment, including both structural changes and specialized equipment for particular activities; and (4) compensatory strategies for impairments in thinking, sensation, or vision. All states require an OT to obtain a license to practice.

Certified Occupational Therapy Assistant

A certified occupational therapy assistant (COTA) works under the direction of an OT. COTAs perform a variety of rehabilitative activities and exercises, as outlined in an established treatment plan. The COTA's minimum educational requirements are described in the current *Essentials and Guidelines of an Accredited Educational Program for the Occupational Therapy Assistant* (AOTA, 1991b).

Speech-Language Pathologist (Speech Therapist)

A speech-language pathologist evaluates speech, language, cognitive-communication, and swallowing skills of children and adults. Speech-language pathologists are required to possess a master's degree or equivalent. The vast majority of states require a speech-language pathologist to obtain a license to practice.

Chiropractor

A Doctor of Chiropractic (DC), or chiropractor, is an individual trained in the science, art, and philosophy of chiropractic. Chiropractic evaluation and treatment are directed at providing a structural analysis of the body's musculoskeletal and neurological systems because, according to chiropractic doctrine, abnormal function of these two systems may affect other systems' function in the body. To practice, chiropractors are usually licensed by a state board. A patient may see a chiropractor and a PT/PTA concurrently.

Certified Orthotist

A certified orthotist (CO) designs, fabricates, and fits orthoses (braces, splints, collars, corsets) prescribed by physicians to patients with disabling conditions of the limbs and spine. A CO must have completed the examination by the American Orthotist and Prosthetic Association (AOPA).

Certified Prosthetist

A certified prosthetist (CP) designs, fabricates, and fits prostheses for patients with a partial or total absence of a limb. A CP must have completed the examination by the AOPA.

Respiratory Therapist

A respiratory therapist evaluates, treats, and cares for patients with breathing disorders. The vast majority of respiratory therapists are employed in hospitals. Patient care activities include performing bronchial drainage techniques, measuring lung capacities, administering oxygen and aerosols, and analyzing oxygen and carbon dioxide concentrations. Education programs for a respiratory therapist are offered by hospitals, colleges, universities, vocational-technical institutes, and the military. The vast majority of states require a respiratory therapist to obtain a license to practice.

Respiratory Therapy Technician Certified (CRRT)

A CRRT is a skilled technician who:

▶ Holds an associate's degree from a 2-year training program accredited by the Committee in Allied Health Education and Accreditation

▶ Has passed a national examination to become registered

▶ Administers respiratory therapy as prescribed and supervised by a physician, including:

■ Pulmonary function tests

■ Treatments consisting of oxygen delivery, aerosols, nebulizers

■ Maintenance of all respiratory equipment

Registered Nurse

A registered nurse is an individual who has graduated from a nursing program at a college or university and has passed a national licensing exam. Historically, many nurses received their education in vocational programs administered by hospitals and were awarded nursing diplomas. Nowadays, most nurses are educated either in 2- to 3-year associate degree programs administered by community colleges or in baccalaureate programs administered by 4-year colleges. A registered nurse is licensed by the state to provide nursing services and is legally authorized or registered to practice as a registered nurse (RN) and use the RN designation. A registered nurse may:

▶ Make referrals to other services under a physician's direction

▶ Supervise other levels of nursing care

▶ Administer medication but cannot change drug dosages

▶ Communicate to the supervising physician any change in the patient's medical or social condition

Rehabilitation (Vocational) Counselor

A rehabilitation counselor helps people deal with the personal, physical, mental, social, and vocational effects of disabilities resulting from congenital disabilities, illness or disease, accidents, or daily life stress. The role of the rehabilitation counselor includes:

▶ An evaluation of the strengths and limitations of individuals

▶ Providing personal and vocational counseling

▶ Arranging for medical care, vocational training, and job placement

Audiologist

An audiologist evaluates and treats individuals of all ages with hearing loss symptoms and other auditory, balance, and related sensory and neural problems.

Athletic Trainer Certified (ATC)

The certified athletic trainer is a professional specializing in athletic healthcare. In cooperation with the physician and other allied health personnel, the athletic trainer functions as an integral member of the athletic healthcare team in secondary schools, colleges and universities, sports medicine clinics, professional sports programs, and other athletic healthcare settings.

Certified athletic trainers have, at a minimum, a bachelor's degree, usually in athletic training, health, physical education, or exercise science.

Social Worker

A social worker helps patients and their families to cope with chronic, acute, or terminal illnesses and attempts to resolve problems that stand in the way of recovery or rehabilitation.

A bachelor's degree is often the minimum requirement to qualify for employment as a social worker; however, a master's degree is often required in the health field. All states have licensing, certification, or registration requirements for social workers.

Massage Therapist

Massage therapy is a regulated health profession with a growing number of states and provinces now requiring a license. Registered massage therapists must uphold specific standards of practice and codes of ethics to hold a valid license. To become a licensed or registered massage therapist, most states and provinces require applicants to pass specific government board examinations, consisting of a written and a practical portion. A registered massage therapist is covered under most health insurance plans.

Acupuncturist

An acupuncturist treats symptoms by inserting very fine needles, sometimes in conjunction with an electrical stimulus, into the body's surface to, theoretically, influence the body's physiological functioning. Typical sessions last between 30 minutes and an hour. At the end of the session, the acupuncturist may prescribe herbal therapies for the patient at home. At the time of writing, 32 states and the District of Columbia use National Certification Commission for Acupuncture and Oriental Medicine (NCCAOM) certification as the main examination criterion for licensure; this takes three to four years to achieve. Each state may also choose to set additional eligibility criteria (usually additional academic or clinical hours). A small number of states have additional jurisprudence or practical examination requirements, such as passing the Clean Needle Technique (CNT) exam.

The Patient

Although often overlooked, the patient is critical to the healthcare team. The population of patients evaluated and treated in physical therapy can vary in age from newborn to elderly.

PRACTICE SETTINGS

PTAs practice in a broad range of inpatient, outpatient, and community-based settings. At a fundamental level, healthcare is divided into three levels: primary, secondary, and tertiary.

▶ *Primary care.* The APTA has endorsed the concepts of primary care set forth by the Institute of Medicine's Committee on the Future of Primary Care,[25] including:[1]

■ Primary care can encompass a myriad of needs that go well beyond the capabilities and competencies of individual caregivers and require varied practitioners' involvement and interaction.

■ Primary care is not limited to the "first contact" or point of entry into the healthcare system.

■ The primary care program is a comprehensive one.

This level of care, which accounts for 80% to 90% of visits to a physician or other caregiver, involves basic or entry-level healthcare, which includes diagnostic, therapeutic (eg, diabetes, arthritis, or hypertension), or preventive services (eg, vaccinations or mammograms) for common health problems. The care is provided across the continuum of activity—acute, rehabilitative, and chronic care management by primary care teams that include PCPs, internists, and pediatricians. The PTA serves a supportive role for the PT and primary care teams by providing reevaluations and physical therapy interventions for musculoskeletal, neuromuscular, cardiovascular/pulmonary, or integumentary disorders. Physical therapy also provides primary care in industrial or workplace settings, in which they manage the occupational health services provided to employees by helping to prevent injury.[1] Finally, through community-based agencies and school systems, physical therapy services coordinate and integrate care provisions to individuals with chronic disorders.[1]

▶ *Secondary care.* In secondary care, individuals with musculoskeletal, neuromuscular, cardiovascular/pulmonary, or integumentary conditions may be treated initially by other practitioners (eg, orthopedists, cardiologists, urologists, or dermatologists) and then referred to physical therapy for secondary care in a wide range of settings, including acute care and rehabilitation hospitals, outpatient clinics, home health, and school systems.[1]

▶ *Tertiary care.* This level of care involves treatment provided by physical therapy in highly specialized, complex, and technology-based settings (eg, heart and lung transplant services, burn units) or in response to the requests of other healthcare practitioners for specialized services that require sophisticated technologies (eg, for individuals with spinal cord lesions, organ transplants, congenital malformations, or closed head trauma).[1]

Hospital

A hospital is an institution whose primary function is to provide inpatient diagnostic and therapeutic services for various medical, surgical, and nonsurgical conditions. Also, most hospitals provide outpatient services, particularly emergency care. Hospitals may be classified in several ways, including by:

▶ Length of stay (short-term or long-term):
  ■ *Acute-care (short-term hospital).* An acute-care hospital can be defined as a facility that provides hospital care to patients who generally require a stay of up to 30 days, and whose focus is on a physical or mental condition requiring immediate intervention and constant medical attention, equipment, and personnel. A hospital's goal is for rapid discharge to the next level of care (to home or another healthcare facility), and a physical therapy recommendation is often very important in discharge planning.
  ■ *Subacute (long-term).* Medical care is provided to medically unstable patients who cannot return home. Required services (medical, nursing, rehabilitative) are provided within a hospital or SNF.

▶ Teaching or nonteaching hospital.
  ■ *Teaching:* a hospital that serves as a teaching site for medicine, dentistry, allied health, nursing programs, or medical residency programs
  ■ *Nonteaching:* a hospital that has no teaching responsibilities or one that serves as an elective site for health-related programs

▶ *Major types of services.* Psychiatric, tuberculosis, burn, general, and other specialties, such as maternity, pediatric, and ear, nose, and throat (ENT).

▶ *Type of ownership or control.* Federal, state, or local government; for-profit or nonprofit.

Long-term Care Facility

Long-term care (LTC) for the elderly or for those with disabilities or illness that require long-term care can be provided at home, in the community, or various types of facilities, such as SNFs, inpatient rehabilitation facilities, long-term acute-care hospitals, or assisted living facilities (ALFs). Each type of long-term care facility provides different services and is, therefore, suitable for different types of patients:

▶ Long-term acute care. These facilities provide care for medically complex or chronically critically ill patients likely to require care for weeks to months. Thus, the provided services can include mechanical ventilation, hemodialysis, and complex wound care.

▶ Inpatient rehabilitation. These facilities provide care for patients recovering from an acute illness, surgery, or trauma. However, to qualify for admission, the patient must tolerate three hours of physical or occupational therapy daily.

▶ Skilled nursing. These facilities provide care for patients that may be chronically ill but are considered medically stable.

Reimbursement for long-term care depends on the income and assets of the individual in need of care and the severity of the care they require:

▶ For low-income elderly individuals and families with limited assets, medical care costs are largely covered by Medicare or Medicaid. However, personal (custodial, nonmedical) care is not covered by Medicare or Medicaid.

▶ Middle-income families often have Medicare Supplement insurance, which provides additional assistance for Medicare co-payments and other gaps.

▶ Higher-income families typically rely on Medicare, Medigap, Supplement Insurance, and private insurance.

Much of the physical therapy provided in LTC facilities is administering appropriate adaptive equipment or assistive devices, promoting prevention activities, and providing health and wellness education.

Home Healthcare

Home healthcare involves the provision of medical or health-related care by a home health agency (HHA), which may be governmental, voluntary, private, nonprofit, or for-profit. Home care services were introduced to reduce the need for hospitalization and its associated costs. An HHA provides part-time and intermittent skilled and nonskilled services and other therapeutic services on a visiting basis to persons of all ages in their homes. Patient eligibility includes:

► Any patient who is homebound or who has great difficulty leaving their home. A person may leave home for medical treatment or for short, infrequent nonmedical absences such as a religious service, dialysis, or a hairdresser/barber.

► *Medicaid Waiver clients.* The Medicaid Waiver for the Elderly and Disabled (E&D Waiver) program is designed to provide services to seniors and the disabled whose needs would otherwise require them to live in a nursing home. The goal is for clients to retain their independence by providing services that allow them to live safely in their own homes and communities for as long as it is appropriate.

► A patient who requires skilled care from one of the following disciplines: nursing, physical therapy, occupational therapy, or speech therapy. The home health services provided by intermittent skilled nursing (< 7 d/wk; < 8 hours a day) include:

■ Observation and assessment

■ Teaching and training

■ Complex care plan management and evaluation

■ Administration of certain medications

■ Tube feedings

■ Wound care, catheters, and ostomy care

■ Nasopharyngeal and tracheostomy aspiration/care

■ Rehabilitation nursing

► *Physician certification.* In the case of an elderly patient, recertification by Medicare is required every 60 days. Medicare only pays for skilled home health services that are provided by a Medicare-certified agency. Medicare defines *intermittent* as skilled nursing care needed or given for less than 7 days each week or less than 8 hours per day throughout 21 days (or less), with some exceptions in special circumstances. A patient must have a face-to-face encounter within 90 days prior or 30 days after the start of home healthcare with a physician, advanced-practice nurse, or physician assistant related to the condition(s) that necessitate home healthcare.

► Patients who continue to demonstrate the potential for progress.

The physical therapy focus includes:

► Environmental safety, including proper lighting, securing scatter rugs, handrails, wheelchair ramps, and raised toilet seats.

► Early intervention (refer to the following section, School System).

► Addressing equipment needs:

■ Equipment ordered in the hospital is reimbursable.

■ Adaptive equipment ordered in the home is not reimbursable except for items such as wheelchairs, commodes, and hospital beds.

► Observing for any evidence of substance or physical abuse:

■ Substance abuse should be reported immediately to the physician.

■ Physical abuse should be immediately communicated to the proper authorities (varies from state to state).

School System

The major goal of physical therapy intervention within the school system is to enhance the child's level of function in the school setting. Recommendations are made for adaptive equipment to facilitate improved posture, head control, and function.

► *Early Intervention Program (EIP).* A national program designed for infants and toddlers with disabilities and their families.

► Congress created the EIP in 1986 under the Individuals with Disabilities Education Act (IDEA). To be eligible for services, children must be less than three years of age and have a confirmed disability, or established developmental delay, as defined by the state, in one or more of the following areas of development: physical, cognitive, communication, social-emotional, and/or adaptive.

Therapeutic and support services include:

► Family education and counseling, home visits, and parent support groups

► Special instruction

► Speech pathology and audiology

► Occupational therapy

► Physical therapy

► Psychological services

► Service coordination

► Nursing services

► Nutrition services

► Social work services

► Vision services

► Assistive technology devices and services

Private Practice

Private practice settings are privately owned and freestanding independent physical therapy practices.

► Practice settings vary from physical therapy and orthopedic clinics to rehabilitation agencies.

► Documentation is required every visit, and reevaluations are required by Medicare every 30 days for reimbursement purposes.

Other healthcare facilities in which a PTA can practice are described in Table 1-1.

TABLE 1-1	Physical Therapist Practice Settings	
Setting	**Characteristics**	**Physical Therapist Role**
Transitional care unit	► Nonmedically-based facility, which may be in a group home or part of a continuum of a rehabilitation center. ► The typical stay is 4-8 months with discharge to home, assisted living facility, or skilled nursing facility (SNF). ► Greater focus placed on compensation versus restoration.	Physical therapy emphasizes improving functional skills for maximum independence to prepare a patient for community reentry or transfer to an assisted living/skilled nursing facility.
Skilled nursing/ Extended care facility (ECF)	► Freestanding facility or part of a licensed hospital and approved by the state (Medicare-certified). ► Eligible individuals receive skilled nursing care and appropriate rehabilitative and restorative services. ► Accepts patients in need of rehabilitation and medical care of a lesser intensity than that received in a hospital's acute/subacute care setting. ► Provides skilled services, including rehabilitation and various other health services (nursing) daily (Medicare defines *daily* as seven days a week of skilled nursing care and five days a week of skilled therapy). ► Physician orders must be rewritten every 60 days.	A SNF must provide 24-hour nursing coverage and the availability of physical, occupational, and speech therapy.
Inpatient rehabilitation facility	► Usually based in a medical setting. ► Provides early rehabilitation, social, and vocational services once a patient is medically stable. ► The primary emphasis is to provide intensive physical and cognitive restorative services in the early months to disabled persons to facilitate their return to maximum functional capacity. ► The typical stay is 3-4 months.	Physical therapy is involved in the coordinated services of medical, social, educational, vocational, and other rehabilitative services (OT, speech).
Chronic/Long-term care facility	► A long-term care facility that is facility- or community-based. ► Sometimes referred to as *extended rehabilitation*. ► Designed for patients with permanent or residual disabilities caused by a nonreversible pathological health condition. Also used for patients who demonstrate slower than expected progress. ► Used as a placement facility—60 days or longer, but not for permanent stays.	The facility has a full range of rehabilitation services (physical, occupational, and speech therapy).
Comprehensive outpatient rehabilitation facility (CORF)	► A nonresidential facility established and operated exclusively to provide outpatient diagnostic, therapeutic, and restorative services to rehabilitate injured, disabled, or sick persons, at a single fixed location, by or under the physician's supervision. Services include physician services; physical, occupational, and respiratory therapy; speech-language pathology services; prosthetic and orthotic devices, including testing, fitting, or training in the use of these devices; social and psychological services; nursing care provided by or under the supervision of a registered professional nurse; drugs and biologicals that cannot be self-administered; and supplies and durable medical equipment. ► CORFs are surveyed every 6 years at a minimum.	Physical therapy (and occupational therapy and speech-language pathology services) may be provided in an off-site location.
Custodial care facility	► Provides medical or nonmedical services that do not seek to cure but are necessary for the patient who cannot care for him/herself. ► Provided during periods when the medical condition of the patient is not changing. ► The patient does not require the continued administration of medical care by qualified medical personnel. ► This type of care is not usually covered under managed-care plans.	Physical therapy involvement is minimal.

(continued)

TABLE 1-1	Physical Therapist Practice Settings (continued)	
Setting	**Characteristics**	**Physical Therapist Role**
Hospice care	▶ A facility or program licensed, certified, or otherwise authorized by law to provide supportive care for the terminally ill. ▶ Focuses on the dying patient and the family's physical, spiritual, emotional, psychological, financial, and legal needs. ▶ Services are provided by an interdisciplinary team of professionals and perhaps volunteers in various settings, including hospitals, freestanding facilities, and homes. ▶ Medicare and Medicaid require that at least 80% of hospice care be provided at home. Eligibility for reimbursement includes: ■ Medicare eligibility. ■ Certification of terminal illness (less than or equal to 6 months of life) by a physician.	Physical therapy may be consulted on an as-needed basis.
Personal care	Optional Medicaid benefit that allows a state to provide services to assist functionally impaired individuals in performing the activities of daily living (eg, bathing, dressing, feeding, grooming).	Physical therapy may be consulted on an as-needed basis.
Ambulatory care (outpatient care)	▶ Includes outpatient preventative, diagnostic, and treatment services provided at medical offices, surgery centers, or outpatient clinics (including private practice physical therapy clinics, outpatient satellites of institutions, or hospitals). ▶ Designed for patients who do not require overnight hospitalization. ▶ More cost-effective than inpatient care, and therefore favored by managed-care plans.	Physical therapy may be consulted on an as-needed basis.

WORKING IN HEALTHCARE

Even though working in healthcare is altruistic, caring for other individuals can prove stressful over time. These stresses can result in a condition known as *caregiver burnout*. The classic symptoms for this condition include the following:

▶ A depletion of physical energy

▶ Emotional exhaustion

▶ Physical withdrawal

▶ An increasingly pessimistic outlook

▶ Increased absenteeism from work

▶ Excessive use of alcohol, medications, or sleeping pills

▶ Difficulty concentrating

Every clinician needs to put time into taking care of him- or herself emotionally and physically. Whenever possible, any caregiving responsibility should be varied or delegated. If necessary, the clinician should strongly consider finding a support group or speaking to someone about getting help. Some activities are beneficial to reduce stress. These include aerobic exercise, meditation, massage, and relaxation techniques.

REFERENCES

1. American Physical Therapy Association. *Guide to Physical Therapist Practice. 3.0.* Alexandria, VA: American Physical Therapy Association; 2014.
2. Menant JC, Gandevia SC. Poliomyelitis. *Handbook of Clinical Neurology*; Philadelphia: Elsevier-Mosby; 2018;159:337-344.
3. American Physical Therapy Association. *A Normative Model of Physical Therapist Professional Education: Version 2004.* Alexandria, VA: American Physical Therapy Association; 2004.
4. American Physical Therapy Association. *Today's Physical Therapist: A Comprehensive Review of a 21st-Century Health Care Profession.* Alexandria, VA: American Physical Therapy Association; 2011.
5. Murphy W. *Healing the Generations: A History of Physical Therapy and the American Physical Therapy Association.* Lyme, Conn: Greenwich Publishing Group, Inc.; 1995.
6. Pinkston D. Evolution of the practice of physical therapy in the United States. In: Scully RM, Barnes MR, eds. *Physical Therapy,* 1st ed. Philadelphia: JB Lippincott; 1989:2-30.
7. Moffat M. The history of physical therapy in the United States. *JOPTE.* 2003; Winter.
8. Moffat M. Three quarters of a century of healing the generations. *Phys Ther.* 1996;76:1242-1252.
9. American Physical Therapy Association. *Professionalism in Physical Therapy: Core Values.* Alexandria, VA: American Physical Therapy Association; 2003.
10. Brunnstrom S. Associated reactions of the upper extremity in adult patients with hemiplegia: an approach to training. *The Physical Ther Rev.* 1956;36:225-236.
11. Bobath K, Bobath B. The facilitation of normal postural reactions and movements in the treatment of cerebral palsy. *Physiotherapy.* 1964;50:246-262.
12. Rood MS. Neurophysiological reactions as a basis for physical therapy. *Phys Ther Rev.* 1954;34:444-449.
13. Knott M, Voss DE. *Proprioceptive Neuromuscular Facilitation.* 2nd ed. New York: Harper & Row Pub Inc.; 1968.
14. *Procedural Interventions Exclusively Performed by Physical Therapists,* HOD P06-00-30-36. House of Delegates standards, policies, positions, and guidelines; 2012.
15. *Minimum Required Skills of Physical Therapist Assistants at Entry-level,* BOD G11-08-09-18. Board of Directors, policies, positions, and guidelines; 2012.
16. *Direction and Supervision of the Physical Therapist Assistant,* HOD P06-05-18-26. House of delegates standards, policies, positions, and guidelines; 2009.
17. Dean E. Physical therapy in the 21st century (Part I): Toward practice informed by epidemiology and the crisis of lifestyle conditions. *Physiother Theory Pract.* 2009;25:330-353.
18. Schmoll BJ. Physical therapy today and in the 21st century. In: Scully RM, Barnes MR, eds. *Physical Therapy,* 1st ed. Philadelphia: JB Lippincott; 1989:31-35.

19. Greenland P, Knoll MD, Stamler J, Neaton JD, Dyer AR, Garside DB, et al. Major risk factors as antecedents of fatal and nonfatal coronary heart disease events. *JAMA*. 2003;290:891-897.

20. Fullinwider RK. Professional codes and moral understanding. In: Coady M, Block S, eds. *Codes of Ethics and the Professions*. Melbourne, Victoria, Australia: Melbourne University Press; 1996:72-87.

21. Frankel MS. Professional codes: Why, how, and with what impact? *J Bus Ethics*. 1989;8:109-115.

22. Swisher LL, Hiller P. The revised APTA code of ethics for the physical therapist and standards of ethical conduct for the physical therapist assistant: Theory, purpose, process, and significance. *Physi Ther*. 2010;90:803-824.

23. Coady M, Block S. *Codes of Ethics and the Professions*. Melbourne, Victoria, Australia: Melbourne University Press; 1996.

24. Purtillo R. Ethical considerations in physical therapy. In: Scully RM, Barnes MR, eds. *Physical Therapy*, 1st ed. Philadelphia: JB Lippincott; 1989:36-40.

25. National Research Council. Defining primary care: An interim report. Washington (DC): The National Academies Press; 1994.

CHAPTER 2

Healthcare Regulations

CHAPTER OBJECTIVES

At the completion of this chapter, the reader will be able to:

1. Describe how the laws, regulations, and policies affect the practice of physical therapy

2. Describe the various methods of insurance reimbursements for healthcare services

3. List the challenges associated with obtaining appropriate access to healthcare within the United States

4. Describe the various associations and organizations that regulate the quality of healthcare

5. Define malpractice and provide examples of patient negligence

6. Describe the impact of the Balanced Budget Act of 1997

7. Have a good understanding of patient rights within the healthcare system

8. Describe how the Health Insurance and Portability and Accountability Act (HIPAA) is designed to protect a patient's privacy

9. Discuss the various legislation that protects a patient within the healthcare system

10. Describe the importance of the Americans with Disabilities Act (ADA) and its impact on society

11. List some of the safety considerations of the home and work environments

OVERVIEW

Over the years, several federal and state laws and regulations have been introduced to protect the public from safety issues, prevent medical fraud, and control reimbursement. There exists a paradox of excess and deprivation in the healthcare system of the United States, in which some individuals are deprived of adequate care because they cannot afford suitable insurance, while others receive an excess of care that is expensive and unnecessary. Healthcare in the United States encompasses a wide spectrum, ranging from the highest quality, most compassionate treatment of those with complex illnesses and well-designed protocols for preventing illness to inappropriate high-risk surgical procedures performed on uninformed patients.[1] For the physical therapist assistant (PTA), embarking on a healthcare career, understanding how healthcare works, including its strengths and inadequacies, is essential.

CLINICAL PEARL

Law: A rule, or system of rules, conduct, or action established by a country or community that regulates the actions of its members and which can be enforced by the imposition of penalties.

Statute: A law passed by a legislature. Statutes impacting the practice of physical therapy can be passed at the federal level (federal statutes) by Congress (see Federal Statutes) or at the state level (state statutes). An example of a state statute is the state Physical Therapy Practice Act, which controls the scope and protection of physical therapy practice.

Policy: A proposed set of ideas or plans that describe a course or principle of action to be taken on a particular issue

Practice act: A physical therapy practice act is a statute defining the scope and practice of physical therapy within the jurisdiction, outlining licensing requirements, and establishing penalties for violating the law.

Regulation: A rule of order prescribed by a superior or competent authority, typically by various federal government departments and agencies with the force of law. Most commonly, at the state level, regulations give further definition to terms in the statutes. Examples of federal agencies that produce regulations include the Social Security Administration, the Internal Revenue Service (IRS), and the Centers for Medicare and Medicaid Services (CMS). An example of state regulation is the Rules of Professional Conduct, the ability to meet professional standards and competently perform the duties of a licensed professional.

Registration: The periodic provision of information by individuals to update public records.

Certification: A legal document that serves as proof that someone is qualified for a particular job by attesting to the individual's status or level of achievement.

Licensure: A permit that allows an individual to perform medical acts and procedures under a scope of practice within a given state and which protects the use of the professional title.

Criminal law: A system of laws concerned with the punishment of an individual who commits a crime that is perceived as threatening, harmful, or otherwise endangering to the property, health, safety, and more aware welfare of people inclusive of one's self.

Civil law: A law that is concerned with the private affairs of citizens or members of a community in such areas as contracts, property, and family law.

Contract law: The existence of an agreement between private parties that stipulates mutual obligations that are enforceable by law.

Risk management: The process of identifying, assessing, and controlling potential threats in advance so that precautionary steps can be taken to reduce occurrences.

FEDERAL STATUTES

A federal statute is a law enacted by Congress with or without the president's approval. These have included the Civil Rights Act of 1964, the Fair Housing and Architectural Barriers Act of 1968, Section 504 of the Rehabilitation Act of 1973, and the Education for All Handicapped Children Act of 1975. The following federal statutes can impact the provision of physical therapy services:

▶ **Americans with Disabilities Act (ADA).**[2] In 1990, the ADA, a wide-ranging civil rights law, marked the first explicit national goal of achieving equal opportunity, independent living, and economic self-sufficiency for individuals with disabilities.[3] The original Act was later amended with the ADA Amendments Act of 2008 (ADAAA), signed into law to give broader protections for disabled workers, with changes effective January 1, 2009. The ADA affords discrimination protections against any American with a disability, similar to the Civil Rights Act of 1964, making it illegal to discriminate based on race, religion, sex, national origin, and other characteristics.

CLINICAL PEARL

The Civil Rights Act of 1991 is a federal law that capped compensatory and punitive damages under Title I of the ADA for intentional job discrimination. The law also amended the ADA's definition of an employee, adding "with respect to employment in a foreign country, such term includes an individual who is a citizen of the United States."

The ADA, which has five titles (Table 2-1), does not function in isolation but is related to other state and federal laws, such as the Family and Medical Leave Act (FMLA) and the Occupational Safety and Health Act (OSHA).

▶ Family and Medical Leave Act (FMLA): The FMLA entitles eligible employees to take unpaid, job-protected leave (up to 12 workweeks of leave in a 12-month period) for specified family and medical reasons (eg, the birth of a child; to care for the employee's spouse, child, or parent who has a serious health condition, etc.) with the continuation of group health insurance coverage under the same terms and conditions as if the employee had not taken leave.

▶ Occupational Safety and Health Act (OSHA): The OSHA goal is to create a safe and healthy working environment for employees. Employers must provide a working environment free from recognized hazards, and employees must adhere to health and safety standards. The National Institute for Occupational Safety and Health (NIOSH) is the research arm of OSHA. NIOSH has developed *Elements of Ergonomics Programs*, a primer based on workplace evaluations of musculoskeletal disorders that is useful in developing a program focusing on ergonomics.

To qualify as a person with a disability, the individual must have a physical or mental impairment that substantially limits the performance of one of life's major activities (Table 2-2).

To fully understand the ADA, it is important to understand the terminology (Table 2-3). Working in concert with the ADA are the Americans with Disabilities Act Accessibility Guidelines (ADAAG; see http://www.access-board.gov/adaag/html/adaag.htm) that detail the technical requirements to be applied during the design, construction, and alteration of buildings and facilities covered by Titles II and III of the ADA to the extent required by regulations issued by federal agencies, including the Department of Justice and the Department of Transportation (Table 2-4).

CLINICAL PEARL

Detailed information about the ADA can be found at http://www.ada.gov/cguide.htm.

▶ **Social Security Act Amendments of 1965.** In 1965, the passage of the Social Security Act Amendments created Medicare, a rudimentary program of hospital insurance for persons aged 65 and older, and Medicaid, a supplementary medical insurance program, funded jointly by the state and federal governments, that provides for states to finance healthcare for individuals who were at, or close to, the public assistance level.

▶ **Emergency Medical Treatment and Labor Act (EMTALA).** In 1986, Congress enacted the Emergency Medical Treatment and Labor Act (EMTALA). Section 1867 of the Social Security Act imposes specific obligations on Medicare-participating hospitals. Specifically, EMTALA, or the Patient Anti-Dumping Law, requires most hospitals to provide medical screening examinations (MSEs) and needed stabilizing treatment, without considering

TABLE 2-1	The Five Titles of the ADA
Title	**Name and Description**
I. Employment	Prohibits employers (an employment agency, labor organization, or joint labor-management committee) from discriminating against a qualified individual with a disability concerning job application procedures, hiring, advancement, and discharge of employees; workers' compensation; job training; and other terms, conditions, and privileges of employment, based on that disability alone. Examples of workplace accommodations include: ▶ Modification of work schedule ▶ Modification of job activities or requirements ▶ Modification to the physical plant ▶ The provision of assistive devices such as a telephone amplifier ▶ Modification of existing furniture or equipment ▶ Access to accessible restrooms, entrances, hallways, doorways, and parking areas. This usually necessitates a review of the application form, process, procedures; selection and hiring procedures; and evaluation, advancement, and training opportunities and activities. Each job description should be written using functional terms (eg, be able to lift 25 pounds and stand for one hour at a time).
II. Public services and transportation	Prohibits disability discrimination by all public entities at the local (school district, municipal, city, and county) and state level. Access includes physical access described in the ADA Standards for Accessible Design and programmatic access that might be obstructed by the entity's discriminatory policies or procedures. Access to a facility or establishment for persons with disabilities, freedom of movement, and access to goods and services should be given immediate attention once inside the facility.
III. Public accommodations	No individual may be discriminated against based on disability with regard to the full and equal enjoyment of the goods, services, facilities, or accommodations of any place of public accommodation by any person who owns, leases (or leases to), or operates a place of public accommodation (most places of lodging [hotel or motel], recreation, transportation, education, dining, stores, care providers, park or zoo, and places of public displays). For existing facilities and those to be constructed, structural physical barriers must be removed or not included. This title usually requires removing, modifying, or altering structural barriers when the changes can be made reasonably and accomplished without significant difficulty or expense. Examples include the installation of ramps, the widening of doorways, the use of door hardware that is more functional than a knob, installation of support bars or rails, auxiliary services and aids for individuals with a vision or hearing impairment (telecommunication display device [TDD]), increased space in restrooms to accommodate a wheelchair, water fountains accessible from the wheelchair, and curb cutouts. Exempted entities include private clubs and establishments exempt from Title II of the Civil Rights Act of 1964, religious organizations or entities controlled by religious organizations, and entities operated by governments exempt from Titles I and II.
IV. Telecommunications	Requires that all telecommunications companies in the United States take steps to ensure functionally equivalent services for consumers with disabilities, notably those who are deaf or hard of hearing and those with speech impairments.
V. Other provisions	Includes technical provisions such as the fact that nothing in the ADA amends, overrides, or cancels anything in Section 504, in addition to an anti-retaliation or coercion provision.

insurance coverage or ability to pay, when a patient presents to an emergency room for attention with an emergency medical condition (EMC), including active labor.

▶ **Health Insurance and Portability and Accountability Act (HIPAA).** This 1996 federal legislation was designed to protect the individual from excessive personal expenditures and protect healthcare-related information.

Under this Act, the financial protections deemed that long-term care (LTC) insurance premiums are tax-deductible if nonreimbursable medical expenses, including part or all of the LTC premiums, exceed 7.5% of an individual's gross income. HIPAA also excludes LTC insurance benefits from taxable income. Not all LTC insurance coverage qualifies for this benefit.

CLINICAL PEARL

Regulatory controls within the US healthcare system include the fraud and abuse provisions included in HIPAA, the Balanced Budget Act of 1997, and those listed in Table 2-5.

HIPAA also issued a Privacy Rule to implement its requirement. The Privacy Rule standards address the use and disclosure of individuals' health information (called "protected health information" or PHI) by organizations subject to the Privacy Rule (called "covered entities"), as well as standards for individuals' privacy rights to understand and control how their health information is used. The Privacy Rule's major

TABLE 2-2	Major Life Activities

Social/Emotional:

► Interaction with others (eg, speech difficulties such as pressured speech, lack of clarity, withdrawal or responding with difficulty or too quickly; self-absorption; inability to relate to or listen to others, including an inability to relate due to paranoia, delusions, hallucinations, obsessive-compulsive ideation, negativity; inability to regulate mood and anxiety; inability to maintain an appropriate distance from others)

► Forming and maintaining relationships with others

► Communication with others (eg, answering questions, following directions, using intelligible speech, recognizing and expressing emotions appropriately, expressing needs, following a sequence)

Cognitive:

► Concentration—as a major life activity itself and also resulting in limitations on other major life activities, such as interaction with others, self-care

► Making decisions

► Complex thinking (eg, planning, reconciling perceptions from different senses [seeing and hearing], sorting relevant from irrelevant details, problem-solving, changing from one task to another)

► Abstract thinking (eg, difficulty generalizing or transferring learning from one setting to another, such as difficulty transferring the skill of cooking in one kitchen to another kitchen)

► Memory—long or short term

► Attention

► Perception

► Distinguishing real from unreal events

► Initiating and completing actions

► Processing information

Physical:

► Taking care of personal needs, such as eating, dressing, toileting, bathing, hygiene, household chores, managing money, following medication or treatment regimens, following safety precautions

► Eating (eg, inability to regulate amounts appropriately or to maintain appropriate diet; the need for strict eating schedule)

► Sleeping (eg, inability to fall asleep, obtain restful sleep, or sleep without interruption; excessive sleeping)

► Reproduction

► Sexual activity

► Traveling

TABLE 2-3	Glossary of ADA Terms

Term	Definition
Accessible	Refers to a site, facility, work environment, service, or program that is easy to approach, enter, operate, participate in, and/or use safely and with dignity by a person with a disability.
Affirmative-action	A set of positive steps that employers use to promote equal employment opportunity and to eliminate discrimination.
Employer	A person engaged in an industry affecting commerce that has 15 or more employees for each working day in each of 20 or more calendar weeks in the current or preceding calendar year, and any agent of such person. Exceptions: The term "employer" does not include the United States, a corporation wholly owned by the government of the United States, or a Native American tribe; or a bona fide private membership club.
Equal Employment Opportunity Commission (EEOC)	A federal agency charged with enforcing Title I of the ADA.
Major life activity	Activities that an average person can perform with little or no difficulty. Major life activities include, but are not limited to: caring for oneself, performing manual tasks, seeing, hearing, eating, sleeping, walking, standing, sitting, reaching, lifting, bending, speaking, breathing, learning, reading, concentrating, thinking, communicating, interacting with others, and working; and the operation of a major bodily function.
Reasonable accommodation	Under Title I, a modification or adjustment to a job, the work environment, or the way things usually are done to enable a qualified individual with a disability to enjoy an equal employment opportunity. A reasonable accommodation is a key nondiscrimination requirement of the ADA.
Undue burden	Concerning complying with Title II or Title III of the ADA, significant difficulty or expense incurred by a covered entity, when considered in light of certain factors. These factors include the nature and cost of the action; the overall financial resources of the site or sites involved; the number of persons employed at the site; and the effect on expenses and resources.

TABLE 2-4	Design Specifications for Accessibility
Ramps	Grade: not greater than 1:12 (8.3%) for new construction, with a vertical rise of not greater than 30 inches. Not greater than 1:10 (10%) for existing sites, with a vertical rise of not greater than 6 inches if space does not permit construction of a grade of 1:12 or less. Not greater than 1:8 (12.5%) for existing sites, with a vertical rise of not greater than 3 inches if space does not permit construction of a grade of 1:12 or less. Minimum width of 36 inches. Must have handrails on both sides. 12 inches of length for each inch of vertical rise. Handrails are required for a rise of 6 inches or more or for horizontal runs of 72 inches or more.
Grade of approach	Not greater than 1:20 (5%) unless requirements for a ramp are met.
Height	Not less than 80 inches vertical clearance. If vertical clearance along an accessible route is less than 80 inches, a warning barrier must be provided.
Doorways	Minimum width of 32 inches. Maximum depth of 24 inches.
Thresholds	Less than ¾ inch for sliding doors. Less than ½ inch for other doors.
Carpet	Requires ½-inch pile or less.
Hallway clearance	36-inch width.
Wheelchair turning radius (U-turn)	60-inch width. 78-inch length.
Forward reach in a wheelchair	Low reach 15 inches. High reach 48 inches.
Side reach in a wheelchair	Reach over an obstruction to 24 inches.
Bathroom sink	Not less than 29-inch height. Not greater than 40 inches from floor to bottom of mirror or paper dispenser. 17 inches minimum depth under the sink to back wall.
Bathroom toilet	17–19 inches from floor to top of the toilet. Grab bars should be 1¼-1½ inches in diameter. 1-inch spacing between grab bars and wall. Grab bar placement 33 to 36 inches up from floor level.
Hotels	Approximately 2% of total rooms must be accessible.
Parking spaces	96 inches wide. 240 inches in length. The adjacent aisle must be 60 inches × 240 inches. Approximately 2% of the total spaces must be accessible.

goal is to ensure that individuals' health information is properly protected while allowing the flow of health information needed to provide and promote high-quality healthcare and protect the public's health and well-being.

▶ The Privacy Rule applies to anyone who transmits health information in electronic form in connection with transactions.

▶ The Privacy Rule protects all "individually identifiable health information" held or transmitted by a covered entity (health plans, healthcare clearinghouses, and any healthcare provider) or its business associate (limited to legal, actuarial, accounting, consulting, data aggregation, management, administrative, accreditation, or financial services), in any form or medium, whether electronic, paper, or oral.

CLINICAL PEARL

According to HIPAA's Privacy Rule, PHI includes all of the following:

▶ Demographic data, which relate to the individual's past, present, or future physical or mental health condition

▶ The provision of healthcare to the individual

▶ The past, present, or future payment for the provision of healthcare to the individual

Individually identifiable health information includes the name, address, date of birth, and Social Security number of the patient.

Further details can be found at http://www.hhs.gov/ocr/hipaa.

TABLE 2-5	Fiscal Regulations within the US Healthcare System
Regulation	**Description**
False Claims Act of 1863	First signed into law in 1863. Underwent significant changes in 1986. It allows citizens to bring lawsuits against groups or other individuals who defraud the government through programs, agencies, or contracts (overbilling for services, "upcoding").
Medicare and Medicaid anti-fraud statutes	Stipulates that an individual who knowingly and willfully offers, pays, solicits, or receives any remuneration in exchange for referring an individual for the furnishing of any item or service (or for the purchasing, leasing, ordering, or recommending of any good, facility, item, or service) paid for in whole or in part by Medicare or a state healthcare program (ie, Medicaid) shall be guilty of a felony. Often referred to as the "anti-kickback" statute.
The Civil Monetary Penalties Law (CMPL)	Authorizes the Secretary of Health and Human Services to impose civil money penalties, an assessment, and program exclusion for various fraud and abuse forms involving the Medicare and Medicaid programs.
Federal self-referral prohibitions	Also known as Stark I and II. The first Self-Referral Prohibitions (Stark I) prohibited physicians from referring lab specimens obtained from Medicare patients to clinical laboratories with which the physician or an immediate family member of the physician had a financial relationship. Also, any clinical laboratory that received a Medicare referral from a physician with which it had a financial relationship could not bill Medicare for that procedure's performance. A financial relationship is defined as either an ownership/investment interest or a compensation relationship. The expanded Physician Self-Referral prohibitions (Stark II), introduced in 1995, prohibits self-referrals (Medicaid and Medicare) of lab services and many other designated health services, including physical therapy.
Pharmaceutical price regulation scheme	A scheme that ensures the national health system has access to good-quality branded medicines at reasonable prices and promotes a healthy, competitive pharmaceutical industry. Includes federal average wholesale price restrictions for Medicaid and state pharmaceutical regulations.
Certificate of Need (CON)	Intended to regulate major capital expenditures that may adversely affect the cost of healthcare services, prevent the unnecessary expansion of healthcare facilities, and encourage the appropriate allocation of resources for healthcare purposes. CON laws became part of almost every state by 1978 after the 1974 National Health Act was passed.

A covered entity must disclose PHI in only two situations:

▶ To individuals (or their representatives) specifically when they request access to, or an accounting of disclosures of, their PHI.

▶ To the Department of Health and Human Services (HHS) when undertaking a compliance investigation or review or enforcement action.

A covered entity is permitted, but not required, to use and disclose PHI, without an individual's authorization, for the following purposes or situations:

▶ To the individual (unless required for access or accounting of disclosures)

▶ Treatment, payment, and healthcare operations

▶ Opportunity to agree or object

▶ Incident to an otherwise permitted use and disclosure

▶ Public interest and benefit activities and Office for Civil Rights (OCR) Privacy Rule Summary

▶ Limited data set: for research, public health, or healthcare operations

CLINICAL PEARL

Suppose the patient feels that a HIPAA violation has occurred. In that case, they can file a complaint with the OCR, which reviews the information and, based on their findings, can either refer the case to the Department of Justice or determine that there was no violation.

Covered entities may rely on professional ethics and best judgments in deciding which of these permitted uses and disclosures to make.

▶ *Workforce training and management.* Workforce members include employees, volunteers, trainees, and other persons whose conduct is under the entity's direct control (whether or not the entity pays them). A covered entity must train all workforce members on its privacy policies and procedures as necessary and appropriate for them to carry out their functions. A covered entity must apply appropriate sanctions against workforce members who violate its privacy policies and procedures or the Privacy Rule.

- *Data safeguards.* A covered entity must maintain reasonable and appropriate administrative, technical, and physical safeguards to prevent intentional or unintentional use or disclosure of PHI in violation of the Privacy Rule and limit its incidental use and disclosure according to otherwise permitted or required use or disclosure. For example, such safeguards might include shredding documents containing PHI before discarding them, securing medical records with lock and key or passcode, and limiting access to keys or passcodes.

- *Documentation and record retention.* A covered entity must maintain, until 6 years after the later date of their creation or last effective date, privacy policies and procedures, privacy practices notices, disposition of complaints, and other actions, activities, and designations that the Privacy Rule requires to be documented.

- *Criminal penalties.* A person who knowingly obtains or discloses PHI in violation of HIPAA faces a fine of $50,000 and up to 1 year imprisonment. The criminal penalties increase to $100,000 and up to 5 years imprisonment if the wrongful conduct involves pretenses, and to $250,000 and up to 10 years imprisonment if the wrongful conduct involves the intent to sell, transfer, or use PHI for commercial advantage, personal gain, or malicious harm.

CLINICAL PEARL

From the clinician's perspective, HIPAA compliance includes the following:

- Ensuring that any conversations about patients do not occur in public areas, such as elevators or cafeterias.

- Only sharing patient information with individuals on a need-to-know basis.

- Securing handwritten or digital documentation from prying eyes.

- **The Patient Protection and Affordable Care Act (PPACA).** The PPACA, commonly known as the Affordable Care Act (ACA), is a federal statute signed into US law in March 2010 and the Healthcare and Education Reconciliation Act of 2010 (also signed into law in March 2010). The statute includes numerous health-related provisions, including:

  - Guaranteed issue and community rating—insurers must offer the same premium to all applicants of the same age, sex, and geographical location regardless of whether the applicant has a preexisting condition.

  - Allows children to remain on their parents' insurance plan until they reach the age of 26.

  - Medicaid eligibility is expanded to include individuals and families up to 133% of the poverty level.

  - New health insurance exchanges in each state must enhance competition by offering a marketplace where individuals and small businesses can compare policy premiums on a like-for-like basis and buy insurance

(with a government subsidy if eligible). Low-income persons and families above the Medicaid level and up to 400% of the poverty level will receive subsidies on a sliding scale if they choose to purchase insurance via a health insurance exchange.

  - Introduction into the tax code of a "shared responsibility payment," which is a fine paid by any large employer (with 50 or more employees) if the government has had to subsidize an employee who bought insurance in the exchange because the employer did not offer a minimum coverage plan or better. Another form of shared responsibility payment or fine is imposed on certain persons who do not have minimum essential coverage for at least one month in the year (individual mandate), though being insured is not mandated by law.

  - Improved benefits for Medicare prescription drug coverage.

  - Establishment of a national voluntary insurance program for purchasing community living assistance services and support.

  - Very small businesses to get subsidies if they purchase health insurance through the exchange.

  - Additional support provided for medical research and the National Institutes of Health (NIH).

The ACA also required all Americans to carry medical insurance that meets federally designated minimum standards or face a tax penalty, although, in some cases, taxpayers may qualify for exemption from the penalty if they were unable to obtain insurance due to financial hardship or other situations.

- The Individuals with Disabilities Education Act (IDEA).* The IDEA is a law that makes available free appropriate public education to eligible children with disabilities throughout the nation and ensures special education and related services (including physical therapy) to those children. Children and youth ages 3 through 21 receive special education and related services under IDEA Part B. Infants and toddlers, birth through age 2, with disabilities and their families receive early intervention services under IDEA Part C. The US Department of Education's OCR provides additional interest resources for individuals with disabilities and their families.

REIMBURSEMENT IN HEALTHCARE

Reimbursement is the method by which healthcare providers are paid by insurance or government payers. While the need for healthcare has not changed, healthcare reimbursement has been a source of frustration for the providers for several decades as insurance companies attempt to balance unaffordable care for certain groups while also trying to control healthcare costs.[4] Reimbursement for physical therapy services varies greatly depending on the practice setting.

---

*https://sites.ed.gov/idea/about-idea/.

Health insurance: A type of insurance covering some, or all, of the cost of an individual's healthcare. Health insurance companies function to offer policies that assume the risk and to process health insurance claims. Employers, the government, and individuals contribute toward the cost of health insurance.

Health insurance premium: A monthly fee paid to a health insurance company, or health plan, to provide health coverage. Other health insurance costs can include deductibles (the amount that the subscriber pays before a health insurer reimburses for all or part of the remaining cost of the covered services), coinsurance (the subscriber is required to assume responsibility for a percentage of the cost of the covered services), and copayments (a fee that the subscriber is required to pay for specific health services at the time of use). Some items related to physical therapy are not typically covered. These include durable medical equipment (DME) where, in most cases, the patient is responsible for the full payment. Examples of DME include a wheelchair, a leg/arm brace, and specialized crutches.

National health insurance (NHI): A universal health insurance system that insures a national population against healthcare costs. Countries with universal healthcare include Austria, Belarus, Croatia, the Czech Republic, Denmark, Finland, France, Germany, Greece, Iceland, Ireland, Italy, Luxembourg, Malta, Moldova, the Netherlands, Norway, Portugal, Romania, Russia, Serbia, Spain, Sweden, Switzerland, Turkey, Ukraine, and the United Kingdom.

Retrospective reimbursement: These payment plans pay healthcare providers based on their actual charges. Examples include fee-for-service (indemnity).

Prospective reimbursement: These payment plans pay healthcare providers based on a fixed payment rate to specific treatments. Examples include diagnostic-related groups (DRGs), the Medicare fee schedule, and the resource-based relative value scale (RBRVS).

CPT codes: Current Procedural Terminology (CPT) codes are numbers assigned to every task and service a medical practitioner may provide to a patient, including medical, surgical, and diagnostic services. CPT codes are developed, maintained, and copyrighted by the American Medical Association (AMA).

HCPCS codes: Healthcare Common Procedure Coding System (HCPCS) codes are used and maintained by the CMS and are used for billing Medicare, Medicaid, and many other third-party payers. There are two levels of codes. Level I codes are based on CPT codes (they are essentially identical) and used for services and procedures usually provided by physicians. Level II codes cover healthcare services and procedures that aren't provided by physicians (eg, physical therapy)

G-codes: Rehab therapy providers initially used G-codes to report to CMS for the Physician Quality Reporting System (PQRS)—a now-defunct quality-reporting program. G-codes were used to fulfill Functional Limitation Reporting (FLR) requirements, a CMS reporting regulation for outpatient rehab providers of Medicare beneficiaries designed to establish an evidence-based connection between rehab therapy treatment and patient progress. To comply with FLR, clinicians had to report functional limitation data in the form of G-codes and the corresponding severity modifiers and therapy modifiers determined at the initial examination, at minimum every tenth visit (or progress note), and at discharge. Eight sets of G-codes generally described SLP functional limitations, while six of the G-code sets generally described PT and occupational therapy (OT) functional limitations. CMS announced the official discontinuation of FLR in the 2019 final rule, citing undue administrative burden and negligible effect on the quality of care. A PTA may still encounter G-codes when reviewing all the documentation if the dates of service occurred when the FLRs were effective, January 1, 2013 through December 31, 2018.

Merit-Based Incentive Payment System (MIPS): Effective January 1, 2017, PQRS was moved into the MIPS, which, in turn, is part of the new Quality Payment Program (QPP) created by the Medicare Access and Children's Health Insurance Program (CHIP) Reauthorization Act of 2015 (MACRA). Within the MIPS, quality performance categories measure healthcare processes, outcomes, and patient experiences of their care.

Advanced alternative payment models (APMs): A payment approach that gives added incentive payments (5%) to provide high-quality and cost-efficient care. APMs can apply to a specific clinical condition, a care episode, or a population.

Reimbursement to healthcare providers can occur in the following ways.

Units of Payment

The methods by which physicians and healthcare services have been reimbursed over the years have varied and range from the simplest to the more complex[5]:

▶ *Fee-for-service with utilization review.* Reimbursement is based on a fee-for-service mechanism, in which the physician or hospital is paid a fee for each office visit, procedure, or supply provided. The third-party payer (whether a private insurance company or a government agency) has the authority to deny payment for expensive or unnecessary medical interventions.

▶ *Payment by an episode of illness.* The entity is paid one sum for all services delivered during one episode of illness. A diagnosis-related group (DRG) is a reimbursement system designed to replace cost-based reimbursement based on the International Classification of

Diseases (ICD) diagnoses, procedures, age, sex, discharge status, and the presence of complications or comorbidities. For example, the federal Medicare program for the elderly typically pays a hospital a flat fee per hospital case, with a different per-case price for each DRG. Today, several different DRG systems have been developed in the United States. They include:

- Medicare DRGs (CMS-DRG & MS-DRG)
- Refined DRGs (R-DRG)
- All Patient DRGs (AP-DRG)
- Severity DRGs (S-DRG)
- All Patient Severity-Adjusted DRGs (APS-DRG)
- All Patient Refined DRGs (APR-DRG)
- International-Refined DRGs (IR-DRG)

The International Conference for the Ninth Revision of the ICD was gathered in 1975 due to an enormous growth of interest in the ICD and to examine the possibility of using a data processing system to evaluate medical care and produce statistics and indexes, and to generate codes based on disease categories. This coding system became the ICD-9 system and was widely used throughout the United States until fairly recently when in 2015, a transition was made to the ICD-10 system to keep up with all of the changes in newer medical diagnoses and a push toward outcome measurement. Since then, a newer version of the ICD, ICD-11, has been released and is scheduled to be implemented in January 2022. Until that time, all HIPAA-covered entities must adhere to the ICD-10 codes, as mandated by the HHS. Based on its predecessor, ICD-9, ICD-10 uses unique alphanumeric codes to recognize the severity of diseases and other health issues to store and retrieve diagnostic information and calculate national mortality and morbidity statistics. While the various medical entities use the vast majority of the ICD-10 codes within the healthcare system, some are used by physical therapy. ICD-10 uses a specific code structure:

- The first character must be an alpha character, excluding "u."
- The second and third characters are numeric.
- The fourth through seventh characters can be a combination of numeric and alpha characters.

The first three characters categorize the injury; whereas the fourth through sixth categories include the anatomical site, severity, and etiology, related to the category; and the seventh character is an extension used to classify the initial or subsequent treatment encounter.

Using right knee patellar tendinopathy as an example, M00 through M99 represent diseases of the musculoskeletal system and connective tissue, M70 through M79 represent other soft tissue disorders, and M76.5 represents patellar tendinopathy of the right knee.

Unfortunately, not all of the physical therapy diagnoses fall under the M category. For example, an injury to the right quadriceps falls under the S category—injuries, poisonings, and certain other consequences of external causes related to a single body region. It has a diagnosis code of S76.101, as S76 represents an injury of muscle, fascia, and tendon at hip and thigh level, and 101 represents an unspecified injury of the right quadriceps muscle, fascia and tendon.

While it is not the PTA's responsibility to initially code a patient's diagnosis, the PTA must understand the coding process basics and the need for specificity in their documentation for correct billing of the patient.

- *Per diem payments.* A hospital is paid for all services delivered to a patient during one day of inpatient care. The levels of these payments are set unilaterally by the state governments or by private insurers. The per diems that private insurers pay hospitals are negotiated annually between each hospital and each insurance carrier.

CLINICAL PEARL

Reimbursement levels are rarely equal to the full charge. For example, private insurers pay hospitals predominantly by per diems or fee-for-service schedules. The profits built into these payments by the hospitals cover the losses incurred by serving Medicare and Medicaid patients, who are billed at high prices but are not reimbursed in full. Also, reimbursements occur with delays, denials, or other complications.

- *Capitation payment.* Capitation is one of several forms of prepaid medical care that differs from a fee-for-service arrangement. Capitation pays a hospital, physician, or group of physicians a set amount for each enrolled person assigned to them, per period, whether or not that person seeks care. In exchange for this fixed rate of reimbursement, physicians essentially become the enrolled patients' insurers, who resolve their patients' claims and assume the responsibility for their unknown future healthcare costs.
- *Payment for all services delivered to all patients within a certain time frame.* This includes a global budget payment of hospitals and salary payment for physicians. Facilities or systems that use a global budget have clear incentives to control costs and to operate efficiently. The major problem with this type of reimbursement is that providers who find themselves in danger of exceeding their budget may respond with "rationing by waiting," resulting in access problems for the patients.
- *Out-of-pocket payments.* This method is used by individuals who have no insurance, whether by choice or financial restrictions.

CLINICAL PEARL

It is the clinician's responsibility to determine the patient's coverage at the beginning of each episode of care and, without compromising patient care, any payment limitation on the part of the patient should be integrated into the plan of care.

TYPES OF HEALTH INSURANCE

At present, individuals can have access to healthcare services through a variety of insurance methods, which include:

▶ *Individual private insurance (generally for self-employed individuals)*. In return for paying a monthly sum, people receive assistance in case of illness.

▶ *Employer-sponsored health (group) insurance.* Employers usually pay most of the premium to purchase health insurance for their employees as one of the employment benefits. In most cases, employment-based plans now require employee contributions and copayments. The government does not treat the health insurance fringe benefits as taxable income to the employee, so the government is, in essence, subsidizing employer-sponsored health insurance. A new form of employment-based private insurance is consumer-driven healthcare (CDH). Defined narrowly, CDH refers to health plans in which individuals have a personal health account, such as a health savings account (HSA) or a health reimbursement arrangement (HRA), from which they pay medical expenses directly. The phrase is sometimes used more broadly to refer to defined-contribution health plans, which allow employees to choose among various plans, often with a fixed dollar contribution from an employer. The characteristics of a CDH include:

- High-benefit options that involve significant employee contributions and deductibles in addition to an employer's contribution *or* lower benefit options that involve fewer employee contributions and deductibles.

- Greater choice and control over one's health plan.

- Economic incentives to better manage care—economic rewards for making good decisions and economic penalties for making ill-advised ones. These economic incentives make patients more likely to investigate medical conditions and treatment options, including information about prices and quality.

▶ *Government financing.* This occurs through government-funded programs, such as Medicare, Medicaid, and the Federal Employees Health Benefits Plans.

- *Medicare.* Administered by the federal government—the CMS. CMS is an agency within the US Department of Health and Human Services, through the extension of title XVIII of the Social Security Act, 1965. Medicare coverage is independent of income or pre-existing conditions.

CLINICAL PEARL

Healthcare Financing Administration (HCFA) was the previous name for the CMS.

CLINICAL PEARL

Medicare currently covers physical therapy services in the following provider settings: skilled nursing facilities (SNFs), home health agencies (HHAs), long-term care hospitals (LTCHs), inpatient rehabilitation facilities (IRFs), acute care hospitals, physical therapy private practice offices, physician's offices, rehabilitation agencies, and comprehensive outpatient rehabilitation facilities (CORFs).[6]

There are four different varieties, or parts, to Medicare:

▶ *Part A.* On reaching the age of 65, people eligible for Social Security are automatically enrolled in Medicare Part A if they are retired. Suppose a person has paid into the Social Security system for ten years. In that case, their spouse is eligible for Social Security.[5] Individuals aged 65 years and older who are still employed and are receiving coverage under an employer's insurance plan must sign up for Medicare Part A by contacting Social Security within eight months of retiring or leaving the company.[7] People who are not eligible for Social Security can enroll in Medicare Part A by paying a monthly premium. Most people do not pay a monthly premium for Part A, but those who do, pay a monthly premium (up to $471 in 2021). People under the age of 65 with permanent disabilities, end-stage renal disease, or amyotrophic lateral sclerosis (ALS) may enroll in Medicare Part A after becoming eligible for Social Security Disability Insurance (SSDI), which usually takes up to 24 months. Part A helps pay for medically necessary inpatient hospital care (limiting the number of hospital days), and, after a hospital stay, limited inpatient care in a skilled nursing facility or limited home healthcare or hospice care (Table 2-6). An individual must enroll for Medicare part A services during a 7-month window around the time they turn 65 (the 3 months before their 65th birthday, the month they turn 65, and 3 months after their 65th birthday).[7] Those who fail to enroll during the enrollment window are permitted to enroll between January 1 and March 31 every year, with coverage beginning July 1 of that year. However, those individuals must pay a monthly penalty of 10% of the premiums for twice the period they were eligible to enroll but did not do so.[7]

CLINICAL PEARL

The Medicare Modernization Act of 2003 made two major changes in the Medicare program:

▶ Medicare Advantage Plan (also known as a Medicare private health plan or Part C): An expansion of the role of private health plans that invigorated the previous Medicare + Choice program by which Medicare beneficiaries could pay an additional premium to enroll in private plans. The most common types of MA programs are health maintenance organizations (HMOs), preferred provider organizations (PPOs), and private fee-for-service (PFFS). Members pay a monthly premium for Part B (and a Part A premium, if applicable) and receive the same benefits offered by original Medicare, but the MA plan may apply different rules, costs, and restrictions.

▶ Medicare Part D: A prescription drug benefit. This program has proved controversial:

TABLE 2-6	Medicare Part A and Part B (2021)		
Medicare Part	**Method of Financing**	**Benefit**	**Medicare Pays**
A	Employers and employees each pay to Medicare 1.45% of wages and salaries into the Social Security system. Self-employed people pay 2.9%.	*Hospitalization* First 60 days 61st to 90th day 91st day and beyond	All but a $1,484 deductible per spell of illness All but $371 per day All but $742 per day per each "lifetime reserve day" after day 90 for each benefit period (up to 60 days over your lifetime)
		Beyond 90 days, if lifetime reserve days are used up	Nothing
		Skilled Nursing Facility (SNF) First 20 days 21st to 100th day Beyond 101 days	 All All but $185.50 per day Nothing
		Home healthcare 100 visits per spell of illness	 100% for skilled care as defined by Medicare regulations
		Medicare-approved amount for durable medical equipment (DME)	20% of the amount
		Hospice care Requires physician certification that individual has a terminal illness	 100% of services, copays for outpatient drugs, and coinsurance for inpatient respite care
B	In part by general federal revenues (personal income and other federal taxes) and in part by Part B monthly premium.	Medical expenses Physician services Physical, occupational, and speech therapy Medical equipment Diagnostic tests	80% of approved amount after a $203 annual deductible
		Preventative care (some Pap smears; some mammogram; hepatitis B, pneumococcal, and influenza vaccinations)	Included in medical expenses, with deductible and coinsurance waived for some services
		Outpatient medications. Partially covered under Medicare Part D	All except for premium, deductible, coinsurance
		Eye refractions, hearing aids, dental services	Not covered

Reproduced with permission from Part A & Part B sign up periods. Medicare.gov https://www.medicare.gov/sign-up-change-plans/how-do-i-get-parts-a-b/part-a-part-b-sign-up-periods.

- There are major gaps in coverage.
- Coverage has been farmed out to private insurance companies rather than administered by the federal Medicare program.
- The government is not allowed to negotiate with pharmaceutical companies for lower drug prices.[5]

▶ *Part B:* Part B (see Table 2-6) is for those eligible for Medicare Part A and who voluntarily elect to pay the Medicare Part B standard premium based on their annual income.[7] Some low-income persons are not required to pay the premium. Part B coverage reimburses for physician visits, outpatient and therapy services (outside those provided in the hospital), and other medical services not covered by Medicare Part A. The enrollment window is the same as for Medicare Part A.

▶ *Part C:* Medicare Part C (Medicare Advantage Plans), often referred to as Part C or MA Plans, replaced Medicare + Choice, or Medicare Part C, and are plans offered by private companies (HMO, PPO, or PFFS) approved by Medicare. Medicare Advantage Plans provide all of the Part A and Part B benefits. Under these plans, Medicare pays a fixed amount for the subscriber's healthcare each month. Some Medicare Advantage Plans also offer extra coverage, like vision, hearing, and dental coverage. In addition to a monthly premium, subscribers may also have to pay out-of-pocket expenses to see a specialist or for doctor's visits. Part C plans can also provide additional benefits or services, including Medicare Part D prescription coverage as long as the patient is enrolled in Part A and Part B.

▶ *Part D:* Part D, enacted as part of the Medicare Prescription Drug Improvement and Modernization Act of 2003, subsidizes the cost of prescription drugs and provides more choices in health coverage (eg, Medicare Advantage) for

Medicare beneficiaries who pay a monthly premium and are enrolled in Part A and Part B.

CLINICAL PEARL

Several factors have negatively impacted Medicare reimbursements, including:

► An overall decrease in the number of workers compared with the number of beneficiaries, leading to a projection that Part A funds will be exhausted by 2030.

► The rising costs of medical care.

► The rising costs of prescription drugs.

► More stringent requirements for reimbursement (limiting physical therapy visits, more frequent reevaluations and updated plans of care [POCs], increasing levels of patient supervision, decreased reimbursement for services provided by a PTA or student therapists).

► *Medicaid.* In all states, Medicaid provides health coverage for some low-income people across various categories: children, pregnant women, parents, seniors, and individuals with disabilities. Medicaid is a federal program mandated by Title XIX of the Social Security Act administered by the states, with the federal government paying between 50% and 76% of the total Medicaid costs. Benefits vary from state to state—the federal contribution is greater in states with lower per capita incomes. Medicaid pays for medical and other services on behalf of certain groups:

■ Low-income families with children who meet certain eligibility requirements.

■ Most elderly, disabled, and blind individuals who receive cash assistance under the federal Supplemental Security Income (SSI) program.

■ Children younger than age 6 and pregnant women whose family income is at or below a percentage of the federal poverty level. In 2020, the federal poverty level was $26,200 for a family of four.

■ School-age children (6–18) whose family income is at or below the federal poverty level.

CLINICAL PEARL

Medicaid services are provided in various settings, including but not limited to home care, intermediate-care facilities for people with intellectual disability (intellectual developmental disorder) (ICF/MR), and schools.[6]

Because of large expenditure growth, the federal government ceded enhanced control of the Medicaid programs to states through Medicaid waivers, which allow states to reduce the number of people on Medicaid, make alterations to the scope of covered services, require Medicaid recipients to pay part of their costs, and obligate Medicaid recipients to enroll in managed care plans.[5]

CLINICAL PEARL

Medicaid waivers are an exception to the usual requirements of Medicaid granted to a state by CMS. The waivers allow states to:

► Waive provisions of the Medicaid law to test new concepts consistent with the Medicaid program's goals. System-wide changes are possible under this provision. Frequently used to establish Medicaid managed care programs.

► Waive freedom of choice. States may require that beneficiaries enroll in HMOs or other managed care programs or select a physician to serve as their primary care case manager.

► Waive various Medicaid requirements to establish alternative, community-based services for (a) individuals who would otherwise require the level of care provided in a hospital or skilled nursing facility and/or (b) persons already in such facilities who need assistance returning to the community. Waivers include older adults, persons with disabilities, persons with intellectual disabilities, persons with chronic mental illness, and persons with acquired immunodeficiency syndrome (AIDS).

► Limit expenditures for nursing facility and home and community-based services for a person 65 years and older so that they do not exceed a projected amount, determined by taking base year expenditure (the last year before the waiver) and adjusting for inflation. Also eliminates requirements that programs be statewide and comparable for all target populations. Income rules for eligibility can also be waived.

In 1997, as part of the Balanced Budget Act (see later), the federal government created the State Children's Health Insurance Program (SCHIP), the largest expansion of taxpayer-funded health insurance coverage for children in the US. SCHIP was replaced by the Children's Health Insurance Program (CHIP), a statutory authority under Title XXI of the Social Security Act. CHIP was designed as a companion program for Medicaid to cover uninsured children (from birth until their 19th birthday) in families with incomes at or below 200% of the federal poverty level, but above the Medicaid income eligibility level.[5] On February 4, 2009, President Obama signed the Children's Health Insurance Reauthorization Act of 2009, expanding the healthcare program to an additional 4 million children and pregnant women, including "lawfully residing" immigrants. States, within broad federal guidelines, are given flexibility in designing their CHIP eligibility requirements and policies.

CLINICAL PEARL

► Primary Care Case Management (PCCM). A Medicaid managed care option is allowed under Section 1915(b) of the Social Security Act, in which each participant is assigned to a single primary care provider who must authorize most other services, such as specialty physician care, before Medicaid can reimburse them.

▶ Medicaid Prudent Pharmaceutical Purchasing Act (MPPPA). Enacted as part of the Omnibus Budget Reconciliation Act of 1990, MPPPA provides that Medicaid must receive the best-discounted price of any institutional purchaser of pharmaceuticals. In doing so, drug companies provide rebates to Medicaid equal to the difference between the discounted price and the price at which the drug is sold. This bill has resulted in cost-shifting throughout the health industry.

In 2018, there were 12.2 million individuals simultaneously enrolled in Medicare and Medicaid.* These dually eligible beneficiaries (lower incomes of all ages) are among the most disabled, chronically ill, and costly in either program. Medicare covers the acute and post-acute care services, while Medicaid covers Medicare premiums and cost-sharing, and—for those beneficiaries below certain income and asset thresholds—long-term care and supportive social services.

▶ *Managed care organizations (MCO).* The MCO plans offer a medical delivery system that attempts to manage the quality and cost of medical services that individuals receive through arrangements with certain physicians, hospitals, and healthcare providers. The plans tend to be the least expensive alternative as they are generally the most restrictive and most directive. There are three major forms of managed care[4]:

■ *Preferred provider organizations (PPOs).* A PPO is a subscription-based MCO that allows members to choose from a limited number of physicians and hospitals (preferred providers) contracted to the PPO. A primary care provider (PCP) is not required for coverage, and a referral is not needed for medical services, but the patient is responsible for copays and annual deductibles. PPOs bill access fees to the insurance company, usually on a discounted fee-for-service basis with utilization review.

■ *Health maintenance organizations (HMOs).* These are organizations that provide healthcare whose patients are required (except in emergencies) to receive their care from a limited number of medical professionals within that HMO who have agreed to provide care within several confines. Members designate an in-network physician to be their primary care provider (PCP). The PCP serves as a gatekeeper for all of the patient's initial care and promotes preventative care.

■ *Point of service (POS).* POS plans are a hybrid of PPOs and HMOs. Members designate an in-network physician to be their primary care provider (PCP) but may go outside of the provider network for healthcare services (and have to pay most of the cost unless the PCP has made a referral to the out-of-network provider).

---

*Medicare-Medicaid Coordination Office, Medicare-Medicaid Dual Enrollment from 2006 through 2018. Available at: https://www.cms.gov/Medicare-Medicaid-Coordination/Medicare-and-Medicaid-Coordination/Medicare-Medicaid-Coordination-Office/Downloads/MMCO_Factsheet.pdf.

CLINICAL PEARL

Managed care plans have had a profound effect on physical therapy concerning reimbursement and delivery of services by establishing limits and other methods to control the utilization and cost of services. These methods include:

▶ Increased documentation requirements with no reimbursement for the time spent by the clinician to produce such documentation.

▶ Discounted fee schedules that pay a percentage of the charge billed by the provider.

▶ Limitations on the number of physical therapy visits.

ACCESS TO HEALTHCARE

Access to healthcare is the ability to obtain health services when needed.[8] The organizational task facing healthcare systems is one of ensuring that the right patient receives the right service at the right time in the right place, and by the right caregiver.[9,10] Health insurance coverage (see Types of Health Insurance, above), whether public or private, is a key factor in making healthcare accessible, and health insurance is often related to employment level. Individuals whose employers choose not to provide health insurance are technically self-employed and must find ways to obtain their health insurance. In 2019, 29.6 million people in the United States were uninsured.[11]

CLINICAL PEARL

A variety of regulations monitor the accessibility of healthcare. These include:

▶ The Health Maintenance Organization Act of 1973.

▶ Anti-discriminatory restrictions (including the Rehabilitation Act of 1973, Pregnancy Discrimination Act of 1978, ADA Act of 1990, and Child Abuse Prevention and Treatment Act Amendments of 1984).

▶ Continuation of coverage requirements (including the Consolidated Omnibus Budget Reconciliation Act [COBRA] of 1986 and state rules).

▶ Mandated health benefits, including mandated standards of care such as bone marrow transplants. There are at present three federally mandated health insurance benefits:

■ The Mental Health Parity Act of 1996.

■ Newborns' and Mothers' Protection Health Act of 1996.

■ Women's Health and Cancer Rights Act of 1998.

Despite health insurance regulation occurring at both the federal and state levels, which monitors such entities as the Blue Cross and Blue Shield carriers (which, if not-for-profit, are often regulated somewhat differently than their commercial counterparts), commercial insurance companies, self-insured plans, and various types of managed care, including HMOs and PPOs, private health insurance coverage continues to decrease. The reasons for this increase in the number of people who are uninsured include:

► The skyrocketing cost of health insurance. The Office of the Actuary in the CMS annually produces projections of healthcare spending for categories within the National Health Expenditure Accounts, which track health spending by source of funds (eg, private health insurance, Medicare, Medicaid), by type of service (hospital, physician, prescription drugs, etc), and by a sponsor (businesses, governments).

► A decrease in the number of highly paid, largely unionized, full-time manufacturing companies with employer-sponsored health insurance.

► An increase in the overall instability and transient nature of employment, resulting in interruptions in coverage.

CLINICAL PEARL

The uninsured suffer worse health outcomes than those with insurance, as they tend to be diagnosed at later stages, receive fewer procedures in emergency departments (EDs), and, on average, are more seriously ill when hospitalized.[11]

Theoretically, the uninsured population is supposed to have access to federal and state healthcare programs such as Medicaid. However, these programs have their limitations; access to care is by no means guaranteed with Medicaid coverage. One of the major reasons for this is that Medicaid pays physicians far less than does Medicare or private insurance, with the result that many physicians do not accept Medicaid patients.[11]

CLINICAL PEARL

Although the number of uninsured people is high, these people do have some access to healthcare:

► Hospital Survey and Construction Act, aka the Hill-Burton Act: Federal legislation enacted in 1946 to support the construction and modernization of healthcare institutions. Hospitals that receive Hill-Burton funds must provide specific levels of charity care. For example, those healthcare institutions that receive tax-exemption, federal Hill-Burton grants, or loans are not allowed to turn away patients because of an inability to pay. However, care is limited to emergency care only. A surcharge on insurance payments covers the costs incurred by this population.

► Individuals who cannot pay for healthcare can receive pro bono or free care through philanthropic donations and services.

Even the so-called insured patients are not guaranteed financial access to healthcare. Many people are underinsured;

that is, their health insurance coverage has limitations restricting access to needed services.[11] For example, many have private health insurance that leaves major expenses uncovered in the event of a serious illness. Other factors that affect the insured are insurance deductibles and copayments, with many plans having high deductibles and substantial copayments.

Finally, in addition to the financial barriers to healthcare, there are several nonfinancial barriers, including:

► *Gender.* In general, females have greater dissatisfaction with healthcare than males.

► *Race.* Because far higher proportions of minorities than whites are uninsured, have Medicaid coverage, or are poor, access problems are amplified for these groups.[11]

► *Lack of prompt access.* Many patients resort to an ED visit because they cannot obtain a timely appointment with their private physician.

► *Shortages in qualified personnel (physicians, pharmacists, nurses).* Patients in rural areas face shortages of all types of healthcare personnel (about 20% of the US population lives in areas that have a shortage of primary healthcare professionals).[11]

► *Lack of drug control.* Although drugs used in the United States must be approved for safety and efficacy, there are no therapeutic duplication or price constraints. Any drug that obtains approval from the US Food and Drug Administration (FDA) may be marketed in the United States, and the distributor has full discretion over the price charged.

► *An increasingly aging population.* The elderly often require a higher percentage of healthcare services, increasing the burden on an already stretched healthcare system.

► *Healthcare fraud.* Healthcare fraud includes medical fraud, health insurance fraud, and drug fraud. According to the National Health Care Anti-Fraud Association (NHCAA),* that conservatively estimates that healthcare fraud costs the nation about $68 billion annually (about 3% of the nation's $2.26 trillion in healthcare spending), the most common types of fraud committed by dishonest providers include: billing for services that were never rendered, billing for more expensive services or procedures than were provided, performing medically unnecessary services solely to generate insurance payments, falsifying a patient's diagnosis to justify tests, accepting kickbacks for patient referrals, or waiving patient copays or deductibles.

CLINICAL PEARL

Socioeconomic status is the dominant influence on health status and healthcare access, although healthcare access does not always guarantee good health.

---

*https://www.nhcaa.org/.

As healthcare costs have increased, efforts to control costs by the government and private entities have reduced the organization's biggest expenses—staffing—by decreasing or replacing the workforce. However, these efforts have the following disadvantages:

► Lower-cost paraprofessionals result in an increased share of the workload being performed by aides and technicians.

► An increase in caseload size results in less time spent with each patient.

QUALITY OF CARE REGULATORS

Some regulations within the US healthcare system attempt to ensure a high quality of care. These include:

► Hospital accreditation and licensure, which includes Medicare conditions of participation (COP), and the Joint Commission (JC, formerly known as Joint Commission on Accreditation of Healthcare Organizations [JCAHO]) (see Voluntary Accrediting Agencies, below)

► State accreditation and licensure, including the Department of Health (DOH)

► Nursing home accreditation and licensure (including the JC, COP, the Nursing Home Reform Act, which was part of the Omnibus Budget Reconciliation Act of 1987, and state regulations)

► Licensure for all other health facilities (see Voluntary Accrediting Agencies, below)

► Peer review, encompassing quality improvement organizations and the Healthcare Quality Improvement Act of 1986

► The Clinical Laboratory Improvement Act of 1967 as amended

► FDA regulation of blood banks

► Blood-borne pathogen requirements imposed by OSHA

► Health outcomes reporting systems mandated by states

VOLUNTARY ACCREDITING AGENCIES

Accreditation of healthcare institutions is a voluntary process by which an authorized agency or organization evaluates and recognizes health services according to a set of standards describing the structures and processes that contribute to desirable patient outcomes. Outpatient centers for comprehensive rehabilitation can be accredited by the JC, AC-MRDD, CORF, and/or CARF.

The Joint Commission (JC)

The JC is a private organization created in 1951 to provide voluntary accreditation to hospitals. Many states rely on JC accreditation as a substitute for their inspection programs. The JC has high standards of quality assurance and a rigorous evaluation process, making it a much-esteemed accreditation agency. Health services certified by the JC are given "deemed status."

TABLE 2-7	The Joint Commission Standards
Patient-focused	
Infection prevention and control	
Medication management	
Provision of care, treatment, and services	
Rights and responsibilities of the individual	
Organization functions	
Management of the environment of care	
Emergency management	
Human resources	
Management of information	
Leadership	
Life safety	
Medical staff	
Nursing	
Performance improvement	
Record of care, treatment, and services	

In the 1990s, the JC revised its standards to reflect the integration of hospital services rather than examining them in isolation and to focus on the patient experience. In 2006, the JC changed the survey process and began unannounced surveys that focused on observations and interviews. Thus, surveys currently involve a "tracer methodology" whereby a survey team enters a facility, selects some patients, and follows those patients' treatment courses throughout the facility. Some of the JC standards that are currently surveyed are listed in Table 2-7. The JC introduced a series of National Patient Safety Goals (NPSGs) in 2002 (effective January 1, 2003) to help accredited organizations address specific areas of concern regarding patient safety. The development and updating of the NPSGs are overseen by the Patient Safety Advisory Group (PSAG), a panel of widely recognized patient safety experts, including nurses, physicians, pharmacists, risk managers, and clinical engineers. The 2021 NPSGs for the hospital program were:

► Identify patients correctly, including the use of at least two patient identifiers (eg, the patient's name and date of birth) when providing care, treatment, and services and eliminating transfusion errors related to patient misidentification. It is important that, at the first treatment session, the clinician introduces him- or herself and confirms that the patient is the one who is supposed to receive the treatment. Patient identification can be confirmed by asking the patient's name or date of birth, checking the patient's identification (ID) bracelet (inpatient), or checking the medical record (ID) number.

► Improve staff communication, including reporting critical results of tests and diagnostic procedures on a timely basis to the right staff person.

► Use medicines safely, including labeling all medications, medication containers, and other solutions on and off the sterile field in perioperative and other procedural settings; reduce the likelihood of patient harm associated with anticoagulant therapy; maintain and communicate accurate patient medication information.

► Use alarms safely, including making improvements to ensure that alarms on medical equipment are heard and responded to on time.

- Prevent infection, including compliance with either the current Centers for Disease Control and Prevention (CDC) hand hygiene guidelines or the current World Health Organization (WHO) hand hygiene guidelines; the implementation of evidence-based practices to prevent healthcare-associated infections due to multidrug-resistant organisms, surgical site(s), indwelling catheter-associated urinary tract infections (CAUTI), and central line-associated bloodstream infections in acute care hospitals.

- Identify patient safety risks, including reducing the risk for suicide, healthcare-associated pressure ulcers, and patient falls.

- Prevent mistakes in surgery, including using a universal protocol to prevent any Wrong-Site, Wrong-Procedure, and Wrong-Person Surgery by conducting a pre-procedure verification process, marking the procedure site, and performing a timeout before the procedure.

CLINICAL PEARL

The JC accredits more than 80% of the nation's hospitals. It also accredits skilled nursing facilities, hospices, and other care organizations that provide home care, mental healthcare, laboratory facilities, ambulatory care, and long-term services.

A typical accreditation process involves:

1. An organization applies for a review.

2. The accrediting agency conducts a survey.

3. The organization conducts a self-study or self-assessment to examine itself based on the accrediting agency standards.

4. An individual surveyor, or a team of surveyors, visits the organization and conducts an on-site review. The whole staff of the organization is involved in the accreditation and reaccreditation process. Tasks include document preparation, hosting the site visit team, and interviews with the accreditors.

5. The accreditation surveyor or team issues a report granting or denying accreditation.

Some disadvantages of accreditation through the JC have been listed and include:

- Hospitals pay for JC surveys, and more than 70% of the JC's revenue comes directly from the organizations it is supposed to inspect.

- Although the JC encourages workers to speak with survey takers, most workers do not have legal protection from retaliation if they do so.

CLINICAL PEARL

The JC surveys a hospital every 3 years. Facilities must demonstrate a 12-month track record for all plans of action at the time of the survey.

Council on Quality and Leadership (CQL)

CQL is a US organization dedicated to defining, measuring, and improving personal and community quality of life for people with disabilities, those with mental illness and substance abuse disorders, and older adults. CQL evolved from the American Association on Mental Deficiency (AAMD; now American Association on Intellectual and Developmental Disabilities—AAIDD). During the 1980s and 1990s, the organization's name evolved from Accreditation Council for Services for Mentally Retarded and Other Developmentally Disabled Persons (ACMRDD) to Accreditation Council on Services for People with Disabilities (ACD), and in 1997, it became the CQL.

Commission on Accreditation of Rehabilitation Facilities (CARF)

CARF is a nonprofit organization designed to recognize standards of excellence in rehabilitation programs across the nation. CARF accreditation standards were developed with the input of consumers, rehabilitation professionals, state and national organizations, and third-party purchasers. CARF is designed to establish standards of quality for freestanding rehabilitation facilities and the rehabilitative programs of the largest hospital systems in the areas of behavioral health; employment (work hardening); community support services and medical rehabilitation (spinal cord injury, chronic pain); and to determine how well an organization is serving its patients, consumers, and the community. Programs accredited by CARF have demonstrated that they meet the national standards for rehabilitation programs.

Comprehensive Outpatient Rehabilitation Facility (CORF)

The CORF accreditation group conducts certification surveys for compliance with federal and state regulations and investigates complaints filed against one of these providers. Certification is achieved by adherence to federal requirements, including:

- Submission of a complete application

- Required documentation

- Successful completion of a survey

Each CORF must be surveyed for certification as directed by the CMS. An application for certification includes submitting a completed application, required documentation, and completing a survey. No fees and no renewal applications are required for certification. The agency imposes no state licensing requirements.

FEDERAL AND STATE HEALTHCARE REGULATIONS

In the United States, healthcare regulation is undertaken to improve performance and quality through various governmental and non-governmental agencies. These entities have varying statutory authority, scope, and remit approaches and outcomes, resulting in a complex, overlapping, duplicative, and sometimes contradictory regulatory environment.

Balanced Budget Act of 1997 (BBA)

This law, enacted by President Clinton and designed to balance the federal budget, made sweeping changes in the Medicare and Medicaid programs. Several of the BBA's significant provisions were payment reductions to healthcare providers, new prospective payment systems for healthcare providers, and reduced healthcare services coverage by the Medicare and Medicaid programs. Some of these payment reductions were reversed by subsequent legislation in 1999 and 2000.

Statutory Laws

Statutes are defined as laws that various state legislatures and Congress passes. These statutes are the basis for statutory law. The legislature passes statutes that are later put into the federal code of laws or pertinent state code of laws. Statutory law consists of legislatures declaring, commanding, or prohibiting something—a particular law established by the government's legislative department. Some statutory laws affect physical therapy:

► *Licensure laws.* Under the US federal government system, each state regulates all healthcare professionals' practice by establishing licensing or regulatory agencies or boards to generate regulations. State licensing statutes establish the minimum level of education and experience required to practice, define the profession's functions, and limit the performance of these functions to licensed persons. These laws:

 ■ Are designed to protect the consumer against professional incompetence and exploitation by opportunists.

 ■ Decide the minimal standards of education. In the case of physical therapy, the minimal standards required include:

   ■ Graduation from an accredited program or its equivalent in physical therapy.

   ■ Successful completion of a national licensing examination. Licensure examination and related activities are the responsibility of the Federation of State Boards of Physical Therapy (FSBPT).

 ■ Determine the ethical and legal standards relating to the continuing practice of physical therapy. Each state determines the criteria to practice and issue a license.

► *Workers' compensation acts.* The rules and regulations of individual state's workers' compensation systems are the primary factors influencing the provision of physical therapy services for patients with work-related injuries. Workers' compensation laws are designed to ensure that employees who are injured or disabled on the job are provided with fixed monetary awards, eliminating the need for litigation. The laws provide a no-fault system that pays all medical benefits and replaces salary (usually at 66%) until recovery occurs. In turn, employees forfeit the right to sue their employers for damages. These rules and regulations also provide benefits for worker's dependents if workers die due to a work-related accident or illness. Some of the rules and regulations also protect employers and fellow workers by limiting the amount an injured employee can recover from an employer and limiting co-workers' liability in most accidents. State workers' compensation statutes establish this framework for most employment. Federal statutes are limited to federal employees or those workers employed in some significant aspect of interstate commerce. The laws vary from state to state, but most states identify four types of disability:

 ■ *Temporary partial*—the injured worker can do some work but is still recuperating from the effects of the injury and is thus temporarily limited in the amount or type of work that can be performed compared to the preinjury work.

 ■ *Temporary total*—the injured worker cannot work during a period when he/she is under active medical care and has not yet reached what is called "maximum medical improvement."

 ■ *Permanent partial*—the injured worker is capable of employment but cannot return to the former job. Benefits are usually paid according to a prescribed schedule for a fixed number of weeks.

 ■ *Permanent total*—the injured worker cannot return to any gainful employment, and lifetime benefits are provided to the employee.

Workers' compensation programs:

 ■ Are financed by covered employers insured or self-insured under property and casualty lines and are mandatory for employers in almost all states.

 ■ Have a limit on the number of visits in some states based on the diagnosis and/or require a pre-approval process to be followed for reimbursement. Other states require the total number of visits or the total number of weeks (duration) and the number of treatments per week (frequency) to be usual, customary, and reasonable.

 ■ Must be offered by all large employers (10 or more employees) or high-risk employers.

► *Malpractice laws.* Malpractice can be defined as a dereliction of professional duty or a failure to exercise an accepted degree of professional skill or learning by one rendering professional services, which results in injury, loss, or damage. Malpractice also encompasses harmful, negligent, or improper practice. PTAs are personally responsible for any act of negligence or other acts that harm a patient through professional-patient relationships.

 ■ Negligence is defined as a failure to do what reasonably competent practitioners would have done under similar circumstances.

 ■ To find a practitioner negligent, harm must have occurred to the patient. Examples could include:

   ■ A burn caused by a hot pack.

- Using defective equipment that results in injury.
- Failing to prevent a patient from falling.
- Causing an injury to a patient through improper exercise.
- Performing any action or inaction that is inconsistent with the Code of Ethics or the Standards of Practice.

CLINICAL PEARL

▶ Every individual (PT, PTA, student P.T., or student PTA) is liable for negligence.

▶ Supervisors or superiors may also be found "vicariously" negligent because of their workers' actions if they provided faulty supervision or inappropriate delegation of responsibilities.

▶ Institutions can be found vicariously negligent if a patient is harmed due to an environmental problem such as a slippery floor or a poorly lit area, or if an employee is deemed incompetent, not properly trained, or not properly licensed.

THE PATIENT

The clinician must always consider a situation from the patient's perspective and understand that all patients have rights within any given healthcare system.

Patient Rights

In 1998, the US Advisory Commission on Consumer Protection and Quality in the Healthcare Industry endorsed the following areas of consumer rights and responsibilities:

I. *Information disclosure.* Consumers have the right to receive accurate, easily understood information, and some require assistance in making informed healthcare decisions about their health plans, professionals, and facilities.

II. *Choice of providers and plans.* Consumers have the right to a choice of healthcare providers that is sufficient to ensure access to appropriate, high-quality healthcare.

III. *Access to specialists.* Consumers with complex or serious medical conditions who require frequent specialty care should have direct access to a qualified specialist of their choice within a plan's network of providers. Authorizations, when required, should be for an adequate number of direct access visits under an approved treatment plan.

IV. *Access to emergency services.* Consumers have the right to access emergency healthcare services when and where the need arises. Health plans should provide payment when a consumer presents to an emergency department with acute symptoms of sufficient severity—including severe pain—such that a "prudent

layperson" could reasonably expect the absence of medical attention to result in placing that consumer's health in serious jeopardy, serious impairment to bodily functions, or serious dysfunction of any bodily organ or part.

V. *Participation in treatment decisions.* Consumers have the right and responsibility to participate in all decisions related to their healthcare and to expect healthcare providers to abide by the informed decisions. Consumers who cannot fully participate in treatment decisions have the right to be represented by parents, guardians, family members, or other conservators.

VI. *Respect and nondiscrimination.* Consumers have the right to considerate, respectful care from all healthcare system members at all times and under all circumstances. An environment of mutual respect is essential to maintain a quality healthcare system.

VII. *Confidentiality of health information.* Consumers have the right to communicate with healthcare providers in confidence and to have the confidentiality of their individually identifiable healthcare information protected. Consumers also have the right to review and copy their medical records and request amendments to their records.

VIII. *Complaints and appeals.* All consumers have the right to a fair and efficient process for resolving differences with their health plans, healthcare providers, and the institutions that serve them, including a rigorous internal review system and an independent system of external review.

IX. *Consumer responsibilities.* In a healthcare system that protects consumers' rights, it is reasonable to expect and encourage consumers to assume reasonable responsibilities. Greater individual involvement by consumers in their care increases the likelihood of achieving the best outcomes and supports quality improvement and a cost-conscious environment.

CLINICAL PEARL

A complete description of the Patient's Bill of Rights can be seen at http://www.opm.gov/insure/archive/health/cbrr.htm.

The Patient Self-Determination Act (PSDA) requires many Medicare and Medicaid providers (hospitals, nursing homes, hospice programs, HHAs, and HMOs) to give adult individuals, at the time of inpatient admission or enrollment, certain information about their rights under state laws, including:

1. The right to participate in and direct their own healthcare decisions.
2. The right to accept or refuse medical or surgical treatment.
3. The right to prepare an advance directive.
4. Information on the provider's policies that govern the utilization of these rights.

The Act also prohibits institutions from discriminating against a patient who does not have an advance directive.

MEDICAL RECORDS

Medical records contain sensitive information, and increasing computerization and other policy factors have increased their privacy threats. Besides information about physical health, these records may include information about family relationships, sexual behavior, substance abuse, and even the private thoughts and feelings that come with psychotherapy. Threats to medical record privacy include the following:

► *Administrative actions.* This includes errors that release, misclassify, or lose information, compromise accuracy, create misuse by legitimate users, and promote uncontrolled access.

► *Computerization.* Although in some situations computerization increases privacy protection (for example, by adding passwords to sensitive areas), it may also decrease privacy protection for the following reasons:

■ Computerization enables the storage of large amounts of data in small spaces. Thus, when an intruder gains access, access is to certain discrete amounts of data and larger collections and perhaps keys to further information.

■ Networked information is accessible from anywhere at any time, allowing access to a larger number of people. This increases the possibility of mistakes or other problems such as misuse or leaks of data.

■ New databases and different types of data sets are more easily created. This both drives demand for new information and makes possible its creation.

■ Information is easily gathered, exchanged, and transmitted. Thus, potential dissemination is theoretically limitless.

■ Access by unrelated parties is possible.

► *Insurance companies.* Insurance companies may check records either before approving treatment or before extending coverage.

► *Financial institutions.* The federal Gramm-Leach-Bliley Act (GLB) allows financial companies such as banks, brokerage houses, and insurance companies to operate independently.

► *Drug companies.* These companies may have deals with doctors and hospitals and may get access to patient lists that can be used for marketing.

► *Employers.* Employers could use sensitive information against employees.

► *Court subpoenas.* Often a patient will be unaware when their records have been subpoenaed. Even worse, unnecessary information is often included when the records are not adequately screened.

Current protections for medical records privacy include:

► Medical ethics.

► The privacy portion of the Hippocratic Oath: "Whatsoever I shall see or hear in the course of my intercourse with men, if it be what should not be published abroad, I will never divulge, holding such things to be holy secrets."

► The 1992 AMA statement that states that medical information must be kept confidential to the greatest possible degree.

► The Privacy Act of 1974 states that no federal agency may disclose information without the person's consent. Agencies must also meet certain requirements for protecting the information.

► *Tort law.* This may include defamation, breach of contract, and other privacy-related torts.

► *HIPAA Privacy Rule*—see the next section.

► *The HHS.*

INFORMED CONSENT

Informed consent is the process by which a fully informed individual can participate in their healthcare choices. It originates from the legal and ethical right the patient has to direct what happens to their body, and from the ethical duty of the physician or healthcare provider to involve the patient in their healthcare.

The most important goal of informed consent is that the patient must have an opportunity to be an informed participant in their healthcare decisions. Basic consent entails checking the patient for any precautions or contraindications, letting them know who you are and what you would like to do, and asking them if it is okay to proceed with the proposed treatment. The more formal process should include a discussion of the following elements:

► The nature of the decision/procedure, including estimated time frames and costs and any associated risk and/or benefit.

► Reasonable alternatives to the proposed intervention.

► The relevant risks, benefits, and uncertainties related to each alternative.

► Assessment of patient understanding.

► The acceptance of the intervention by the patient.

MEDICAL ERRORS

The importance of patient safety cannot be overstated, but medical/clinical errors continue to occur even with the best intentions. The two main causes of medical error are:

- An intervention does not go according to plan. Examples include surgical errors and improperly functioning or poorly maintained equipment. From a rehabilitation perspective, activities that place the patient at risk, such as ambulation, aerobic exercise, and transfers, should always be performed with caution:
  - Diminished skin integrity can lead to skin breakdown during transfers, positioning, or exercise.
  - A decrease in bone density can result in a fracture during transfers, manual techniques, and ambulation.
- An incorrect intervention. Examples include errors in medication prescriptions or regimens and laboratory report inaccuracies. An adverse drug error (ADE) is an example of a medication error. The three most common types of medication errors are a failure to administer an ordered medication; a deviation in the prescribed dose, strength, or quantity of a drug; and the dispensing or administering of the incorrect drug. In rehabilitation, an incorrect intervention could include using an incorrectly high amount of resistance for a patient's exercise.

CLINICAL PEARL

The six rights of the drug administration, used by nurses when administering drugs, include:

- Right individual
- Right medication
- Right dose
- Right time
- Right route
- Right documentation

The consequences of a medical error run the gamut from causing the patient no harm to causing the patient's death.

Several agencies work cooperatively to develop strategies and standards that are designed to reduce medical errors. These agencies include:

- The Institute of Medicine (IOM)
- The Agency for Health Research and Quality (AHRQ)
- The JC

The focus of these agencies is to examine and analyze policies and procedures within the institution that have the potential to cause harm, including:

- The complexity of the healthcare delivery system. In large institutions, it is easy for a patient to become a number rather than a person.
- The number of caregivers involved in the patient's care. The more caregivers involved in a patient's care, the greater the chance of an error.
- Flaws in the design of systems or equipment. These flaws can be inherent in the equipment design or the physical layout of the treatment area. One of the most common problems is the overcrowding of equipment, which does not permit sufficient space for safe negotiation. Another common problem is the physical location of one department to another. Systems and departments should be designed to enhance patient flow.
- Improper or faulty installation and maintenance of equipment. All electrical equipment must be checked annually for safety. For example, extension cables should not be used, and neither should portable heaters.
- Incorrect design of a treatment area. In many cases, areas are used for a specialty when they were designed for another specialty.

The JC categorizes a medical error as either a sentinel (adverse) event or a potential adverse event:

- Sentinel event: An unexpected occurrence that involves death or serious injury, or the risk thereof, which may have been avoided through appropriate care or alternative interventions. Such events are called sentinel events because they signal the need for immediate investigation and response. Examples of a sentinel event are provided in Table 2-8.
- Potential adverse event: no actual harm occurs.

TABLE 2-8	Examples of a Sentinel Event

- Any patient death, paralysis, coma, or other major permanent loss of function (eg, loss of a limb) associated with a medication or procedural error
- Any suicide of a patient in a setting where the patient is housed around-the-clock, including suicides following elopement from such a setting
- Any elopement, that is, unauthorized departure, of a patient from an around-the-clock care setting resulting in a temporally related death (suicide or homicide) or major permanent loss of function
- Any procedure on the wrong patient, wrong side of the body, or the wrong organ
- Any intrapartum (related to the birth process) maternal death
- Any perinatal death unrelated to a congenital condition in an infant having a birth weight greater than 2500 grams
- Assault, homicide, or other crime resulting in patient death or major permanent loss of function
- A patient fall that results in death or major permanent loss of function as a direct result of the injuries sustained in the fall
- Hemolytic transfusion reaction involving major blood group incompatibilities

The terms *sentinel event* and *medical error* are not synonymous; not all sentinel events occur because of an error, and not all errors result in a sentinel event.

The JC reviews organizations' activities in response to sentinel events. Healthcare providers must alert the JC and state licensing authorities of all sentinel events and include a review of any risk factors, preventative measures, and a root cause analysis (RCA). The RCA is designed to determine what happened, why or how it happened, and what could be done to prevent the event's recurrence.

MATERIAL SAFETY DATA SHEET

The various products used by a clinical facility, especially cleaning chemicals, can cause a patient injury. In the United States, OSHA requires a material safety data sheet (MSDS) or safety data sheet (SDS) to be available to employees for potentially harmful substances in the workplace under the Hazard Communication Regulation. The MSDS is also required to be made available to local fire departments and local and state emergency planning officials under Section 311 of the Emergency Planning and Community Right-to-Know Act. Table 2-9 lists some safety recommendations (see also Chapter 5).

THE HOME AND WORK ENVIRONMENTS

Treating the injured worker or person with a disability requires that the PTA must be knowledgeable regarding the following[12]:

▶ An understanding of all aspects of the patient's community, home, and work. This includes the physical environment in which an individual functions, including both built and natural objects.

▶ The psychosocial issues and cultures of the patient's environment.

▶ *Accessibility:* the degree to which an environment affords the use of its resources for an individual's level of function.

▶ *Universal design (lifespan design):* this design concept emphasizes social inclusion by creating environments that are usable by a wide range of individuals of different ages, stature, sizes, and abilities and addresses the changing needs of humans across the lifespan.[13]

▶ *Environmental barriers:* defined as physical impediments to prevent individuals from functioning optimally in their surroundings. Environmental barriers can be external or internal.[13,14]

  ■ *Exterior barriers.* External barriers include sidewalks, driveways, garage/carport accessibility, access to the

TABLE 2-9	Recommended Safety Precautions
Hand hygiene	This is the single most important procedure to prevent the spread of infection and cross-contamination and should be performed before and after each treatment session.
Staff competency	All personnel who provide patient care should be trained, qualified, and competent in their assigned duties.
Patient protection	As appropriate, the patient should be protected with safety straps, bed rails, and so forth according to established regulatory state and federal guidelines. Patient transfers should not be attempted unless sufficient staff is present.
Sufficient space	The clinician should always plan ahead so that sufficient space to maneuver any equipment or to perform a task is available.
Treatment area	Remove any clutter, including equipment that is not being used or is blocking a walkway, electrical cords, loose rugs/floor mats, and any water spills.
Equipment	All equipment should be regularly assessed to ensure that it functions properly.
Preparation	The clinician should obtain any equipment or supplies needed before a patient arrives for treatment so that the patient will not be left unattended.

grounds, and entry into the accommodation. Exterior access routes include the frequency and mode of transportation typically used to reach the destination, parking, lighting in the parking area, and safety traveling to the entrance. Outside steps should have a maximum height of 7 inches and depth of at least 11 inches and should not have tread lip projections.[13] If the patient has to use a ramp for home or work, the clinician should ensure that the patient can safely ascend and descend it and that it is soundly built. For safety and ease of use, a ramp should ideally have an incline of at least 1 foot in length for each inch of rising (1:12 ratio). For example, a 6-inch step leading into the home/building requires a 6-foot ramp.[14] Handrails should be fitted for patients who ambulate with difficulty and those with impaired balance, especially on any steps and ramps.

  ■ *Interior barriers.* Interior access routes should be checked to ensure that there is enough space for basic mobility in and out of rooms with any assistive device the patient requires. The clinician should make a note of the type and resistance of any floor coverings. Doorways must be at least 32 inches wide for a standard wheelchair to pass and ideally 1 to 2 inches wider than this to account for inaccurate maneuvering and the usual oblique approach to doors.[14] The clinician should check that lighting in all areas is bright enough for safe task performance, and that light switches can be reached by the patient or the lights come on automatically as the patient enters the environment.[14] Also, it is important to note the height of and access to electrical outlets/switches, the size and space available in each room, the location and access to communication units such as telephones and computers, the location and access to heating/cooling controls, and the location and access to safety devices (smoke/carbon monoxide detectors, circuit breaker panel, etc.).

Guidelines for a wheelchair-accessible home are described in Table 2-10.

CLINICAL PEARL

Rather than individual joint motion, the functional range of motion (ROM) is generally most relevant to environmental barriers. Similarly, functional muscle testing, such as whether the individual has the strength to operate levers, lift, carry, push, and pull objects as required by the expected roles, is more useful than an examination of strength by measurement of individual muscle performance with manual muscle testing or other approaches.[14]

CLINICAL PEARL

The Multidirectional Reach Test is an effective test used in physical therapy to determine the functional ROM.[15,16] Another measure of functional ROM is a map of the patient's reach zones, which look like semicircles extending in front of and to the patient's side.[14] These items can be classified as primary, secondary, or tertiary. Objects are then placed in the zones according to their frequency of use.

► *Primary zone:* Frequently used objects, which can be used while keeping elbows at the side of the body.
► *Secondary zone:* All objects used 4 to 10 times an hour can be reached without the elbow moving further forward than the anterior portion of the rib cage.
► *Tertiary zone:* Infrequently used objects that can be reached without exceeding full elbow extension or 90 degrees of shoulder flexion.

TABLE 2-10 Guidelines for a Wheelchair-Accessible Home

Full Access
► Clearance of 30″ × 48″ in front of and adjacent to any fixtures or workspaces, and appliance.
► The height of any fixture/control is not to exceed 48″ above the floor.
Feedback
► Those with vision or hearing impairments use clicks, beeps, and lights to verify a switch is activated.
Comfort Zone
► The reach zone in which a person can comfortably perform a task. The standard reach zone for a standing adult is from 28″ to 75″. The standard reach zone for a seated adult is from 20″ to 44″.
Neutral Handedness
► Placement of fixtures, workspaces, and appliances so they can be approached from the left- and right-hand sides.
Site/Foundation
► The site's contours allow all entrances to be at the same level as the driveway, for no-step entrances.
Walkways
► 5′ wide, flat, smooth, and firm.
► All approaches from the street, including from the curb to the entrance.
► Mailboxes to be located beside walkways and within the comfort zone.
Garage
► There should be an electric door with 9′ height clearance to accommodate the van.
► Interior measurements account for 5′ clearance on each side of vehicles for chair lifts.
Entryways
► Walkways to extend a minimum of 25′ beyond the latch side of the door.
► Thresholds are to be flush and a minimum of 3′ wide.
► Guest entrances are to have a doorbell installed 36″ from the ground and have two peepholes (one at 40″ one at 60″).
► Gated entries need 36″ thresholds and easy-open latches.
Doors/Hardware
► All doors to have flush thresholds and must be 36″ wide with an 18″ clearance on the latch side.
► Doorknobs to be lever handle type.
► Locks must be easily operated with one hand.
► Knobs and locks installed below 36 and to be of the immediate feedback style if required.
Windows/Hardware
► Casement and vertical sliding sash windows are the preferred styles.
► Lock hardware should have large levers and be easy to operate.
► Lifts, pulls, cranks, and locks should be large and accessible.

(continued)

TABLE 2-10   Guidelines for a Wheelchair-Accessible Home (continued)

Floors/Carpet

▶ Smooth, hard finishes (wood, linoleum) with matte surfaces are preferred.
▶ Carpet to be firm, ½" (or less) cut pile.
▶ The tile is to have a nonslip surface.

Electrical

▶ Service panels must be located in a prominent, fully accessible area.
▶ All controls to be rocker type with feedback.
▶ Thermostats, outlets, and controls are to be accessible and between 18" and 48" off the floor.
▶ Extra outlets and controls placed in bedrooms if required by the buyer.

Grab Bars

▶ 1.25" to 1.5" in diameter with a spacing of 1.5" between wall and bar.

Gas

▶ Meters with earthquake shutoff valves or full access to the meter for emergency shutoff are a must.

Telephone

▶ Phone jacks are to be in all rooms.

Smoke and Carbon Monoxide Detectors

▶ Smoke and carbon monoxide detectors are to be placed in the kitchen and in the hall outside sleeping areas.

Bathrooms

▶ Walls to be sheathed in ¾" plywood to allow grab bar installation anywhere.
▶ The door is to either open outward or be pocket type (a door that slides into a hollow cavity).
▶ Clear floor space around each fixture is required for full accessibility.
▶ Outlets to have ground-fault circuit interrupters.
▶ Sinks mounted to walls or sitting vanity styles should have insulation covers on pipes or plumbing shields.
▶ Bowls with a front depth of 3" and sloping back to 6" are recommended.
▶ Faucets with lever handles are the easiest to operate for both water and temperature control.
▶ Drain stops that are rubber plugs on a chain are preferred over plunger controls located behind the spout.
▶ The toilet is to have an 18" seat height for ease in lateral transfer and be fully accessible.
▶ Toilet paper dispenser to be installed within the buyer's comfort zone.
▶ Grab bars and handholds should be placed anywhere needed.
▶ Tubs to be a minimum of 30" × 60" × 18" deep.
▶ Roll-in showers to be a minimum of 30" × 60".
▶ Showers to be a minimum of 36" × 36" and have built-in seats.
▶ Cabinets should be accessible, frameless, and have doors that easily open with one hand.
▶ Wet rooms need to be tiled in slip-proof tile and be sloped for drainage.
▶ Heat lamps should be included.

Kitchens

▶ Counters and workspaces are to be offered at different heights (32"-34"-36") and various depths (16"-19"-24").
▶ Appliances should be fully accessible. Braille and large-print dials should be offered.
▶ Cabinets should be accessible and frameless with "D" style pulls.
▶ Cooktops need smooth surfaces with staggered burners and controls that are easy to operate.
▶ Ovens that are built-in with side hinges are the best design to use.
▶ Microwave ovens need to be mounted within the comfort zone.
▶ Pullout shelves underneath ovens and cooktops add convenience.
▶ Sink to have a height between 32" and 36" and depth between 8" and 5" with drains and disposals in the rear. Plumbing shields installed in the knee recesses prevent burns.
▶ Faucets that control the temperature and flow of water and have retractable hose sprays should be used.
▶ Dishwasher to have push-button controls and to be located within the comfort zone.
▶ Outlets for small appliances are to be located within the comfort zone.
▶ Controls for disposals/fans to be located within the comfort zone.

Laundry

▶ Easy access to front-loading machines.
▶ Counters, poles, and ironing areas to be accessible and within the comfort zone.

Stairway

▶ It should be at least 48" wide with handrails on both sides.
▶ The landings at both the top and bottom should be no smaller than 36" × 36".
▶ Chair and seat lifts can traverse curves and corners; motors can be located in remote locations (closets) or at the top or bottom of stairs.
▶ If the chair and seat lifts are inadequate, elevators can be constructed. Home elevators need a floor space area of at least 4 × 6 square feet on each floor to accommodate the elevator car.

Hallways

▶ A width of 40" is required for easy movement through halls.

Data from Lema AR: Simplified disabled housing, 2006. http://www.freepatentsonline.com/y2006/0059797.html.

REFERENCES

1. Bodenheimer TS, Grumbach K. Introduction: the paradox of excess and deprivation. In: Bodenheimer TS, Grumbach K, eds. *Understanding Health Policy: A Clinical Approach*, 5th ed. New York: McGraw-Hill; 2009:1-3.

2. Americans with Disabilities Act of 1989. 104 Stat 327. 1989:101-336, 42 USC 12101 s2 (a) (8).

3. Waddell G, Waddell H. A review of social influences on neck and back pain disability. In: Nachemson AL, Jonsson E, eds. *Neck and Back Pain: The Scientific Evidence of Causes, Diagnosis, and Treatment*. Philadelphia: Lippincott Williams and Wilkins; 2000:13-55.

4. Bodenheimer TS, Grumbach K. Reimbursing healthcare providers. In: Bodenheimer TS, Grumbach K, eds. *Understanding Health Policy: A Clinical Approach*. 5th ed. New York: McGraw-Hill; 2009:31-41.

5. Bodenheimer TS, Grumbach K. Paying for healthcare. In: Bodenheimer TS, Grumbach K, eds. *Understanding Health Policy: A Clinical Approach*. 5th ed. New York: McGraw-Hill; 2009:5-16.

6. American Physical Therapy Association. *Today's Physical Therapist: A Comprehensive Review of a 21st-Century Health Care Profession*. Alexandria, VA: American Physical Therapy Association; 2011.

7. Bodenheimer TS, Grumbach K. Access to healthcare. In: Bodenheimer TS, Grumbach K, eds. *Understanding Health Policy: A Clinical Approach*, 5th ed. New York: McGraw-Hill; 2009:17-30.

8. Rodwin VG. *The Health Planning Predicament*. Berkeley, CA: University of California Press; 1984.

9. Bodenheimer TS, Grumbach K. How health care is organized. In: Bodenheimer TS, Grumbach K, eds. *Understanding Health Policy: A Clinical Approach*, 5th ed. New York: McGraw-Hill; 2009:43-57.

10. Cha AE, Cohen RA. *Reasons for Being Uninsured Among Adults Aged 18-64 in the United States, 2019*. NCHS data brief. 2020:1-8.

11. Lechner D, Daly J, Maltchev K, McKelvy B, Fadel S. The work-injured population. In: Boissonnault WG, ed. *Primary Care for the Physical Therapist: Examination and Triage*. St Louis: Elsevier Saunders; 2005: 271-287.

12. Schmitz TJ. Examination of the environment. In: O'Sullivan SB, Schmitz TJ, eds. *Physical Rehabilitation*, 5th ed. Philadelphia: FA Davis; 2007:401-467.

13. Paterson M, Mets T. Environmental assessment: Home, community, and work. In: Cameron MH, Monroe LG, eds. *Physical Rehabilitation: Evidence-Based Examination, Evaluation, and Intervention*. St. Louis, MO: Saunders/Elsevier; 2007:918-936.

14. Guide to Physical Therapist Practice. Third Edition. American Physical Therapy Association. 2014; http://guidetoptpractice.apta.org

15. Mackenzie M. A simplified measure of balance by functional reach. *Physio Res Int*. 1999;4:233-236.

16. Duncan PW, Weiner DK, Chandler J, Studenski S. Functional reach: a new clinical measure of balance. *J Gerontol*. 1990;45:M192-M197.

CHAPTER 3

Evidence-Informed Practice and Clinical Decision-Making

CHAPTER OBJECTIVES

At the completion of this chapter, the reader will be able to:

1. Provide a historical perspective on the evolution of evidence-informed practice (EIP)

2. Discuss the importance of EIP

3. List some of the reasons why EIP became important in healthcare

4. Describe the various research designs and their advantages and disadvantages

5. Differentiate among the experimental, quasi-experimental, and nonexperimental research designs

6. Differentiate between the form and uses of the null and research hypotheses

7. Differentiate among and discuss the roles of independent, dependent, and extraneous variables

8. Discuss the concept of research validity of a study

9. List the various threats to validity

10. Describe the different types of reliability and the roles they play in EIP

11. Discuss the various hierarchies of evidence

12. Discuss how EIP can be used in clinical decision-making

OVERVIEW

An important component of the Vision 2020 statement set forth by the American Physical Therapy Association (APTA) is achieving direct access through independent, self-determined, professional judgment and action.[1] In light of the APTA's movement toward realizing Vision 2020, an operational definition of *autonomous practice* and the related term *autonomous physical therapist practitioner* is given by the APTA's board as follows:

▶ "Autonomous physical therapist practice is practice characterized by independent, self-determined professional judgment and action."

▶ "An autonomous physical therapist practitioner within the scope of practice defined by the *Guide to Physical Therapist Practice* provides physical therapy services to patients who have direct and unrestricted access to their services, and may refer as appropriate to other healthcare providers and other professionals and for diagnostic tests."[2]

Evidence is used comprehensively in clinical decision-making within the healthcare professions. The physical therapy profession has expressed a commitment to the development and use of evidence through various initiatives, including the APTA's introduction of a periodic feature in their journal, "Evidence in Practice," and a database of research articles, "Hooked on Evidence." Evidence-informed practice (EIP) refers to a practice that is associated with epidemiological evidence and healthcare needs.[3]

CLINICAL PEARL

The production of evidence to support physical therapy services is only truly effective when practitioners integrate evidence into their practice.

EIP refers to integrating the best available evidence with clinical expertise and patient values and circumstances to produce specific evidence-supported interventions.[4] This contrasts with the old-fashioned reliance on knowledge gained from authority, hearsay, habit, or tradition.

CLINICAL PEARL

The goals of using EIP in physical therapy are to:
▶ Improve the quality of care
▶ Standardize certain facets of care
▶ Achieve the best patient outcomes

The relatively recent interest in the use of EIP has resulted from some issues, including[5-12]

▶ The continued increase in healthcare costs.

- Extensive documentation of apparently unexplained practice variations in the management of a variety of conditions.

- An increase in publicity surrounding medical errors.

- The identification of potential or actual harm resulting from previously approved medications or techniques.

- Recent trends in technology assessment and outcomes research.

- The rapid evolution of Internet technology.

- The need for proof of the efficacy of a particular treatment or technique to commercial and government insurance payers.

Ultimately, physical therapy practitioners are movement specialists, and task analysis forms the basis of their diagnosis.[13] Clinical decision-making requires deliberate thought and sound judgment, both of which involve a degree of expertise. Although a physical therapist assistant (PTA) is not responsible for determining a patient's diagnosis or the design of the patient's plan of care (POC), a PTA spends a large proportion of their working day making decisions about a patient's clinical progression based on an interpretation of the treatment plan designed by the physical therapist (PT), while attending to patients' needs. Clinical knowledge of anatomy, physiology, and treatment concepts, supplemented with EIP, is essential to provide the most effective clinical interventions so that the patient achieves the best outcomes. For example, the PTA must effectively communicate with the patient about the rationale of a specific intervention, its risks and benefits, and the evidence supporting its use. It is also within the scope of the PTA's duties to offer suggestions or recommendations to the supervising PT if a patient under their care is not responding as expected.

EVIDENCE-INFORMED PRACTICE

Research involves a controlled, systematic approach to obtain an answer to a question.[14] A search for relevant evidence to answer the question is then followed by a critical appraisal of its qualities, applicability, and conclusions. This approach requires knowledge of the evidence appraisal process, access to the evidence, and the ability to discriminate between stronger and weaker evidence.

CLINICAL PEARL

EIP is best supported by research that is relevant and advances knowledge in the professional field.[15]

Also, some criteria must be met, including[16]:

- The credibility of the research in terms of its design and execution. Some research designs are outlined in Table 3-1. Research designs can be viewed as a continuum in terms of their usefulness.

TABLE 3-1	Research Designs
Type of Design	**Description**
Experimental	Purposeful manipulation of subjects who have been randomly assigned to two or more groups with measurement of their resulting behavior. Experimental designs are the most restrictive in terms of the amount of control imposed on study participants and conditions. The classic experimental study design is the randomized controlled trial (RCT).
Quasi-experimental	Maintains the purposeful manipulation of the experimental design but involves no randomization of subjects to groups or has only one subject group to evaluate. Often used when researchers have difficulty obtaining sufficient numbers of subjects or when group membership is predetermined by a subject characteristic (whether or not the subject received a particular medical or surgical intervention). Single-system designs can be used to investigate the usefulness of an intervention.
Nonexperimental or observational	Researchers are simply observers who collect information about the phenomenon of interest; there is no experimental manipulation of subjects. These designs have less control than quasi-experimental studies, as they have similar limitations concerning their groupings.
Physiologic studies	Focus only on cellular, anatomical, or physiological systems and not on personal level function.
Case report	Describes what occurred with a patient/client.
Case-control studies	A retrospective approach in which subjects known to have the diagnosis of interest are compared to a control group known to be free of the diagnosis.
Cohort design	Refers to a group of subjects who are followed over time and usually share a common characteristic such as gender, occupation, or diagnosis.
Narrative review	A summary of prior research on a particular topic without using a systematic search and critical appraisal process.
Systematic review	A narrative review that addresses a specific research question. Includes detailed inclusion and exclusion criteria for selecting studies to review and preestablished quality criteria to rate the value of the individual studies, usually applied by blinded reviewers.

CLINICAL PEARL

► Qualitative research: A research approach that assumes that truth is subjective and relative to each individual, such that multiple realities exist, the measurement of which is influenced by the interdependence of researchers and the subjects.[17] Data are provided in words rather than in numbers through interviews, surveys, or other mechanisms.

► Quantitative research: A research approach that assumes that an objective reality exists that can be measured using standardized numerical measures that can be evaluated to determine cause-and-effect relationships by researchers independent of the subjects.[17]

► Whether or not the research article is peer-reviewed.

► The relevance of the findings for the field and/or the specific journal. Ideally, the study should address the specific clinical question the clinician is trying to answer, and the subjects in the study should have characteristics that are similar to the patient/client in question.[16] The standard for assessing the efficacy and value of a test or intervention is the clinical trial, that is, a prospective study assessing the effect and value of a test or intervention against a control in human subjects.[18]

► The contribution to the body of knowledge about the topic.

► The date of the publication.

The gathering of evidence must occur in a systematic, reproducible, and unbiased manner to select and interpret the findings.[19] The EIP process generally occurs in 5 steps[20]:

1. Formulating a clinical question, including details about the patient type or problem, the intervention being considered, a comparison intervention, and the outcome measure to be used.

2. Searching for the best evidence, including a literature search on Ovid, EMBASE, PubMed, PEDro, or other medical search engine databases using the clinical question keywords.

3. Critical appraisal of the evidence. In general, there are two types of clinical studies—those that analyze primary data and those that analyze secondary data.[21]

   ■ Primary data include case reports and series, case-control, cross-sectional, cohort (both prospective and retrospective), and randomized controlled trials (RCTs) (Table 3-2).[21]

TABLE 3-2	Randomized Controlled Trials, Systematic Reviews, and Clinical Practice Guidelines
Randomized controlled trials (RCTs)	Experimental designs that focus on treatment efficacy. Involve experiments on people. Less exposed to bias. Ensures comparability of groups. Typically, volunteers agreed to be randomly allocated to groups receiving one of the following: ► Treatment and no treatment ► Standard treatment and standard treatment plus a new treatment ► Two alternate treatments The common feature is that the experimental group receives the treatment and the control group does not. At the end of the trial, the outcomes of subjects in each group are determined—the difference in outcomes between groups provides an estimate of the size of the treatment effect. Best suited to answer questions about whether an experimental intervention has an effect and whether that effect is beneficial or harmful to the subjects.
Systematic reviews	Reviews of the literature conducted in a way that is designed to minimize bias. It can be used to assess the effects of health interventions, the accuracy of diagnostic tests, or the prognosis for a particular condition. Usually involve criteria to determine which studies will be considered, the search strategy used to locate studies, the methods for assessing the quality of the studies, and the process used to synthesize the findings of individual studies. Particularly useful for busy clinicians who may be unable to access all the relevant trials in an area and may otherwise need to rely on their incomplete surveys of relevant trials.
Clinical practice guidelines	Recommendations for the management of a particular clinical condition. Involve the compilation of evidence concerning the needs and expectations of the recipients of care, the accuracy of the diagnostic tests, and the effects of any therapy and the prognosis. Usually necessitates the conduct of one or sometimes several systematic reviews. It can be presented as a clinical decision algorithm. It can provide a useful framework on which clinicians can build clinical practice methods.

Data from Boyling JD, Jull GA: Grieve's Modern Manual Therapy: The Vertebral Column. Philadelphia, PA. Churchill Livingstone; 2004 and Petticrew M. Systematic reviews from astronomy to zoology: myths and misconceptions, BMJ 2001 Jan 13;322(7278):98-101.

- Secondary data analysis occurs in systematic reviews or meta-analyses for pooling or synthesizing data to answer a question that is perhaps not practical or answerable within an individual study.[21]

Another way to broadly categorize studies is *experimental*, where treatment is introduced to subjects, or *observational*, in which no active treatment is introduced to the subjects.[21]

4. Applying the evidence to the patient. Once the evidence has been critically appraised, the clinician must consider the evidence in the context of his or her clinical expertise and the patient's values and preferences or goals.

5. Evaluation of the outcome. The outcome is the end product of the patient/client management process and is distinguished from treatment effects. An outcome reflects the patient/client's goals for the physical therapy episode of care from the patient/client's perspective.

Research Article

Each research article consists of some elements, which include[22]:

- *Title.* The purpose of the title is to identify the major variables studied and provide clues about whether the research purpose is a description, relationship analysis, or difference analysis.

- *Abstract.* This element briefly summarizes the purpose of the research, the methods, and the results.

- *Introduction.* This element defines the study's broad problems, states the study's specific purposes, and places the problem and purposes into any previous work's theoretical context.

- *Method.* This portion is usually subdivided into Subjects (the method used for their selection, inclusion and exclusion criteria, methods used to assign them to various groups, and any other significant features of the subjects, including mean age and sex), Dependent Variables, Design, Instruments, Procedures, and Data Analysis sections—see later.

- *Results.* This element presents the results without commenting on their meaning.

- *Discussion.* The purpose of the discussion is to present the authors' interpretation of the results and their assessment of study limitations and future research directions.

- *Conclusions.* As its name suggests, this element concisely restates the research's important findings and presents a conclusion for each purpose outlined in the introduction.

- *References.* List of references cited in the text of the article.

Hypotheses

Most research begins with a question or purpose statement. For example, does age predict whether a patient will be discharged to home or inpatient rehabilitation following a total knee replacement? A hypothesis attempts to offer a prediction. In the previous example, the prediction may be, "Yes, age does predict whether a patient will be discharged to home or inpatient rehabilitation following a total knee replacement."

There are two types of statistical hypotheses for each situation: the null hypothesis (H_0) and the alternative hypothesis (H_A).

- *Null hypothesis (H_0):* A hypothesis stating that there will be no difference between the groups or variables.[23] The null hypothesis is also referred to as the statistical hypothesis. This study type's premise is that the results may be due to the chance rather than the experiment or phenomenon of interest.[15]

- *Alternative (research) hypothesis (H_A):* A hypothesis stating that there will be a difference between the groups or variables.[23] The alternative hypothesis is also referred to as the *research hypothesis*. This study type's premise is that the results include directional statements such as more/less than and positive/negative.[15]

Subject Selection

Whenever clinical research is performed, data are collected from people, specifically, a target population based on the research question or purpose—for example, all athletes who undergo rotator cuff surgery. Unfortunately, not every member of these target populations may be accessible to the researchers, so the researchers use a collection of subjects called a *sample* that best represents the population from which they are drawn.

CLINICAL PEARL

- A population consists of all subjects (human or otherwise) that are being studied.

- A sample is a group of subjects selected from a population. One of the challenges facing researchers is to achieve an adequate sample size to avoid an incorrect conclusion.

To avoid any biasing occurring with the collected information, samples must be collected systematically. Sampling can occur using a probabilistic method or a nonprobabilistic method.

Probabilistic methods include:

- *Random sampling:* All items have the same chance of selection, thereby minimizing sampling bias—for example, drawing numbers out of a hat.

- *Systematic sampling:* In which potential subjects are organized according to an identifier such as birth date, Social Security number, or medical record number.

- *Stratified sampling:* Sometimes called *proportional* or *quota* random sampling, involves dividing the population into homogeneous subgroups called strata and then taking a simple random sample from each subgroup to highlight a specific subgroup. Thus, stratified sampling ensures that the overall population will be well-represented by key subgroups. For example, the most common strata used to formulate subgroups include age, gender, religion, educational achievement, socioeconomic status, and nationality.

- *Cluster sampling:* Involves dividing the population into groups or clusters (such as geographic boundaries), then randomly selecting sample clusters and using all members of the selected clusters as subjects of the samples. For example, it may not be possible to list all of the patients of a chain of physical therapy clinics. However, it would be possible to randomly select a subset of clinics (stage 1 of cluster sampling) and then interview a random sample of patients who visit those clinics (stage 2 of cluster sampling).

Non-probabilistic methods include[24]:

- *Convenience sampling:* Researchers recruit easily available individuals who meet the study criteria—for example, requesting students to volunteer.
- *Snowball sampling:* The researchers start with a few subjects and then recruit more via word of mouth from the original participants.
- *Purposive sampling:* The researchers make specific choices about who will serve as subjects in this study by handpicking individuals with certain characteristics.

Variables

Studies about a diagnostic test require information about the specific test performed and the diagnoses obtained, whereas studies about an intervention require information about the interventions provided and their effects.[25] The tests, diagnoses, interventions, and effects are referred to generically as variables.[25]

CLINICAL PEARL

A variable is a measurement of phenomena that can assume more than one value or more than one category.[14] The two traits of a variable that should always be achieved include:

- Each variable should be *exhaustive*: it should include all possible answerable responses.
- Each variable should be *mutually exclusive*: no respondent should be able to have two attributes simultaneously.

Dependency refers to the role of the variable in the experiment or study. Different study designs require different types of variables. Two common types of variables include the independent variable and dependent variable:

- *Independent variable*: The variable is purposely manipulated by the researcher; independent variables are controlled or fixed to observe their effect on dependent variables. An example of an independent variable would be the type of treatment received by a subject.
- *Dependent variable:* The variable that is the outcome of interest in a study. Using pain as an example, if a study examines the effects of iontophoresis on pain levels, the iontophoresis is the independent variable, and the measurement of pain levels is the dependent variable.

CLINICAL PEARL

An extraneous variable is a factor other than the independent variable set to influence or confound the dependent variable.[26] Examples of extraneous variables include subjects, equipment, and environmental conditions.

Measurement of Variables

Variables can be classified by how they are categorized, counted, or measured. This type of classification uses measurement scales. The four classic scales (or levels) of measurement include[27]:

- *Nominal (classificatory, categorical):* Classifies data into mutually exclusive, exhausting categories in which no order or ranking can be imposed. Examples include arbitrary labels, such as zip codes, religion, and marital status.
- *Ordinal (ranking):* Classifies data into categories that can be ranked, although precise differences between the ranks do not exist. Examples include letter grades (A, B, C, etc.) and body builds (small, medium, large).
- *Interval:* Ranks data where precise differences between units of measure exist, although there is no meaningful zero. Examples include temperature (degrees Celsius, degrees Fahrenheit), IQ, calendar dates.
- *Ratio:* Possesses all the characteristics of interval measurement, and there exists a true zero. Examples include height, weight, age, and salary.

Validity

Research or test validity is defined as the degree to which a test measures what it purports to measure and how well it correctly classifies individuals with or without a particular condition.[28-30]

CLINICAL PEARL

A test is considered to have diagnostic accuracy if it can discriminate between patients with and without a specific disorder.[31]

There are several forms of measurement that may be evaluated to determine the potential validity of a study:

- *Construct validity.* Construct validity, a theoretical form of validity refers to a test's ability to represent the underlying construct (the theory developed to organize and explain some aspects of existing knowledge and observations). For example, a test of motor function—based on a particular construct of what "motor function" means—should correlate highly with other tests that measure similar concepts of motor function, such as tests for dexterity and coordination.[2]
- *Face validity.* Face validity refers to the degree to which the questions or procedures incorporated within a test make sense to the users. The assessment of face validity is

based on the notion that the finding is valid "on the face of it." For example, if a weighing scale indicates that a normal-sized person weighs 2000 pounds, that scale does not have face validity. In contrast, goniometric measurements have face validity as measurements of joint position.[2]

▶ *Content validity*. Content validity refers to whether the test used is fully representative of what it aims to measure—the content of the test method must cover all relevant parts of the subject it aims to measure because if some aspects are missing (or if irrelevant aspects are included), the validity is threatened. For example, suppose you want to develop a test of patient function that covers every form of function. If some function measures are omitted from the function test, then the test results may not be an accurate indication of the patient's function.

CLINICAL PEARL

It is important to remember that there are no perfect studies because of the reciprocal nature of many of the threats to validity.

Several factors can threaten the validity of a research project. The most common threats to validity include:

▶ *Ambiguity*—when a correlation is taken for causation.

▶ *Subject assignment*—subject age, gender, ethnic and racial background, educational level, and presence of comorbidities can all threaten the validity unless randomization is used.

▶ *Errors of measurement*—random errors or systematic errors.

▶ *History*—when some critical event occurs between the pretest and posttest results.

▶ *Instrumentation*—when the researcher changes the measuring device.

▶ *Maturation*—when people change or mature physically, psychologically, emotionally, or spiritually over the research period.

▶ *Attrition*—when people die or drop out of the research project.

▶ *Testing*—subjects may appear to demonstrate improvement based on their growing familiarity with the testing procedure or based on different instructions and cues provided by the person administering the test.

▶ *The John Henry Effect*—when groups compete to score well.

▶ *The Hawthorne Effect*—a tendency of research subjects to act atypically due to their awareness of being studied.

Validity is directly related to the notion of sensitivity and specificity. Sensitivity is the test's ability to pick up what it is testing for, and specificity is the test's ability to reject what it is not testing for.

▶ Sensitivity represents the proportion of patients with a disorder who test positive. A test that can correctly identify every person who has the disorder has a sensitivity of 1.0. *SnNout* is an acronym that when a symptom or sign's

sensitivity is high, a *negative* response rules *out* the target disorder. Thus, a so-called highly sensitive test helps to rule out a disorder. The positive predictive value is the proportion of patients with positive test results who are correctly diagnosed.

▶ Specificity is the proportion of the study population without the disorder that tests negative.[32] A test that can correctly identify every person who does not have the target disorder has a specificity of 1.0. *SpPin* is an acronym that when *s*pecificity is extremely high, a *p*ositive test result rules *in* the target disorder. Thus, a so-called highly specific test helps rule in a disorder or condition.

CLINICAL PEARL

Interpretation of sensitivity and specificity values is easiest when their values are high.[33] A test with very high sensitivity but low specificity, or vice versa, is of little value, and the acceptable levels are generally set at between 50% (unacceptable test) and 100% (perfect test), with an arbitrary cutoff at about 80%.[32]

Reliability

Numerous physical therapy tests are designed to help the clinician rule out some of the many possible diagnoses. Regardless of which test is chosen, the test must be performed reliably by the clinician to be a valuable guide. Reliability describes the extent to which a test or measurement is free from error. A test is considered reliable if it produces precise, accurate, and reproducible information.[34] Two types of reliability are often described:

▶ *Interrater*. This type of reliability determines whether two or more examiners can repeat a test consistently.

▶ *Intrarater*. This type of reliability determines whether the same single examiner can repeat the test consistently.

Reliability is quantitatively expressed through an agreement index, with the simplest index being the percentage agreement value. The statistical coefficients most commonly used to characterize the reliability of the tests and measures are the intraclass correlation coefficient (ICC) and the kappa statistic (κ), both of which are based on statistical models[35]:

▶ The ICC is a reliable coefficient calculated with variance estimates obtained through an *analysis of variance* (Table 3-3).[36] The advantages of the ICC over a correlation coefficient are that it does not require the same number of

TABLE 3-3	Intraclass Correlation Coefficient Benchmark Values	
Value	**Description**
<0.75	Poor-to-moderate agreement
>0.75	Good agreement
>90	Reasonable agreement for clinical measurements

Data from Portney L, Watkins MP. Foundations of Clinical Research: Applications to Practice. Norwalk, CT: Appleton & Lange; 1993.

raters per subject, and it can be used for two or more raters or ratings.[36]

▶ The kappa statistic (κ) overcomes the problem of chance agreement when used with nominal and ordinal data.[37] Theoretically, κ can be negative if the agreement is worse than chance. Practically, in clinical reliability studies, κ usually varies between 0.00 and 1.00.[38] The κ statistic does not differentiate among disagreements; it assumes that all disagreements are of equal significance.[38]

The standard error of measurement (SEM) reflects the reliability of the response when the test is performed many times and indicates how much change there might be when repeated.[38] If the SEM is small, then the test is stable, with minimal variability between tests.[38]

CLINICAL PEARL

To determine if a test is reliable and valid, the test must be examined in a research study and, preferably, multiple studies.

Once a test's specificity and sensitivity are established (see Validity, above), the predictive value of a positive test versus a negative test can be determined if the prevalence of the disease/dysfunction is known. For example, when the disease's prevalence increases, a positive test is more likely to indicate the disease is present (a false negative is less likely). A negative result of a highly sensitive test will probably rule out a common disease, whereas if the disease is rare, the test must be much more specific for it to be clinically useful.

The likelihood ratio (LR) is the index measurement that combines sensitivity and specificity values and can gauge the performance of a diagnostic test, as it indicates how much a given diagnostic test result will lower or raise the pretest probability of the target disorder.[32,39]

CLINICAL PEARL

Diagnostic tests are used for discovery, confirmation, and exclusion.[40] Tests for discovery and exclusion must have high sensitivity for detection, whereas confirmation tests require high specificity.[41]

Four measures contribute to sensitivity and specificity (Table 3-4):

▶ *True-positive.* The test indicates that the patient has the disease or dysfunction, and the gold-standard test confirms this.

▶ *False positive.* The clinical test indicates that the disease or dysfunction is present, but the gold-standard test does not confirm this.

▶ *False negative.* The clinical test indicates the disorder's absence, but the gold-standard test shows that the disease or dysfunction is present.

▶ *True negative.* The clinical and gold-standard tests agree that the disease or dysfunction is absent.

These values are used to calculate the statistical measures of accuracy, sensitivity, specificity, negative and positive predictive values, and negative and positive LRs, as indicated in Table 3-5. Another way to summarize diagnostic test performance is to use Table 3-4 through the diagnostic odds ratio (DOR): DOR = true/false = $(a \times d)/(b \times c)$. A DOR value ranges from 0 to infinity, with higher values indicating better discriminatory test performance. A score of 1 means a test does not discriminate between patients with the disorder and those without.

CLINICAL PEARL

The DOR value rises steeply when sensitivity or specificity becomes near perfect.

The quality assessment of studies of diagnostic accuracy (QUADAS)[42] is an evidence-based quality assessment tool currently recommended for use in systematic reviews of diagnostic accuracy studies. The QUADAS tool is a list of 14 questions that should each be answered "yes," "no," or "unclear" (Table 3-6). A score of 10 or more "yes" answers is indicative of a higher quality study, whereas a score of fewer than 10 "yes" answers suggests a poorly designed study.

USING EVIDENCE

The methodologic hierarchy or rating of scientific studies is well documented in the literature (Table 3-7). Clinicians must constantly remind themselves that without information gathered from controlled clinical trials, they have a limited scientific basis for their tests or interventions.[43]

When integrating evidence into the clinical, an understanding of how to appraise the quality of clinical studies' evidence is important. One of the major problems in evaluating studies is that the volume of information makes it difficult for the busy clinician to obtain and analyze all of the evidence.[34] The other problem involves deciding whether the literature results are definite enough to indicate an effect other than chance. Judging the strength of the evidence becomes an important part of making clinical decisions.

CLINICAL PEARL

Clinical prediction rules (CPRs) are tools designed to assist clinicians when caring for patients. However, although there is a growing trend toward designing several CPRs for physical therapy, few presently exist.

TABLE 3-4	2 × 2 Table		
		Disease/Outcome	
		Present	**Absent**
Test	Positive (+ve)	a (true +ve)	b (false +ve)
	Negative (−ve)	c (false −ve)	d (true −ve)

TABLE 3-5	Definition and Calculation of Statistical Measures	
Statistical Measure	**Definition**	**Calculation**
Accuracy	The proportion of people who were correctly identified as either having or not having the disease or dysfunction	$(TP + TN)/(TP + FP + FN + TN)$
Sensitivity	A pretest probability to determine the proportion of people with the disease or dysfunction who will have a positive test result	$TP/(TP + FN)$
Specificity	A pretest probability to determine the proportion of people without the disease or dysfunction who will have a negative test result	$TN/(FP + TN)$
Positive predictive value	A posttest probability to determine the proportion of people who truly have the disease or dysfunction when the test is positive	$TP/(TP + FP)$
Negative predictive value	A posttest probability to determine the proportion of people who truly do not have the disease or dysfunction when the test is negative	$TN/(FN + TN)$
Positive likelihood ratio	How likely a positive test result is in people who have the disease or dysfunction as compared to how likely it is in those who do not have the disease or dysfunction	Sensitivity$/(1 - $specificity$)$
Negative likelihood ratio	How likely a negative test result is in people who have the disease or dysfunction as compared to how likely it is in those who do not have the disease or dysfunction	$(1 - $sensitivity$)/$specificity

TP, true positive; TN, true negative; FP, false positive; FN, false negative.

Reproduced with permission from Leibold MR, Huijbregts PA, Jensen R: Concurrent criterion-related validity of physical examination tests for hip labral lesions: a systematic review, J Man Manip Ther 2008;16(2):E24-E41.

TABLE 3-6	The QUADAS Tool			
Item		**Yes**	**No**	**Unclear**
1.	Was the spectrum of patients representative of the patients who will receive the test in practice?	( )	( )	( )
2.	Were selection criteria clearly described?	( )	( )	( )
3.	Is the reference standard likely to correctly classify the target condition?	( )	( )	( )
4.	Is the time between the reference standard and index test short enough to be reasonably sure that the target condition did not change between the two tests?	( )	( )	( )
5.	Did the whole sample, or a random selection of the sample, receive verification using a reference standard of diagnosis?	( )	( )	( )
6.	Did patients receive the same reference standard regardless of the index test result?	( )	( )	( )
7.	Was the reference standard independent of the index test (ie, the index test did not form part of the reference standard)?	( )	( )	( )
8.	Was the execution of the index test described in sufficient detail to permit replication of the test?	( )	( )	( )
9.	Was the execution of the reference standard described in sufficient detail to permit its replication?	( )	( )	( )
10.	Were the index test results interpreted without knowledge of the results of the reference standard?	( )	( )	( )
11.	Were the reference standard results interpreted without knowledge of the results of the index test?	( )	( )	( )
12.	Were the same clinical data available when test results were interpreted as would be available when the test is used in practice?	( )	( )	( )
13.	Were uninterpretable/intermediate test results reported?	( )	( )	( )
14.	Were withdrawals from the study explained?	( )	( )	( )

Reproduced with permission from Whiting P, Rutjes AW, Reitsma JB, et al. The development of QUADAS: a tool for the quality assessment of studies of diagnostic accuracy included in systematic reviews. BMC Med Res Methodol. 2003 Nov 10:3;25.

TABLE 3-7   A Hierarchy of Evidence Grading

	Level of Evidence Grading = 1a	Level of Evidence Grading = 1b	Level of Evidence Grading = 1c	Level of Evidence Grading = 2a	Level of Evidence Grading = 2b	Level of Evidence Grading = 2c	Level of Evidence Grading = 3a	Level of Evidence Grading = 3b	Level of Evidence Grading = 4	Level of Evidence Grading = 5
Type of Study	A systematic review of randomized clinical trials that do not have a statistically significant variation in the direction or degrees of results	An individual randomized clinical trial with a narrow confidence interval	An all-or-none study (a study in which some or all patients died before treatment became available, and then none died after the treatment)	A systematic review of cohort studies that do not have a statistically significant variation in the direction or degrees of results	Individual cohort study (including low-quality randomized clinical trial)	Nonexperimental research (correlational, observational)—commonly used to evaluate outcomes of care in *real-world* clinical conditions	Nonrandomized trial with concurrent or historical controls / Study of sensitivity and specificity of a diagnostic test / Population-based descriptive study	Individual case-control study	Cross-sectional study / Case series study-Case report	Expert consensus / Clinical experience

Data from Sackett D: Rules of evidence and clinical recommendations on the use of antithrombotic agents, Chest 1986 Feb;89 (2 Suppl):2S-3S; and the Oxford Center for Evidence-based Medicine (www.cebm.net).

The best evidence for making decisions comes from randomized controlled trials, systematic reviews, and evidence-based clinical practice guidelines.[44] At the other end of the continuum is the unsystematic collection of patient/client data. In between the two ends of the continuum are the study designs outlined in Table 3-1, with quasi-experimental designs being the strongest and narrative reviews being the weakest.

It may also be possible to discriminate between high- and low-quality trials by asking three simple questions[44]:

1. Were subjects randomly allocated to conditions? Random allocation implies that a nonsystematic, unpredictable procedure was used to allocate subjects to conditions.

2. Was there blinding of assessors and patients? Blinding of assessors and patients minimizes the risk of the placebo effect and the Hawthorne effect.[45]

3. Was there an adequate follow-up? Ideally, all subjects who enter the trial should subsequently be followed up to avoid bias. In practice, this rarely happens. As a general rule, losses to follow-up of less than 10% avoid serious bias, but losses to follow-up of more than 20% cause potential for serious bias.

Patients may be referred to physical therapy with a nonspecific diagnosis, an incorrect diagnosis, or no diagnosis at all.[46] A diagnosis can only be made when all potential causes for the signs and symptoms have been ruled out.

CLINICAL DECISION-MAKING

The clinical decision-making process is a multifaceted, fluid process that combines tacit knowledge with accumulated clinical experience.[47] To be a successful clinician, one has to apply the PTA curriculum's academic content to the clinical setting, which takes time to develop. For example, the PT's treatment plan may include using electrical stimulation to enhance a patient's quadriceps strength to help with the patient's functional activities. Based on this information, the PTA must make a clinical decision about the type of electrical stimulation and the parameters to be used. Over time, such decisions become easier. According to Kahney,[48] the expert seems to do less problem solving than the novice because the former has already accumulated solutions to many of the clinical problems previously encountered.[49] Thus, the clinician's knowledge base is critical in the process.[50] However, the PTA must always be aware of those clinical decisions that they can safely make and those that require consultation with the supervising PT. Indeed, the PTA must understand what their role adds to the overall POC for a patient. Conversely, the PT, who is responsible for the PTA and patient management, must know the PTA's education and experience level in order to delegate safely.

As described in Chapter 1, the PTA can modify both the approach and the sequencing of any specific intervention as long as such decisions are within the POC written by the supervising PT. This decision-making may require communication with the supervising PT if, for example:

▶ The POC includes a specific intervention that the PTA is insufficiently trained in.

▶ The PTA has a question about the POC in terms of clarity.

▶ The PTA notices a change in the patient's status that might require a reassessment of the patient by the supervising PT.

▶ A patient has met one or more goals outlined in the POC.

▶ A patient has an adverse reaction to a particular intervention listed in the POC.

▶ A patient is not making progress toward the goals despite the PTA's modifications within the POC.

The state practice act, which varies from state to state, often dictates what a PTA can do. For example, in some states, PTAs can perform joint mobilizations and a sharp debridement of wounds, whereas, in other states, only a PT can perform these tasks. In those states that allow only a PT to perform these tasks, the reasoning is that these types of interventions require "immediate and continuous examination and evaluation throughout the intervention."[51] However, on the subject of joint mobilizations, the 2013 position on Physical Therapy Assistant (PTA) Education and Joint Mobilization put forth by the Commission on Accreditation of Physical Therapy Education (CAPTE) questioned this rationale.[52] Specifically, CAPTE supported the addition of *grade I and II peripheral joint mobilization techniques* to the PTA curriculum. CAPTE felt that these techniques do not require manual force at the end range of tissue restriction that may produce an adverse patient response, and that these types of peripheral joint mobilization techniques are often included in a patient's home program, which a PTA may be asked to teach or monitor.[52] Needless to say, both the PT and PTA must know what their state practice act allows. Complicating matters is that some payer regulations can dictate whether a patient is delegated to a PTA, as some payers have specific requirements regarding supervision, while others pay less or nothing for PTA interventions.[53]

It is worth noting that some clinical decisions are based on knowledge acquired outside of the PTA curriculum. For example, it is easy to conclude that a pyramid is far more stable when placed in its normal position than when placed upside down. One does not need to know the terms "base of support" and "center of gravity" to understand why one of the two is the more stable, and it is not difficult to extrapolate how a standard walker provides more stability for a patient than a standard cane.

Various frameworks have been applied to clinical practice to guide clinical decision-making and provide structure to the healthcare process.[54-60] Whereas the early frameworks were based on disablement models, the more recent models have focused on enablement perspectives using algorithms. An algorithm is a systematic process involving a finite number of steps that solve a problem. Algorithms used in healthcare allow for clinical decisions and adjustments to be made during the clinical reasoning and decision-making process because they are not prescriptive or protocol-driven.[47]

From the PTA's perspective, the established treatment goals, which can be either short-term or long-term, drive patient care (see Chapter 4). To maintain a sufficient level of progress toward the treatment goals requires a combination of clinical decision-making and effective communication with the supervising PT. The PTA must also remember that every patient is unique and can respond differently to any given treatment. Although the PTA cannot change the POC, the PTA can alert the supervising PT. For example, suppose there is no change in a patient's manual muscle grade after a sufficient period of resisted exercises, or the patient is unable to tolerate an increase in resistance. In that case, the PTA must notify the supervising PT so that an alteration in the POC can be made, or the patient can be referred to another healthcare professional for further evaluation. There are also occasions when the POC is not specific. For example, the PT may write, "Use modalities to decrease pain." In this case, the PTA could use their clinical knowledge to decide whether to use ice, heat, electrical stimulation, or a combination of these, provided that their decision-making is based on sound clinical practice. Doing so does not involve making a change to the POC. Conversely, if the PT wrote, "Quad strengthening using short arc quads," the PTA could not decide to use wall slides to strengthen the quads. Using another example of a nonspecific POC, the PT may write, "Use progressive balance activities to enhance gait." Suppose the PTA would like to generate some evidence-based ideas for balance training

exercises. In that case, they could do an online search of peer-reviewed journals or PubMed* using their knowledge of the hierarchy of evidence (Table 3-7) to find the most effective exercises based on the type of research study.

The patient can serve as an adjunct to the clinical decision-making process, so establishing effective communication with every patient is critical. For example, a patient must feel comfortable to relate any changes in his or her symptoms and to ask any questions about their treatment.

Clinical decision-making is ultimately based on comfort level, understanding one's limitations, emotional intelligence, a willingness to ask questions and self-evaluate, and being open-minded, creative, and flexible.[61] The template in Table 3-8 outlines some of the diagnosis-dependent thought processes that the PTA should use when seeing a patient for the first time. Table 3-9 provides information on making clinical decisions about a patient's progress once the PTA has been treating a patient for a few sessions.

---

*www.pubmed.com.

TABLE 3-8	Clinical Decision-Making Process for the PTA
Topic	**Factors to Consider**
Diagnosis	What is the medical diagnosis?
	What structure(s) is/are involved?
	What is the estimated stage of healing (postsurgical/acute, subacute, or chronic)?
	What signs and symptoms will you expect from the patient based on the diagnosis?
	What are some of the potential adverse signs and symptoms that could occur with the diagnosis?
Physician/Nursing Notes	Are there any abbreviations you don't know the meanings of?
	Is there any medical vocabulary you don't understand?
	Are there any nursing restrictions?
	Are there any needs for personal protective equipment (PPE) or other precautions?
	Are restraints being used on the patient?
	Are there any tests planned that might impact the treatment session or the scheduled time for the session?
	What other disciplines are treating the patient (OT, speech, dialysis, etc.)?
Past Medical History (PMH)	Are there any diagnoses in the PMH that may impact a physical therapy intervention?
Medications	What is the purpose of the prescribed medications?
	What are the potential side effects of the prescribed medications?
Laboratory Results	What are the normal levels and ranges for each of the tests and results?
	What is the relevance of each of the results that are not within the normal ranges?
Physical Therapist Findings	What are the patient's impairments and functional limitations?
	Are there any key findings in ROM, strength, balance?
	What is the patient's level of independence?
	Does the patient require any type of assistive device?
	Are there any specialized techniques (breathing, percussion, wound care, mobilization, modalities, etc) included in the POC, and what is your comfort level with them?
Plan of Care (POC)	What questions will you ask the patient during your first session?
	How do you plan to explain your intervention to the patient?
	What activities and exercises are you planning for the first session based on the POC?
	How do you plan to order your activities and exercises in the first session?
	What are your anticipated goals for the first session?

TABLE 3-9	Clinical Decision-Making Process for Patient Progress
Topic	**Factors to Consider**
Subjective and objective	What subjective reports would make you change your treatment plans?
	Is the patient motivated?
	When is the patient's next physician appointment (if an outpatient)?
	What objective findings would make you change your treatment plans?
	Are there any cultural or communication issues that you become aware of when you meet the patient?
Tests and measures	Which tests and measures do you use to assess the patient's response to the treatment?
	Which tests and measures do you use to assess the patient's progress?
Assessment of treatment session	Were there any observations or findings during the session that caused sufficient concern for you to hold treatment or check with the nursing staff, supervising physical therapist, or physician?
	Was the patient compliant?
Documentation	What are the most important observations or findings to document?
	How do you plan to document the findings and results of the session?
Plan	Was there anything in the treatment session that altered your perception of the patient's prognosis?
	How do you plan to continue implementing the goals of the POC?
	Are you going to change the resistance grade of the exercises?
	Do you have an estimation about any gains (ROM, gait, function, etc) the patient might make in the next session?
	What exercises/activities do you want the patient to perform/practice in between sessions?
Future sessions	If the patient did not respond well to the treatment session, what changes do you plan to make?
	If the patient responded well to the treatment session, what changes do you plan to make?
	Do you plan to seek some ideas to tweak the exercises or activities?

REFERENCES

1. American Physical Therapy Association House of Delegates. *Vision 2020.* HOD 06-00-24-35. Alexandria, VA: American Physical Therapy Association; 2000.
2. American Physical Therapy Association. *Guide to Physical Therapist Practice. 3.0.* Alexandria, VA: American Physical Therapy Association; 2014.
3. Dean E. Physical therapy in the 21st century (Part I): toward practice informed by epidemiology and the crisis of lifestyle conditions. *Physiother Theory Pract.* 2009;25:330-353.
4. Sackett DL, Strauss SE, Richardson WS, et al. *Evidence Based Medicine: How to Practice and Teach EBM,* 2nd ed. Edinburgh: Churchill Livingstone; 2000.
5. Jewell DV. Introduction. *Guide to Evidence-based Physical Therapy Practice.* Sudbury, MA: Jones and Bartlett; 2008:5-18.
6. Sheth SA, Kwon CS, Barker FG, 2nd. The art of management decision making: From intuition to evidence-based medicine. *Otolaryngol Clin North Am.* 2012;45:333-351, viii.
7. Saitz R. Evidence-based design: Part of evidence-based medicine? *Evid Based Med.* 2012;18:1.
8. Rosner AL. Evidence-based medicine: Revisiting the pyramid of priorities. *J Bodyw Mov Ther.* 2012;16:42-49.
9. Rhee JS, Daramola OO. No need to fear evidence-based medicine. *Arch Facial Plast Surg.* 2012;14:89-92.
10. Matthews DR. Wisdom-based and evidence-based medicine. *Diabetes Obes Metab.* 2012;14 Suppl 1:1-2.
11. Mansi IA, Banks DE. Evidence-based medicine for clinicians. *South Med J.* 2012;105:109.
12. Mansi IA, Banks DE. The challenge of evidence-based medicine. *South Med J.* 2012;105:110-113.
13. Schenkman M, Deutsch JE, Gill-Body KM. An integrated framework for decision making in neurologic physical therapist practice. *Phys Ther.* 2006;86:1681-1702.
14. Underwood FB. Clinical research and data analysis. In: Placzek JD, Boyce DA, eds. *Orthopaedic Physical Therapy Secrets.* Philadelphia: Hanley & Belfus, Inc.; 2001;130-139.
15. Jewell DV. Questions, theories, and hypotheses. *Guide to Evidence-based Physical Therapy Practice.* Sudbury, MA: Jones and Bartlett; 2008:81-95.
16. Jewell DV. General characteristics of desirable evidence. *Guide to Evidence-based Physical Therapy Practice.* Sudbury, MA: Jones and Bartlett; 2008:19-34.
17. Domholdt E, Carter R, Lubinsky J. Qualitative research. *Rehabilitation Research: Principles and Applications.* St. Louis, MO: Elsevier Saunders; 2010:157-173.
18. Friedman LM, Furberg CD, DeMets DL. *Fundamentals of Clinical Trials,* 2nd ed. Chicago: Mosby-Year Book; 1985: 2, 51, 71.
19. Sackett DL, Haynes RB, Tugwell P. *Clinical Epidemiology: A Basic Science for Clinical Medicine.* Boston: Little, Brown and Co.; 1985.
20. Straus SE, Richardson WS, Glasziou P, Haynes RB. Evidence-Based Medicine. University Health Network, http://www.cebm.utoronto.ca/; 2006 [cited 2006].
21. Fisher C, Dvorak M. Orthopaedic research: What an orthopaedic surgeon needs to know. *Orthopaedic Knowledge Update: Home Study Syllabus.* Rosemont, IL: American Academy of Orthopaedic Surgeons; 2005:3-13.
22. Carter RE, Lubinsky J, Domholdt E. Evaluating evidence one article at the time. In: Carter RE, Lubinsky J, eds. *Rehabilitation Research: Principles and Applications.* 4th ed: PA: Elsevier Saunders; 2011:341-358.
23. Bluman AG. Hypothesis testing. In: Bluman AG, ed. *Elementary Statistics: A Step by Step Approach,* 4th ed. New York: McGraw-Hill; 2008: 387-455.
24. Jewell DV. Research subjects. *Guide to Evidence-based Physical Therapy Practice.* Sudbury, MA: Jones and Bartlett; 2008:127-143.
25. Jewell DV. Variables and their measurement. *Guide to Evidence-based Physical Therapy Practice.* Sudbury, MA: Jones and Bartlett; 2008:145-167.
26. Domholdt E, Carter R, Lubinsky J. Variables. *Rehabilitation Research: Principles and Applications.* St. Louis, MO: Elsevier Saunders; 2010: 67-74.
27. Bluman AG. The nature of probability and statistics. In: Bluman AG, ed. *Elementary Statistics: A Step by Step Approach,* 4th ed. New York: McGraw-Hill; 2008:1-32.
28. Feinstein AR. *Clinimetrics.* Westford, MA: Murray Printing Company; 1987.
29. Marx RG, Bombardier C, Wright JG. What we know about the reliability and validity of physical examination tests used to examine the upper extremity. *J Hand Surg.* 1999;24A:185-93.

30. Roach KE, Brown MD, Albin RD, et al. The sensitivity and specificity of pain response to activity and position in categorizing patients with low back pain. *Phys Ther*. 1997;77:730-738.

31. Schwartz JS. Evaluating diagnostic tests: What is done—what needs to be done. *J Gen Intern Med*. 1986;1:266-267.

32. Van der Wurff P, Meyne W, Hagmeijer RHM. Clinical tests of the sacroiliac joint, a systematic methodological review. Part 2: validity. *Man Ther*. 2000;5:89-96.

33. Davidson M. The interpretation of diagnostic tests: A primer for physiotherapists. *Aust J Physiother*. 2002;48:227-233.

34. Cleland J. Introduction. *Orthopedic Clinical Examination: An Evidence-based Approach for Physical Therapists*. Carlstadt, NJ: Icon Learning Systems, LLC; 2005:2-23.

35. Wainner RS. Reliability of the clinical examination: How close is "close enough"? *J Orthop Sports Phys Ther*. 2003;33:488-491.

36. Huijbregts PA. Spinal motion palpation: A review of reliability studies. *J Man & Manip Ther*. 2002;10:24-39.

37. Laslett M, Williams M. The reliability of selected pain provocation tests for sacroiliac joint pathology. *Spine*. 1994;19:1243-1249.

38. Portney L, Watkins MP. *Foundations of Clinical Research: Applications to Practice*. Norwalk, CT: Appleton & Lange; 1993.

39. Jaeschke R, Guyatt G, Sackett DL. User's guides to the medical literature. III. How to use an article about a diagnostic test. B. What are the results and will they help me in caring for my patients? *JAMA*. 1994;27:703-707.

40. Feinstein AR. Clinical biostatistics XXXI: on the sensitivity, specificity & discrimination of diagnostic tests. *Clin Pharmacol Ther*. 1975;17:104-116.

41. Anderson MA, Foreman TL. Return to Competition: Functional Rehabilitation. In: Zachazewski JE, Magee DJ, Quillen WS, eds. *Athletic Injuries and Rehabilitation*. Philadelphia: WB Saunders; 1996:229-261.

42. Whiting P, Rutjes AW, Reitsma JB, Bossuyt PM, Kleijnen J. The development of QUADAS: a tool for the quality assessment of studies of diagnostic accuracy included in systematic reviews. *BMC Medical Research Methodology*. 2003;3:25.

43. Schiffman EL. The role of the randomized clinical trial in evaluating management strategies for temporomandibular disorders. In: Fricton JR, Dubner R, eds. *Orofacial Pain and Temporomandibular Disorders (Advances in Pain Research and Therapy, Vol. 21)*. New York: Raven Press; 1995:415-463.

44. Maher CG, Herbert RD, Moseley AM, Sherrington C, Elkins M. Critical appraisal of randomized trials, systematic reviews of randomized trials and clinical practice guidelines. In: Boyling JD, Jull GA, eds. *Grieve's Modern Manual Therapy: The Vertebral Column*. Philadelphia: Churchill Livingstone; 2004:603-614.

45. Wickstrom G, Bendix T. The "Hawthorne effect"—What did the original Hawthorne studies actually show? *Scand J Work Environ Health*. 2000;26:363-367.

46. Clawson AL, Domholdt E. Content of physician referrals to physical therapists at clinical education sites in Indiana. *Physical Ther*. 1994;74:356-360.

47. Hoogenboom BJ, Voight ML. Clinical reasoning: An algorithm-based approach to musculoskeletal rehabilitation. In: Voight ML, Hoogenboom BJ, Prentice WE, eds. *Musculoskeletal Interventions: Techniques for Therapeutic Exercise*. New York: McGraw-Hill; 2007:81-95.

48. Kahney H. Problem solving: current issues. Buckingham: Open University Press; 1993.

49. Coutts F. Changes in the musculoskeletal system. In: Atkinson K, Coutts F, Hassenkamp A, eds. *Physiotherapy in Orthopedics*. London: Churchill Livingstone; 1999:19-43.

50. Jones MA. Clinical reasoning in manual therapy. *Physical Ther*. 1992;72:875-884.

51. *Procedural interventions exclusively performed by physical therapists*, HOD P06-00-30-36. House of Delegates Standards, Policies, Positions, and Guidelines, 2012.

52. Position Statement: PTA Education and Peripheral Joint Mobilization [database on the Internet], 2012 [cited 3/6/2021].

53. Reynolds EL, Kerber KA, Hill C, De Lott LB, Magliocco B, Esper GJ, et al. The effects of the Medicare NCS reimbursement policy: Utilization, payments, and patient access. *Neurology*. 2020;95:e930-e935.

54. Higgs J, Jones M, eds. *Clinical Reasoning in the Health Professions*. 2 ed. London: Butterworth-Heinemann; 2000.

55. Rothstein JM, Echternach JL, Riddle DL. The Hypothesis-Oriented Algorithm for Clinicians II (HOAC II): a guide for patient management. *Physical Ther*. 2003;83:455-470.

56. Echternach JL, Rothstein JM. Hypothesis-oriented algorithms. *Physical Ther*. 1989;69:559-564.

57. Rothstein JM, Echternach JL. Hypothesis-oriented algorithm for clinicians. A method for evaluation and treatment planning. *Physical Ther*. 1986;66:1388-1394.

58. Schenkman M, Butler RB. A model for multisystem evaluation, interpretation, and treatment of individuals with neurologic dysfunction. *Physical Ther*. 1989;69:538-547.

59. Schenkman M, Butler RB. A model for multisystem evaluation treatment of individuals with Parkinson's disease. *Physical Ther*. 1989;69:932-943.

60. Schenkman M, Donovan J, Tsubota J, Kluss M, Stebbins P, Butler RB. Management of individuals with Parkinson's disease: rationale and case studies. *Physical Ther*. 1989;69:944-955.

61. Facione NC, Facione PA. *Critical Thinking and Clinical Reasoning in the Health Sciences: An International Multidisciplinary Teaching Anthology*. Millbrae, CA: The California Academic Press/Insight Assessment; 2008.

Clinical Documentation

CHAPTER 4

CHAPTER OBJECTIVES

At the completion of this chapter, the reader will be able to:

1. Discuss the various types of clinical documentation

2. Describe the normal sequence and order used in clinical documentation

3. Describe the purpose and importance of clinical documentation

4. Understand the common medical abbreviations used in healthcare

5. Understand how the legal requirements for cosigning by the supervising PT varies from state to state

OVERVIEW

Communication between the physical therapist (PT) and physical therapist assistant (PTA) is critical to ensure that the patient/client receives safe, appropriate, comprehensive, efficient, person-centered, and high-quality health-care services from initial evaluation through discharge.[1] Together with verbal communication, written communication in the form of documentation forms the strong collaborative process that is essential between the PT and PTA.

Documentation in healthcare includes any entry into the patient/client record. As the record of client care, documentation also provides useful information for the other healthcare team members and for third-party payers. This documentation, considered a legal document, becomes a part of the patient's medical record. As such, a clinician should never enter an endnote or sign an entry for someone else and should not ask someone else to perform such acts. Documentation is a mark of a clinician's credibility, honesty, and intent, and any breaches of documentation rules can lead to charges of incompetence, negligent behavior, poor judgment, or prosecution.

CLINICAL PEARL

Clinical documentation serves to:

▶ Inform other healthcare providers as to the status of the patient

▶ Describe what and how the patient performed

▶ Provide necessary information for payer sources

▶ Protect the clinician in case of patient complaint or injury

APTA GUIDELINES

Whenever possible, documentation should follow the APTA's *Guidelines: Physical Therapy Documentation.*[*]

▶ An initial note is written after the first patient visit and documents the results from the examination, the subsequent evaluation, diagnosis, prognosis, and plan of care.

▶ A progress note is written after each subsequent visit and documents the results of any reexamination and reevaluation and any change in the prognosis and plan of care as appropriate.

▶ A discharge note is completed when therapy is discontinued and occurs after the final examination and evaluation are performed.

---

[*]American Physical Therapy Association Board of Directors. Guidelines: Physical Therapy Documentation of Patient/Client Management (BOD G03-05-16-41). Available at: http://www.apta.org/uploadedFiles/APTAorg/About_Us/Policies/Practice/DocumentationPatientClientManagement.pdf. Accessed February 28, 2014.

NOTE FORMATS

Several types of format are commonly used for writing notes:

- Problem-oriented medical record (POMR): a traditional form of documentation developed in the 1960s by Dr. Lawrence Weed. The POMR has four phases: formation of a database which includes current and past information about the patient; development of a specific, current problem list which includes problems to be treated by various practitioners; identification of a specific treatment plan developed by each practitioner; and assessment of the effectiveness of the treatment plans.

- Subjective, objective, assessment, plan (SOAP): a progression of the POMR note format introduced in the 1970s and now used by each clinician involved in the patient's care to address each of the patient's problems. Several variations of the SOAP format have been developed over the years.

- Patient/client management based on *The Guide to Physical Therapist Practice*, initially published in 1997, with the second edition publishing a Documentation Template for use in both inpatient and outpatient settings in 2014.[1]

- Electronic health record (EHR): many facilities use documentation software that has strengths and weaknesses. For example, the software's documentation fields are quite rigid and do not always allow for a detailed narrative. Also, they remove some of the conversational interaction between the patient and the clinician and therefore hinder relationship building. However, EHR, including oral dictations into recorders, can improve productivity and efficiency.

Whatever format is used, the clinician should attempt to complete a patient's documentation during the session or as soon as possible after the patient interaction, as this will improve accuracy and speed up reimbursement.

The purposes of documentation are as follows[2]:

- To document what the clinician is doing to manage the individual patient's case.

- To record examination findings, patient status, the intervention provided, and the patient's response to treatment.

- To communicate with all other healthcare team members; this helps provide consistency among the services provided, including communication between the PT and the PTA.

- To provide information to third-party payers, such as Medicare and other insurance companies, who decide about reimbursement based on the quality and completeness of the physical therapy received and the documentation that verifies the intervention.

- To help the PT/PTA organize his/her thought processes involved in patient care.

- To document the patient's functional outcome or outcomes through objective and measurable terms, language, or data. Strength and range-of-motion data should be linked to the person's ability to perform functional tasks such as dressing, lifting, reaching, eating, and personal hygiene.

- To serve as a source of data for quality assurance, peer and utilization review, and research.

SOAP Format

In addition to documenting a patient's progress, SOAP notes encourage clinical reasoning using a step-by-step approach.

- *Subjective:* information about the condition reported by the patient, family member, significant other, another healthcare provider or is read from the medical chart. This information includes the patient's chief complaint, other complaints, how the symptoms occurred, and how the current condition impacts the patient's function and lifestyle. One of three acronyms can be used to organize this section: OLDCARTS, PQRST, and SOCRATES

OLDCARTS

Onset: When did the symptoms begin?
Location: Where are the symptoms located?
Duration: How long have the symptoms been felt since the last session?
Characterization: How does the patient describe the symptoms?
Alleviating and aggravating factors: What makes the symptoms better/worse?
Radiation: Do the symptoms move or stay in one location?
Temporal factor: Are the symptoms worse/better at a certain time (morning, night, after eating, etc.)?
Severity: Using a scale of 1 to 10, 1 being the least, 10 being the worst, how does the patient rate the symptoms?

PQRST

P: Provocative or palliative (what make the symptoms better or worse?)
Q: Quality or quantity (what are the symptoms like?)
R: Region or radiation (where are the symptoms, where do they radiate?)
S: Severity (how bad are the symptoms?)
T: Timing (when did the symptoms start, and how often do they occur?)

SOCRATES

S: Site
O: Onset
C: Character
R: Radiation
A: Associated symptoms
T: Timespan/duration
E: Exacerbating and relieving factors
S: Severity

The clinician also notes whether the patient has any preconceived goals that he/she hopes to achieve from physical therapy.

▶ *Objective:* everything that the clinician witnessed, performed, or measured during the treatment session, including signs (womb description, vital signs, etc) and tests and measures (range of motion, strength, quality of movement, level of independence, adaptive equipment, etc).

▶ *Assessment:* analysis and interpretation of the subjective and objective data (overall status, pain rating following the session, strength, progress toward goals, time of exercises or activities in seconds and minutes, etc), the treatment effectiveness, and goal completion collected during the encounter. The PT makes this assessment following the initial examination, whereas the PTA uses this section to report any progress the patient has made toward the treatment goals and any recommended modifications. Sometimes this section is referred to as *the problem list* as it can be used to outline any impediments to a patient's progress. Any comments documented in this section must be objective. For example, "the patient did well with his

activities" does not provide the reader with any objective information. Better would be: "the patient was able to ambulate unassisted for two minutes compared with 90 seconds in the previous session."

▶ *Plan:* the specific plan (geared toward the POC goals) for the next treatment session. The plan includes when the next session is scheduled, when the next supervisory visit by the PT is scheduled, any instructions given to the patient, the number of treatment sessions the patient has remaining, and any updating of goals based on discussion with the supervising physical therapist. The PT completes this section after the initial examination and provides details about the expected goals (measurable and include a timeframe), the treatment plan designed to achieve the expected goals, and the anticipated measurable and functional outcomes, including a list of exercises and activities. The PTA completes this section in the daily progress note.

- The PT will see the patient for a supervisory visit on 4/6/21.
- Will focus on hip abductor strengthening through standing exercises and balance activities to improve gait stability.
- The patient will perform PROM and AROM exercises to the right shoulder at bedside, and the exercises will be followed with an ice pack to the right shoulder for 15 min.

Patient/Client Management Format

- *Examination:* the information gathered during the initial examination by the PT is organized according to the nature of the data into History, Review of Systems (ROS), and Tests and Measures.
- *Evaluation:* this information is divided into two sections: Diagnosis and Prognosis.
  - The diagnosis attempts to relate the patient's functional deficits to the patient's impairment.
  - The prognosis section includes the predicted level of improvement (rehabilitation potential) that the patient will achieve and the amount of time it will take to achieve that improvement level.
- *Plan of Care:* The *plan of care* (POC) consists of statements that specify the goals, predicted level of optimal improvement, specific interventions to be used, and proposed duration and frequency of the interventions that are required to reach the goals and outcomes (see Next Section).[1]

Long-term (Expected Outcomes) Goals. Long-term goals are the final product of a therapeutic intervention. The purposes of long-term goals are the same as those for short-term goals. Long-term goals typically use functional terms rather than items such as degrees of range of movement (ROM) or muscle strength grades.

PLAN OF CARE

The POC written by the PT consists of a blend of consultation, education, and intervention combined with the patient's aspirations and patient-identified problems, and those problems identified by the clinician.[3] The POC is typically guided by the short- and long-term goals designed by the PT, which are dynamic, so that they can be altered as the patient's condition changes, and strategies to achieve those goals based on the patient's stage of healing.

Short-term (Anticipated) Goals. Short-term goals are the interim steps along the way to achieving the long-term goals. The purposes of the short-term goals include:

- To set the priorities of an intervention.
- To direct the intervention based on the specific needs and problems of the patient.
- To provide a mechanism to measure the effectiveness of the intervention.
- To communicate with the PTA and other healthcare professionals.
- To explain the rationale behind the goal to third-party payers.

The PT must include the following information within the POC based on the anticipated goals.

- Frequency of treatments, including how often the patient will be seen per day or week.
- What interventions the patient will receive, including any modalities, therapeutic exercise, and any specialized equipment.
- Plans for discharge, including patient and family education, equipment needs, and referral to other services as appropriate.

When writing goals, the clinician should use the following guidelines:

- **Who.** This refers to the individual involved. Almost always, this is the patient, but it can be a family member.
- **What.** This refers to what the individual will accomplish functionally and to the level of ability. For example, the patient will demonstrate independence with ambulation using a cane for a distance of 100 feet.
- **When.** This refers to an estimate of the time needed to accomplish the goal, which is usually expressed in days or

weeks, depending on the patient's diagnosis and general condition. The time frame may be a function of the clinical setting. For example, in an acute care setting, where the patient may be seen for only 3 to 5 days, the focus will be on short-term goals, and the time frame can be based on the next time the patient will be seen. In contrast, in a long-term care setting, where the patient may be seen for months, more focus is placed on the long-term goals.

▶ *How.* This refers to the circumstances under which the functional task will be completed or the circumstances necessary for the functional task to be completed. The *how* includes the amount of assistance a patient requires to perform a task or any necessary assistive devices.

The documented goals should be listed based on priority, with the most important or more vital functional activities listed first.

MEDICAL NECESSITY

Medicare and other insurance companies have varying criteria for determining whether a given procedure is medically necessary. In essence, a procedure is considered medically necessary if it is a procedure that a clinician, exercising prudent judgment, feels is reasonable and necessary for a patient. For example, a physical therapist must justify why a patient needs a skilled therapeutic intervention for reimbursement purposes. This justification is usually made based on evidence that the patient continues to demonstrate improvement in their functional level. As per the APTA,[*] physical therapy treatment is medically necessary if:

▶ A licensed PT determines it is so based on an evaluation;

▶ It minimizes or eliminates impairments, activity limitations, and/or participation restrictions;

▶ It is provided throughout the episode of care by the physical therapist under his or her direction and supervision;

▶ It requires the knowledge, clinical judgment, and abilities of the therapist;

▶ It is not provided exclusively for the patient's convenience;

▶ It is provided using evidence of effectiveness and applicable standards of practice; and

▶ The type, amount, and duration of the therapy help a patient improve function, minimize loss of function, or decrease the risk of injury (or disease).

GUIDELINES FOR DOCUMENTATION

Clinical documentation must be provided promptly. In these days of increased cost efficiency, time spent documenting is nonreimbursable. Thus, the emphasis in medical record entries is on brevity, clarity, and accuracy.

---

[*]https://www.apta.org/siteassets/pdfs/policies/guidelines-documentation-patient-client-management.pdf

▶ *Brevity:* the clinician must learn to use concise sentences while adhering to the clinical facility's style. Facility-recognized abbreviations can be used to aid in brevity (see Medical Abbreviations and Terminology).

▶ *Clarity:* the clinician must learn to write legibly and in a style that clarifies the documentation's meaning. Facility-recognized abbreviations can be used to aid in clarity.

▶ *Accuracy:* the medical record is a permanent, legal document, and so the information contained within it must be accurate and factual. There should be no blank or empty lines between one entry and another. If an error is made, a felt marker, correction fluid, or tape should not be used. Instead, the clinician should put a line through the error (making certain that the deleted material remains legible), write the date, and place his or her initials above the error. Also, in the margin, the clinician should state why the correction is necessary. Black ink should be used for all corrections and entries. There are currently many software programs available for EHR specific to rehabilitation that can indicate when an entry has been altered and identify the person responsible for the entry. Any corrections within an EHR typically require the completion of an addendum.

CLINICAL PEARL

The use of punctuation within a clinical facility varies, and the following are just guidelines:

▶ Hyphens (-) should be used with care because of their confusion with the minus sign.

▶ The colon (:) can often be used instead of "is." For example, "shoulder abduction: 0–110°."

▶ The semicolon (;) can often be used to connect two related statements. For example, "able to sleep on the stomach; pain not felt during the night."

On occasion, a physician may give a verbal order. In such instances, the clinician documents the order's date and time and the order's details—the abbreviation *v.o.* is typically used, followed by the physician's name and the clinician's signature.

Every entry into the medical record must be signed using a legal signature followed by the initials that indicate the clinician's status as a PT or PTA. The professional designator to be used after the therapist's signature is currently under debate. In the 1970s and 1980s, RPT (Registered Physical Therapist) or LPT (Licensed Physical Therapist) were used. It was then decided in the 1980s and early 1990s to use PT—a physical therapist could not practice without being licensed or registered, so using "R" or "L" was redundant. There is currently a debate about whether to change the designator to DPT, although the same redundancy argument could be used for the letter "D." The need for different types of notes to be cosigned by the supervising PT varies from state to state.

The PTA must remember that documentation is not just a formality or a time-consuming activity. Documentation can provide information about a patient's progress or lack of progress toward the assigned goals. This measurement of progress is referred to as outcome measurement and is becoming increasingly important for third-party payers. It is also important as a means of assessing how successful the current interventions are and can help in the clinical decision-making process (see Chapter 3).

PATIENT REFUSAL

Every patient has the right to refuse treatment for any reason. Such a situation can place the PTA in an awkward position. Sometimes the refusal is a one-off because the patient is going through a difficult time or the scheduled time is not convenient, so the PTA must try to determine a reason for the refusal and whether the refusal is for the current session or includes any future treatment sessions. The PTA must also try to explain the benefits of the treatments to the patient and the potential consequences of not receiving the treatment. If the patient still refuses the treatment, the PTA must document the refusal and the reason for the refusal in the patient's medical record and notify the supervising PT.

INCIDENT/OCCURRENCE REPORTING

Incident/occurrence reporting is the process of documenting all injuries, illnesses, accidents, damage to equipment, and any near misses that could have resulted in injury, death, or property damage. The purpose of incident/occurrence reporting is for the risk management department to understand the underlying/contributing conditions that led to, or contributed to, the occurrence of a safety incident; identify appropriate corrective actions that must be taken to address these underlying/contributing conditions here, and implement timely and effective corrective actions. In most institutions, there is a time within which the incident report must be submitted (usually 24 hours to 3 days following the incident). An incident/occurrence report typically contains the following information:

▶ The name or description of the incident/occurrence. Attention should be paid to making the report simple, clear, and inclusive.

▶ Time and date of incident/occurrence.

▶ First and last names and titles of persons involved, if appropriate. If the patient is involved, an additional form of identification is needed (medical record number, date of birth, address, admission date, etc).

▶ A brief description of the incident/occurrence location.

▶ A brief factual description of the actual incident. A simple, chronological narrative that does not express an opinion as to the cause works best. All of the information provided must have been witnessed firsthand by the reporter.

▶ A description of the circumstances surrounding the incident and the condition of the involved individual following the incident.

▶ Information about any steps that were taken after the incident in terms of whether treatment was received by the involved individual and/or where the individual was transported to.

▶ What is being done and/or will be done to prevent a recurrence.

▶ Other departments involved or to become involved in the incident (emergency services, physician, etc), as appropriate.

▶ The name and title of the person submitting the report. The PTA must notify the supervising PT of the incident and supply the completed report to the PT. No discussion about the incident should take place with the patient or any uninvolved personnel.

The incident report, which is considered confidential and administrative, is not considered part of the medical record and is therefore filed in a separate location. Also, in most instances, even though the incident is documented in the patient's medical record, no mention is made about the completion of an incident report.

MEDICAL ABBREVIATIONS AND TERMINOLOGY

To read and understand a medical record, the clinician must be familiar with the abbreviations and medical terminology commonly used. Many of the terms are derived from Greek or Latin words. A medical term is a word or phrase made up of elements to express a specific idea:

▶ *Root element*: the main subject or topic of a medical term, commonly a body part. For example, *osteo-* (bone).

▶ *Prefix element*: used at the beginning of a medical term to change the medical term's meaning or make it more specific. For example, *hemi-* (half).

▶ *Suffix element*: used at the end of a medical term to describe a body part's condition or an action to a body part. For example, *porosis* (a porous condition), as of the bones—osteoporosis.

▶ Examples of these elements of medical terminology are provided in Table 4-1.

TABLE 4-1   **Commonly Used Abbreviations**

A	Assessment	CBC	Complete blood count
AAA	Abdominal aortic aneurysm	CC	Chief complaint
A&O	Alert and oriented	CF	Cystic fibrosis
AAROM	Active assisted range of motion	CGA	Contact guard assist
abd	Abduction	CHF	Congestive heart failure
ABG	Arterial blood gases	CHI	Closed head injury
ACL	Anterior cruciate ligament	c/o	Complains of
add	Adduction	CNA	Certified nursing assistant
ADL	Activities of daily living	CNS	Central nervous system
Ad lib	At discretion	CO	Cardiac output
AE	Above elbow	COPD	Chronic obstructive pulmonary disease
A.fib	Atrial fibrillation	CP	Cerebral palsy
AFO	Ankle foot orthosis	CPM	Continuous passive motion
AIDS	Acquired immunodeficiency syndrome	CR	Contract-relax
AIIS	Anterior inferior iliac spine	CRF	Chronic renal failure
AK	Above knee	CTLSO	Cervical-thoracic-lumbar-sacral orthosis
ALS	Amyotrophic lateral sclerosis	CTR	Carpal tunnel release
amb	Ambulation	CXR	Chest X-ray
AMA	Against medical advice	DDD	Degenerative disk disease
ANS	Autonomic nervous system	DF	Dorsiflexion
A-P (AP)	Anterior-posterior	DJD	Degenerative joint disease
ARF	Acute renal failure	DOB	Date of birth
AROM	Active range of motion	DOE	Dyspnea on exertion
ASAP	As soon as possible	DTR	Deep tendon reflex
A-V	Arteriovenous	DVT	Deep venous thrombosis
AVM	Arteriovenous malformation	Dx	Diagnosis
Bid (BID)	Twice a day	d/c (D/C)	Discontinued or discharged
BK	Below knee	DIP	Distal interphalangeal
b/l	Bilateral	EENT	Ear, eyes, nose, throat
BMI	Body mass index	EOB	Edge of bed
BOS	Base of support	E-stim	Electrical stimulation
BP	Blood pressure	EMG	Electromyogram
bpm	Beats per minute	ER	External rotation or emergency room
BR	Bed rest	$\bar{x}$	Except
CA	Cancer	ex	Exercise
CABG	Coronary artery bypass graft	ext	Extension
CAD	Coronary artery disease	Ft	Feet

(continued)

TABLE 4-1   Commonly Used Abbreviations (continued)

FUO	Fever, unknown origin	LP	Lumbar puncture
Flex	Flexion	Lt	Left
Fx	Fracture	LTG	Long-term goal
FWW	Front wheeled walker	MCL	Medial collateral ligament
FWB	Full weight-bearing	MCP	Metacarpophalangeal
FES	Functional electrical stimulation	MI	Myocardial infarction
GB	Gallbladder	MMT	Manual muscle test
GCS	Glasgow Coma Scale	MVA	Motor vehicle accident
GI	Gastrointestinal	N/A	Not applicable
GSW	Gunshot wound	NAD	No apparent distress/No abnormality detected
GTT	Glucose tolerance test	N&V	Nausea and vomiting
HB	Heart block	NIDDM	Noninsulin-dependent diabetes mellitus
HEP	Home exercise program	NKA	No known allergies
HNP	Herniated nucleus pulposus	NVD	Nausea, vomiting, and diarrhea
HOB	Head of bed	NWB	Nonweight-bearing
HP	Hot pack	OA	Osteoarthritis
HR	Heart rate or hold-relax	OOB	Out of bed
HTN	Hypertension	OP	Outpatient
HVD	Hypertensive vascular disease	OR	Operating room
Hx	History	ORIF	Open reduction and internal fixation
IADL	Instrumental activities of daily living	OT (OTR)	Occupational therapy
ICU	Intensive care unit	PCL	Posterior cruciate ligament
IDDM	Insulin-dependent diabetes mellitus	PEEP	Positive end expiratory pressure
IND	Independent	PF	Plantarflexion
IPPB	Intermittent positive pressure breathing	PIP	Proximal interphalangeal
IR	Internal rotation	PMH	Past medical history
IV	Intravenous	PNF	Proprioceptive neuromuscular facilitation
JRA	Juvenile rheumatoid arthritis	PO	By mouth, orally (from the Latin *per os*, meaning by mouth)
Jt	Joint	Post-op	Postoperative
KAFO	Knee-ankle-foot orthosis	PRE	Progressive resistive exercises
LBP	Low back pain	PRN	As needed
LCL	Lateral collateral ligament	PROM	Passive range of motion
LE	Lower extremity	PSH	Past surgical history
LMN	Lower motor neuron	PWB	Partial weight-bearing
LOB	Loss of balance	q	Every
LOC	Loss of consciousness	qd	Every day
LOS	Length of stay	qh	Every hour

TABLE 4-1   Commonly Used Abbreviations (continued)

qid	Four times a day	THA	Total hip arthroplasty
qn	Every night	TID/Tid	Three times a day
RA	Rheumatoid arthritis	TKA	Total knee arthroplasty
RD	Respiratory distress	TKE	Terminal knee extension
reps	Repetitions	TMJ	Temporomandibular joint
r/o	Rule out	TO	Telephone order
ROM	Range of motion	TPR	Temperature, pulse, and respiration
Rt	Right	TTWB	Toe-touch weight-bearing
RTC	Rotator cuff	Tx	Traction
Rx	Treatment, prescription	UE	Upper extremity
SCI	Spinal cord injury	US	Ultrasound
$\bar{s}$	Without (From the Latin *sine* meaning without)	UTI	Urinary tract infection
SLR	Straight leg raise	VC	Vital capacity
SLS	Single-leg stance	VO/v.o.	Verbal order
SOB	Shortness of breath	VS	Vital signs
SPV	Systolic pressure variation	WB	Weight-bearing
STG	Short-term goal	WBAT	Weight-bearing as tolerated
SVP	Small volume parenteral	$\bar{c}$	With (From the Latin *cum* meaning with)
TAH	Total abdominal hysterectomy	WFL	Within functional limits
TB	Tuberculosis	WNL	Within normal limits
TBI	Traumatic brain injury	W/O	Without
TDWB	Touchdown weight-bearing	y/o	Year(s) old
TENS	Transcutaneous electrical nerve stimulation		

REFERENCES

1. American Physical Therapy Association. *Guide to Physical Therapist Practice. 3.0.* Alexandria, VA: American Physical Therapy Association; 2014.
2. Kettenbach G. Background information. In: Kettenbach G, ed. *Writing SOAP Notes with Patient/Client Management Formats*, 3rd ed. Philadelphia: FA Davis; 2004:1-5.
3. Schenkman M, Deutsch JE, Gill-Body KM. An integrated framework for decision making in neurologic physical therapist practice. *Phys Ther.* 2006;86:1681-1702.

CHAPTER 5

Preparation for Patient Care

CHAPTER OBJECTIVES

At the completion of this chapter, the reader will be able to:

1. Discuss the differences between values and beliefs

2. List some of the most common negative biases of healthcare workers

3. Provide some examples of nonverbal communication

4. Define *empathy*

5. Discuss the importance of health equity and cultural competency among healthcare providers

6. Describe what health disparity is

7. List the five steps to achieving cultural competence

8. Discuss the importance of infection control in healthcare

9. Describe some of the microorganisms that can be encountered in healthcare and their various modes of transmission

10. List some of the precautions that must be used with special populations

OVERVIEW

Patient care is a partnership between a patient and the clinician—it is something a clinician does *with* a patient, not *to* a patient. The primary focus of patient care is to enhance a patient's function through positive interactions, with each interaction having an objective. In some cases, this involves helping a patient to regain former skills, whereas in other cases, it may involve teaching a patient ways to compensate for the loss of a physical or mental attribute. Generally speaking, most interventions aim to increase either a patient's mobility or a patient's stability. Determining the focus or objective requires clinical decision making (see Chapter 3) and preparation.

CLINICAL PEARL

Essential for patient care preparation is the knowledge of several general principles, so that patient and clinician safety is ensured. For example, having to leave a patient unguarded to retrieve a piece of equipment must be avoided at all times. All equipment is required to be inspected before use. Suppose a piece of equipment is found to be malfunctioning. In that case, correct procedures must be followed: labeling the piece of equipment as defective and reporting the defect to the appropriate personnel, such as the clinical engineering department.

THE HEALTHCARE TEAM

Often, a healthcare team, made up of many different professions, plays a role in reviewing a patient's condition and making decisions (see Chapter 1). This patient-centered interprofessional collaboration, which is more common outside the outpatient work areas, enhances problem-solving and care coordination. In most cases, team conferences involving members from each discipline (nursing, social services, etc.) are held on the patient's behalf. In addition to these discussion meetings, it is not unusual for fellow professionals to cotreat a patient. For example, a patient who has undergone hip replacement is often cotreated by physical therapy and occupational therapy. The advantage of cotreatment is that it reduces duplication of treatments, enhances input from different professionals, and often results in interventions for complex problems that exceed what an individual profession could accomplish. Another example of cotreatment occurs when a physical therapist (PT) and a physical therapist assistant (PTA) work together with the same patient. The PT examines the patient, provides a plan of care (POC), establishes the goals or desired outcomes, and determines the therapeutic interventions to be used. The PTA performs the treatment activities for which he or she is qualified and frequently communicates, both orally and in writing, with the supervising PT, who evaluates the results of the treatment and the patient's responses to it so that alterations or adjustments to the POC can be made as necessary.

INITIAL PREPARATION

A significant component of the clinician-patient interaction occurs before the clinician ever comes into contact with the patient. Before starting any procedure, the clinician must prepare for the steps ahead, both mentally and physically. For example, the treatment area must be organized with safety in mind and for efficient use. Preparation of the treatment area may include removing any obstacles, adjusting the height of the treatment table, or checking the availability of a particular piece of equipment. Enough room must be allowed for unimpeded movement. Before meeting the patient, the clinician should perform a comprehensive review of the patient's medical record or chart, including all of the following:

▸ Diagnosis or reason for admittance

▸ Past medical history

▸ Past surgical history

▸ Current history and physical findings

▸ Imaging test results, as appropriate

▸ Laboratory test results, as appropriate

▸ Prescribed medications

▸ Contents of the POC

▸ Confirmation that orders for physical therapy are current

After the chart review, the clinician enters the patient's room, performs a personal introduction, and then reminds the patient why physical therapy has been ordered. This can include the treatment goals, the desired outcomes, and a review of any pertinent precautions (eg, physician-ordered restrictions of motion). The patient should be asked if they have any questions before the clinician proceeds.

Listening with empathy involves understanding the ideas being communicated and the emotion behind the ideas. In essence, empathy acknowledges the other person's viewpoint so that a deep and true understanding of what the person is experiencing can be obtained. The term *patient-centered* refers to an interviewing technique that provides a method to understand better the environment in which the patient resides, their worldview, and the unique conditions that affect their health. It is an approach that requires the clinician to become familiar with the personality beneath the presenting problem. The interview style should be altered from patient to patient, as understanding and answering ability vary between each individual. In general, the interview should flow as an active conversation, not as a question-and-answer session. The following points are recommended to make the interview process as effective as possible:

▸ Eliminate physical barriers, such as desks and tables—the clinician and patient should be at a similar eye level, facing each other, with a comfortable space between them (approximately 3 feet) (Figure 5-1) so that the patient feels the clinician is interested and paying attention. Compare

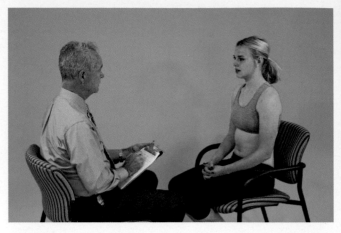

FIGURE 5-1 Clinician-patient interaction. (Reproduced with permission from Dutton M: Introduction to Physical Therapy and Patient Skills, 2nd ed. New York, NY: McGraw Hill; 2014.)

Figure 5-1 with Figure 5-2 and note the contrasting body language and degree of attention afforded to the patient.

▸ Make *content* and *process* observations. This skill involves not focusing solely on the content of what is being said but being able to read the nonverbal cues and gestures made by the patient. For example, the patient may say, "Everything is fine" (content) while fidgeting with his or her hands (process), to which the clinician might respond, "But you do seem a little nervous today." Thus, process observation is about "stating, not rating" behaviors and using the observations as a springboard for inquiry and discussion.

▸ Use active and nonjudgmental listening. The clinician should ask questions that demonstrate that he or she has been listening to the patient by reflecting the patient's feelings. For example, stating, "You seem worried or anxious about this," demonstrates to the patient that the clinician has some insight into the emotional overtones behind the words being spoken.

▸ Demonstrate a caring approach by conveying concern and support through both verbal responses and body language. Methods include maintaining eye contact, nodding at appropriate times, not moving around or being

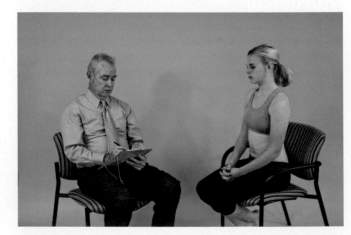

FIGURE 5-2 Clinician-patient interaction with incorrect posture and positioning. (Reproduced with permission from Dutton M: Introduction to Physical Therapy and Patient Skills, 2nd ed. New York, NY: McGraw Hill; 2014.)

distracted, using encouraging verbalizations, mirroring body postures and language, and leaning forward.

A transfer of accurate information must occur between the patient and the clinician. A successful learning process requires the clinician to have patience, focus, and self-criticism.[1]

The clinician should provide the patient with encouraging responses, such as a nod of the head. Leading questions such as "Does it hurt more when you walk?" should be avoided. A more neutral question would be, "What activities make your symptoms worse?"

APPEARANCE

During each encounter, the patient is consciously or subconsciously making an opinion about the clinic environment, including cleanliness, and the entire clinical staff from the receptionist to all team members. These observations continue throughout each session irrespective of whether a staff member interacts directly with the patient or communicates with another patient or staff member. Thus, the clinician's appearance should always convey an air of professionalism (Figure 5-1). Professionalism is not restricted to the conduct, aims, or qualities while in the clinic but should be a way of life. In addition to appearance, it is important to project such qualities as a polite and well-spoken demeanor, reliability, competence, etiquette, accountability, and ethical behavior. The development of professionalism begins as a student.

Most institutions have a dress code in addition to a mandatory name tag that should be adhered to. The dress code is designed to project a professional image to patients or other members of the healthcare team and typically includes instructions on how:

▶ To prevent overexposure of the clinician's body. For example, most clinics do not allow the staff to wear clothing that exposes their midriff or armpits, and some clinics have strict guidelines for the number and location of

exposed piercings and tattoos, hair color, and the use of nail polish.

▶ To prevent injury to a patient or staff member from jewelry such as dangling earrings, necklaces, or bracelets.

▶ To prevent infection. For example, while wearing a simple finger band and unchipped nail polish may be acceptable, removing all finger and wrist jewelry and wearing no nail polish may be the safest option to prevent infection transmission in most healthcare settings.[2]

COMMUNICATION

Based on the APTA's Section on Administration (SOA) that published the Leadership, Administration, and Management Preparation (LAMP) document in early 1999 (see Chapter 1),[3] a Delphi study by Lopopolo and colleagues[4] concluded that the top 5 LAMP skills in order of importance were communication, professional involvement and ethical practice, delegation/supervision, stress management, and reimbursement sources.

Thus, much about becoming a clinician relates to effectively communicating with the patient, the patient's family, and the other healthcare team members. Communication between the clinician and the patient, which involves interacting with the patient using terms they can understand, begins when the clinician first meets the patient and continues throughout any future sessions. One of the aims of any interaction is to create an efficient and effective exchange and develop a rapport between the clinician and the patient.

Patient-clinician interactions can occur in several environments, including hospital rooms, outpatient clinics, and the home, and at many levels. Given the melting-pot society that we now live in, patients are likely to come from diverse cultural and ethnic backgrounds, influenced by individual factors related to the psychological and socioeconomic conditions that affect health, behavioral practices, and access to care.

A patient's ability to communicate depends largely on the setting, their background, and their medical status. For example, some patients have cognitive, visual, or hearing deficits, do not speak English, or cannot verbalize effectively. In extreme cases, the patient may have difficulty due to poor levels of arousal or attention.

It is important to remember that listening is often more critical than speaking. Even when performing a dependent mobility task, the clinician can engage the patient both physically and cognitively to some degree.

Attention to nonverbal cues, including gestures, touch, and distance between speakers, is especially important because they are often performed subconsciously and misinterpreted. Examples of such nonverbal cues include:

▶ *Facial expression.* The facial expression should be one of interest and concern.

▶ *Voice volume.* The voice volume should be at a level that is sufficient for the patient to hear. Avoid speaking loudly when possible, especially to those who are hard of hearing.

▶ *Posture.* An upright and attentive posture is preferable (see Figure 5-1).

▶ *Touch.* Based on respect of the patient's cultural preferences and personal boundaries, the clinician should use a confident and firm touch.

▶ *Gestures.* Gestures should be limited to those describing a particular activity.

▶ *Physical closeness.* Comfort with physical closeness varies according to culture. In the United States, a distance of 18 inches to 4 feet is considered normal for a professional distance.

▶ *Eye contact.* Maintaining eye contact enhances trust and demonstrates attentiveness (see Figure 5-1).

▶ *Eye level.* Whenever possible, the clinician should alter his or her position so that the patient and clinician's eye level is the same. For example, if the patient is sitting, the clinician should assume a sitting position (see Figure 5-1).

CLINICAL PEARL

Learn to be a good listener by:

▶ Looking at the person who is talking and give him or her your full attention

▶ Making appropriate eye contact

▶ Showing understanding by summarizing and asking for confirmation

▶ Letting the speaker finish the point they were making

▶ Showing interest

▶ Being respectful

CLINICAL PEARL

A patient's privacy and dignity should be maintained at all times. Privacy includes the patient's personal space. Whenever appropriate, the clinician should ask the patient's permission before carrying out an action (moving the patient's belongings off the bedside table, sitting down, etc).

Given the nature of the physical therapy profession, PTAs frequently interact with people with disabilities. When writing or speaking about people with disabilities, it is important to put the person first. Group designations such as "the blind" or "the disabled" are inappropriate because they do not reflect the individuality, equality, or dignity of people with disabilities. Similarly, words such as "normal person" imply that the person with a disability is not normal, whereas "person without a disability" is descriptive but not negative. Etiquette that is considered appropriate when interacting with people with disabilities is based primarily on respect and courtesy. Outlined next are tips to help when communicating with persons with disabilities, provided by the Office of Disability Employment Policy; the Media Project, Research and Training Center on Independent Living, University of Kansas, Lawrence, KS; and the National Center for Access Unlimited, Chicago, IL.

General Tips

When introduced to a person with a disability, it is appropriate to offer to shake hands. People with limited hand use or who wear an artificial limb can usually shake hands (shaking hands with the left hand is an acceptable greeting). If you offer assistance to a person with a disability, wait until the offer is accepted, then listen to, or ask for, any instructions. Address people who have disabilities by their first names only when extending the same familiarity to all others.

Communicating with Individuals Who Are Blind or Visually Impaired

The clinician should speak to the individual when approaching him or her and speak in a normal tone of voice. When conversing in a group, remember to identify yourself and the person to whom you are speaking. The clinician should not attempt to lead the individual without first asking; allow the person to hold your arm and control her or his movements. Direct action should be given using descriptive words, giving the person verbal information that is visually obvious to individuals who can see. For example, if you are approaching a series of steps, mention how many steps there are. If you are offering a seat, gently place the individual's hand on the chair's back or arm so that the person can locate the seat. At the end of the session, the clinician should tell the individual that they are leaving.

Communicating with Individuals Who Are Deaf or Hard of Hearing

The clinician should gain the patient's attention before starting a conversation (eg, tap the person gently on the shoulder or arm), and then look directly at the individual, face the light, speak clearly, in a normal tone of voice, and keep the hands from obstructing the mouth. Short, simple sentences should be used. If the patient uses a sign language interpreter, the clinician should speak directly to the person, not the interpreter. If the clinician places a phone call, he or she should let the phone ring longer than usual. If a Text Telephone (TTY) is not available, the clinician should dial 711 to reach the national telecommunications relay service, which will facilitate the call.

Communicating with Individuals with Mobility Impairments

Whenever possible, the clinician should position themselves at the wheelchair user's eye level without leaning on the wheelchair or any other assistive device. Never patronize people who use wheelchairs by patting them on the head or shoulder. Do not assume that an individual wants to be pushed—ask first.

Communicating with Individuals with Speech Impairments

If the clinician does not understand something the patient said, they should not pretend that they did. Instead, they should ask the individual to repeat what was said and then repeat it back. To help the patient, the clinician should try to ask questions that require only short answers or a nod of the head. The clinician should not speak for the individual or attempt to finish her or his sentences. If the clinician is having difficulty understanding the individual, writing should be considered an alternative means of communicating, but only after asking the individual if it is acceptable.

Communicating with Individuals with Cognitive Disabilities

Whenever possible, the clinician and patient should communicate in a quiet or private location, and the clinician should be prepared to repeat what is said, orally or in writing. The clinician must be patient, flexible, and supportive. The clinician should wait for the individual to accept an offer of assistance; do not "over-assist" or be patronizing.

At the end of the first visit, and at subsequent visits, the clinician should ask if there are any questions. Each session should have closure, which may include a handshake, if appropriate.

SOCIAL NETWORKING IN THE WORKPLACE

Social media is everywhere, including the workplace, and while it can serve as a free promotional tool for an organization, the lines between personal and professional use have become increasingly blurred, introducing the need to regulate these communications. For example, the APTA's House of Delegates has developed standards of conduct in the use of social media for PTs, PTAs, and physical therapy students.* Based on these standards and others, the clinician should adhere to the following recommendations:

▶ Strictly adhere to the company's social media policy and regulations and what is and is not permitted.

▶ Be professional and accurate in any communications.

▶ Avoid interacting with patients and supervisors on social media. Such familiarity may create not only awkward situations but also the potential for liability.

▶ Avoid creating separate personal and professional social media profiles.

▶ Do not misrepresent the APTA, other organizations, educational institutions, clinical sites, or employers.

▶ Avoid posting comments or photos on an account that identify you as an employee of a company.

▶ Do not post any confidential information, trade secrets, or customer data that is not public knowledge.

▶ Demonstrate appropriate conduct per the Standards of Ethical Conduct for the Physical Therapist Assistant.

▶ Do not engage in social media (Facebook, Twitter, Instagram, etc.) while at work. Many employers block any access to unnecessary sites from computers.

VALUES AND BELIEFS

Every individual has an internalized system of values and beliefs that they have developed throughout life. Consciously or otherwise, a clinician brings a set of values and beliefs to every patient interaction. Values and beliefs guide actions and behavior and help to form attitudes toward different things and situations. Prior experiences have honed these values and beliefs.

▶ *Values.* Values are characteristics that are deemed important to an individual. Examples include honesty, effort, perseverance, and loyalty. Numerous studies have demonstrated that both conscious and unconscious values can have an impact on interactions with others.

▶ *Beliefs.* Beliefs are assumptions that are made based on life's experiences. Examples include religion, gender bias, and racial equality. Belief bias occurs when someone's evaluation of an argument's logical strength is biased by their belief in the truth or falsity of the conclusion. People tend to accept conclusions that fit in with their systems of belief. A bias can be negative or positive. The most common negative biases of healthcare workers involve:

- *Race/ethnicity.* In the United States, patients of racial and ethnic minorities tend to receive healthcare interventions that are inferior to those received by Caucasian patients even when income and insurance levels are similar.

- *Gender.* Research is commonly conducted on male subjects, and the conclusions from this research have been generalized and applied to women without consideration of structural or biochemical differences.

- *Ageism.* Older patients are often considered senile, hard of hearing, frail, lonely, and incapable of learning new things.

- *Obesity.* Assumptions are made that this population is lazy, lacking in self-discipline and motivation, and ugly, and that they have brought their weight problems on themselves.

*https://www.apta.org/uploadedFiles/APTAorg/About_Us/Policies/Ethics/StandrdsConductSocialMedia.pdf

- *Disability.* Although patients with disabilities are often viewed positively, they are often treated with pity.
- *Substance abuse.* It is a generally held belief that substance abuse is the individual's fault because of a lack of willpower.

As clinicians, we are likely to interact frequently with individuals whose values and cultural practices differ from our own. These differences can result in a judgmental response that will either validate or invalidate those values and cultural practices. It is important that the judgmental response is not critical, biased, or one of disapproval, but that every conscious effort be made to accept differences as long as those differences serve the patients' well-being.

CLINICAL PEARL

The following behaviors are associated with negative beliefs:

- ▶ Avoiding or minimizing patient interactions.
- ▶ Using derogatory terms or nicknames when describing a patient.
- ▶ Ignoring patient requests or needs.
- ▶ Treating a patient without compassion, commitment, or respect.
- ▶ Referring to the patient as a number and not using his or her name.

CULTURAL COMPETENCY

In today's healthcare, a clinician will encounter people of racial, ethnic, and cultural minorities, immigrant and refugee communities, those with disabilities, and lesbian, gay, bisexual, and transgender populations. Also, within these populations can be economically and socially disadvantaged groups. One of the US government's goals is to create health equity and promote cultural competency among healthcare providers to increase positive outcomes for all people.

CLINICAL PEARL

A health disparity is a difference in rates of illness, disease, or conditions among different populations and a difference in these populations' health outcomes. Some of these health disparities result from poverty, acculturation, behavior and lifestyle, nutrition, access to healthcare services, genetic predisposition, education level, discrimination, differing levels of insurance coverage, and differing access to high-quality networks of preventive and primary care.

In 2010, according to the US Census Bureau, about 30% of the nation's population identified themselves as members of racial or ethnic minority groups. By 2050, these groups are expected to account for almost half of the country's population.

It is widely accepted that racial and ethnic minority populations, on average, receive lower levels of care and have higher rates of certain conditions and diseases than Caucasians. It has also become clear that the economic and social conditions under which people live can affect their health and well-being. The World Health Organization (WHO) recently published a final report and recommendations for creating health equity through action on the social determinants of health (http://www.who.int/social_determinants/en).

A precise definition of *culture* has been widely debated and broadly described, with certain common characteristics, including an integrated pattern of learned beliefs and behaviors that can be shared among groups. Included in the pattern are thoughts, communication styles, ways of interacting, views on roles and relationships, values, practices, and customs. In essence, culture serves to help individuals to shape and explain their values and to provide meaning. Different cultures are too often considered "exotic" or about "other people" and have been associated with socioeconomic status, religion, gender, and sexual orientation.

CLINICAL PEARL

A cultural continuum of five points has been designed that ranges from cultural proficiency to cultural destructiveness with various possibilities between these two extremes.[5-8] The continuum indicates how people see and respond to difference:

- ▶ Cultural Destructiveness. The most negative end of the continuum, represented by attitudes, approaches, and practices that are destructive to cultures.
- ▶ Cultural Incapacity. Unintentionally destructive, but lack the capacity to help minorities.
- ▶ Cultural Blindness. Well-intentioned, but too ethnocentric.
- ▶ Cultural Pre-competence. Characterized by appropriate responses of acceptance and respect for difference.
- ▶ Cultural Competence and Proficiency. Holds culture in high esteem. Conducts research and develops new therapeutic approaches based on culture.

Cultural competency can be viewed as a set of congruent behaviors, attitudes, and policies that blend to form effective interactions within a cross-cultural framework. To be culturally competent, an individual must be aware of, respect, and accept different cultures and resist the temptation to make assumptions about people and situations.

CLINICAL PEARL

The five steps to achieving cultural competence include:

- ▶ Awareness
- ▶ Acknowledgment
- ▶ Validation
- ▶ Negotiation
- ▶ Accomplishment

Examples of how culture can affect healthcare include differences in languages and nonverbal communication patterns; cultural differences in the perception of illness, disease, medical roles and responsibilities; and cultural preferences to treat illnesses. Overcoming these barriers requires the cooperation of the patient, the organization, and the clinician.

CLINICAL PEARL

Ways to improve interpersonal communication with culturally diverse patients or those with limited English proficiency or low health literacy include:

1. Slowing down the rate of speaking, rather than speaking loudly.
2. Using or drawing pictures.
3. Limiting the amount of information provided and using simple, nonmedical language.
4. Using the "teach-back" or "show-me" technique.

Wherever possible, questions should be asked to help patients and families from culturally diverse backgrounds. Such questions can include:

► Can you tell me the languages that you understand and speak?
► Do you use any traditional health remedies to improve your health?
► In addition to yourself, is there someone with whom you want us to discuss your medical condition?
► Are there certain healthcare procedures and tests that your culture prohibits?
► Are there any situations where you would prefer to be treated by a clinician of a specific gender?

To minimize the difficulty encountered by patients with limited or no English proficiency, system-wide procedures or resources can be put in place. Resources to support this capacity may include:

► Trained interpreters
► Bilingual/bicultural or multilingual/multicultural staff
► Materials developed for specific cultural, ethnic, and linguistic groups, including culturally and linguistically appropriate signage

The National Standards on Culturally and Linguistically Appropriate Services (CLAS) (http://clas.uiuc.edu/) are directed at healthcare organizations. The 14 CLAS standards are organized by themes: culturally competent care, language access services, and organizational supports for cultural competency.

PATIENT RELATED INSTRUCTION

Patient/family/client-related instruction forms the cornerstone of every physical therapy session. During the physical therapy visits, the clinician and the patient work to alter the patient's perception of their functional capabilities. Together, the patient and clinician discuss the parts of the patient's life that they can and cannot control and then consider how to improve those parts that can be changed. The clinician must spend time educating the patient about his or her condition so that they can fully understand the importance of their role in the rehabilitation process and become an educated consumer. Educating the patient about strategies to adopt to prevent recurrences and self-manage their condition is also very important. Discussions about intervention goals must continue throughout the rehabilitative process and must be mutually acceptable.

Often, the physician relies on physical therapy to give a broader explanation about the condition and to answer questions and concerns related to the rehabilitative process. Patient education aims to create independence, not dependence, and foster an atmosphere of learning in the clinic. A detailed explanation should be given to the patient in a language that he or she can understand. This explanation should include:

► The name of the structure(s) involved and the cause of the problem. Whenever possible, an illustration of the offending structure should be shown to the patient. Anatomic models can be used to explain biomechanical principles in layperson's terms.

► Information about any interventions that are planned.

► The estimated prognosis of the problem and a discussion about the patient's functional goals. An estimation of the healing time is useful for the patient to not become frustrated at a perceived lack of progress.

► What the patient is permitted to do to help themselves, including the correct use of the involved joint or area and a brief description about the relevant stage of healing. This information makes the patient aware and more cautious when performing activities of daily living (ADLs), recreational activities, and the home exercise program. Emphasis should be placed on dispelling the myth of "no pain, no gain," and patients should be encouraged to respect pain. Patients often have misconceptions about when to use heat and ice, and it is the clinician's role to clarify such issues.

► Home exercise program. Before prescribing a home exercise program, the clinician should consider the time needed to perform the program. Also, the level of tolerance and motivation for exercise varies among individuals and is based on their diagnosis and healing stage. A short series of exercises performed more frequently during the day should be prescribed for patients with poor endurance or when the emphasis is on functional reeducation. Longer programs performed less frequently are aimed at building strength or endurance. Each home exercise program needs to be individualized to meet the patient's specific needs.

There are probably as many ways to teach as there are to learn. The clinician needs to be aware that people may have very different preferences for how, when, where, and how often to learn. Patient adherence and compliance are vitally important in the healing process. Whereas *compliance* can be defined as engaging in a behavior as instructed or prescribed,[9] *adherence* can be defined as choosing to engage in behaviors. The latter term has gained more acceptance because it indicates a more proactive approach from the patient.

Both compliance and adherence are related to motivation. Anecdotally, unmotivated patients may progress more slowly. Much literature has conceptualized or reported poor motivation in rehabilitation as secondary to patient-related factors, including depression, apathy, cognitive impairment, low self-efficacy (eg, low confidence in one's ability to rehabilitate successfully), fatigue, and personality factors.[10] Therefore, when implementing the POC, the clinician must consider the patient's stage of learning, the best approach in terms of the structure of the tasks, the type of practice to be used, and the type of feedback given. Litzinger and Osif[11] organized individuals into four main types of learners, based on instructional strategies:

1. *Accommodators.* This type looks for the significance of the learning experience. These learners enjoy being active participants in their learning and will ask many questions, such as, "What if?" and "Why not?"

2. *Divergers.* This type is motivated to discover a given situation's relevance and prefers to have information presented in a detailed, systematic, and reasoned manner.

3. *Assimilators.* This type is motivated to answer the question, "What is there to know?" These learners like accurate, organized delivery of information, and they tend to respect the expert's knowledge. They are perhaps less instructor-intensive than some other types of learners and will carefully follow prescribed exercises, provided a resource person is available and able to answer questions.

4. *Convergers.* This type is motivated to discover the relevancy, or "how," of a situation. The instructions given to this type of learner should be interactive, not passive.

Another way of classifying learners incorporates three common learning styles:

1. *Visual.* As the name suggests, the visual learner assimilates information by observation, using visual cues and information such as pictures, anatomic models, and physical demonstrations. Written materials can be used to provide detailed information but are made more user-friendly with diagrams and illustrations.

2. *Auditory.* Auditory learners prefer to learn by having things explained to them verbally. When providing verbal instructions, it is important to choose the vocabulary that is appropriate for the patient. The use of layman's terms is often preferable to using medical vocabulary.

3. *Tactile.* Tactile learners, who learn through touch and interaction, are the most difficult of the three groups to teach. Close supervision is required with this group until they have demonstrated to the clinician that they can perform the exercises correctly and independently. PNF techniques, with their emphasis on physical and tactile cues, often work well with this group.

A patient's learning style can be identified by asking how he or she prefers to learn. For example, some patients will prefer a simple handout with pictures and instructions; others will prefer to see the exercises demonstrated and then have supervision while performing the exercises. Some may want to know why they are doing the exercises, which muscles are involved, why they are doing three sets of a particular exercise, and so on. Others will require less explanation. Whatever method is preferred, the clinician must provide the information at a pace that the patient can digest. The most critical information should be provided first.

PATIENT COMFORT AND SAFETY

The patient's well-being is always the central focus of any interaction or procedure. Treatment tables, mats, or beds should be prepared with linens and pillows before the patient arrives in the treatment area. Additional sheets may be required as pull sheets for transfers or draping. Pillows can be used for patient positioning and/or comfort. Call bells must be within reach of patients in areas where patients will be left unattended. Finally, the clinician should always emphasize cleanliness, particularly hand hygiene (see Infection Control).

INFECTION CONTROL

A major focus of healthcare is the prevention of the spread of infection by fostering a clean environment. The degree of cleanliness required depends on the level of the contamination threat. A pathogen, commonly referred to as a germ, is a microorganism that causes disease in (infects) its host. Some healthcare environments and situations can increase the potential for infection. These infections are responsible for about 20,000 deaths per year in the United States.[12]

CLINICAL PEARL

Nosocomial infections are those that originate or occur in a hospital or hospital-like setting. A healthcare-associated infection (HAI) refers to an infection acquired in any healthcare setting.

Approximately 10% of American hospital patients (about 2 million every year) acquire a clinically significant nosocomial infection.[12] Nosocomial infections are due to several factors occurring in tandem:

▶ A high prevalence of pathogens

▶ A high prevalence of immunocompromised hosts

▶ High potential of the chains of transmission from patient to patient

Although a hospital's purpose is to corral the sick and injured into one place to treat them efficiently, this environment increases the potential for transmitting pathogens from individual to individual via various routes. In addition to the higher likelihood of pathogen transmission, the high prevalence of pathogens provides an environment for the potential evolution of new microorganisms resistant to conventional treatment methods. As a method to counteract the increasing rate of HAIs, Medicare ceased payment for some HAIs beginning October 1, 2008, following provisions in the Medicare Modernization Act of 2003 and implemented a policy on October 1, 2008, that penalized hospitals if a Medicare patient acquired any of several conditions during their inpatient stay, including surgical site infections, urinary tract infections (UTIs), pneumonia, pressure injuries, hip fracture, deep vein thrombosis, and foreign objects left in surgical sites.[13]

Hospitals or hospital-like settings are hosts to several opportunistic microorganisms. An opportunistic microorganism takes advantage of certain opportunities (eg, compromised host) to cause disease. Compromised hosts include:

► Those with broken skin or mucous membranes (wounds)
► The immunocompromised

The most common sites of nosocomial infections are as follows:

► Urinary tract
► Surgical wounds
► Respiratory tract
► Skin (especially after a serious burn)
► Blood (bacteremia)
► Gastrointestinal (GI) tract
► Central nervous system

Infection is the process by which this microorganism establishes a parasitic relationship with its host. The invasion and multiplication of microorganisms produce an immune response and subsequent signs and symptoms.[14]

For an infection to occur, a chain of events that involves several steps must occur in chronological order (Table 5-1). These steps include the infectious agent encountering a reservoir (host), entering a susceptible reservoir, exiting the reservoir, and then being transmitted (by a vehicle) to a new host. Examples of how the infectious agent can exit the reservoir include:

► The nose
► The mouth and throat
► The eyes
► The intestinal tract
► The urinary tract
► Multiple body fluids

TABLE 5-1	The Chain of Infection
Element	**Description**
Pathogen reservoir	A pathogen can be found in food, water, people, and inanimate objects.
	An individual may carry a pathogen without showing any signs or symptoms of the disease. Also, healthcare workers who are sick can put both coworkers and patients at risk and so may be required to wear a face mask.
	A common pathogen reservoir is the nails of the hand, including artificial nails. The CDC recommends keeping natural nail length to less than one-quarter of an inch.
	Visitors can be significant pathogen reservoirs. Good hand hygiene is encouraged and, on occasion, the use of face masks.
Portal of exit	Pathogens can exit their host through bodily excretions and secretions through openings in the skin.
Means of transmission	Pathogens are transmitted primarily by three modes:
	► *Contact* (direct and indirect). Direct-contact transmission involves the physical transfer of pathogens directly from one person to another through physical contact. Indirect transmission occurs when an uninfected person comes into contact with pathogens on a person or object and then passes those pathogens on to another person through physical contact.
	► *Droplet.* This involves large pathogenic particle droplets coming into contact with either the host's conjunctivae or the nose or mouth's mucous membranes, usually through coughing or sneezing.
	► *Airborne.* This involves small pathogenic particle droplets being either inhaled or deposited on a susceptible host.
Mode of entry	The most common entry modes are the nose's mucous membranes, the eyes, and openings in the skin.
Susceptibility	The risk of infection increases based on both the virulence of the pathogen and the host's susceptibility.

Examples of the vehicle of transmission include the following:

- *Air*: droplets of body fluid from a cough or sneeze
- *Indirect contact*: occurs when an uninfected person comes into contact with pathogens on a person or object (eg, clothing, equipment, patient care items, toys)
- *Direct contact*: with another person's skin, body fluids such as blood, semen, and saliva, and eating utensils

Without this transmission, the infection cannot take place. Once the infectious agent has left the host, it must enter another host for the infection to spread. An infectious agent can enter a host through a break in a person's skin barrier, mucous membranes, eyes, mouth, nose, or genitourinary tract.

CLINICAL PEARL

The body has several natural defense mechanisms to prevent the entry of an infectious agent:

- Intact skin is the primary barrier to infection, as it is relatively resistant to the absorption of microorganisms and the loss of many body fluids.
- The respiratory tract is lined with cilia, minute hair-like organelles that function to filter and trap microorganisms and prevent them from entering other areas of the lungs.

Entry into a host does not guarantee that the infection will spread. For that to occur, the host must be susceptible, or the organism must be difficult to destroy. Multidrug-resistant organisms (MDROs) are organisms that have developed resistance to one or more antibiotics. Most healthy individuals are not susceptible to most infections, but those who are sick, at either end of the life span, malnourished, or immunocompromised are at a greater risk.

CLINICAL PEARL

- The majority of microorganisms proliferate best in a dark, warm, moist environment.
- The majority of microorganisms cannot multiply in a cool, dry, light, or extremely cold environment.

Many microorganisms are responsible for infectious diseases, including fungi (yeast and molds), helminths (eg, tapeworms), viruses, bacteria, protozoa, and prions.

- *Fungi.* Certain types of fungi (such as *Candida*) are commonly present on body surfaces or in intestines. Although generally innocuous, these fungi sometimes cause aggressive local infections of the skin and nails, vagina, mouth, or sinuses in immunocompromised individuals—spreading quickly to other organs and often proving fatal.

CLINICAL PEARL

Fungal diseases in humans are called mycoses.

Some fungal infections (for example, blastomycosis and coccidioidomycosis) can have serious outcomes even in otherwise healthy people.

- *Bacteria.* Bacteria are microscopic, single-celled organisms encountered in the environment, on the skin, in the airways, in the mouth, and in the digestive and genitourinary tracts of people and animals.

Bacteria can be classified according to shape (cocci [spherical], bacilli [rod-like], and spirochetes [spiral or helical]), their use of oxygen (aerobes, those that can live and grow in the presence of oxygen, and anaerobes, those that can tolerate only low levels of oxygen such as those found in the intestine or in decaying tissue), or by color after a particular chemical (Gram) stain is applied (the bacteria that stain blue are called gram-positive, whereas those that stain pink are called gram-negative). Gram-positive and gram-negative bacteria differ in the types of infections they produce and the types of antibiotics required to manage them.

- *Gram-positive bacteria.* These bacteria are usually slow to develop antibiotic resistance, but some (eg, *Bacillus anthracis* and *Clostridium botulinum*) can produce toxins that cause serious illness. Disease-causing anaerobes include clostridia, peptococci, and peptostreptococci, the latter two of which are part of the mouth's, upper respiratory tract's, and large intestine's normal bacterial population (flora).

- *Gram-negative bacteria.* These bacteria possess a unique outer membrane rich in molecules called lipopolysaccharides (endotoxins) that make them more resistant to antibiotics than gram-positive bacteria. The lipopolysaccharides can potentially cause high fever and a life-threatening drop in blood pressure. Gram-negative bacteria have a great facility for mutation—the capacity to exchange genetic material (DNA) with other strains of the same species and even with different species.

CLINICAL PEARL

Bacteremia is the presence of viable bacteria in the circulating blood. Most bacteria that enter the bloodstream are rapidly removed by white blood cells. However, if the bacteria become viable, they may establish a focal infection, or the infection may progress to septicemia; the possible sequelae of septicemia include shock, disseminated intravascular coagulation, multiple organ failure, and death.[15]

- *Mycoplasmas.* Mycoplasmas are unusual, self-replicating bacteria that have no cell wall component and very small genomes.[14] For this reason, antibiotics that are active against bacterial cell walls do not affect mycoplasmas.[14]

- *Clostridia.* Clostridia, which normally inhabit the human intestinal tract, soil, and decaying vegetation, are toxin-producing anaerobes that can cause tetanus, botulism, and tissue infections. Clostridia, particularly *Clostridium perfringens*, also infect wounds. Clostridial wound infections, including skin gangrene, muscle gangrene (clostridial myonecrosis), and tetanus, are rather uncommon but may be fatal.

- *Rickettsiae.* Rickettsiae are small, gram-negative, intracellular organisms that cause several diseases, including Rocky Mountain spotted fever and epidemic typhus. Like viruses, rickettsiae require a host for replication and cannot survive independently in the environment. In humans, rickettsiae infect the cells lining the small blood vessels, causing the blood vessels to become inflamed or choked, or bleed into the surrounding tissue. The various types of rickettsial infections produce similar symptoms, including fever, severe headache, a characteristic skin rash, and a general feeling of malaise. As the rickettsial disease progresses, a person typically experiences confusion and severe weakness—often with cough, dyspnea, and sometimes vomiting and diarrhea. In some people, the liver or spleen enlarges, the kidneys fail, and blood pressure falls dangerously low. Death can occur.

Because ticks, mites, fleas, and lice transmit rickettsiae, a report of a bite from one or more of these vectors is a helpful clue—particularly in geographic areas where the rickettsial infection is common.

- *Ehrlichioses.* Ehrlichioses are similar to rickettsiae: they are microorganisms that can live only inside an animal or person's cells. Unlike rickettsiae, however, ehrlichioses inhabit white blood cells (such as granulocytes and monocytes). Ehrlichioses occur in the United States and Europe but are most common in the midwestern, southeastern, and south-central United States. Ehrlichioses are most likely to develop between spring and late fall when ticks are most active.

▶ *Virus.* A virus is a subcellular organism made up only of a ribonucleic acid (RNA) or a deoxyribonucleic acid (DNA) nucleus covered with proteins.[14] Viruses are completely dependent on host cells and cannot replicate unless they invade a host cell and stimulate it to participate in forming additional virus particles.[14] The virus can either kill the cell it enters or alter its function. Some viruses leave their genetic material in the host cell, where it remains dormant for an extended time (latent infection, eg, herpesviruses). Viruses are not susceptible to antibiotics and cannot be destroyed by pharmacologic means.[14] However, antiviral medications can mitigate the course of the viral illness.[14]

Probably the most common viral infections are upper respiratory infections. In small children, viruses also commonly cause croup, laryngitis, bronchiolitis, or bronchitis.

Some viruses (for example, rabies, West Nile virus, and several encephalitis viruses) infect the nervous system. Viral infections may also develop in the skin, sometimes resulting in warts or other blemishes.

▶ *Prions.* Prions are newly discovered proteinaceous, infectious particles consisting of proteins but without nucleic

acids.[14] These particles are transmitted from animals to humans and are characterized by a long, latent interval in the host. Examples include Creutzfeldt-Jakob disease and bovine spongiform encephalopathy or "mad cow disease."[14]

▶ *Parasite.* A parasite is an organism that resides on or inside another organism (the host) and causes harm to the host. Parasitic infections are common in rural parts of Africa, Asia, and Latin America and less prevalent in industrialized countries.

Parasites enter the body through the mouth or skin. Parasites that enter through the mouth are swallowed and can remain in the intestine or burrow through the intestinal wall and invade other organs. Parasites that enter through the skin bore directly through the skin or are introduced through the bites of infected insects (the vector). Some parasites enter through the soles of the feet when a person walks barefoot or through the skin when a person swims or bathes in water where the parasites are present.

The diagnosis of a parasitic infection can be made from samples of blood, tissue, stool, or urine for laboratory analysis.

Some parasites, particularly those that are single-celled, reproduce inside the host. Other parasites have complex life cycles, producing larvae that spend time in the environment or as an insect vector before becoming infective. If egg-laying parasites live in the digestive tract, their eggs may be found in the person's stool when a sample is examined under a microscope. Antibiotics, laxatives, and antacids can substantially reduce the number of parasites, making their detection in a stool sample more difficult.

Food, drink, and water are often contaminated with parasites in areas with poor sanitation and unhygienic practices.

CLINICAL PEARL

▶ *Sanitization:* the cleaning of pathogenic microorganisms from public eating utensils and objects.

▶ *Decontamination:* to remove, inactivate, or abolish blood-borne pathogens (BBPs) on a surface or object to the point where the BBPs are no longer capable of transmitting infectious particles, and the surface or object is rendered safe for handling, use, or disposal.

▶ *Disinfection:* refers to a reduction in the number of viable microorganisms present in a sample. Not all disinfectants are capable of sterilizing. Many disinfectants are used alone or in combinations (eg, hydrogen peroxide) in the healthcare setting. These include alcohols, chlorine and chlorine compounds, formaldehyde, glutaraldehyde, peracetic acid, and quaternary ammonium compounds.

▶ *Sterilization:* any process that abolishes all forms of microbial life, including transmissible agents (eg, fungi, bacteria, or viruses) present on a surface, within a fluid, in medication, or a biological culture medium. The surface of an object is either sterile or nonsterile; there are no gradations in sterility. Sterilization can be accomplished using various methods, including heat, chemicals, physical cleaning, and forced air purification.

Controlling the Transmission of Infection

Contamination refers to any instance when an object, surface, or field comes into contact with anything that is not sterile. The most effective ways of preventing contamination and the spread of infection include effective personal and hand hygiene and effective cleaning and handling techniques.

CLINICAL PEARL

A *fomite* is any inanimate object or substance such as clothing, book, or furniture that is capable of carrying an infectious organism.

The best way of preventing or controlling the transmission of infection is through the use of sterile techniques and an emphasis on cleanliness.

CLINICAL PEARL

Depending on the clinical setting, the PTA may be required to interact with patients who have open wounds, are immunocompromised, or require the use of medical or surgical aseptic techniques.

▶ *Medical asepsis:* any practice that helps to reduce the number and spread of microorganisms. The practice of medical asepsis includes patient isolation in cases of tuberculosis or hepatitis.

▶ *Surgical asepsis:* the complete removal of microorganisms and their spores from the surface of an object. The surgical asepsis procedure begins with cleaning the object in question, using medical asepsis principles, followed by a sterilization process. Although physical therapy departments do not typically use surgical aseptic techniques, they prepare and use sterile fields and gloves, particularly with wound care.

In 1985, the Centers for Disease Control and Prevention (CDC) introduced Universal Precautions to protect healthcare workers and reduce disease transmission.

The CDC has since revised its previous information and currently recommends using Standard Precautions by healthcare workers when they have contact with any patient's body fluid (secretions or excretions) or blood (Table 5-2), and Transmission-Based Precautions (Table 5-3) when in contact with special patient populations that have highly transmissible pathogens.

CLINICAL PEARL

Universal Precautions apply to the following body fluids: blood, semen, and vaginal, tissue, cerebrospinal, synovial (joint cavity), pleural, peritoneal, pericardial, and amniotic fluids. The CDC has stated that Universal Precautions also apply to feces, nasal secretions, sputum, sweat, tears, urine, and vomitus.[16]

In addition to these recommendations, most institutions and agencies have enacted additional policies and procedures to control infection and disease (Table 5-4). These policies and procedures emphasize good hand hygiene, good respiratory hygiene, a clean environment, the correct disposal of soiled articles (eg, patient linens, wound dressings), and the safe disposal of needles and other sharps (Table 5-5).

Standard Precautions

Standard Precautions (Table 5-2) are required when working with all patients and clients in any healthcare setting, including the patient's home. Generally, the clinician should:

▶ Avoid direct contact with patients, fomites, or, especially, body fluids.

TABLE 5-2   Standard Precautions

Handwashing

1. Wash hands after touching blood, body fluids, secretions, excretions, and contaminated items, whether or not gloves were worn.
2. Wash hands immediately after removing gloves, between patient contacts, and when otherwise indicated to reduce transmission of microorganisms.
3. Wash hands between tasks and procedures on the same patient to prevent cross-contamination of different body sites.
4. Use plain (nonantimicrobial) soap for routine handwashing.
5. An antimicrobial agent or a waterless antiseptic agent may be used for specific circumstances (hyperendemic infections) as defined by infection control.

Gloves

1. Wear gloves (clean, unsterile gloves are adequate) when touching blood, body fluids, secretions, excretions, and contaminated items; put on clean gloves just before touching mucous membranes and nonintact skin.
2. Change gloves between tasks and procedures on the same patient after contact with materials containing high concentrations of microorganisms.
3. Remove gloves promptly after use, before touching uncontaminated items and environmental surfaces, and before going on to another patient; wash hands immediately after glove removal to avoid the transfer of microorganisms to other patients or environments.

Mask and Eye Protection or Face Shield

1. Wear a mask and eye protection or a spray shield to protect mucous membranes of the eyes, nose, and mouth during procedures and patient care activities that are likely to generate splashes or sprays of blood, body fluids, secretions, and excretions.

Gown

1. Wear a gown (a clean, unsterile gown is adequate) to protect skin and prevent soiling of clothing during procedures and patient care activities that are likely to generate splashes or sprays of blood, body fluids, secretions, and excretions.
2. Select a gown appropriate for the activity and the amount of fluid likely to be encountered.
3. Remove a soiled gown as soon as possible and wash hands to avoid transferring microorganisms to other patients or environments.

Patient Care Equipment

1. Handle used patient-care equipment soiled with blood, body fluids, secretions, and excretion in a manner that prevents skin and mucous membrane exposures, contamination of clothing, and transfer of microorganisms to other patients or environments.
2. Ensure that reusable equipment is not used for another patient's care until it has been cleaned and reprocessed appropriately.
3. Ensure that single-use items are discarded properly.

Environmental Control

1. Follow hospital procedures for the routine care, cleaning, and disinfection of environmental surfaces, beds, bed rails, bedside equipment, and other frequently touched surfaces.

Linen

1. Handle, transport, and process used linen soiled with blood, body fluids, secretions, and excretion in a manner that prevents skin and mucous membrane exposures and contamination of clothing and avoids transfer of microorganisms to other patients or environments.

Occupational Health and Blood-Borne Pathogens

1. Prevent injuries when using needles, scalpels, and other sharp instruments or devices, when handling sharp instruments and procedures; when cleaning used instruments; and when disposing of used needles.
2. Never recap used needles, or otherwise manipulate them using both hands, or use any other technique that involves directing the needle's point toward any part of the body; rather, use either a one-handed "scoop" technique or mechanical device designed for holding the needle sheath.
3. Do not remove used needles from disposable syringes by hand, and do not bend, break, or otherwise manipulate used needles by hand.
4. Place used disposable syringes and needles, scalpel blades, or other sharp items in an appropriate puncture-resistant container for transport to the reprocessing area.
5. Use mouthpieces, resuscitation bags, or other ventilation devices as an alternative to mouth-to-mouth resuscitation.

Patient Placement

1. Use a private room for a patient who contaminates the environment or who does not (or cannot be expected to) assist in maintaining appropriate hygiene or environmental control.
2. Consult Infection Control if a private room is not available.

Data from Centers for Disease Control and Prevention, Hospital Infection Control Practices Advisory Committee. Part II. Recommendations for Isolation Precautions in Hospitals. February 2007.

▶ Wear barriers such as gloves when contact is necessary or expected.

▶ Avoid puncturing himself or herself with anything and therefore should minimize exposure to sharp instruments, especially body fluid–contaminated sharp instruments.

▶ Avoid exposing patients to any body fluids (or substances, eg, "weeping dermatitis") of others, such as that of health-care workers.

The most basic standard precaution is hand hygiene. There are two primary methods of hand hygiene: hand rubbing and handwashing.

▶ *Hand rubbing.* This technique uses an alcohol-based (60% to 95% alcohol [isopropyl, ethanol, *n*-propanol]) and skin conditioner product (to prevent skin irritation and dryness) dispensed from a wall-mounted unit or an antimicrobial/antiseptic hand wipe. Hand rubbing is used to decontaminate hands instead of handwashing. After performing several hand rubs, the hands may become sticky, and handwashing should be used to cleanse them.

CLINICAL PEARL

A typical hand rubbing procedure involves:

▶ The removal of all jewelry from the hands and wrists.

▶ The cleansing agent is applied from the dispenser to one palm and the hands are rubbed vigorously together using friction or rubbing motions, covering all surfaces of both hands.

▶ The rubbing is continued until the hands are dry, taking 25 to 30 seconds, depending on the product.

TABLE 5-3	Transmission-Based Isolation Precautions

Airborne Precautions

In addition to Standard Precautions, use Airborne Precautions, or the equivalent, with all patients known or suspected to be infected with serious illness transmitted by airborne droplet nuclei (small-particle residue) that remain suspended in the air and that can be dispersed widely by air currents within a room or over a long distance (for example, *Mycobacterium tuberculosis*, measles virus, chickenpox virus).

1. Respiratory isolation room.
2. Wear respiratory protection (mask) when entering the room.
3. Limit movement and transport of the patient to essential purposes only. Mask a patient when transporting out of the area.

Droplet Precautions

In addition to Standard Precautions, use Droplet Precautions, or the equivalent, for patients known or suspected to be infected with a serious illness due to microorganisms transmitted by large-particle droplets that can be generated by the patient during coughing, sneezing, talking, or the performance of procedures (eg, mumps, rubella, pertussis, influenza).

1. Isolation room.
2. Wear respiratory protection (mask) when entering the room.
3. Limit movement and transport of a patient to essential purposes only. Mask a patient when transporting out of the area.

Contact Precautions

In addition to Standard Precautions, use Contact Precautions, or the equivalent, for specified patients known or suspected to be infected or colonized with serious illness transmitted by direct patient contact (and/or skin-to-skin contact) or contact with items in the patient's environment.

1. Isolation room. Complete isolation precaution policies can be found in a healthcare facility's infection control manual.
2. Wear gloves when entering the room; change gloves after having contact with infective material; remove gloves before leaving patient's room; wash hands immediately with an antimicrobial agent or waterless antiseptic agent. After glove removal and handwashing, ensure that hands do not touch contaminated environmental items.
3. Wear a gown when entering the room if you anticipate your clothing will have substantial contact with the patient, environmental surfaces, or items in the patient's room, or if the patient is incontinent or has diarrhea, ileostomy, colostomy, or wound drainage not contained by the dressing. Remove gown before leaving patient's room; after gown removal, ensure that clothing does not contact potentially contaminated environmental surfaces.
4. Single patient use equipment.
5. Limit movement and transport of a patient to essential purposes only. Use precautions when transporting a patient to minimize the risk of transmitting microorganisms to other patients and contamination of environmental surfaces or equipment.

Data from Guideline for Isolation Precautions in Hospitals. Part II. Recommendations for isolation precautions in hospitals. Hospital Infection Control Practices Advisory Committee. 2008.

▶ *Handwashing.* According to the CDC, handwashing with soap and water is necessary before and after preparing food; before eating; when organic material such as blood or dirt is visible; before and after treating a patient with an infection; before and after performing wound care; after visiting the bathroom or assisting patients with post-toileting hygiene; after changing a diaper; after touching garbage; following nose-blowing, coughing, or sneezing; after handling animals, pet food, or animal waste; or after multiple hand rubbing applications.[*] It is important to avoid touching any potentially contaminated surface during or after the handwashing process. It is important to remember that the sink, soap dispenser, and towel container are considered to be contaminated.

CLINICAL PEARL

Handwashing procedure:

▶ All jewelry is removed from the hands and wrists.

▶ The faucet is adjusted (**Figure 5-3**) until the water is warm, and then the wrists and hands are immersed.

▶ Soap is applied (**Figure 5-4**), water is applied (**Figure 5-5**), and the hands are washed vigorously using rubbing

(**Figure 5-6**) or friction (**Figure 5-7**) motions for approximately 20 to 30 seconds (approximately the time it takes to sing "Happy Birthday" twice), or approximately 60 seconds if the hands have contacted body fluids, an infected wound, or a contaminated surface, making sure that all areas of the hands and wrists (between the fingers [**Figure 5-8**], under the nails, the dorsum of the hands, and the thumbs) are included.

▶ The hands and then wrists (moving from proximal to distal) are rinsed thoroughly while the hands are directed downward, maintaining no contact with the sink rim or basin (**Figures 5-9** and **5-10**). Avoid shaking the hands off in the sink to get them dryer.

▶ Once the soap lather has been completely removed from all surfaces, the hands are dried with a disposable paper towel while the water continues to flow (**Figures 5-11** through **5-13**).

▶ The towels used to dry the hands are discarded, and a clean, dry towel is used to turn off the faucet (**Figures 5-14** and **5-15**) before also being discarded.

Transmission-Based Precautions

Transmission-based precautions (Table 5-3) are required for patients known to be at risk for the presence of pathogens. Transmission-based precautions are standard precaution

---

[*]https://www.cdc.gov/handwashing/when-how-handwashing.html. Updated November 24, 2020. Accessed February 28, 2021.

TABLE 5-4	Basic Precautions
Hand hygiene	The single most effective way to protect the patient and the caregiver. Every caregiver and hospital visitor should perform it before or after a treatment or contact with a patient. Hand rubbing: advantages include less time to use, is more effective than soap and water, is more accessible than sinks, significantly reduces bacterial counts on hand, and causes less damage to the skin than soap and water. Handwashing: not the most effective method to decontaminate the hands except when hands are visibly dirty, soiled, or considered to be contaminated. The soap typically includes an antimicrobial or germicidal agent. Many handwashing stations have knee- or foot-operated controls for the faucet. Warm water promotes lather and is less irritating than hot or cold water.
Respiratory hygiene	Often referred to as "cough etiquette." Includes: ► Covering of the mouth and nose with a tissue during a cough or sneeze. ► Coughing or sneezing into the upper sleeve or elbow rather than into the hands if no tissue is available. ► Hand hygiene after contact with respiratory secretions. ► Maintaining a distance of more than 3 feet from persons with respiratory infections in common waiting areas. ► Wearing a face mask on entering a healthcare facility if one has increased production of infectious respiratory secretions.
Clean environment	► Treatment tables or mat tables require regular cleaning, ideally between each use (except when linen covering or paper sheet is used). ► Linens, including sheets, pillowcases, and towels, should be changed after each use and properly laundered and stored. ► Equipment that comes into contact with a patient or with a contaminated area, including such things as goniometers, ambulation devices, ankle weights, and exercise machines, must be cleaned regularly. ► Toys are common clinical items that can serve as pathogen reservoirs; therefore, only toys that can be easily cleaned and disinfected should be provided (avoid the use of stuffed or furry toys). Containers should be designated for toys that have been cleaned and for those that require cleaning.
Disposal of soiled items	All items that have been used by or with a patient are considered soiled, even if no contamination is visible. Linens should be placed in an appropriate laundry container, and gloves should be worn when handling soiled items. Soiled items that have come in contact with the patient's blood or suspected infectious material require special handling and should be disposed of in specially labeled biohazard containers. Hand hygiene should always be performed after disposing of used and soiled items.
Sharps containers	Any instrument capable of puncturing the skin, such as needles and scalpels, must be discarded in a specific container, typically referred to as a *sharps container*.

TABLE 5-5	Correct Disposal of Clinical Items
Item	**Disposal Method**
Instruments and equipment	Cleaned or disposed of according to institutional or agency policies and procedures. ► Contaminated reusable equipment should be placed carefully in a container, labeled, and returned to the appropriate department for sterilization. ► Contaminated disposable items should be placed carefully in a container, labeled, and discarded. Staff members who handle contaminated instruments or equipment should wear gloves and wash or rub the hands before and after the gloves have been applied and removed.
Needles, scalpels, and other sharp instruments	Should be placed in puncture-proof containers. No attempt should be made to bend or break the needle before it is discarded according to institutional or agency policies and procedures.
Departmental stethoscope	The ear tips should be wiped with alcohol before and after each use.
Contaminated or soiled linen	Should be disposed of with minimal handling, sorting, and movement according to institutional or agency policies and procedures.
Contaminated dressings, bandages, and other disposable materials	Should be properly placed in a nonporous container or bag, labeled, and discarded according to institutional or agency policies and procedures.

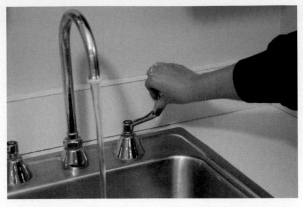

FIGURE 5-3 Handwashing procedure—adjusting the faucet to correct temperature.

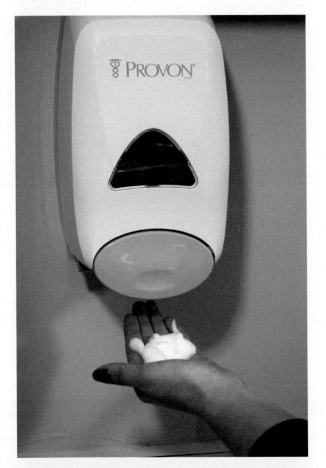

FIGURE 5-4 Handwashing procedure—applying the soap.

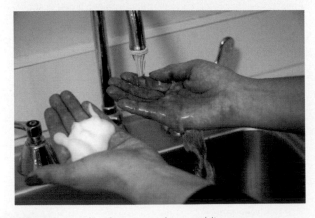

FIGURE 5-5 Handwashing procedure—adding water.

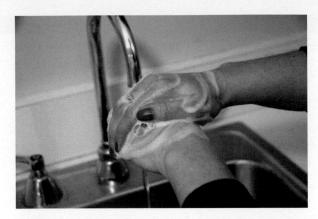

FIGURE 5-6 Handwashing procedure—rubbing motions.

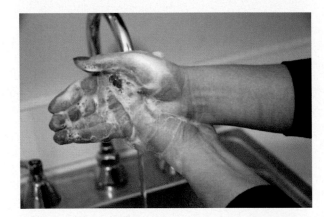

FIGURE 5-7 Handwashing procedure—friction motions.

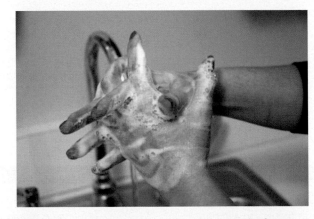

FIGURE 5-8 Handwashing procedure—between the fingers.

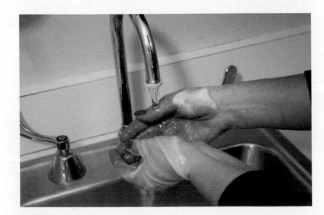

FIGURE 5-9 Hand rinsing procedure—hands are directed downward.

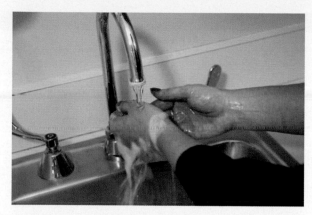

FIGURE 5-10 Hand rinsing procedure—maintaining no contact with the sink rim or basin.

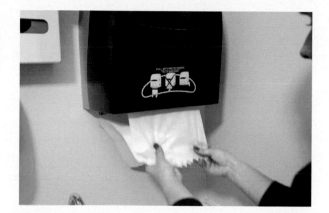

FIGURE 5-11 Hand drying using a paper towel dispenser.

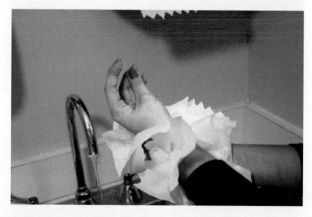

FIGURE 5-12 Hand drying with a paper towel starting at the wrists.

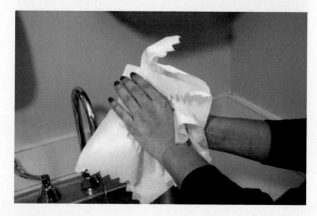

FIGURE 5-13 Hand drying the front and back of the hands.

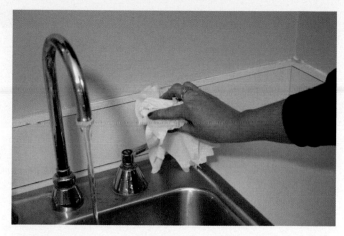

FIGURE 5-14 Using the paper towel to touch the faucet after hand drying.

procedures that include additional practices specific to the infectious microorganism's transmission mode.

CLINICAL PEARL

The transmission of microorganisms in a healthcare setting is generally a consequence of either accidental or deliberate disregard of established protocols designed to minimize transmission between patients or from hospital workers to patients. Such protocols include aseptic handwashing, following the correct isolation procedures for specific infectious diseases, and donning the appropriate personal protective equipment (PPE) (Table 5-6).

Personal Protective Equipment

Personal protective equipment (PPE) may be necessary to protect the clinician from the patient, although patients can wear PPE in some cases. The amount and type of PPE worn are determined by the likelihood of encountering body fluids and contaminated areas, and the modes in which known or suspected pathogens are transmitted. The various types of PPE are described in Table 5-6. Special procedures must

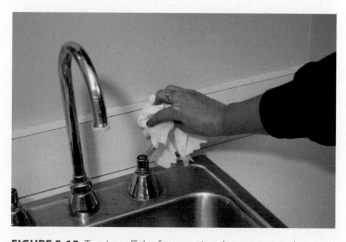

FIGURE 5-15 Turning off the faucet using the paper towel.

TABLE 5-6	Personal Protective Equipment	
Equipment	**Description of Use**	**Purpose and Precautions**
Gloves	Two types: ▶ Exam—the gloves are clean but have not undergone sterilization. Dispensed singly from a box. ▶ Sterile—have been treated to remove microorganisms. Packaged in pairs and sealed to prevent contamination. Used when there is a potential for coming in contact with a patient's body fluids, direct contact with someone who has an infection, handling equipment or touching surfaces that may be contaminated, or when there is a cut, wound, or break in the skin.	To prevent pathogens from entering small cuts, wounds, or breaks in the skin. Latex sensitivity is common in healthcare workers. Nonlatex and nonvinyl gloves are available for those who have a latex sensitivity.
Gowns	Disposable gowns that are designed to cover the arms and the front of the clinician's body to at least the mid-thigh.	Used to protect the clinician's skin and clothing from possible contact with pathogens.
Face protector	These come in a variety of designs: ▶ Face mask: fits over the clinician's nose and mouth. ▶ Goggles: often worn with face masks. ▶ Face shield: a combination of a face mask and goggles.	Face masks help protect against the spray of body fluids and secretions and prevent the dispersal of potentially infectious respiratory particles. Goggles protect the eyes against splashes from body fluids or chemicals.
Particulate respirator	Fully disposable or reusable face masks designed to filter particulate matter in the air at a higher level than standard surgical masks. The CDC recommends N95 (95% filter with no resistance to oils).	It is typically used in the presence of tuberculosis (TB) and severe acute respiratory syndrome (SARS).

be followed when donning and doffing PPE so that the items are donned and doffed in a particular order to avoid contamination.

CLINICAL PEARL

A common axiom used when donning and doffing PPE is "clean to clean and dirty to dirty." When a patient is in protective isolation, the order in which garments are donned is extremely critical, whereas the garment doffing sequence is less critical. Conversely, when the clinician is to be protected from the patient, the common donning sequence is less critical, whereas the garment doffing sequence is extremely critical. In either scenario, the clinician should perform hand hygiene after removing the gloves and clothing and avoid contact until this has been performed thoroughly.

Hand hygiene should be performed before donning PPE and immediately after removal of PPE. Although each facility has its specific protocols related to donning and doffing of PPE, an example of such a method follows.

▶ *Donning and doffing gloves.* If exam gloves are donned, no specific techniques are required (Figures 5-16 through 5-22). However, if sterile gloves are being used, a specific (clean) technique must be used (see Clinical Pearl). In either situation, if a tear develops while donning a glove, it should be disposed of and replaced with a new one. Depending on the procedure, the clinician may go through several pairs of sterile gloves in one session. For

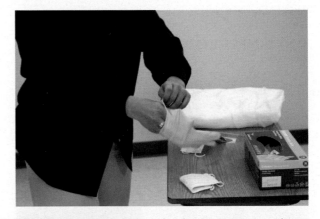

FIGURE 5-16 Donning nonsterile gloves using minimal contact with the outside of the glove.

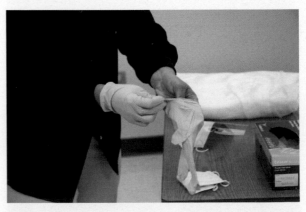

FIGURE 5-17 Donning nonsterile gloves using the gloved hand and minimal contact with the outside of the glove.

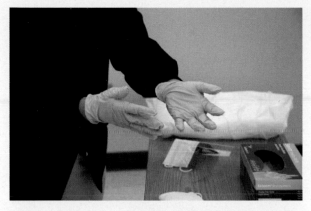

FIGURE 5-18 Both gloves successfully donned onto both hands.

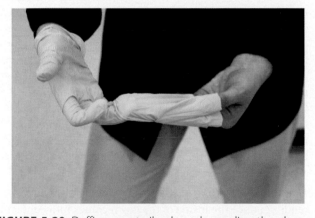

FIGURE 5-19 Doffing nonsterile gloves by hooking the gloved finger under the edge of the glove.

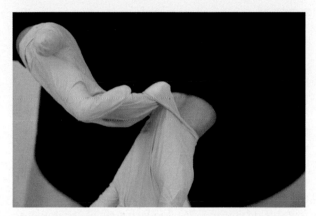

FIGURE 5-20 Doffing nonsterile gloves by peeling the glove off the hand while turning it inside out.

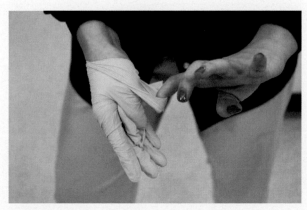

FIGURE 5-21 Doffing nonsterile gloves by hooking the nongloved finger on the edge of the glove.

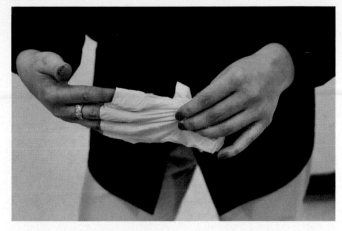

FIGURE 5-22 Doffing nonsterile gloves by peeling the glove off the hand while turning it inside out.

CLINICAL PEARL

To don a sterile pair of gloves, the clinician creates a clean field by clearing a surface at least 1 to 2 feet away from other objects. The clear surface is then covered with a clean item such as a towel or disposable patient protective barrier, and all items to be used are placed on the clean area. If a sterile field is required, a sterile covering is placed on the work surface by holding only the tips of the edges. Any tape that may be needed to secure dressings is prepared ahead of time by ripping the strips and hanging them from the edge of the work surface before cleaning the hands again and donning new gloves before proceeding.

Once the area has been prepared, the clinician—while taking care not to touch the sterile surface with the hands—opens the inner packet containing the gloves like a book, with the flaps facing the clinician, and without touching the outside of the gloves with the bare hands. Each glove has a cuff rolled back about 2 inches. The clinician picks up one glove by the inside of the glove, using one hand, which is still inside the gown cuff (see above) or bare. The glove is placed palm down on its proper hand so that the thumb of the glove rests on the thumb of the hand, and the fingers of the glove are directed toward the elbow.

Grasping the cuff of the glove by the hand or through the cuff of the gown, the clinician covers the cuff over the hand to seal or enclose the hand within the glove cuff, and then gently maneuvers the fingers and hand into the glove, while the other hand remains within the gown sleeve. The other glove is donned in the same manner. Once both gloves have been donned completely, they are held above waist level and should not be allowed to touch the gown or other objects in order to maintain sterility. If necessary, a sterile towel can be wrapped over the gloved hands to protect them until it is time to treat the patient.

example, one pair must be used to remove the soiled dressings, then a new set is needed to examine and treat the wound, and then a further pair is used to apply a new dressing. Each separate wound is treated as a separate treatment site to prevent cross-contamination.

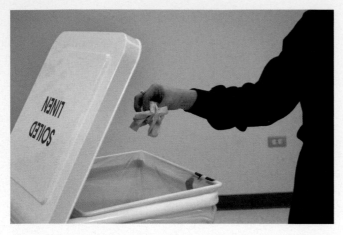

FIGURE 5-23 Disposing of gloves.

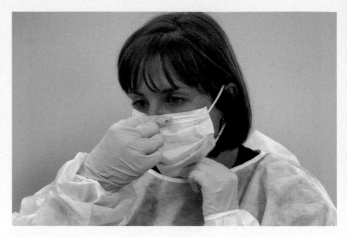

FIGURE 5-25 Pressing on the nose piece to contour it for a better fit.

After treating the patient, the gloves can be removed in any sequence, after which good hand hygiene is performed. The most common method to remove gloves is as follows (**Figures 5-16** through **5-22**): using one gloved hand to pull the opposite glove away from the hand, then placing the fingers of the bare hand under the remaining glove and using them to remove the glove without touching the outside of the gloves with the bare hands. The gloves are then disposed in the appropriate receptacle (**Figure 5-23**).

CLINICAL PEARL

Never leave a patient's room while still wearing gloves. Gloves should be removed before leaving the patient's room and washing the hands.

▶ ***Donning and doffing a face mask or respirator.*** If a face mask or respirator is used, the clinician applies it while holding it by its ties or edges (**Figure 5-24**). The mask or respirator should be positioned on the face to fit over the nose and under the chin. The upper ties are tied at the middle of the back of the head. The lower ties are tied at the neck while ensuring that the neck or cap is not touched as the mask is being tied. If the mask has a flexible piece designed to fit on the bridge of the nose, the

clinician can gently press on the nose piece to contour it for a better fit once the face mask has been donned (**Figure 5-25**). A mask or respirator can be removed by carefully untying each of the ties and then handling it by the ties while avoiding touching the center of the mask with the hands before disposing of it in an appropriate receptacle.

▶ ***Donning and doffing eye or face shields.*** If eye protection is necessary, the clinician can apply goggles or a face shield (**Figure 5-26**). Modern goggles are similar to glasses and are worn accordingly, but some goggles have elastic straps that fit snugly around the head. The goggles must be comfortable, provide good peripheral vision, and ensure a secure fit. In place of a face mask and goggles, a chin-length face shield may be used, although it is important to remember that face shields do not protect against airborne transmission and, therefore, often have to be used in conjunction with a surgical mask or respirator. Goggles are removed by handling the earpieces or headbands and not the front of the goggles. Face shields are removed similarly by touching only the earpieces or headbands at the side of the head before they are disposed of in an appropriate receptacle (**Figure 5-27**).

▶ ***Donning and doffing a disposable gown.*** If a gown is required, once the inside of the gown comes into contact

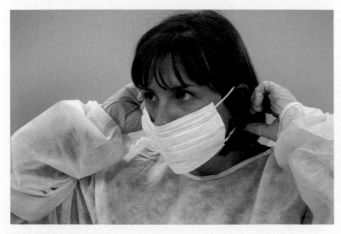

FIGURE 5-24 Applying a face mask.

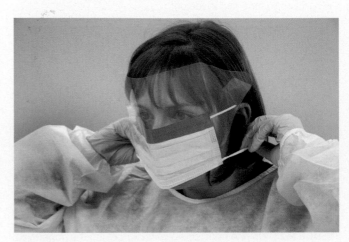

FIGURE 5-26 Donning a face shield.

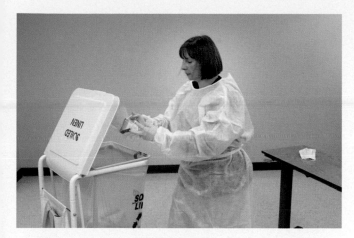

FIGURE 5-27 Disposing of a face shield.

with the clinician's clothing, it is considered contaminated. The clinician picks up the gown with one hand by grasping the gown's center or neck and allows it to unfold without letting it touch the body (Figure 5-28). The clinician may need to shake the gown so that it opens fully. Once opened fully, the clinician inserts one hand and arm through one sleeve inside the gown (Figure 5-29), maintaining gown-to-gown contact but not allowing the

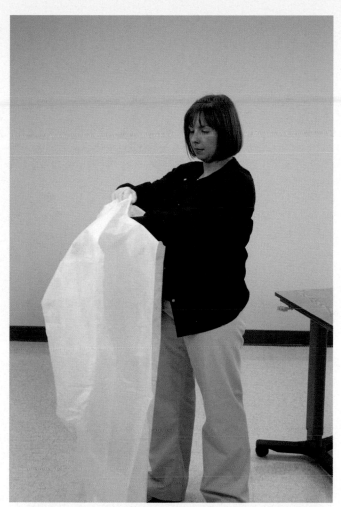

FIGURE 5-29 Inserting one hand into one sleeve inside the gown.

hand to extend through the gown cuff (if a closed glove technique is to be used) (Figure 5-30). The clinician then places the other arm through the other sleeve in the gown (Figure 5-31), again maintaining gown-to-gown contact and keeping that hand inside the cuff (if a closed glove technique is to be used). Once the clinician has checked to be sure that the gown covers the arms on the front of the body to at least mid-thigh level (Figure 5-32), the straps are tied behind the clinician at the neck (Figures 5-33 through 5-35) and waist (Figures 5-36 and 5-37). After treating the patient, the gown can usually be removed in any sequence, such as the one outlined in Figures 5-38 through 5-46, and then good hand hygiene is performed. To remove a gown following isolation precautions, the clinician unties the gown's waist tie and then carefully unties the tie at the neck while avoiding touching the gown's neck, cap, or outer side. The clinician then slips both hands under the gown at the neck and shoulders and peels the gown away from the body, turning the sleeves inside out. Each arm is pulled out of the gown by grasping the cuffs one at a time by slipping the fingers underneath each of them. Then, while holding the gown's inside surface at the shoulders, the clinician folds or rolls the gown in on itself so that the gown's inner surface is exposed and the contaminated surfaces are contained within. The gown is then discarded into an appropriate receptacle.

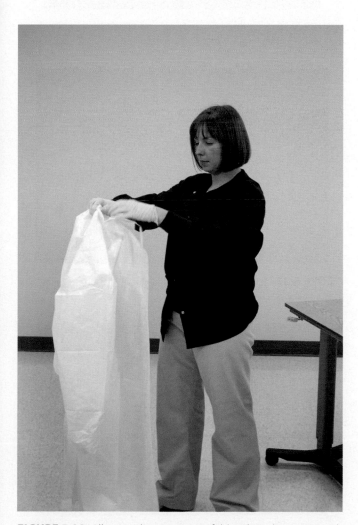

FIGURE 5-28 Allowing the gown to unfold without letting it touch the body.

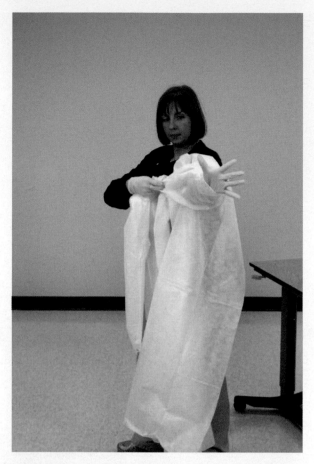

FIGURE 5-30 Placing the arm through the sleeve in the gown.

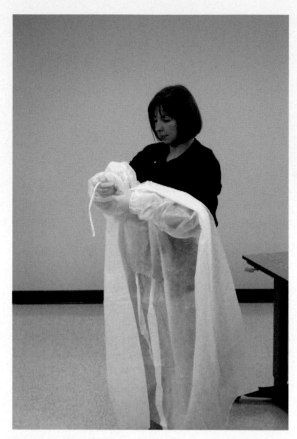

FIGURE 5-32 Sequence of applying and tying the straps behind the clinician at the neck—locate the tie strings.

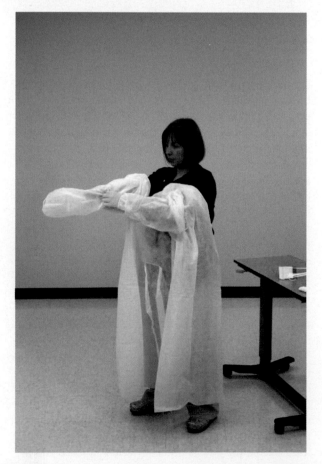

FIGURE 5-31 Ensuring that the gown covers the arms on the front of the body.

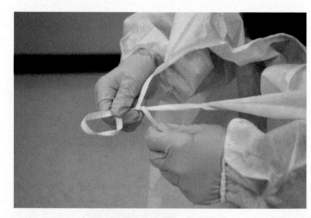

FIGURE 5-33 Sequence of applying and tying the straps behind the clinician at the neck—tying a bow.

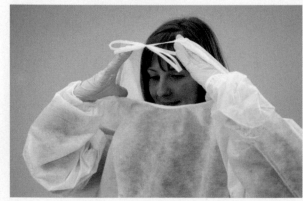

FIGURE 5-34 Sequence of applying and tying the straps behind the clinician at the neck—moving the bow over the head.

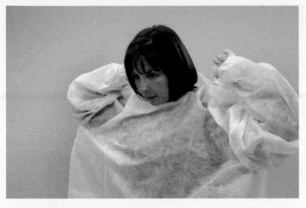

FIGURE 5-35 Sequence of applying and tying the straps behind the clinician at the neck—placing the bow behind the head.

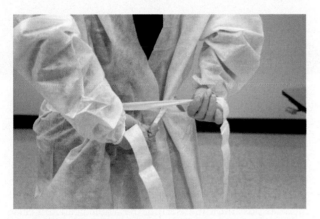

FIGURE 5-36 Crossing the straps at the waist.

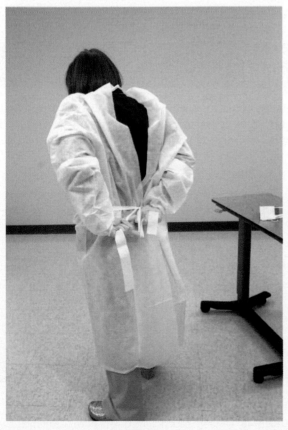

FIGURE 5-37 Tying the straps at the waist.

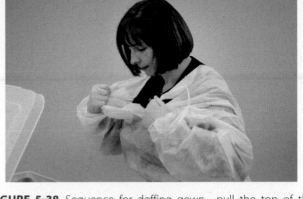

FIGURE 5-38 Sequence for doffing gown—pull the top of the gown forward.

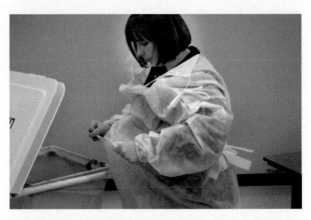

FIGURE 5-39 Sequence for doffing gown—pull the bottom of the gown forward.

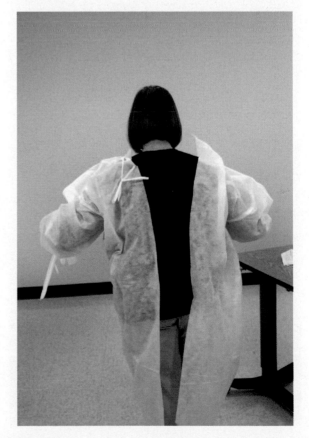

FIGURE 5-40 Sequence for doffing gown—neck and waist straps disengaged.

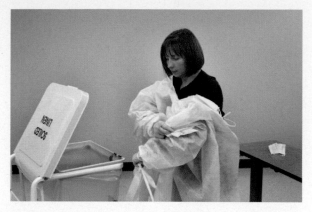

FIGURE 5-41 Sequence for doffing gown—start pulling the gown off one shoulder.

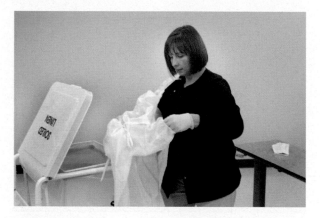

FIGURE 5-42 Sequence for doffing gown—pull the gown off one arm.

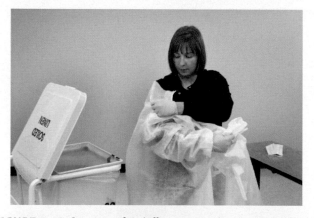

FIGURE 5-43 Sequence for doffing gown—begin removing the gown from the other arm.

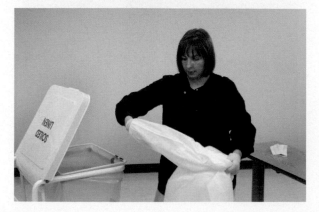

FIGURE 5-44 Sequence for doffing gown—remove the gown from the arm.

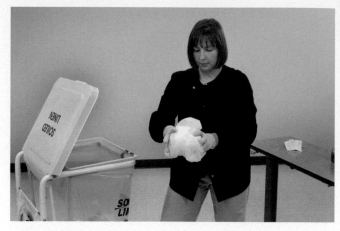

FIGURE 5-45 Sequence for doffing gown—scrunch the discarded gown into a ball.

► *Donning and doffing a cap.* If a cap is to be used, the clinician should don it before donning the gown. The cap should be donned while avoiding touching the head as much as possible and inserting the whole head and ears in the cap. To remove a cap, the clinician handles it by its ties or gently grasps the center at the top and lifts it from the head.

PRECAUTIONS FOR SPECIAL POPULATIONS

Certain populations with impaired resistance to infection require extra precautions to protect the patient. These populations include patients who are transplant recipients,

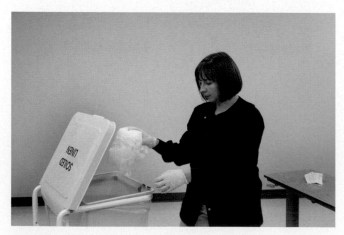

FIGURE 5-46 Sequence for doffing gown—dispose of the gown in the appropriate receptacle.

including bone marrow transplants, and those undergoing chemotherapy. These precautions include but are not limited to[17]:

- Placing a patient in a private room with the air pressure positive compared to the corridor outside.
- Performing good hand hygiene using an antimicrobial soap before entering the patient's room or providing direct patient care.
- Permitting only essential personnel and visitors to enter the patient's room and preventing anyone who is ill or feels like they may be getting sick from entering.
- Permitting no live plants, fresh fruits, or uncooked vegetables without the approval of the attending physician.
- Allowing the patient to leave their room only for essential purposes with the attending physician's permission. If allowed to leave, the patient must wear a surgical mask.

In addition to those populations already mentioned, pediatric and geriatric patients bring their own set of challenges because these populations tend to be at higher risk of infection, especially when they have weakened immune systems due to an acquired or congenital health problem. Key precautions with these populations in addition to standard precautions include the implementation of respiratory hygiene and cough-etiquette strategies for patients with suspected influenza or infection with another respiratory-tract pathogen to the extent feasible; separation of infected, contagious children from uninfected children when feasible; and appropriate sterilization, disinfection, and antisepsis.

CLINICAL PEARL

To help prevent nosocomial infection and to break the chain of transmission, the clinician should:

- Observe an aseptic technique. In physical therapy, aseptic techniques can include the use of PPE.
- Frequently perform handwashing, especially between patients
- Perform careful handling, cleaning, and disinfection of fomites
- Where possible, use single-use disposable items
- Enforce patient isolation
- Avoid, where possible, any medical procedures that can lead to nosocomial infection

THE CRITICAL CARE ENVIRONMENT

Critical care environments have different names depending on the area of specialization:

- ICU—intensive care unit or intermediate care unit
- CCU—coronary care unit or critical care unit
- MICU—medical intensive care unit
- SICU—surgical intensive care unit

- NICU—neurologic intensive care unit or neonatal intensive care unit
- PACU—Postanesthesia care unit

PTAs who practice in these critical care settings face a variety of complex challenges. The amount of preparation required to treat patients in this environment is more than for a typical hospital setting. Critically ill patients have limited mobility because of tenuous hemodynamic status, multiple central catheters, life-support monitors, artificial airways, sedative medication, impaired levels of alertness, electrolyte imbalances, multiple medical problems, deconditioning, sleep disturbances, and muscle weakness. The benefits of early mobilization of this population include weaning from mechanical ventilation, improving tissue perfusion, promoting better rest periods, improving emotional state, decreasing the incidence of acquired pressure ulcers, restoring function and mobility, relieving pain, and decreasing the length of stay (thereby reducing healthcare costs). However, mobilizing patients in this environment is not without risk. Catheters and supportive equipment attached to patients can become dislodged and cause injury, and reinsertion of catheters can increase infection risk and cause unwanted stress and pain for patients and families.[18] The treating clinician may find the highly technical environment somewhat daunting, especially as the stakes are high. However, provided that the clinician approaches these situations logically, a degree of comfort level will be reached fairly quickly.

In most cases, orientation is provided to new clinicians, which includes a formal introduction to the nursing staff and other key members of the healthcare team, as well as information regarding the equipment and the various treatment protocols. Most critical care environments consist of a series of individualized cubicles, with one patient in each cubicle. Typically, before entering an intensive care unit, the clinician reviews the patient's medical record for any changes in the patient status, any procedures that are scheduled, any special precautions that need to be taken (eg, respiratory isolation), or any changes in the orders for the patient.

The medical chart contains laboratory values, which provide information about the patient's blood chemistry, blood gases, and urinalysis, depending on the patient's diagnosis. Reference laboratory values are provided in Table 5-7.

It is also worth noting whether the patient has a do not resuscitate (DNR) directive in the medical record.

CLINICAL PEARL

In general, if a patient has a DNR status, no attempt is made to administer chest compressions, insert an artificial airway, administer resuscitative drugs, defibrillate, provide respiratory assistance (other than suctioning the airway and administering oxygen), initiate resuscitative IV, or initiate cardiac monitoring. However, the following procedures are generally accepted as part of the DNR status: suctioning the airway, administering oxygen, positioning the patient for comfort, splinting or immobilization, controlling bleeding, providing pain medication, providing emotional support, and contacting other appropriate

TABLE 5-7 Reference Laboratory Values

Profile	Component	Related Physiology	Reference Value	Significance
Arterial blood gases (ABGs)	Arterial PaO$_2$	Reflects the dissolved oxygen level based on the pressure it exerts on the bloodstream.	80–100 mm Hg	A decrease indicates pulmonary dysfunction, eg, hypoventilation.
	Arterial PaCO$_2$	Reflect the dissolved carbon dioxide level based on the pressure it exerts on the bloodstream.	35–45 mm Hg	Indicates pulmonary dysfunction—hypoventilation leads to an elevation.
	Arterial pH	Reflects the free hydrogen ion concentration.	7.35–7.45	<7.35 = acidosis >7.45 = alkalosis Collectively this test and the arterial PO$_2$ and arterial PCO$_2$ tests help reveal the acid-base status and how well oxygen is being delivered to the body.
	Oxygen saturation (SAO$_2$)	Usually, a bedside technique (pulse oximetry) is used to indicate the level of oxygen transport.	95%–98%	During exercise or physical activity, a minimum of 90% saturation should be maintained to avoid hypoxemia.
Fluids and electrolytes	Sodium (Na)	Major extracellular cation that serves to regulate serum osmolality, fluid, and acid-base balance; maintains the transmembrane electric potential for neuromuscular functioning.	135–145 mEq/L	*Increased* values found with excessive sweating, hypothalamus disease, diabetes insipidus, hypoadrenalism, excess sodium intake. *Decreased* values found with diuretic medication, kidney disease, congestive heart failure, diabetic ketoacidosis, sweating, severe vomiting and diarrhea.
	Potassium (K)	Major intracellular cation: maintains normal hydration and osmotic pressure.	3.5–5.0 mEq/L	*Increased* values with tissue damage, urinary obstruction, primary adrenal insufficiency, diabetes mellitus. *Decreased* values with prolonged vomiting and diarrhea, diuretic medication, corticosteroid excess.
	Calcium (Ca)	Transmission of nerve impulses, muscle contractility; cofactor in enzyme reactions and blood coagulation.	8.5–10.8 mg/dL; inversely related to phosphorus level	*Increased* values with hyperparathyroidism, carcinoma metastatic to bone, multiple myeloma; loss of neuromuscular excitability and muscle weakness may be seen. *Decreased* values with vitamin D deficiency, malabsorption, kidney disease, hypoparathyroidism; muscle tetany may be observed.
	Phosphorus (PO$_4$)	Integral to the structure of nucleic acids, in adenosine triphosphate energy transfer, and in phospholipid function. Phosphate helps to regulate calcium levels, metabolism, base balance, and bone metabolism.	2.6–4.5 mg/dL; inversely related to calcium level	*Increased* values with renal disease, hypoparathyroidism, hyperthyroidism. *Decreased* values with malabsorption, hyperparathyroidism.
Blood enzymes	Creatine kinase (CK)	An enzyme found predominantly in the heart, brain, and skeletal muscle. Aids in protein catabolism. Can be separated into subunits or isoenzymes, each derived from a specific tissue; CPK-MB = cardiac CPK-MM = skeletal muscle. Blood levels of CPK-MB typically rise within 2 to 6 hours after a heart attack, reach their highest levels within 12 to 24 hours, and fall to normal levels within 3 days.	CK-Total = 25–255 μL/L CK-MB = 0–5.9 mL/L CK-MM = 5–70 μL/L	CK-Total: severe hypokalemia, carbon monoxide poisoning, seizures, pulmonary and cerebral infarctions. CPK-MB: myocardial infarction (an ongoing high level of CPK-MB levels after 3 days may mean that an MI is progressing and more heart muscle is being damaged), postcardiac surgery, muscular dystrophies, polymyositis. CPK-MM: trauma, muscular dystrophy, dermatomyositis, hypothyroidism, seizures.

			Reference values	Indications
	Lactate dehydrogenase (LDH)	Present in all body tissues and is abundant in red blood cells. Acts as a marker for hemolysis. Isoenzymes are LDH 1–5.	105–333 IU/L	LDH 1–2: myocardial infarction, myocarditis, shock, hemolytic and sickle cell anemia. LDH 3: shock, pulmonary infarction. LDH 4: shock. LDH 5: congestive heart failure, shock, hepatitis, cirrhosis, liver congestion.
	Alkaline phosphatase	An enzyme most effective in an alkaline environment. Associated with bone metabolism/calcification and lipid transport.	Adults: 20–140 IU/L Infants to adolescents: Up to 104 IU/L	*Increased* = severe biliary obstruction, cirrhosis, hepatitis. Indicates increased osteoblastic activity:150–250 IU/L indicates a fracture.350–700 IU/L indicates active heterotrophic ossification. Used as an indicator for Paget disease, bone metastasis, osteomalacia, and hyperparathyroidism. *Decreased* = the healing of bone has ceased (nonunion fracture), or normal finding indicating bone growth has stopped with skeletal maturity.
Cellular blood elements	White blood cells (WBCs)	Produced in bone marrow; provide defense against foreign agents/organisms.	$4.3–10.8 \times 10^9$/L	*Increased* values with infection (bacterial), most illnesses, inflammation, allergic reactions, parasitic infections, leukemias, stress overall stimulation of bone marrow. *Decreased* values with chemotherapy, bone marrow failure, viral infections, alcoholism, AIDS.
	Red blood cells (RBCs)	Produced in bone marrow, carry oxygen to tissues.	$4.6–6.2 \times 10^{12}$/L (male) $4.2–5.4 \times 10^{12}$/L (female)	*Increased* values with lack of oxygen, smoking, exposure to carbon monoxide, long-term lung disease, diseases of kidney, heart, bone marrow; dehydration, vomiting, diarrhea, sweating, severe burns, diuretics. *Decreased* values with anemia from blood loss (colon cancer), decreased in RBC production (tumor, medication, lack of nutrients), increased RBC destruction (sickle cell disease).
	Hemoglobin (Hgb)	Reflects oxygen-carrying capacity.	14–18 g/dL (male) 13–16 g/dL (female)	Values of 8–10 g/dL typically result in decreased exercise tolerance, increased fatigue, and tachycardia, conditions that may contraindicate aggressive therapeutic measures, including strength and endurance training.
	Hematocrit	The measure of the ratio of packed red blood cells to whole blood.	40–54 mL/dL (male) 37–48 mL/dL (female)	By dividing the hematocrit level by 3, one can approximate the hemoglobin level.
	Platelet count	Reflects the potential to address injury to vessel walls, thus regulating homeostasis.		*Increased* values with severe bleeding, infection, strenuous exercise, pregnancy, splenectomy, iron deficiency, rheumatoid arthritis, leukemia. *Decreased* values with infection, vitamin B_{12} or folic acid deficiency, severe internal bleeding, cancer, and autoimmune conditions.

healthcare providers. Recently, varying degrees of DNR have been introduced:

► *DNR comfort care:* permit comfort care only both before and during a cardiac or respiratory arrest. Resuscitative therapies are not administered before an arrest. This order is generally regarded as appropriate for patients who have a terminal illness, short life expectancy, little chance of surviving CPR, and a desire to let nature take its course in the face of an impending arrest.

► *DNR comfort care–arrest:* Resuscitative therapies will be administered before an arrest but not during an arrest.

Once the medical record has been reviewed, the clinician then communicates with the nursing staff to get the most recent update on the patient and to inform the nurse responsible for the patient about the activities planned for the patient.

CLINICAL PEARL

Generally speaking, the more acute the patient's condition, the less intense the treatment and the shorter the treatment duration.

Upon entering the patient's cubicle, the clinician should systematically observe the equipment on the bed, on the wall, and floor. The clinician should also observe the patient and determine the patient's level of arousal and overall condition before proceeding. In most cases, the patient's vital signs will be displayed on a monitor.

CLINICAL PEARL

The most common ICU monitor, the vital sign monitor, can display values of any of the following:

► Cardiac rhythm patterns

► Blood pressure

► Respiration rate

► Oxygen saturation level

► Blood gases

► Temperature

The monitor activates an alarm if unacceptable parameters or ranges for the above physiological indicators occur. The clinician should pay attention to this monitor during patient activities to observe the patient's responses. Portable versions of the vital monitor are also available.

If the patient is conscious, the clinician should introduce themselves, explain the purpose of the visit, and describe what the patient can expect.

The following sections describe the most common types of equipment and devices found in the critical care environment.

CLINICAL PEARL

A common treatment goal for patients in a critical care environment is minimizing or preventing the adverse effects of inactivity and immobility through a gradual progression of functional activities that the patient can tolerate.

Bed Type

Standard Adjustable. The standard hospital bed has two motors: one for the legs and one for the back. These beds can also have a third motor as an option that allows the whole bed to go up and down. The lower portion of the bed is typically hinged, so it can be adjusted to provide knee flexion/hip flexion (Fowler's position). The average size for this type of bed is 36 inches wide × 80 inches long. In the interest of safety, these beds are fitted with side rails that can be lifted until a locking mechanism is engaged and lowered to allow the patient to get out of bed. If a side rail is to be lifted or lowered, the clinician must check that such a movement will not compress or stretch any line, lead, or tube that is connected to the patient, and whenever the patient is returned to the bed, the clinician should ensure that the side rail is in its correct position.

The majority of these beds have a device (call button) attached to the side rail that can be used to contact nursing personnel, or a similar device, attached to an electrical cord, is provided for the patient. These beds come with a standard vinyl-covered innerspring or foam mattress, but designs are available for skin shear, reinforced borders to help a patient get in and out of bed, and several layers of foam for circulation, cushioning, pressure relief, and comfort. These beds are typically used with patients who do not require specialized equipment, such as those in the late stages of dementia (bed rails can be used as a restraint method for short periods) and postsurgery patients. The benefits of this type of bed are that they ease caregiving, enhance patient comfort, are adjustable, and can help relieve various conditions, including:

► Respiratory difficulties

► Patients susceptible to aspiration

► Patients with digestive problems such as reflux

► Cardiac patients

The ability to raise the upper part of the bed aids with activities of daily living such as:

► *Sitting up in bed.* A person is more likely to slip down when in a sitting position in bed if a pillow or wedge is not under his/her knees.

► Eating/drinking using a bed tray.

► Brushing teeth.

If the patient frequently sits up in bed, the clinician should ensure that the patient is educated on correct body alignment and posture. If the patient cannot self-support good body alignment, the clinician can use pillows to help prop him/her up. A small pillow placed under the head can also increase comfort.

Bariatric. These hospital beds are electrically operated beds with reinforced frames and decks designed for people from 600 to 1000 lb, depending on the design. The dimensions can be 42 inches wide (600 lb), 48 inches wide (750 lb), and 54 inches wide (1000 lb).

Air Fluidized (Clinitron). These beds contain 1600 lb of silicone-coated glass beads called microspheres through which heated and pressurized air flows through to suspend a polyester cover that supports the patient. The airflow, combined with the microspheres, develops the properties associated with fluids and provides contact pressure to the patient's body of only 11 to 15 mm Hg. The indications for this type of bed include patients with several infected lesions, obese patients with risk of skin deterioration, patients who require skin protection, and patients whose position cannot be altered easily (those with extensive skin grafts and those who require prolonged immobilization). The advantages of using this type of bed include:

▶ Reduced need for topical medication and dressings because the microclimate is favorable for the healing process

▶ Ability to control the temperature of the bed

▶ Reduction in overall skin pressure

When the unit is turned off, the polyester cover becomes a firm surface, which may benefit certain nursing procedures (turning a patient during dressing changes).

In addition to being very expensive, the disadvantages of using this type of bed include:

▶ The polyester cover can be easily punctured.

▶ The air flowing across the patient's skin may cause dehydration.

▶ Tall or obese persons may be uncomfortable in this bed.

▶ The height of the bed surface from the floor is fixed.

▶ These beds tend to be very noisy.

Circular Turning Frame (Circ-O-Lectric Bed or Stryker Wedge). This type of bed has an anterior/posterior frame attached to two circular supports, which can move a patient vertically from supine to prone as the circular supports rotate through 180° around a short axis. At any point within their half-circle range during the rotation, the circular supports can be stopped. This type of bed is indicated when skeletal stability and alignment are required. The advantages of using this type of bed include:

▶ One person can safely and easily turn or position a patient.

▶ It provides easy access for a variety of therapeutic interventions.

▶ Attachments can be added to provide traction (cervical) or immobilization.

▶ The unit can be elevated to several heights.

▶ Various patient positioning options are available (eg, hip and knee flexion, and semirecumbent). It is also possible to position a patient in a fully upright position to allow them to step off the bed onto the floor.

The disadvantages of using this type of bed include:

▶ The amount of space required to allow the frames to rotate.

▶ A doorway must be over 7 feet high to allow the bed to pass through.

▶ Increased axial compressive pressure through the patient as they are moved into the vertical position during the transition.

This bed's use is contraindicated for unhealed, unstable vertebral fractures, any patient whose skin is susceptible to shearing and pressure, and any patient who suffers from motion sickness, vertigo, nausea, or orthostatic hypotension.

Posttrauma Mobility (Keane, Roto-rest). This type of bed is designed to maintain a seriously injured patient in a stable position and maintain proper postural alignment through adjustable bolsters. The bed, which is designed to oscillate from side to side in a cradle-like motion to reduce the amount of prolonged pressure on the patient's skin, is indicated for patients with restricted respiratory function, advanced or multiple pressure sores, severe neurologic deficits, and those who require stabilization and skeletal alignment after extensive trauma (spinal injuries, with or without the complication of paraplegia or quadriplegia, and also for head injuries and certain orthopedic cases to help manage patients at risk for pulmonary complications as a result of immobility).

The side-to-side motion provided by the bed improves upper respiratory function, reduces the need to turn the patient, provides environmental stimulation for the neurologically impaired patient, reduces urinary stasis, and improves bowel function. However, there are several disadvantages associated with this type of bed, including:

▶ The constant motion of the bed may induce motion sickness.

▶ Exercising may be restricted by bolsters and alignment supports.

▶ The bed requires a lot of room to oscillate.

Low Air Loss (Alternating Pressure) Therapy. These mattresses feature airflow throughout the sacral and torso areas to minimize skin maceration by reducing excess moisture under the patient. These mattress systems are available to fit all standard hospital beds, including pediatric, geriatric, and bariatric configurations, and are a proven way to help prevent and treat pressure ulcers by suspending the patient on several segmental air-filled cells while circulating air across the skin to reduce moisture and help maintain a constant skin interface pressure. The user can electronically adjust the amount of air pressure in each cell and electronically adjust the bed to several different positions, including hip and knee flexion, sitting, or a semirecumbent position. This type of bed is indicated for patients who require prolonged immobilization, patients who are at high risk of developing pressure ulcers or who have existing ulcers, patients who are obese, and those whose condition requires frequent elevation of the trunk. This type of bed has sensors that measure the patient's weight in the bed, and the air bladders are inflated or deflated automatically to distribute the patient's weight correctly. The disadvantages of this type of bed include:

▶ The air cells can be punctured or torn by sharp objects.

▶ The patient's position must be frequently altered to prevent pressure ulcers.

Lines, Leads, and Tubes

Intravenous (IV) Line. IV lines are used for several purposes:

▶ To infuse fluids, nutrients, electrolytes, and medications via a plastic bag that measures the number of drops of fluid administered per minute

▶ To obtain venous blood samples

▶ To insert catheters into the central circulatory system

IVs are most commonly placed in the forearm or back of the hand. Complications associated with IV administration include cellulitis, phlebitis, thrombosis, sepsis, air embolus, and pulmonary thromboembolism.

Nasogastric (NG) Tube. A flexible tube connected to an electric pump is passed through the nose and down through the nasopharynx and esophagus into the stomach, which provides access to the stomach for diagnostic and therapeutic purposes (feeding and administering drugs and other oral agents directly into the GI tract). Before treating a patient on an NG tube, the pump must be stopped. The patient is positioned in an upright or semi-upright position for at least 30 minutes (1 hour for pediatric patients) before supine activities.

Enterostomy Feeding Tube. A flexible feeding tube (percutaneous endoscopic gastrostomy/jejunostomy [PEG/PEJ]) that is inserted by endoscopic or a small surgical opening in the abdomen so that nutritional solutions can be conveyed directly into the stomach or jejunum through a tube. The main difference between a PEG and a PEJ is that the physician inserts the PEG tube percutaneously into the stomach with an endoscope, whereas the PEJ tube is inserted into the intestine to the jejunum.

Endotracheal Tube. An endotracheal tube is a specific type of artificial airway for a patient who cannot oxygenate/ventilate independently. A large-diameter flexible tube can be inserted through the mouth (orotracheal) or nose (nasotracheal). Verification of correct placement is done by X-ray. Once correctly placed, the tube must not be moved unless there is a physician's written order.

Chest Tube (Pleur-Evac). This is a flexible plastic tube that is surgically inserted through an incision on the side of a patient's chest and into the pleural space. It is used to remove air (pneumothorax) if placed in the anterior or lateral chest wall, fluid (pleural effusion, blood, chyle) if placed inferiorly and posteriorly, or pus (empyema) from the intrathoracic space, using mediastinal tubes. The chest tube is connected to one to three large bottles, which are responsible for collecting air/fluid without permitting the lung to collapse. The clinician should avoid activities that pull on these tubes, because if they are accidentally dislodged or disconnected from the bottle, the patient's lung will collapse completely.

Jackson-Pratt Drain. A drainage device, which consists of a surgical tube connected to a suction bulb that is used to pull excess fluid from the body by constant suction.

Autofusion Surgical Drain (Hemovac or Autovac). A disposable, self-contained postsurgical drain used to remove pus, blood, or other fluids from a wound. Before a treatment session, the clinician should ask the nursing staff to empty any drain that is more than half full.

Patient-controlled Analgesia (PCA). PCA is commonly assumed to imply on-demand, intermittent IV administration of opioids under patient control—a sophisticated microprocessor-controlled infusion pump delivers a preprogrammed dose of opioids when the patient pushes a demand button.

Catheters

Central Venous Catheter. A central venous line catheter is most often used for the administration of chemotherapy or other medications, measurement of central venous pressure, or blood withdrawal.

Hickman Catheter. Hickman, also known as an indwelling right atrial catheter, has both an entry and exit point. The entry is usually through the jugular vein in the neck, and the catheter is then run through part of the body until it reaches the tip of the right atrium. It emerges from there and is attached to two or three tubes that are exterior to the chest. This type of catheter is used for drawing blood, providing nutrition/fluids, and administering medications. As with most permanent IV lines or catheters, the Hickman can be prone to infection. Because the line is inserted into the major veins, this can be very serious.

Indwelling Urinary (Foley) Catheter. This type of catheter is inserted into the bladder via the urethra. Urinary catheters are used to drain the bladder in cases of:

▶ Urinary incontinence (leaking urine or being unable to control urination)

▶ Urinary retention (being unable to empty the bladder on demand)

▶ Surgery on the prostate or genitals

▶ Other medical conditions such as multiple sclerosis, spinal cord injury, or dementia

An indwelling urinary catheter is one that is left in the bladder. It is held in place in the bladder by a small balloon. The urine drains through plastic tubing into a collection bag, bottle, or urinal. Complications associated with urinary catheters include infection of the urinary tract or bladder, development of a urethral fistula, and kidney failure. Before starting a treatment session, the clinician should drain urine from the catheter tubing. During treatment sessions, the clinician should ensure that the collection bag is always placed below the bladder's level. Any signs of foul-smelling urine, cloudy dark urine, or urine with blood in it should be reported to the patient's physician or nurse.

Suprapubic Catheter. This type of catheter is inserted directly into the bladder through a small incision in the stomach and the bladder. Indications for a suprapubic catheter include:

▶ A failed trial using a urethral catheter

▶ Long-term use (if left in for long periods, urethral catheters can lead to acquired hypospadias and recurrent/chronic urinary tract infections [UTIs])

Contraindications include:

▶ Lower abdominal incisions, which can lead to adhesions

▶ Pelvic fracture

Complications associated with this type of catheter include:

▶ UTIs

▶ Blockages

▶ Bladder stones

▶ Bladder cancer

The clinician should use caution to avoid placing a gait or transfer belt directly over the insertion site.

Colostomy Bag. A colostomy is a surgical procedure in which a stoma is formed by drawing the healthy end of the large intestine or colon through an incision in the anterior abdominal wall and suturing it into place via an ostomy. In conjunction with the attached stoma appliance, this opening provides an alternative channel for feces to leave the body. People with colostomies must wear an ostomy-pouching system to collect intestinal waste. Ordinarily, the pouch must be emptied or changed a couple of times a day depending on the frequency of activity; in general, the further from the anus (ie, the further "up" the intestinal tract) the ostomy is located, the greater the output and more frequent the need to empty or change the pouch.

Rectal Tube. A rectal tube aims to remove gas from the lower intestines or remove or contain fecal matter. The collection bag should be kept below the level of the tube.

Life-Support Equipment

Mechanical Ventilator. A machine that generates a controlled flow of gas into a patient's airways using positive pressure from oxygen and air received from cylinders or wall outlets. The incoming gas is pressure-reduced and blended according to the prescribed inspired oxygen tension (FiO_2), accumulated in a receptacle within the machine, and delivered to the patient using one of many available modes of ventilation. Flow is either volume-targeted and pressure-variable, or pressure-limited and volume-variable. There are two phases in the respiratory cycle, high lung volume and lower lung volume (inhalation and exhalation). Gas exchange occurs in both phases. Inhalation serves to replenish alveolar

gas. Prolonging the higher volume cycle duration enhances oxygen uptake while increasing intrathoracic pressure and reducing the time available for CO_2 removal. A variety of mechanical ventilators exist, including:

▶ *Positive pressure.* These ventilators require an artificial airway (endotracheal or tracheostomy tube) and use positive pressure to force gas into a patient's lungs. Inspiration can be triggered either by the patient or the machine. There are four types of positive-pressure ventilators:

■ *Volume-cycled.* This type, which is the most commonly used in critical care environments, delivers a preset tidal volume, then allows passive expiration. This is ideal for patients with acute respiratory distress syndrome (ARDS) or bronchospasm, since the same tidal volume is delivered regardless of the amount of airway resistance.

■ *Pressure-cycled.* These ventilators, which are also commonly used in the critical care environment, deliver gases at a preset pressure, then allow passive expiration. The benefit of this type is a decreased risk of lung damage from high inspiratory pressures, which is particularly beneficial for neonates who have a small lung capacity. The disadvantage is that the tidal volume delivered can decrease if the patient has poor lung compliance and increased airway resistance. This type of ventilation is usually used for short term therapy (less than 24 hours). Some ventilators can provide both volume-cycled and pressure-cycled ventilation.

■ *Flow-cycled.* This type delivers oxygenation until a preset flow rate is achieved during inspiration.

■ *Time-cycled.* This type delivers oxygenation over a preset time period. These types of ventilators are not used as frequently as the volume-cycled and pressure-cycled ventilators.

▶ *Negative pressure.* Negative-pressure ventilation is typically only used in a few situations. These units allow negative pressure to be applied only to the patient's chest by using a combination of a form-fitted shell and a soft bladder. Rather than connecting to an artificial airway as with the more modern ventilators, these ventilators were designed to enclose the body from the outside so that when the gas is pulled out of the ventilator chamber, the resulting negative pressure causes the chest wall to expand, which pulls air into the lungs. For exhalation to occur, cessation of the negative pressure causes the chest wall to fall. These devices can be used for patients with neuromuscular disorders, especially those with some residual muscular function, because they do not require a tracheostomy with its inherent problems.

Modes of Ventilation

The mode of ventilation refers to how a machine ventilates a patient compared to the patient's respiratory efforts (http://www.enotes.com/ventilators-reference/ventilators).

Control Ventilation (CV). CV, which delivers the preset volume or pressure regardless of the patient's own inspiratory efforts, is used for patients who cannot initiate their breath. If used with spontaneously breathing patients, they must be sedated and/or pharmacologically paralyzed, so they do not breathe out of synchrony with the ventilator.

Assist-control Ventilation (AC) or Continuous Mandatory Ventilation (CMV). AC or CMV, which delivers a preset volume or pressure in response to the patient's inspiratory effort, initiates the breath if the patient does not do so within a preset amount of time. This mode is used for patients who can initiate a breath but who have weakened respiratory muscles. The patient may need to be sedated to limit the number of spontaneous breaths, as hyperventilation can occur in patients with high respiratory rates.

Synchronous Intermittent Mandatory Ventilation (SIMV). SIMV, which delivers a preset volume or pressure and a preset respiratory rate while allowing the patient to breathe spontaneously, initiates each breath in synchrony with the patient's breaths. SIMV is used as a primary mode of ventilation as well as a weaning mode. (During weaning, the preset rate is gradually reduced, allowing the patient to slowly return to breathing independently.) The disadvantage of this mode is that it may increase the effort of breathing and cause respiratory muscle fatigue. (Breathing spontaneously through ventilator tubing has been compared to breathing through a straw.)

Positive-end Expiratory Pressure (PEEP). PEEP, which is positive pressure that is applied by the ventilator at the end of expiration and does not deliver breaths, but is used as an adjunct to CV, AC, and SIMV to improve oxygenation by opening collapsed alveoli at the end of expiration. Complications from the increased pressure can include decreased cardiac output, lung rupture, and increased intracranial pressure.

Constant Positive Airway Pressure (CPAP). CPAP is similar to PEEP, except that it works only for patients who are breathing spontaneously. The effect of CPAP (and PEEP) is compared to inflating a balloon but not letting it completely deflate before inflating it again. The second inflation is easier to perform because resistance is decreased. CPAP can also be administered using a mask and CPAP machine for patients who do not require mechanical ventilation but who need respiratory support (eg, patients with sleep apnea).

Pressure Support Ventilation (PSV). PSV is preset pressure that augments the patient's spontaneous inspiration effort and decreases the work of breathing. The patient completely controls the respiratory rate and tidal volume. PSV is used for patients with a stable respiratory status and is often used with SIMV during weaning.

Independent Lung Ventilation (ILV). This method is used to ventilate each lung separately in patients with unilateral lung disease or a different disease process in each lung. It requires a double-lumen endotracheal tube and two ventilators. Sedation and pharmacologic paralysis are used to facilitate optimal ventilation and increase comfort for the patient in whom this method is used.

High-frequency Ventilation (HFV). HFV delivers a small amount of gas rapidly (as many as 60 to 100 breaths per minute). It is used when conventional mechanical ventilation compromises hemodynamic stability, during short-term

procedures, or for patients at high risk for lung rupture. Sedation and/or pharmacologic paralysis are required.

Inverse Ratio Ventilation (IRV). The normal inspiratory: expiratory ratio is 1:2, but this is reversed during IRV to 2:1 or greater (a maximum of 4:1). This method is used for patients who are still hypoxic, even with the use of PEEP. Longer inspiratory time increases the amount of air in the lungs at the end of expiration (the functional residual capacity) and improves oxygenation by reexpanding any collapsed alveoli. The shorter expiratory time prevents the alveoli from collapsing again. This method requires sedation and therapeutic paralysis because it is very uncomfortable for the patient.

Monitoring Equipment

Arterial Line. The arterial line (A-line) is connected to a pressure transducer that provides a way to constantly measure a patient's blood pressure and also provides access for frequent blood sampling, thereby avoiding repeated needle punctures. An A-line is typically inserted into one of four arteries: radial, femoral, dorsal pedal, or axillary. Arterial lines are usually changed every 4 to 5 days to decrease the risk of infection. Accidental displacement of an A-line is a life-threatening emergency, as significant blood loss can occur very quickly unless direct pressure is promptly applied to the insertion site.

Cardiac Leads. A series of 12 leads connected to the anterior chest to monitor the heart's electrical activity.

Pulse Oximeter. A noninvasive method allowing the monitoring of the saturation of a patient's hemoglobin levels in the blood. Usually, an external clip is attached to the patient's fingertip or earlobe.

Pulmonary Artery Catheterization (Swan-Ganz). Initially developed for the management of acute myocardial infarction, this catheter has gained widespread use in managing a variety of critical illnesses and surgical procedures such as the diagnosis of idiopathic pulmonary hypertension, valvular disease, intracardiac shunts, cardiac tamponade, and pulmonary embolus (PE). The catheter is inserted into the internal jugular or the femoral vein and is then glided into the basilic or subclavian vein before being passed into the right atrium of the heart, the right ventricle, and then out through the pulmonary artery. The catheter, designed to provide accurate and continuous pulmonary artery pressure measurements, can detect even subtle changes in right-sided heart pressure and the lung arteries. The catheter can also be used to draw blood samples. Normal readings are as follows[19]:

► Right atrium: 0-8 mmHg

► Right ventricle: 15-25/0 mmHg

► Pulmonary artery: 15-25/5-15 mmHg

► Pulmonary capillary wedge pressure: 9-23/1-12 mmHg

Accidental displacement of this device creates a life-threatening emergency for the patient, as significant blood loss can occur quickly unless direct pressure is promptly applied to the insertion site.

Intracranial Pressure (ICP) Monitor. Cerebrospinal fluid (CSF) is a colorless, clear fluid produced by the highly vascular choroid plexus in the lateral third and fourth ventricles that functions as a cushion for the brain and spinal cord. ICP monitoring, which calculates the pressure exerted against the skull by brain tissue, blood, or CSF, is a common practice when treating intracranial pathology with risk for elevated ICP, including patients who have sustained a closed head injury, a cerebral hemorrhage, or an overproduction of CSF. Normal values are between 5-15 mmHg, and anything greater than 20 mmHg is considered abnormal. When the brain suffers an insult or injury, changes occur that affect cerebral hemodynamics, including changes in ICP, cerebral blood flow, and oxygen delivery. ICP data are very useful to help predict outcomes and worsening intracranial pathology, such as cerebral edema or hemorrhage. Intraventricular catheters, which are antibiotic-impregnated and coated ventricular catheters to prevent infections, are considered the gold standard for measuring ICP because they are placed directly into the ventricle and are attached to a pressure transducer. An external ventricular device can assist with controlling increased ICP by allowing for therapeutic CSF drainage.

CLINICAL PEARL

Extreme care must be taken with patients who have an ICP inserted when raising the head of the bed (increases the drainage, thereby lowering the ICP) or lowering the head of the bed below 30° (increases the ICP). Also, activities such as isometric exercises and the Valsalva maneuver have been shown to increase ICP and should therefore be avoided. Other precautions include:

▶ Avoiding hip flexion greater than 90°

▶ Avoiding head-chest neck flexion

▶ Avoiding placing the patient in the prone or Trendelenburg position

▶ Avoid lowering the patient's head more than 15° below horizontal

Oxygen Delivery Systems

Nasal Cannula. A device with two plastic prongs, inserted into each of the patient's nostrils, which delivers supplemental oxygen or airflow to a patient who requires low to moderate oxygen concentrations.

Oronasal Mask. A triangular plastic device covered with small vent holes that covers the patient's nose and mouth and allows exhaled air to be expelled.

Tracheotomy/Tracheostomy. This is a method to provide a semi-permanent, or permanent, oxygen delivery system to a patient via an incision on the anterior aspect of the neck to form a direct connection with the trachea and to allow a patient to breathe without the use of his or her mouth or nose. The tracheostomy is a 2- to 3-inch-long (51- to 76-mm) curved metal or plastic tube connected to a wall unit via a long plastic tube inserted into a tracheostomy stoma to maintain a patent airway. This type of procedure is usually not used unless the patient has had an endotracheal tube in for an extended period and cannot be weaned from the ventilator. Indications in the acute setting include severe facial trauma, head

and neck cancers, and large congenital tumors of the head and neck. Indications in the chronic setting include the need for long-term mechanical ventilation and tracheal hygiene.

THE GRIEVING PROCESS

It is not uncommon for a healthcare provider to encounter a patient who has suffered the loss of someone or something close to them (loved one, pet, a job, or possibly a role—entering retirement). Grief is a normal and natural response to a loss, so it is important to realize that acknowledging the grief promotes the healing process. There are various ways in which individuals respond to loss, some healthy and some that may hinder the grieving process.

CLINICAL PEARL

Factors that can hinder the grieving process include:

▶ Avoidance or minimization of one's emotions.

▶ Use of alcohol or drugs to self-medicate.

▶ Use of work (over-function at the workplace) to avoid feelings,

Healthy responses to grief include:

▶ Allowing sufficient time to experience thoughts and feelings openly to oneself.

▶ Acknowledging and accepting all feelings, both positive and negative.

▶ Using a journal to document the healing process.

▶ Confiding in a trusted individual.

▶ Expressing feelings openly. Crying offers a release.

▶ Identifying any unfinished business and attempting to come to a resolution.

▶ Attending bereavement groups that can provide an opportunity to share grief with others who have experienced a similar loss.

Invariably an individual passes through a series of stages during the grieving process. These stages reflect various reactions that may surface as an individual makes sense of how a loss affects them. Experiencing and accepting all feelings remains an important part of the healing process. Elizabeth Kubler Ross[20] identified several stages that occur during the grieving process:

▶ *Stage 1:* Shock, numbness, and denial.

  ▪ Shock usually occurs as the initial reaction to psychological trauma or severe and sudden physical injury.[21] During stressful situations, individuals express themselves through physiologic and emotional responses. These reactions serve to protect the individual from an overwhelming experience.

  ▪ Numbness is a normal reaction to an immediate loss and should not be confused with lack of caring.

  ▪ Denial is often used as a defense mechanism to alleviate anxiety and pain associated with a disability or illness.[21]

Denial and feelings of disbelief occur as a specific phase early in the adaptation process and serve to protect the person from having to confront the overwhelming implications of illness or injury at once.[21] Denial and disbelief will diminish as the individual slowly acknowledges the impact of this loss and accompanying feelings.

It is common for people to avoid making decisions or taking action at this point.

▶ *Stage 2:* Anger. This reaction usually occurs when an individual feels helpless and powerless. Anger may result from feeling abandoned, occurring in cases of loss through death. Feelings of resentment may occur toward one's higher power or life in general for the injustice of this loss. After an individual acknowledges anger, guilt may surface because of expressing these negative feelings.

Making decisions at this point is difficult because an individual's energy is focused on emotion rather than on problem-solving.

▶ *Stage 3:* Depression and detachment. After recognizing the true extent of the loss, some individuals may experience depressive symptoms. Sleep and appetite disturbance, lack of energy and concentration, and crying spells are some typical symptoms. Feelings of loneliness, emptiness, isolation, and self-pity can also surface during this phase, contributing to this reactive depression. For many, this phase must be experienced to begin reorganizing one's life.

▶ *Stage 4:* Dialogue and bargaining. People become more willing to explore alternatives after expressing their feelings. At times, individuals may ruminate about what could have been done to prevent the loss. Individuals can become preoccupied with ways that things could have been better, imagining all the things that will never be. This reaction can provide insight into the impact of the loss; however, intense feelings of remorse or guilt may hinder the healing process if not properly resolved. This phase may be marked by externalized hostility toward other people or objects in the environment.

▶ *Stage 5:* Acceptance. Time allows the individual an opportunity to resolve the range of feelings that surface. Acknowledgment is the first sign that the patient has accepted or recognized the condition's permanency and its future implications.[21] Decisions are much easier to make because people have found new purpose and meaning as they have begun to accept the loss. Adjustment is the final phase in adaptation and involves the development of new ways of interacting successfully with others and one's environment.[21]

Physical Therapy Approach During the Grieving Process

▶ Discuss quality-of-life issues with patient/family.

▶ Make time for grief work.

▶ Focus on the positive: realize and maximize all clinical opportunities.

▶ Learn to deal with the patient's or family's anger during the discharge crisis.

▶ Realize the importance of comfort measures and pain management to patient/family.

▶ Work with appropriate pastoral supports.

▶ Try to engage the patient's interest in things.

▶ Respect the needs of privacy, independence, and decathexis (the gradual weakening and separating of emotional ties) of the patient.

REFERENCES

1. Corrigan B, Maitland GD. *Practical Orthopaedic Medicine.* Boston: Butterworth; 1985.
2. Cimon K, Featherstone R. *Jewellery and Nail Polish Worn by Health Care Workers and the Risk of Infection Transmission: A Review of Clinical Evidence and Guidelines.* Ottawa, Ontario, Canada: Canadian Agency for Drugs and Technologies in Health; 2017.
3. Kovacek P, Powers D, Iglarsh ZA, et al. Task force on leadership, administration, and management preparation (LAMP). *The Resource.* 1999;29:8-13.
4. Lopopolo RB, Schafer DS, Nosse LJ. Leadership, administration, management, and professionalism (LAMP) in physical therapy: A Delphi study. *Phy Ther.* 2004;84:137-150.
5. Abrishami D. The need for cultural competency in health care. *Radiol Technol.* 2018;89:441-448.
6. Desapriya E, Mehrnoush V, Bandara AN. Cultural competency and culturally safe clinical care. *CMAJ.* 2018;190:E84.
7. Gergely SW. Cultural Competency matters: Calling for a deeper understanding of healthcare disparities among murse leaders. *J Nursing Adm.* 2018;48:474-477.
8. Pullen P, Moore HM. Cultural competency in health care. *Tenn Med.* 2009;102:31.
9. Brawley LR, Culos-Reed SN. Studying adherence to therapeutic regimens: Overview, theories, recommendations. *Control Clin Trials.* 2000;21:156S-1563S.
10. Lenze EJ, Munin MC, Quear T, Dew MA, Rogers JC, Begley AE, et al. The Pittsburgh Rehabilitation Participation Scale: Reliability and validity of a clinician-rated measure of participation in acute rehabilitation. *Arch Phys Med Rehabil.* 2004;85:380-384.
11. Litzinger ME, Osif B. Accommodating diverse learning styles: Designing instruction for electronic information sources. In: Shirato L, ed. *What Is Good Instruction Now? Library Instruction for the 90s.* Ann Arbor, MI: Pierian Press; 1993:26-50.
12. Decoster A, Grandbastien B, Demory MF, Leclercq V, Alfandari S. A prospective study of nosocomial-infection-related mortality assessed through mortality reviews in 14 hospitals in northern France. *J Hosp Infect.* 2012;80:310-315.
13. Monegro AF, Muppidi V, Regunath H. Hospital Acquired Infections. [Updated 2020 Sep 3]. In: StatPearls [Internet]. Treasure Island (FL): StatPearls Publishing; 2021 Jan. Available from: https://www.ncbi.nlm.nih.gov/books/NBK441857/ StatPearls. Treasure Island, FL; 2021.
14. Goodman CC, Kelly Snyder TE. Infectious disease. In Goodman CC, Boissonnault WG, Fuller KS, eds. *Pathology: Implications for the Physical Therapist,* 2nd ed. Philadelphia: Saunders; 2003:194-235.
15. Bass JW, Wittler RR, Weisse ME. Social smile and occult bacteremia. *Pediatr Infect Dis J.* 1996;15:541.
16. Black JG. Epidemiology and nosocomial infections. *Microbiology Principles and Applications,* 7th ed. Upper Saddle River, NJ: Prentice Hall; 2008:426-462.
17. University of North Carolina hospitals: understanding isolation precautions. http://www.unc.edu/~rlensley/tb2.htm#PROTECTIVE. UNC Hospitals' Precautions for the Prevention of Disease Transmission: Protective Precautions; updated August 10, 2012.
18. Adler J, Malone D. Early mobilization in the intensive care unit: A systematic review. *Cardiopulm Phys Ther J.* 2012;23:5-13.
19. Rodriguez Ziccardi M, Khalid N. *Pulmonary Artery Catheterization.* StatPearls. Treasure Island (FL); 2021.
20. Kübler-Ross E. *On Death and Dying.* New York: Macmillan; 1969.
21. Precin P. Influence of psychosocial factors on rehabilitation. In O'Sullivan SB, Schmitz TJ, eds. *Physical Rehabilitation,* 5th ed. Philadelphia: F. A. Davis; 2007:27-63.

CHAPTER 6

Monitoring Vital Signs

OVERVIEW

The triad of pulse, respiration rate, and blood pressure is often considered as a baseline indicator of a patient's health status, which is why each is called a *vital* or *cardinal sign*. All four practice patterns in the *Guide to Physical Therapist Practice*[1] include measuring pulse, blood pressure, and respiration as a routine part of any physiologic examination. Temperature is not included because physical therapist assistants (PTA) do not routinely assess it. However, as a temperature can often provide an important clue to the severity of the patient's illness, particularly the presence of infection, it is discussed in this chapter. Additional physiologic status measurements, which are not universally considered vital signs, include assessing perceived exertion ratings, pain, and pulse oximetry.

Clinical indicators that highlight the need to monitor vital signs include dyspnea, hypertension, fatigue, syncope, chest pain, irregular heart rate, cyanosis, intermittent claudication, nausea, diaphoresis, and pedal edema. Certain patient populations also warrant a vital sign assessment, including elderly patients (older than 65 years), very young patients (younger than two years), debilitated patients, patients with a history of physical inactivity, and patients recovering from a recent trauma. The measurement of vital signs can also assess a patient's response to activity.

It is worth remembering that several variables can influence the results of the vital signs measurements. These include caffeine consumption, alcohol consumption, tobacco use, physical activity level, medications, and the use of illegal drugs.[2] The other variables that can influence the results are outlined in Table 6-1.

CLINICAL PEARL

▶ Pulse oximetry (**Figure 6-1**) is an important related measure, as it provides information on arterial blood oxygen saturation levels.

▶ Pain is considered by many to be a vital symptom.[3-12]

HEART RATE

When the heart muscle of the left ventricle contracts, blood is ejected into the aorta, and the aorta stretches. At this point, the distention wave (pulse wave) is most pronounced and can be detected as a pulse at certain points around the body. The pulse rate (or frequency) is the number of pulsations (peripheral pulse waves) per minute.

CLINICAL PEARL

In most people, the pulse is an accurate measure of heart rate. However, in certain cases, including arrhythmias, the heart rate can be (much) higher than the pulse rate. In these cases, the heart rate should be determined by auscultation of the central pulse at the heart apex (fifth interspace, midclavicular vertical line, also known as the apical pulse or point of maximal impulse [PMI]). The pulse deficit

Figure 6-1 to Figure 6-7, Figure 6-10 to Figure 6-19 are all reproduced with permission from Dutton M: Introduction to Physical Therapy and Patient Skills, 2nd ed. New York, NY: McGraw Hill; 2014.

TABLE 6-1	Variables That Can Influence Vital Signs Data
Hormonal status	
Age	
Stress	
Obesity	
Diet	
Gender	
Family history	
Time of day	
Menstruation	
General health status	
Pain	

(the difference between heartbeats and pulsations at the periphery) is determined by simultaneous palpation at the radial artery and auscultation at the heart apex. Except in cardiac disease or peripheral arterial disease, the apical and radial pulse rates will be equal. Suppose there is a difference between the apical and radial pulse rates. In that case, only the apical pulse should be used to assess the patient, and the differences should be noted in the patient's medical record.

The pulse, measured in beats per minute (bpm), is taken to obtain information about the cardiovascular system's resting state and its response to activity or exercise and recovery.[13] Such information includes the resting heart rate, the pulse quality, the pulse amplitude, and any irregularities in the rhythm.[13]

▶ *Resting heart rate:* the normal adult heart rate is 70 bpm, with a range of 60 to 80 bpm. A rate greater than 100 bpm is referred to as tachycardia. Normal causes of tachycardia include anxiety, stress, pain, caffeine, dehydration, or exercise. A rate of less than 60 bpm is referred to as bradycardia. Athletes may normally have a resting heart rate lower than 60 bpm. The normal range of resting heart rate in children is between 80 and 120 bpm. The rate for a newborn is 120 bpm (normal range 70 to 170 bpm).

▶ *Pulse quality:* a pulse's quality refers to the amount of force created by the ejected blood against the arterial wall

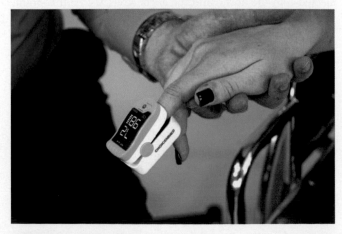

FIGURE 6-1 Pulse oximeter.

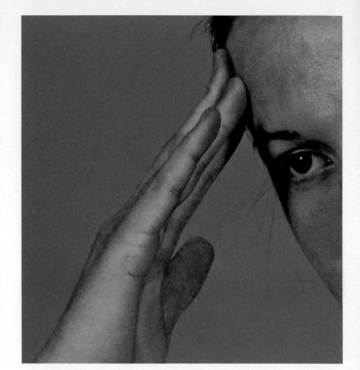

FIGURE 6-2 Pulse point—temporal.

during each ventricular contraction.[14] The quality can be described as thready (a weak and irregular heart rate), weak (poor force), strong (good force), regular (even beats), or irregular (both strong and weak beats or uneven beats).

▶ *Pulse amplitude:* the pulse amplitude indicates the heart's efficiency in pushing blood into the arteries and placing pressure on the vessel's walls. A high volume may result in a bounding pulse, whereas a low volume may present as a weak or thready pulse.

▶ *Rhythm irregularities:* the pulse rhythm is the pattern of pulsations and the intervals between them.[14] In a healthy individual, the rhythm is regular and indicates that the time intervals between pulse beats are essentially equal. Arrhythmia or dysrhythmia refers to an irregular rhythm in which pulses are not evenly spaced.[14]

As the pulse travels toward the peripheral blood vessels, it gradually diminishes and becomes faster.

The pulse can be taken at several points, including the temporal (Figure 6-2), carotid (Figure 6-3), brachial (Figure 6-4), radial (Figure 6-5), femoral (within the femoral triangle), popliteal (Figure 6-6), dorsal pedal (Figure 6-7), and posterior tibial artery (Table 6-2).

CLINICAL PEARL

The most accessible pulse points are usually the radial or carotid pulse. The radial pulse is normally used when the patient is alert and active, whereas the carotid pulse is used when detecting the pulse is critical.

On occasion, a specific pulse point site is chosen based on the patient's condition. For example, points in the lower

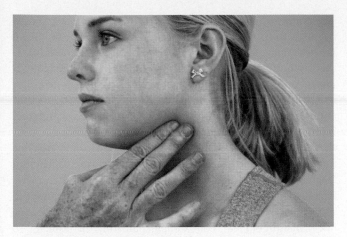

FIGURE 6-3 Pulse point—carotid.

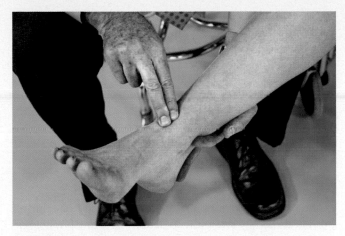

FIGURE 6-7 Pulse point—dorsal pedal.

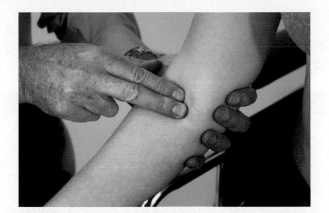

FIGURE 6-4 Pulse point—brachial.

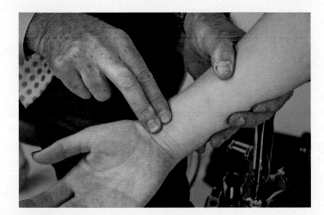

FIGURE 6-5 Pulse point—radial.

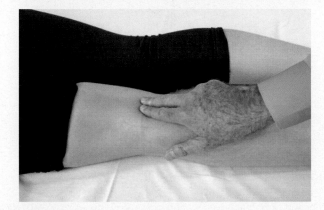

FIGURE 6-6 Pulse point—popliteal.

extremity may be used with a patient who has peripheral vascular disease—if there is an arterial occlusion of the knee, the groin's pulse will be stronger than the pulse palpated at the foot.

CLINICAL PEARL

The carotid artery should be palpated gently to avoid stimulating the baroreceptors, which can provoke severe bradycardia or even stop the heart in some sensitive persons.

For enhanced patient comfort, the clinician should stand on the same side as the carotid artery being assessed.

At no time should both carotid arteries be palpated simultaneously, as this can potentially cut off blood supply to the brain.

TABLE 6-2	Palpation Sites for Pulse Reading
Pulse	**Location**
Radial	The distal radial artery is located on the lateral (thumb) side of the wrist's anterior surface.
Carotid	The carotid artery is located to the side of the larynx and medial to the sternocleidomastoid muscle.
Brachial	In an adult, the brachial artery is located in the antibrachial fossa, just medial to the biceps brachii tendon. In an infant, the brachial artery can be located in the middle of the upper arm.
Temporal	The temporal artery is located at a point anterior and adjacent to the ear.
Femoral	The femoral artery is located at the femoral triangle, slightly lateral and anterior to the inguinal crease.
Popliteal	The popliteal artery is located at the midline of the posterior knee crease, between the tendons of the hamstring muscles.
Dorsal pedal	The dorsal pedal artery is located along the midline or slightly medial on the foot's posterior aspect.
Posterior tibial	The posterior tibial artery is located on the foot's medial aspect, inferior to the medial malleolus.

One should avoid using the thumb when taking a pulse, as it has its own pulse that can interfere with the detection of the patient's pulse. When taking a pulse, the fingers must be placed near the artery and pressed gently against a firm structure, usually a bone.

The main objective in taking a patient's pulse rate during a physical therapy session is to determine if any physiologic response occurs during activity. The response can vary greatly depending on the patient's condition and activity intensity. In addition to activity level, several factors can affect the pulse rate. These include:

▶ *Medications.* Medications can cause the pulse rate to either increase or decrease.

▶ *Pacemaker.* Pacemakers are designed to maintain the heart rate within a specific range, irrespective of other factors.

▶ *Emotional status.* The pulse rate typically increases during episodes of high stress, anxiety, and fear. For example, the patient may be nervous being in a medical facility.

▶ *Age.* Adolescents and younger people typically exhibit an increased rate, whereas those older than 65 may exhibit a decreased rate.

▶ *Gender.* Male pulse rates are usually slightly lower than female rates.

▶ *The temperature of the environment.* A pulse rate tends to increase with higher temperatures and decrease with lower temperatures.

▶ *Pathology.* A high resting pulse rate, a marker of sympathetic overactivity, is associated with coronary artery disease, stroke, sudden death, and noncardiovascular diseases.[15,16] Also, an active infection with an associated fever can increase the pulse rate.

▶ *Physical conditioning.* Individuals who perform frequent, sustained, and vigorous aerobic exercise tend to exhibit a lower than normal pulse rate.

Abnormal responses to an increase in activity level include the following:

▶ The pulse rate does not increase or only increases slowly.

▶ The pulse rate declines before the intensity of the activity declines.

▶ The rate of the pulse increase exceeds the level expected for a particular activity.

▶ The pulse rate demonstrates an abnormal rhythm.

Procedure. The clinician washes his or her hands, obtains a timepiece that measures seconds, and explains the procedure to the patient. The patient is typically seated but may also be recumbent or standing. The clinician selects an arterial site and gently places two fingertips over the artery. Gentle pressure is applied to the point when the patient's pulse can be detected.

The count, which is performed silently in the head, typically begins with the first beat after a time interval. For example, if the interval begins when a digital counter is at 0 seconds, "1" is the first beat felt after the 0 starting point. Alternatively, the clinician starts the time frame when the first beat is felt. The length of time for taking the pulse depends on the patient's situation. For example, the clinician can palpate for 15 seconds and multiply by 4 (or 30 seconds and multiply by 2) with a regular rhythm (evenly spaced beats), or 60 seconds for a baseline measurement, or in the presence of a regularly irregular rhythm (regular pattern overall with "skipped" beats) or irregularly irregular rhythm (chaotic, no real pattern). It is important to remember that the shorter duration of palpation produces a larger margin of error. For example, palpating the beats for 10 seconds and multiplying by six results in a 6 beats/min margin of error, whereas palpating the beats for 30 seconds and multiplying by two only results in a 2 beats/min margin of error. The clinician documents the findings regarding the location used, the number of beats per minute, the patient position, and any variation in the rhythm or volume.

Although the simplest way to assess the heart rate is by measuring the pulse, the most accurate way to examine heart rhythm is to use an electrocardiogram (ECG or EKG).[17] This method is used frequently in the inpatient setting. By placing 4-12 electrodes on the skin near the patient's heart, a typical ECG can provide information about the heart's electrical activity by tracing the rate, rhythm, and waveform of a normal heartbeat. This tracing is represented by a P wave, QRS complex, and T wave (Figure 6-8). Each of these characteristics represents a portion of the cardiac cycle (Figure 6-9). In addition to

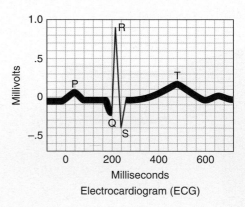

FIGURE 6-8 Electrocardiogram tracing showing PQRST waves. (Reproduced with permission from Van de Graaff KM, Fox SI: Concepts of human anatomy and physiology, 5th ed. New York, NY: McGraw Hill; 1999.)

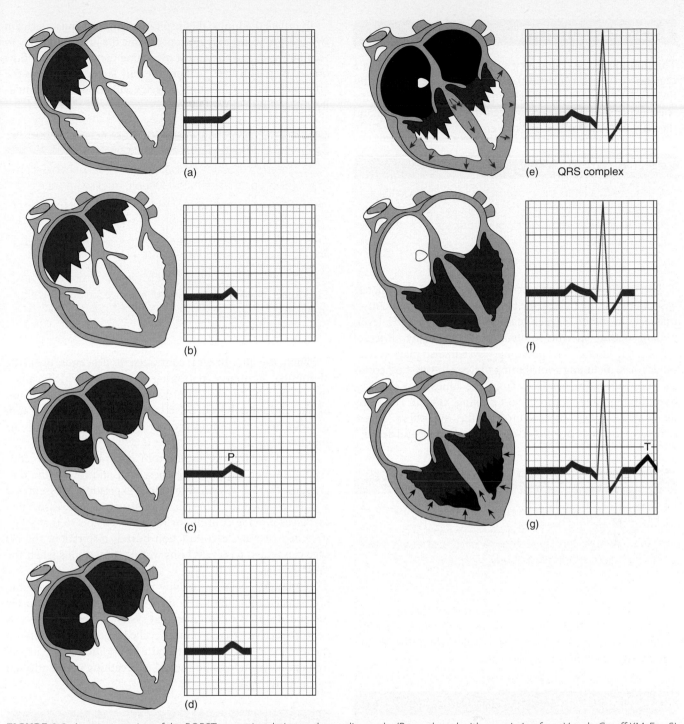

(a)

(b)

(c) P

(d)

(e) QRS complex

(f)

(g) T

FIGURE 6-9 A representation of the PQRST waves in relation to the cardiac cycle. (Reproduced with permission from Van de Graaff KM, Fox SI: Concepts of human anatomy and physiology, 5th ed. New York, NY: McGraw Hill; 1999.)

the more familiar P, QRS, and T waveforms, the J point, which occurs at the end of the QRS complex and the beginning of the ST segment, is also commonly documented, as it represents the end of depolarization and the beginning of repolarization. Although it is not within the scope of practice for a PTA to interpret an ECG's findings, it is important to know what each waveform represents when reading medical records.

The heart rate can also be monitored during a patient's activities of daily living (ADLs) through the use of a Holter monitor, a small device attached to the patient's belt that monitors the patient's heart rate through a series of electrodes placed on the patient's chest.

CLINICAL PEARL

Many recreational and serious athletes, who want to monitor cardiac activity during exercise, use a chest strap monitor with a watch-like receiver that displays a continuous reading of heart rate. These monitors can alert the user if the heart rate falls outside the desired range during exercise. Although these monitors provide an easy method of monitoring a heart rate, most cannot detect heart rate disorders (arrhythmias) or abnormal heart rhythms (dysrhythmias), and they may vary in their validity and reliability[18,19]

107

RESPIRATION RATE

The pulmonary or respiratory system is contained within a cagelike structure, consisting of the sternum, 12 pairs of ribs, the clavicle, and the thoracic spine's vertebrae. The normal chest expansion difference between the resting position and the fully inhaled position is 2 to 4 cm.

CLINICAL PEARL

Any factor that limits the movement of the rib cage results in limited respiration. Such factors include body position and posture and pathologic conditions such as scoliosis and osteoporosis.

The respiratory system's primary function is to exchange gases between the tissues, the blood, and the environment so that arterial blood oxygen, carbon dioxide, and pH levels remain within specific limits throughout many different physiologic limits.[20] The pulmonary system also plays several other roles, including contributing to temperature homeostasis via evaporative heat loss from the lungs and filtering, humidifying, and warming or cooling the air to body temperature.[20] This process protects the respiratory system structures from damage caused by dry gases or harmful debris.[20]

CLINICAL PEARL

- *External respiration:* the exchange of gases between the atmosphere and the blood
- *Internal respiration:* the exchange of gases between the blood and the cells of the body

For inspiration to occur, the lungs must be able to expand when stretched—they must have high compliance. For expiration to occur, the lungs must get smaller when this tension is released—they must have elasticity.

CLINICAL PEARL

- *Ventilation:* the movement of air through the conducting airways
- *Respiration:* a term used to describe the gas exchange within the body

The diaphragm, innervated by the phrenic nerve, is the primary muscle of inspiration, with the ribs serving as levers. The 11 internal and external intercostals, which connect one rib to the next, serve to elevate the ribs and increase thoracic volume.[21]

- The external intercostals function to elevate the ribs and to increase thoracic volume.
- The internal intercostals function to lower the ribs, thereby decreasing thoracic volume.[19]

To inflate the lungs, the inspiratory muscles must perform two types of work: they must overcome the lung's tendency to recoil inward, and they must overcome the resistance to flow offered by the airways.[22] Therefore, any factor that affects the efficiency of the respiratory muscles will also affect the quality and quantity of respiration.

CLINICAL PEARL

The accessory muscles of inspiration are used when a more rapid or deep inhalation is required or in disease states.

- The scalenes and sternocleidomastoid raise the upper two ribs.
- The levator costarum and serratus raise the remaining ribs.

  Also, by fixing the shoulder girdle, the trapezius, pectorals, and serratus anterior can become inspiration muscles.

When the diaphragm contracts, it descends over the abdominal contents, flattening the dome, which causes the lower ribs to move outward, resulting in protrusion of the abdominal wall. Also, the contracting diaphragm causes a decrease in intrathoracic pressure, which pulls air into the lungs.[21]

Normal inspiration results from inspiratory muscle contraction, which expands the chest wall and lowers the diaphragm. During relaxed breathing, expiration is essentially a passive process.[14] The rib cage structure and associated cartilages provide continuous inelastic tension so that when stretched by muscle contraction during inspiration, the rib cage can return passively to its resting dimensions when the muscles relax.[22]

Respiratory muscle activity involves multiple neural, mechanical, and chemical control components and is closely integrated with the cardiovascular system.[14] The spontaneous neuronal activity that produces cyclic breathing originates in the respiratory centers in the brain. In addition to the neural influences, the automatic control of breathing is also affected by chemoreceptors.[20]

CLINICAL PEARL

Three chemical levels in particular play a critical role in controlling respiration: the blood acid-base balance (pH—related to the concentration of free-floating hydrogen ions within the body), the partial pressure of carbon dioxide within the arterial blood bicarbonate (PaCO$_2$), and the number of bicarbonate ions within the arterial blood (HCO$_3^-$).

Other factors that influence respiration include[14]:

- *Age:* the newborn's resting rate is between 25 and 50 breaths per minute, a rate that gradually slows until adulthood when it ranges between 12 and 16 breaths per minute.

► *Body size and stature:* men generally have a larger vital capacity than women, and adults larger than adolescents and children. Tall, thin individuals generally have a larger vital capacity than stout or obese individuals.

► *Exercise:* resting rate and debt increase with exercise due to increased oxygen demand and carbon dioxide production.

► *Body position:* the recumbent position can significantly affect respiration by compressing the chest against the supporting surface and pressure from abdominal organs against the diaphragm.

► *Environment:* exposure to pollutants such as gas and particle emissions, asbestos, chemical waste products, or coal dust can diminish the ability to transport oxygen.

► *Emotional stress:* can result in an increased rate and depth of respirations.

► *Pharmacologic agents:* any drug that depresses central nervous system (CNS) function will result in respiratory depression. Examples include narcotic agents and barbiturates. Conversely, bronchodilators decrease airway resistance and residual volume with a resultant increase in vital capacity and airflow.

► *Pathology:* several conditions can impact the respiratory system of which there are two main categories:

■ Restrictive. This category results from an inability of the lungs to fully expand. Diseases within this category include pneumonia, tuberculosis, pulmonary fibrosis, and sarcoidosis, but there are also structural causes such as scoliosis, kyphosis, and obesity.

■ Obstructive. This category results from an inability to exhale fully. Diseases within this category include chronic obstructive pulmonary disease (COPD), cystic fibrosis, emphysema, and asthma.

Monitoring the respiratory system involves measuring the rate, rhythm, depth, and character of the patient's breathing using observation and palpation.

► *Rate:* the rate of breathing refers to the number of breaths per minute. Respiration rates over 25 breaths per minute or under 10 breaths per minute (when at rest) may be considered abnormal. An expiration is normally approximately twice as long as an inspiration. The opposite occurs in conditions such as COPD.

► *Rhythm:* The breathing rhythm refers to the breathing pattern's regularity and the interval between each breath.

CLINICAL PEARL

The following breathing patterns are characteristic of disease[23]:

► Cheyne–Stokes respiration, characterized by a periodic, regular, sequentially increasing depth of respiration, occurs with serious cardiopulmonary or cerebral disorders.

► Biot's respiration, characterized by irregular spasmodic breathing and periods of apnea, is almost always associated with hypoventilation due to CNS disease.

► Kussmaul's respiration, characterized by deep, slow breathing, indicates acidosis as the body attempts to blow off carbon dioxide.

► Apneustic breathing is an abnormal pattern of breathing characterized by a postinspiratory pause. The usual cause of apneustic breathing is a pontine lesion.

► Paradoxical respiration is an abnormal breathing pattern in which the abdominal wall is sucked in during inspiration (it is usually pushed out). Paradoxical respiration is due to paralysis of the diaphragm.

► *Depth:* the depth of breathing refers to the amount of air exchange (volume of air being exchanged in the lungs) with each respiration. Deep breathing is associated with greater thoracic expansion, whereas shallow breathing is associated with minimal chest expansion. The clinician should compare both the anterior-posterior diameter and the transverse diameter during rest and at full inhalation.

► *Character:* the character of breathing refers to a deviation from normal, resting, or quiet respiration. A normal breathing response would be an increase in the respiratory rate and depth with exercise. The Borg scale of Rate of Perceived Exertion (RPE) is commonly used to assess breathing intensity based on activity (Table 6-3). An abnormal breathing response would be a difficulty with breathing (dyspnea) in a patient at rest. Also, normal breathing is barely audible. Abnormal breathing can be associated with some distinguishing characteristics (Tables 6-4 and 6-5).

Several pieces of equipment are required to assess the respiration rate, including a timing device and a tape measure.

TABLE 6-3	Rating of Perceived Exertion	
Traditional Scale	**Verbal Rating**	**Revised 10-Grade Scale**
6	No exertion at all	0
7	Very, very light	0.5
8		
9	Very light	1.0
10		
11	Light	
12	Fairly light	2.0
13	Moderate	3.0
14	Somewhat hard	4.0
15	Hard (heavy)	5.0
16		6.0
17	Very hard	7.0
18		8.0
19	Very, very (extremely) hard	9.0
20	Maximal (exhaustion)	10.0

Data from Borg GA: Psychophysical basis of perceived exertion. *Med Sci Sports Exerc.* 1982:14(5);377–381; *Borg's Perceived Exertion and Pain Scales.* Champaign, IL: Human Kinetics;1998.

TABLE 6-4	Abnormal Breathing Patterns
Pattern	**Description**
Cheyne-Stokes	A common and bizarre breathing pattern, characterized by alternating periods of apnea and hyperpnea. Typically, over 1 minute, a 10- to 20-second episode of apnea or hypopnea is observed, followed by respirations of increasing depth and frequency. The cycle then repeats itself. Despite periods of apnea, significant hypoxia rarely occurs. This breathing pattern occurs in congestive heart failure, encephalitis, cerebral circulatory disturbances, and drug overdose, manifesting as a lesion of the bulbar center of respiration. However, the breathing pattern may also be present as a normal finding in children, healthy adults following fast ascension to great altitudes, or during sleep.
Kussmaul's breathing	Rhythmic, gasping, and very deep respiration with normal or reduced frequency. Associated with severe diabetes or renal acidosis or coma. Also known as air hunger syndrome.
Hyperventilation	Rapid breathing, often due to anxiety.
Biot (ataxic) breathing	Breathing that is irregular in timing and depth. It is indicative of meningitis or medullary lesions.
Apneustic breathing	An abnormal pattern of breathing that is characterized by a postinspiratory pause. The usual cause of apneustic breathing is a pontine lesion.
Paradoxical respiration	An abnormal breathing pattern in which the abdominal wall is sucked in during inspiration (it is usually pushed out). Paradoxical respiration is due to paralysis of the diaphragm.
Sleep apnea	Sleep apnea is defined as the cessation of breathing during sleep. There are three different types of sleep apnea: ▶ *Obstructive:* the most common. This is characterized by repetitive pauses in breathing during sleep due to the obstruction and/or collapse of the upper airway (throat), usually accompanied by a reduction in blood oxygen saturation, followed by an awakening to breathe—called an apnea event. The respiratory effort continues during the episodes of apnea. ▶ *Central:* a neurologic condition causing cessation of all respiratory effort during sleep, usually with decreases in blood oxygen saturation. The person is aroused from sleep by an automatic breathing reflex, so they may end up getting very little sleep at all. ▶ *Mixed:* a combination of the previous two.

TABLE 6-5	Abnormal Breath Sounds
Sound	**Description**
Crackles	Crackles are discontinuous, explosive, "popping" sounds that originate within the airways. They are heard when an obstructed airway suddenly opens, and the pressures on either side of the obstruction suddenly equilibrate, resulting in transient, distinct vibrations in the airway wall. The dynamic airway obstruction can be caused either by an accumulation of secretions within the airway lumen or airway collapse caused by pressure from inflammation or edema in surrounding pulmonary tissue. Crackles can be heard during inspiration when intrathoracic negative pressure results in the opening of the airways or expiration when positive thoracic pressure forces a collapsed or blocked airway to open. Crackles are heard more commonly during inspiration than expiration. They are significant as they imply either accumulation of fluid secretions or exudate within airways or inflammation and edema in the pulmonary tissue.
Wheezes	Continuous musical tones that are most commonly heard at end inspiration or early expiration. Result when a collapsed airway lumen gradually opens during inspiration or gradually closes during expiration. As the airway lumen becomes smaller, the airflow velocity increases, resulting in the airway wall's harmonic vibration and musical tonal quality. It can be classified as either high-pitched or low-pitched wheezes. It can be monophonic (a single pitch and tonal quality heard over an isolated area) or polyphonic (multiple pitches and tones heard over a variable area of the lung). Wheezes are significant because they imply decreased airway lumen diameter caused either by thickening of reactive airway walls or by the collapse of airways due to pressure from surrounding pulmonary disease.
Stridor	Intense continuous monophonic wheezes heard loudest over extrathoracic airways that can often be heard without the aid of a stethoscope. These extrathoracic sounds are often referred down the airways and can often be heard over the thorax. They are often mistaken as pulmonary wheezes. Tend to be accentuated during inspiration when extrathoracic airways collapse due to lower internal lumen pressure. Stridor is significant and indicates upper airway obstruction.
Stertor	A poorly defined and inconsistent term that describes harsh discontinuous crackling sounds heard over the larynx or trachea. Also described as a snoring sound heard over extrathoracic airways. Stertor is significant because it is suggestive of the accumulation of secretions within extrathoracic airways.
Rhonchi	Abnormal dry, leathery sounds in the lungs, which indicate inflammation of the bronchial tubes.

A full assessment of a patient's respiration rate includes all of the following:

- Observation for signs or symptoms of abnormal respiration, including the breathing quality in relation to the patient's activity level.
- Palpation of the patient's radial pulse and a recording of the pulse rate.
- Observation of the patient's rate of breathing. The rate is usually measured when a person is at rest and simply involves counting the number of breaths for 30 seconds and multiplying it by 2. If the total appears abnormal, the clinician should count the breaths for one minute.
- Measurement of chest expansion with inspiration compared to the relaxed state.

CLINICAL PEARL

Pulse oximetry provides a simple way of partly assessing a patient's breathing by measuring arterial blood's oxygen saturation (SpO_2). A two-sided sensor, which monitors the oxygenation of the patient's hemoglobin, is placed on a thin part of the patient's body, usually a fingertip (see Figure 6-1) or earlobe. Factors such as fingernail polish, bright lighting, poor circulation, or temperature can affect the reading. Light consisting of two different wavelengths is passed between one sensor and the other. Depending on the blood's color, these two wavelengths are absorbed differently, and a ratio of the two wavelengths is represented on the digital display as a percentage of oxygen saturation. Oxygen saturation is not affected by age. Acceptable normal ranges for SpO_2 are from 95% to 99%, whereas saturation levels between 88% and 94% indicate hypoxia and highlight a possible pulmonary or cardiovascular disease.

Procedure. The clinician washes his or her hands, obtains a timepiece that measures seconds, and explains the procedure to the patient. The patient is typically seated but may also be recumbent or standing. The clinician gently places two fingertips over the radial artery at the wrist. The clinician then counts either the inspirations or the expirations. The count, which is performed silently in the head, typically begins with the first breath after a time interval. For example, if the interval begins when a digital counter is at 0 seconds, "1" is the first breath noted after the 0 starting point. Alternatively, the clinician starts the time frame when the first breath is noted. The length of time for counting breaths depends on the patient's situation, but the usual method is to count for 30 seconds and multiply by 2. The clinician documents the findings regarding the number of breaths per minute, the patient position, and any variation in the depth, rhythm, or character (Tables 6-4 and 6-5).

CLINICAL PEARL

Within the inpatient environment, it is not uncommon for a patient to be prescribed supplemental oxygen to maintain their SpO_2 levels. For example, oxygen is typically prescribed to achieve a target saturation of 94–98% for most acutely ill patients or 88–92% for those at risk of respiratory failure. The prescription should include a diagnosis of the condition requiring the use of oxygen, the oxygen flow rate in liters per minute, and an estimate of the frequency and duration of use (eg, 3 liters per minute, 50 minutes per hour, 12 hours per day). There are no regulations that prohibit PTAs from using oxygen for patients, provided that the oxygen has been prescribed and the parameters based on the physician's orders are being adhered to. If a patient should become hypoxic during a treatment session, the PTA should run through a quick checklist before declaring a medical emergency. This checklist includes assessing whether one or all of the following reduces the hypoxia:

- If the patient is supine, raise the head of the bed.
- If the patient is already on supplemental oxygen, ensure equipment is turned on and set at the required flow rate and is connected to an oxygen supply source. If a portable tank is being used, check the tank's oxygen level and confirm that the patient's nasal cannula is fitted properly.
- If deep breathing and coughing techniques help patients effectively, clear their airway and improve their oxygen levels.
- If the patient uses an inhaler and, if so, its location.
- If adjusting the oxygen level (within the parameters set by the physician) provides relief.

BLOOD PRESSURE

Every single beat of the heart involves a sequence of interrelated events known as the cardiac cycle. The cardiac cycle consists of three major stages: atrial systole, ventricular systole, and complete cardiac diastole.

- The atrial systole consists of the contraction of the atria. This contraction occurs during the last third of diastole and complete ventricular filling.
- The ventricular systole consists of the ventricular contraction and the flow of blood into the circulatory system. Once all the blood empties from the ventricles, the pulmonary and aortic semilunar valves close.
- The complete cardiac diastole involves relaxation of the atria (atrial diastole) and ventricles (ventricular diastole) in preparation for refilling with circulating blood. End diastolic volume is the amount of blood in the ventricles after diastole, about 120 mL.

CLINICAL PEARL

- The heart has a two-step pumping action. One action is involved in the pumping of blood from the right half of the heart through the lungs and back to the left half of the heart (pulmonary circulation); the other action is involved with pumping blood from the left half of the heart through all the tissues of the body (except, of course, the lungs) and back to the right half of the heart (systemic circulation).

▶ The ventricles are the pumps that produce the pressures that drive the blood through the entire pulmonary and systemic vascular systems and back to the heart by contracting and relaxing.

Blood pressure (BP), a product of cardiac output and peripheral vascular resistance, is defined as the pressure exerted by the blood on the walls of the blood vessels, specifically *arterial blood pressure* (the pressure in the large arteries).

▶ Peak pressure in the arteries occurs during contraction of the left ventricle (systole) and provides the clinician with the systolic pressure measurement.

▶ The lowest pressure in the arteries occurs during cardiac relaxation when the heart is filling (diastole) and provides the clinician with the diastolic pressure measurement.

The difference between systolic and diastolic pressure is called *pulse pressure*. To withstand and adapt to various pressures, arteries are surrounded by varying smooth muscle thicknesses with extensive elastic and inelastic connective tissues.[13]

The assessment of BP provides information about the heart's effectiveness as a pump and blood flow resistance. It is measured in mm Hg and is recorded in two numbers. The systolic pressure is the pressure exerted on the brachial artery when the heart is contracting, while the diastolic pressure is the pressure exerted on the artery during the cardiac cycle's relaxation phase.[13] BP is documented as the systolic pressure over the diastolic pressure, for example, 120/80.

CLINICAL PEARL

A useful tool in assessing a patient with claudication is the ankle-brachial index (ABI), which is calculated as the ratio of systolic blood pressure at the ankle to the arm. A normal ABI is 0.9 to 1.1. However, any patient with an ABI less than 0.9, by definition, has some degree of arterial disease.

A category of prehypertension has established more aggressive guidelines for medical intervention of hypertension. The normal values for resting BP in adults are:

▶ *Normal:* systolic blood pressure < 120 mm Hg and diastolic blood pressure < 80 mm Hg

▶ *Prehypertension:* systolic blood pressure 120 to 129 mm Hg or diastolic blood pressure ≤ 80 mm Hg

▶ *Stage 1 hypertension:* systolic blood pressure 130 to 139 mm Hg or diastolic blood pressure 80 to 89 mm Hg

▶ *Stage 2 hypertension:* systolic blood pressure ≥ 140 mm Hg or diastolic blood pressure 90 mm Hg

▶ *Hypertensive crisis:* systolic blood pressure ≥ 180 mm Hg or diastolic blood pressure ≥ 120 mm Hg

The normal values for resting blood pressure in children are:

▶ *Systolic:* birth to 1 month, 60 to 90 mm Hg; up to 3 years of age, 75 to 130 mm Hg; and over 3 years of age, 97 to 120 mm Hg

▶ *Diastolic:* birth to 1 month, 30 to 60 mm Hg; up to 3 years of age, 45 to 90 mm Hg; and over 3 years of age, 57 to 80 mm Hg

CLINICAL PEARL

Ideally, BP should be determined in both arms. Causes of marked asymmetry in blood pressure of the arms include the following: errors in measurements, a marked difference in arm size, thoracic outlet syndromes, embolic occlusion of an artery, dissection of an aorta, external arterial occlusion, coarctation of the aorta, and atheromatous occlusion.[23]

Hypertension is one of the most common worldwide diseases afflicting humans and is an important public health challenge. Regulation of normal blood pressure is a complex process. Persistent hypertension can result in organ damage to the aorta and small arteries, heart, kidneys, retina, and CNS.

Many physical factors influence blood pressure:

▶ *Age:* the normal systolic range generally increases with age. BP normally rises gradually after birth and reaches a peak during puberty. By late adolescence (18 to 19 years), adult BP is reached.[14] In older adults, the rise in blood pressure is primarily because of the degenerative effects of arteriosclerosis.[14]

▶ *Rate of pumping (heart rate):* the rate at which blood is pumped by the heart—the higher the heart rate, the higher (assuming no change in stroke volume) the blood pressure.

▶ *The volume of blood:* the amount of blood present in the body. The more blood present in the body, the higher the amount of blood returned to the heart and the resulting cardiac output.

▶ *Dehydration:* a significant decrease of body fluids may cause low blood pressure.

▶ *Cardiac output:* the rate and volume of flow—a product of the heart rate, or the rate of contraction, multiplied by the stroke volume, the amount of blood pumped out from the heart with each contraction—the efficiency with which the heart circulates the blood throughout the body.

▶ *The resistance of the blood vessel walls (peripheral vascular resistance):* the higher the resistance, the higher the blood pressure; the larger the blood vessel, the lower the resistance. Factors that influence peripheral vascular resistance include arteriolar tone, vasoconstriction, and to a lesser extent, blood viscosity.

▶ *Viscosity, or thickness, of the blood:* if the blood gets thicker, it increases blood pressure. Certain medical conditions can change the viscosity of the blood. For instance, low red blood cell concentration, anemia, reduces viscosity, whereas increased red blood cell concentration increases viscosity.

▶ *Body temperature:* an increase in body temperature causes the heart rate to increase. Conversely, a decrease in body temperature causes the heart rate to decrease.

▶ *Arm position:* BP may vary as much as 20 mm Hg by altering arm position.[14] The pressure should be determined in both arms (see later).

▶ *Exercise:* physical activity will increase cardiac output, with a consequent linear increase in blood pressure. Greater increases are noted in systolic pressure owing to proportional changes in the pressure gradient of peripheral vessels.[14] Systolic readings greater than 250 mm Hg or diastolic readings greater than 115 mm Hg during exercise or other high-level activity should serve as serious warnings. Similarly, a drop in systolic pressure of more than 10 mm Hg from baseline, or a failure of the systolic pressure to increase with an increasing workload, should cause concern.

▶ *Valsalva maneuver:* An attempt to exhale forcibly with the glottis, nose, and mouth closed.[14] This results in:

  ▪ An increase in intrathoracic pressure with an accompanying collapse of the veins of the chest wall

  ▪ A decrease in blood flow to the heart and a decreased venous return

  ▪ A drop in arterial blood pressure

When the breath is released, the intrathoracic pressure decreases, and venous return is suddenly reestablished as an *overshoot* mechanism to compensate for the drop in blood pressure. This causes a marked increase in heart rate and arterial blood pressure.[14]

▶ *Orthostatic hypotension:* defined as a drop in systolic blood pressure within three minutes of assuming an upright position—a decrease in BP below normal (a systolic blood pressure decrease of at least 20 mm Hg or a diastolic blood pressure decrease of at least 10 mm Hg) to the point where the pressure is not adequate for normal oxygenation of the tissues.[13] Orthostatic hypotension can occur as a side effect of antihypertensive medications, and in cases of low blood volume in patients who are postoperative or dehydrated, and in those with dysfunction of the autonomic nervous system, such as that which occurs with a spinal cord injury or postcerebrovascular accident.[13] Activities that may increase the chance of orthostatic hypotension, such as application of heat modalities, hydrotherapy, pool therapy, moderate-to-vigorous exercise using the large muscles, sudden changes of position, and stationary standing, should be avoided in susceptible patients.[13]

There are several ways that BP can be measured. The most accurate method involves placing a cannula into a blood vessel and connecting it to an electronic pressure transducer. The less accurate but also less invasive method is the auscultation method, which uses manual measurement using a sphygmomanometer, an inflatable (Riva Rocci) cuff (Figure 6-10) placed around the upper arm, at roughly the same vertical height as the heart in a sitting person, using the brachial artery. BP measurements are usually taken on the left arm because it is physically located nearer the aorta, but the right arm can also be used (Figure 6-10).

The chosen cuff must be the proper size to obtain an accurate measurement to prevent erroneous readings. The ideal cuff has a bladder length that is approximately 80% of the arm circumference, and the width of the bladder should be approximately 40% of the circumference of the midpoint of the limb.

The patient should be allowed to sit quietly for approximately 5 minutes before the measurements are taken and should not have been exercising for 15 to 30 minutes.

Procedure

The clinician washes his or her hands and obtains a clean stethoscope and a sphygmomanometer. The procedure is explained to the patient while the patient is positioned in sitting with the forearm supported approximately at the heart level, and the feet are on the floor with the legs uncrossed. The clinician exposes the antecubital space of the patient's arm, while making sure that any clothing that is rolled up does not create additional constriction, and then palpates the brachial pulse (see Figure 6-4) for future placement of the cuff and stethoscope diaphragm. The deflated cuff is applied to the arm with the center of the bladder over the medial aspect of the arm (approximately 2 to 3 cm or 1½ fingerbreadths

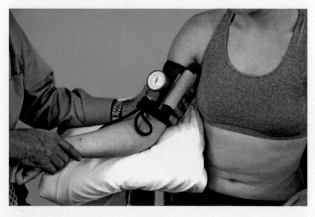

FIGURE 6-10 Sphygmomanometer.

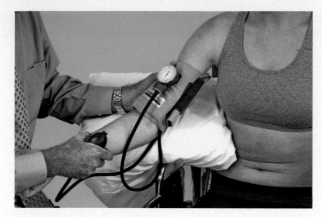

FIGURE 6-11 Placement of cuff.

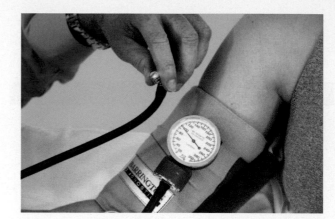

FIGURE 6-13 Inflation of cuff.

above the antecubital space) so that it will occlude the artery when it is inflated (Figure 6-11). The clinician applies the stethoscope to his or her ears with the earpieces directed forward and places the diaphragm on the skin where the brachial artery was palpated. Firm but gentle pressure is applied to the diaphragm (Figure 6-12). The clinician ensures that all of the air is out of the cuff bladder, the valve on the pump is closed, and the pressure gauge reading is zero. While listening with the stethoscope, the clinician uses the same hand to slowly inflate the blood pressure cuff by squeezing the bladder (Figure 6-13). The clinician uses the other hand to palpate the patient's radial pulse while inflating the cuff to 70-80 mm Hg in increments of 10 mm Hg. The cuff is further inflated until the radial pulse is not palpable and then inflated further to the point when the pressure level reaches either 20 to 30 mm Hg above the first Korotkoff sound (see Clinical Pearl), or 30 mm Hg above the point at which the radial pulse disappears. Some consider 200 mm Hg as the upper limit of inflation, but this can lead to a measurement error in patients with hypertension. At this point, the clinician uses the thumb and index finger of the hand used to squeeze the pump to slowly open the valve and release the pressure in the cuff (Figure 6-14). At the point when the clinician begins to hear a "whooshing" or pounding sound (first Korotkoff sound), the pressure reading (systolic) is noted. The cuff pressure is further released until a muffling sound can be heard (fourth Korotkoff sound), indicating the diastolic blood pressure reading. The clinician records the

BP readings, including the patient's position and the upper extremity used. If it is necessary to repeat the measurements, the cuff is completely deflated, and the patient is permitted to sit quietly for one to two minutes before proceeding again. Once the measurements are completed, the clinician cleans the equipment in preparation for future use.

CLINICAL PEARL

Korotkoff described five phases of sounds:

1. The first clear, rhythmic tapping sound that gradually increases in intensity represents the highest pressure in the arterial system during ventricular contraction and is recorded as the systolic pressure. The clinician should be alert for the presence of an auscultatory gap, especially in patients with hypertension. An auscultatory gap is the temporary disappearance of sound normally heard over the brachial artery between phase 1 and phase 2 and may cover a range of 0-40 mm Hg.[14] Not identifying this gap may lead to an underestimation of systolic pressure and overestimation of diastolic pressure.[14]

2. This phase represents the murmur or swishing sound heard as the artery widens and more blood flows through the artery. This sound is heard for most of the time between the systolic and diastolic pressures.

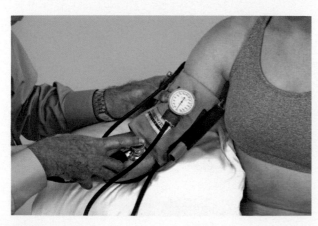

FIGURE 6-12 Diaphragm over the brachial pulse.

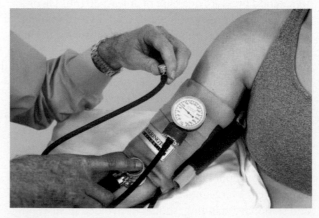

FIGURE 6-14 Controlled deflation of cuff.

3. During this phase, the sounds become crisp, more intense, and louder.

4. The fourth phase is characterized by a distinct sound that has a soft muffling quality. At pressures within 10 mm Hg above the diastolic blood pressure (in children less than 13 years old, pregnant women, and in patients with high cardiac output or peripheral vasodilation), the muffling sound should be used to indicate the first diastolic reading, but both the muffling (phase 4) and the sound disappearance (phase 5) should be recorded.

5. The last sound that is heard, which is traditionally recorded as the second diastolic reading.

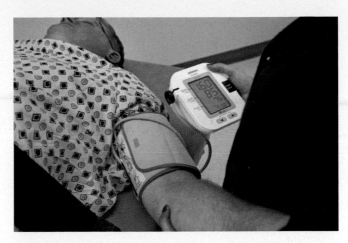

FIGURE 6-15 Automated digital blood pressure monitor.

Although the systolic blood pressure is commonly taken to be the pressure at which the first Korotkoff sound is first heard, and the diastolic blood pressure reading is taken at the point at which the fourth Korotkoff sound is just barely audible, there has recently been a move toward the use of the fifth Korotkoff sound (ie, silence) as the actual diastolic blood pressure, as this has been felt to be more reproducible.[27-32] However, during pregnancy, the fifth phase may not be identifiable, in which case the fourth is used.[33-35]

CLINICAL PEARL

Any error that occurs during a blood pressure reading can result in highly inaccurate interpretations, especially because the cutoff levels for hypertension categories are close together, making the distinction between normal and hypotensive BP very slight. The most common errors include:

▶ The failure to accurately determine the first Korotkoff sound

▶ Use of inappropriate cuff size

▶ Incorrect patient positioning (unsupported tested arm, arm not level with the heart, legs crossed while sitting, and unsupported sitting)

▶ Incorrect placement of stethoscope

▶ Too rapid deflation of the cuff

CLINICAL PEARL

Many medical facilities currently use automated digital monitors to measure blood pressure. Similar units are also the most common devices used for at-home self-monitoring (Figure 6-15). The patient setup is the same as for the auscultation method. After the cuff is placed on the patient's upper arm, the cuff automatically inflates to a pressure higher than the systolic pressure using oscillometry. An electronically operated pump and valve gradually release the pressure, and a transducer senses the periodic expansion and contraction of the brachial artery wall. The device uses this information to calculate the systolic and diastolic pressures, which are displayed digitally. Although these devices are less susceptible to human error, their accuracy varies widely based on the manufacturer and model.

Recently, ultrasonic BP measuring devices have been introduced. These new devices work by using mathematically based software to measure blood flow and vein or artery wall distention as the heart beats, based on images generated by the ultrasound device. The patient setup is similar to that used by the auscultation method, but instead of using a stethoscope, ultrasonic waves are reflected off the brachial artery distal to the cuff.

TEMPERATURE

Body temperature, a balance between the heat produced and lost in the body, is one indication of an individual's metabolic state. Temperature measurements provide information on the basal metabolic state, possible presence or absence of infection, and metabolic response to exercise.[13] For example, an infection or systemic illness can result in an increased body temperature. The "normal" core body temperature of an adult, measured in the pulmonary artery, is generally considered to be 98.6°F (37°C). However, a temperature in the range of 96.5 to 99.4°F (35.8 to 37.4°C) is not at all uncommon. Fever or pyrexia refers to any temperature exceeding 100°F (37.7°C).[23] Hyperpyrexia refers to any extreme elevation of temperature above 41.1°C (or 106°F),[13] whereas hypothermia refers to an abnormally low temperature (below 35°C or 95°F).

In most individuals, there is a daily variation in body temperature of 0.5 to 2°F (1°C), with the low temperature occurring before waking and the high temperature occurring about 12 hours after waking. Menstruating women have a well-known temperature pattern that reflects the effects of ovulation, with the temperature increasing slightly (0.25°C-0.5°C measured in the morning) around ovulation.[23] In both aging and fit individuals, there is more temperature variation during the day. Finally, whereas ingestion of meals can slightly elevate or lower core temperature, alcohol ingestion slightly lowers core temperature.

CLINICAL PEARL

It is worth noting that in adults over 75 years of age and in those who are immunocompromised (eg, transplant recipients, corticosteroid users, persons with chronic renal insufficiency, or anyone taking excessive antipyretic medications), the fever response may be blunted or absent.[13]

The clinical measurement of temperature is merely an estimate of the true core temperature. Several sites can be used, including the ear canal (tympanic), oral cavity, axilla, and rectum (Table 6-6).

▶ *Rectal or tympanic measurements:* commonly used with infants and unconscious patients because of the difficulty of maintaining the thermometer position at the other sites. Although there are concerns about the accuracy of tympanic measurements across all age groups,[36,37] studies have shown them to be reliable.[38,39]

▶ *Axillary measurement:* only used when the other sites cannot be used because of its decreased accuracy.

CLINICAL PEARL

Rectal temperatures tend to be the highest and closest to the actual core temperature, whereas axillary temperatures tend to be the lowest and furthest from true core temperature.[36]

Oral Procedure. The oral temperature is generally taken by placing a probe thermometer under the patient's tongue. The thermometer can be a standard one (Figure 6-16) or a battery-operated electronic thermometer (Figure 6-17). After washing his or her hands, the clinician inserts a clean probe into the patient's mouth, positioned under the tongue, and held in place by the lips (not with the teeth). The patient is asked to breathe through the nose. Typically, the probe remains in place for 30 to 90 seconds. Electronic devices emit an audible alarm when the temperature reaches its final value. The clinician notes the value and then removes the probe from the patient's mouth, discards the probe cover, and turns the unit off. The clinician then washes his or her hands before recording the result.

TABLE 6-6	Normal Temperatures Based on Site
Rectal	36.6°C–38°C (97.9°F–100.4°F)
Tympanic	35.8°C–38°C (96.4°F–100.4°F)
Oral	35.5°C–37.5°C (95.9°F–99.5°F)
Axillary	34.7°C–37.3°C (94.5°F–99.1°F)

Tympanic Procedure. The tympanic measurement involves placing a specially designed electronic monitor into the ear canal that reads the infrared energy emitted from the tympanic membrane (eardrum), detects when the maximum temperature has been reached, and then provides a liquid crystal display (LCD) of the temperature. The electronic monitor uses disposable, single-use probe covers. Newer designs of these monitors convert the tympanic temperature to an estimated core temperature. Several precautions must be taken when using a tympanic device. Ideally, the clinician should[40,41]:

▶ Ensure that there is no excessive earwax present.

▶ Confirm that the patient's ear has not been resting against a pillow or similar object. If it has, the clinician should wait for 2 to 3 minutes before taking a reading.

▶ Take readings from both ears, as measurements can vary between sides. Alternatively, the clinician can take a reading from one ear and document which ear was used.

To take a tympanic temperature, the clinician washes his or her hands before applying a clean lens filter. As appropriate, the clinician selects the correct setting (some units have both an "oral" and a "rectal" setting) and then gently but firmly pulls on the patient's ear to straighten the ear canal. The ear is pulled straight back for an infant, whereas, for anyone older than one year, the ear is pulled up and back. The clinician then inserts the thermometer lens cone, with its clean filter applied, into the ear opening, rocking it back and forth gently to insert it far enough to seal the ear canal. The clinician then depresses and holds the activation button for one second until the temperature reading appears in the display window and mentally records the value. The lens cone is then removed from the patient's ear and discarded. Depending on the facility, the lens filter is discarded or thoroughly washed before being used again. The clinician washes his or her hands and records the temperature reading.

Rectal Procedure. Specifically designed rectal thermometers are used to record rectal temperatures. After washing his or her hands, the clinician applies a lubricant to the thermometer probe, and with the patient in a side-lying position with the hips and knees flexed, the clinician inserts the thermometer into the rectum far enough for the probe to be within the cavity but not so far as to push into tissue resistance. The thermometer remains in place for three minutes or until the electronic device indicates completion and the temperature reading is noted. The clinician then removes and cleans the probe, washes his or her hands, and then records the temperature.

CLINICAL PEARL

Ingestible telemetric body core temperature sensors, which measure approximately ¾ of an inch in length, have recently been introduced to measure and monitor the temperature of athletes. The "thermometer pill" has a silicone-coated exterior and microminiaturized circuitry on the interior, including a quartz crystal temperature

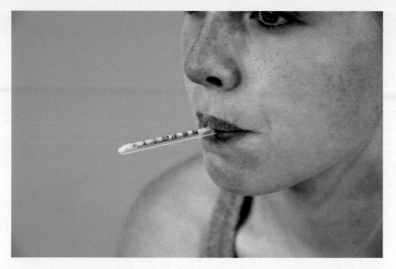

FIGURE 6-16 Standard thermometer.

sensor, and is powered by a miniature battery. As the pill is swallowed, the temperature sensor vibrates at a frequency relative to the body's temperature, transmitting a harmless and low-frequency signal through the body, which an external receiver can record. After 18 to 30 hours, the pill passes safely from the digestive system.

THE ASSESSMENT OF PAIN

Many clinical environments consider pain as the fifth vital sign, although strictly speaking, pain is a symptom rather than a sign. Pain, always an abnormal finding, is felt by everyone at some point or other and is considered an emotional experience that is highly individualized and extremely difficult to evaluate. Also, pain perception and the response to the painful experience can be influenced by various cognitive processes, including anxiety, tension, depression, past pain experiences, and cultural influences.[42]

Perhaps the simplest descriptors for pain are acute and chronic.

Acute pain can be defined as "the normal, predicted physiological response to an adverse chemical, thermal, or mechanical stimulus . . . associated with surgery, trauma, and acute illness."[43] This type of pain usually precipitates a visit to a physician because it has one or more of the following characteristics[44]:

▶ It is new and has not been experienced before.

▶ It is severe and disabling.

▶ It is continuous, lasting for more than several minutes, or recurs very frequently.

▶ The site of the pain may cause alarm (eg, chest or eye).

▶ In addition to the sensory and affective components, acute pain is typically characterized by anxiety. This may produce a fight-or-flight autonomic response, which is normally used for survival needs. This autonomic reaction is also associated with an increase in systolic and diastolic blood pressure, a decrease in gut motility and salivatory flow, increased muscle tension, and papillary distention.[45,46]

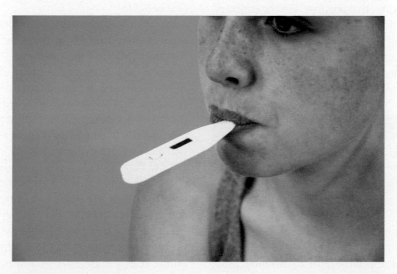

FIGURE 6-17 Battery-operated electronic thermometer.

CLINICAL PEARL

▶ Hyperalgesia is an increased response to a noxious stimulus. Primary hyperalgesia occurs at the site of injury, whereas secondary hyperalgesia occurs outside the site of injury.

▶ Allodynia is defined as pain in response to a previously innocuous stimulus.

▶ Referred pain is a site adjacent to or at a distance from the site of an injury's origin. Referred pain can occur from muscle, joint, and viscera. For example, during myocardial infarction, the pain felt in the neck, shoulders, and back rather than in the chest, the injury site.

Acute pain following trauma, or the insidious onset of a musculoskeletal condition, is typically chemical in nature. Although motions aggravate the pain, they cannot be used to alleviate the symptoms. In contrast, cessation of movement (absolute rest) tends to alleviate the pain, although not necessarily immediately. The structures most sensitive to chemical irritation in order of sensitivity are:

▶ The periosteum and joint capsule
▶ Subchondral bone, tendon, and ligament
▶ Muscle and cortical bone layer
▶ The synovium and articular cartilage

CLINICAL PEARL

The aching type of pain associated with degenerative arthritis and muscle disorders is often accentuated by activity and lessened by rest. Pain that is not alleviated by rest and that is not associated with acute trauma may indicate the presence of a serious disorder such as a tumor or aneurysm. This pain is often described as deep, constant, and boring and is apt to be more noticeable and more intense at night.[47]

Chronic pain. Unlike acute pain, chronic pain does not serve a useful biological, protective purpose. On the contrary, it often limits our capacity for physical activity and participation in social undertakings.[48,49] The symptoms of chronic pain typically behave in a mechanical fashion, in that they are provoked by activity or repeated movements and reduced with rest or a movement in the opposite direction.

CLINICAL PEARL

Referred pain, which can be either acute or chronic, must be verified by the clinician by determining its cause and whether the cause is within the scope of practice.

In general, as a condition worsens, the pain distribution becomes more widespread and distal (peripheralizes). As the condition improves, the symptoms tend to become more localized (centralized).

CLINICAL PEARL

It must be remembered that the location of symptoms for many musculoskeletal conditions is quite separate from the source. For example, a cervical disk protrusion can produce symptoms throughout the upper extremity. The term *radiating pain* is used to describe symptoms with their origin at a spinal nerve but felt within the nerve's distribution into either the upper or lower extremity.

Although pain measurement does not directly measure a patient's physiologic status, it can provide important information to aid in diagnosis, prognosis, and intervention planning. Although largely subjective, pain assessment can be made more quantitative by using various visual and verbal pain scales. For example, a simple body map can be used where the patient marks the location and type of pain on a diagram (Figure 6-18). One of the easiest methods to quantify the intensity of pain is to use a 10-point visual analog scale (VAS). The VAS is a numerically continuous scale that requires the pain level to be identified by asking a patient to make a pencil mark on a 100-mm/10-cm line. The patient is asked to rate their present pain compared with the worst pain ever experienced, with 0 representing no pain, 1 representing minimally perceived pain, and 10 representing pain that requires immediate attention.[51] Alternatively, the patient can circle the appropriate number on a 0-to-10 series (Figure 6-18).[50] The clinician needs to describe the purpose of the pain rating and how the rating works. It is also important that the clinician obtain information about whether the patient is currently on pain medication and when the last dose was taken.

CLINICAL PEARL

The Joint Commission (JC) requires an appropriate assessment of the patient's pain as an element of standard care.

Also, the Pain Disability Index can be used to rapidly assesses the severity of pain and its impact on functioning (Table 6-7).

Because pain is variable in its intensity and quality, describing it is often difficult for the patient. The McGill Pain Questionnaire (MPQ),[52] designed in 1971 to use verbal descriptors to assess the intensity and quality of the patient's symptoms, is now widely used in pain research and practice (see Table 6-8). A patient first selects a single word from each group that best describes his or her pain, and then reviews the list to select three words from groups 1 to 10 that best reflect their pain, two words from groups 11 to 15, a single word from group 16, and then a single word from groups 17 to 20. Upon completion, the patient will have selected seven words that best describe his or her pain.[53] The implication is that each word chosen reflects a particular sensory quality of pain.

A similar scale to the MPQ is the modified somatic perception questionnaire (MSPQ), a simple 13-item, 4-point self-report scale (Table 6-9), which is used to measure somatic and autonomic perception. The MSPQ has a minimum score

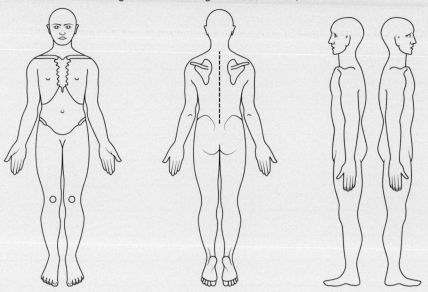

Name: _____

Date: _____   Signature: _____

Please use the diagram below to indicate where you feel symptoms right now. Use the following key to indicate different types of symptoms.

KEY: Pins and Needles = 000000   Stabbing – ///////   Burning = XXXXX   Deep Ache = ZZZZZZ

Please use the three scales below to rate your pain over the past 24 hours. Use the upper line to describe your pain level right now. Use the other scales to rate your pain at its worst and best over the past 24 hours.

RATE YOUR PAIN: 0 = NO PAIN. 10 = EXTREMELY INTENSE

1.	Right now	0	1	2	3	4	5	6	7	8	9	10
2.	At its worst	0	1	2	3	4	5	6	7	8	9	10
3.	At its best	0	1	2	3	4	5	6	7	8	9	10

FIGURE 6-18 Body map for describing the location and type of pain.

of zero and a maximum score of 39. The higher the score, the greater the somatic symptoms.

Several pain rating scales exist for use with infants and children. The pain of infants can be assessed using a tool such as the FLACC (face, legs, activity, cry, and consolability), an observational scale assessing pain behaviors quantitatively with preverbal patients. Physiologic and behavioral responses to nociceptive or painful stimuli can also be used.[54] Physiologic manifestations of pain include increased heart rate, heart rate variability, blood pressure, and respiration, with evidence of decreased oxygenation (cyanosis).[54]

CLINICAL PEARL

The assessment of pain in children is somewhat challenging, and the choice of approach depends on the child's age and abilities. The 3 main approaches to measuring pain intensity in children are as follows[55]:

▶ *Physiological.* Physiological indicators (eg, increased heart rate, blood pressure, sweating) are associated with a generalized (nonspecific) stress reaction and more strongly associated with distress and anxiety than self-report pain measures. For this reason, physiological indicators should not be used in isolation to estimate the presence, quality, or intensity of pain.

▶ *Observations of behavior.* Observational measures involve observing an individual's nonverbal behavior (eg, crying, facial expression, torso and limb movements) and interactions (eg, social, appetite). Observational measures are particularly useful for assessing pain in children aged less than 4 years, who do not have the language skills necessary to communicate pain.

▶ *Self-report.* A child's ability to understand and report the presence and intensity of pain requires cognitive skills, including receptive language and understanding, knowledge and memory of pain, executive function (eg, cognitive flexibility, working memory), and the ability to understand and estimate magnitudes and symbolic processing.

For the assessment of children, two common scales are currently used:

▶ *Faces Pain Rating Scale.*[56] This 0-to-5 scale consists of a series of six pictures of cartoonlike faces expressing various facial expressions from crying (Hurts worst—5) to smiling (No hurt—0). The child is asked to point to the face that best describes his or her pain.

▶ *The Oucher Scales.*[57] There are two ethnically based self-report Oucher scales; a (0 to 100) number scale for older

119

TABLE 6-7	The Pain Disability Index

The rating scales below are designed to measure the degree to which several aspects of your life are presently disrupted by chronic pain. In other words, we would like to know how much your pain is preventing you from doing what you would normally do or from doing it as well as you normally would. Respond to each category by indicating the *overall* impact of pain in your life, not just the pain at its worst.

For each of the 7 categories of life activity listed, please circle the number on the scale that describes the level of disability you typically experience. A score of 0 means no disability at all, and a score of 10 signifies that all of the activities in which you would normally be involved have been totally disrupted or prevented by your pain.

(1) FAMILY/HOME RESPONSIBILITIES

This category refers to activities related to the home or family. It includes chores or duties performed around the house (eg, yard work) and errands or favors for other family members (eg, driving children to and from school).

0	1	2	3	4	5	6	7	8	9	10

No disability   Total disability

(2) RECREATION

This category includes hobbies, sports, and other similar leisure-time activities.

0	1	2	3	4	5	6	7	8	9	10

No disability   Total disability

(3) SOCIAL ACTIVITY

This category refers to activities that involve participation with friends and acquaintances other than family members. It includes parties, theater, concerts, dining out, and other social functions.

0	1	2	3	4	5	6	7	8	9	10

No disability   Total disability

(4) OCCUPATION

This category refers to activities that are a part of or directly related to one's job. This includes nonpaying jobs as well, such as that of a housewife or volunteer worker.

0	1	2	3	4	5	6	7	8	9	10

No disability   Total disability

(5) SEXUAL BEHAVIOR

This category refers to the frequency and quality of one's sex life.

0	1	2	3	4	5	6	7	8	9	10

No disability   Total disability

(6) SELF-CARE

This category includes activities that involve personal maintenance and independent daily living (eg, taking a shower, driving, getting dressed, etc).

0	1	2	3	4	5	6	7	8	9	10

No disability   Total disability

(7) LIFE-SUPPORT ACTIVITY

This category refers to basic life-supporting behaviors such as eating, sleeping, and breathing.

0	1	2	3	4	5	6	7	8	9	10

No disability   Total disability

Data from Pollard CA. Preliminary validity study of pain disability index, Percept Mot Skills. 1984 Dec;59(3):974.

TABLE 6-8 Modified McGill Pain Questionnaire

Patient's Name _____ Date _____

Directions: Many words can describe pain. Some of these words are listed below. If you are experiencing any pain, check (√) next to every
word that describes your pain.

A. Flickering

    Quivering

    Pulsing

    Throbbing

    Beating

    Pounding

B. Jumping

    Flashing

    Shooting

C. Pricking

    Boring

    Drilling

    Stabbing

D. Sharp

    Cutting

    Lacerating

E. Pinching

    Pressing

    Gnawing

    Cramping

    Crushing

F. Ugging

    Pulling

    Wrenching

G. Hot

    Burning

    Scalding

    Searing

H. Tingling

    Itchy

    Smarting

    Stinging

I. Dull

    Sore

    Hurting

(continued)

TABLE 6-8   Modified McGill Pain Questionnaire (continued)

	Aching	
	Heavy	
J.	Tender	
	Taut	
	Rasping	
	Splitting	
K.	Tiring	
	Exhausting	
L.	Sickening	
	Suffocating	
M.	Fearful	
	Frightful	
	Terrifying	
N.	Punishing	
	Grueling	
	Cruel	
	Vicious	
	Killing	
O.	Wretched	
	Blinding	
P.	Annoying	
	Troublesome	
	Intense	
	Unbearable	
Q.	Spreading	
	Radiating	
	Penetrating	
	Piercing	
R.	Tight	
	Numb	
	Drawing	
	Squeezing	
	Tearing	
S.	Cool	
	Cold	
	Freezing	
T.	Nagging	
	Nauseating	
	Agonizing	

(continued)

TABLE 6-8	Modified McGill Pain Questionnaire (continued)
Dreadful	
Torturing	

KEY TO PAIN QUESTIONNAIRE
Group A: Suggests vascular disorder
Groups B–H: Suggests neurogenic disorder
Group I: Suggests musculoskeletal disorder
Groups J–T: Suggests emotional disorder

SCORING GUIDE: ADD UP TOTAL NUMBER OF CHECKS (√):
Total: 4–8 = NORMAL
    8–10 = Focusing too much on pain
    10–16 = May be helped more by a clinical psychologist than by a physical therapist
    >16 = Unlikely to respond to therapy procedures

TABLE 6-9	Modified Somatic Perceptions Questionnaire (MSPQ)

Please describe how you have felt during the PAST WEEK by marking a checkmark (√) in the appropriate box. Please answer all questions. Do not think too long before answering.

	Not at All	A Little, Slightly	A Great Deal, Quite a Bit	Extremely, Could Not Have Been Worse
Heart rate increase				
Feeling hot all over				
Sweating all over				
Sweating in a particular part of the body				
Pulse in neck				
Pounding in head				
Dizziness				
Blurring of vision				
Feeling faint				
Everything appearing unreal				
Nausea				
Butterflies in stomach				
Pain or ache in the stomach				
Stomach churning				
Desire to pass water				
Mouth becoming dry				
Difficulty swallowing				
Muscles in neck aching				
Legs feeling weak				
Muscles twitching or jumping				
Tense feeling across the forehead				
Tense feeling in jaw muscles				

Reproduced with permission from Main C, Wood P, Hillis S, et al. The Distress and Risk Assessment Method. A simple patient classification to identify distress and evaluate the risk of poor outcome. *Spine*. 1992 Jan;17(1):42-52.

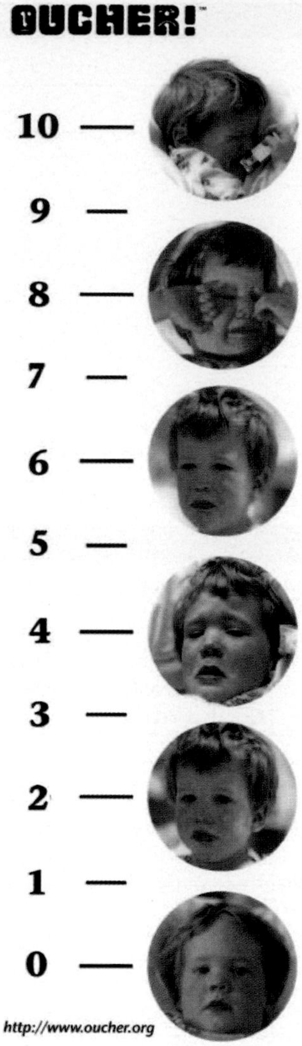

OUCHER!™

http://www.oucher.org

FIGURE 6-19 Caucasian Oucher scale to measure pain.

children and a photographic scale for younger children (aged 3 to 5) (Figure 6-19). Children who can count to 100 by ones or tens and understand, for example, that 72 is more than 45, can use the numerical scale. Children who do not understand numbers should use the picture scale. The Oucher picture scale has three versions—Caucasian, African American, and Hispanic—suitable for children. Although this covers a wide variety of patients, females are not represented, nor are several other cultures. The scale uses six photographs of a child's face representing "no hurt" to "biggest hurt you can ever have" and includes a vertical scale with numbers from 0 to 10.

Reducing a patient's pain to zero may be unrealistic, depending on its cause. The physical therapist (PT) may use the reduction of pain as part of the plan of care. For example, a goal may be to have the patient rate their pain level at 3/10 while transferring from sitting to standing following back surgery, when the pain was rated as 6/10 at the initial examination. Often, a patient's pain level is governed by the stage of healing where pain levels are typically higher in the earlier stages but should lessen as the healing progresses. Suppose the patient reports a relatively sudden increase in their pain or symptoms from one session to another or during a session. In that case, the PTA must consult with the supervising PT to ascertain the possible reasons for this change.

EMERGENCY FIRST AID

An emergency, whether characterized by unresponsiveness, an acute medical condition, drug intoxication, or trauma, demands a rapid response and management. A logical, sequential priority system must be implemented immediately. All healthcare employees involved in patient care should be aware of the facility's emergency procedures in which they work and should be qualified to provide first aid in the case of an emergency. Most healthcare facilities have a series of emergency codes to indicate the occurrence of an emergency. For example:

▶ Code blue may represent a flood.

▶ Code amber may represent child abduction.

▶ Code red may represent a fire.

▶ Code black may represent a cardiac arrest.

CLINICAL PEARL

At the very minimum, all healthcare employees should know how to contact and request emergency assistance (eg, the use of 911 or the equivalent number to contact the police, fire, or emergency services).

These days, it is not uncommon for patients to wear a medical alert bracelet or necklace, which informs others of any medical conditions, allergies, health history, medication needs, and so forth.

CLINICAL PEARL

A crash cart or code cart is a set of trays/drawers/shelves on wheels used in hospitals for transporting and dispensing emergency medication/equipment at the site of a medical/surgical emergency. The contents of a crash cart vary from institution to institution but typically include the tools and drugs needed to treat a person in or near cardiac arrest. These include but are not limited to:

▶ Defibrillators and suction devices

▶ Advanced cardiac life support (ACLS) drugs

▶ First-line drugs for treatment of common problems (anaphylactic shock, deep venous thrombosis [DVT], etc)

▶ Drugs for rapid sequence intubation, endotracheal tubes, and other intubating equipment

▶ Drugs for peripheral and central venous access

▶ Pediatric equipment

▶ Other drugs and equipment as required by the facility

PTAs must be able to recognize the signs and symptoms that are associated with a medical emergency, including:

▶ Difficulty breathing, shortness of breath.

▶ Chest or upper abdominal pain or pressure lasting two minutes or more.

TABLE 6-10	Typical Contents of an Environmental, Employee, and Patient Safety Manual

Employee job duties, descriptions, and responsibilities

Supervisor relationships, organization table, and the chain of command

Plans for the evacuation and care of patients and the expected function of all personnel at the time of an emergency

Security measures for patient and employee valuables and procedures for items that are lost or found

The establishment of equipment inspection, repair, and maintenance records

The process and procedures for general infection control and handling of toxic materials

The application and use of personal protective equipment (PPE), the handling of body fluids, and the management of patients who are placed in isolation

▶ Loss of consciousness, fainting, unexplained nausea, sudden dizziness, or sudden weakness.

▶ Seizure. Any patient who convulses without a known cause should be evaluated and treated carefully.

▶ Incontinence of bowel or bladder without a known cause.

▶ Signs of a major burn.

▶ Reports of vision changes.

▶ Difficulty speaking.

▶ Confusion or changes in mental status, unusual behavior, difficulty awakening.

▶ Any sudden or severe pain.

▶ Head pain that lasts longer than five minutes.

▶ Uncontrolled bleeding.

▶ Shock symptoms, such as confusion; disorientation; and cool/clammy, pale skin.

▶ Severe or persistent vomiting or diarrhea.

▶ Coughing or vomiting blood.

▶ Unusual abdominal pain.

▶ Suicidal or homicidal feelings.

▶ Certain patient populations, such as the elderly, debilitated persons, and persons with cognitive deterioration, spinal cord injury, chronic respiratory condition, an acute/chronic cardiac condition, or acute/chronic diabetes.

CLINICAL PEARL

The "Good Samaritan" law provides certain protection from lawsuits to people who give first aid or other emergency care or treatment to someone suffering an injury or sudden illness. The care or treatment must be given at the scene of an emergency outside of a hospital, doctor's office, or another medical facility. The law protects volunteers who help when someone becomes ill or is injured in places such as on the street or highway; in parks, restaurants, or businesses; or even private residences. If someone is already at a hospital or other medical facility, the law does not apply.

Each physical therapy department has several policies and procedures regarding environmental, employee, and patient safety included in the unit's policy/procedure or safety manual. The typical contents of this manual are outlined in Table 6-10.

The initial response by the PTA should be an assessment of the patient's physiologic status performed in a sequence referred to as the ABCs (airway, breathing, circulation) for babies and CABs (circulation, airway, breathing) for every other age group. The letters D (disability—neurologic status) and E (exposure—expose the sites of all injuries) follow (Table 6-11).

TABLE 6-11	Situations That Require First Aid and Appropriate Action	
Situation	**Description**	**Appropriate Action**
Anaphylaxis	A life-threatening allergic reaction that can cause shock, a sudden drop in blood pressure, and trouble breathing.	Immediately call 911 or the facility's emergency number. Ask the person if he or she is carrying an epinephrine autoinjector to treat an allergic attack. Have the person lie still on their back and loosen tight clothing and cover the person with a blanket. Don't give the person anything to drink. If there's vomiting or bleeding from the mouth, turn the person on their side to prevent choking. If there are no breathing, coughing, or movement signs, begin cardiopulmonary resuscitation (CPR).
Autonomic hyperreflexia	Occurs in individuals with a relatively recent complete injury to the cervical and upper thoracic portions of the spinal cord down to the T6 cord level. Signs and symptoms include severe hypertension, bradycardia, and profuse diaphoresis above the cord lesion level.	Immediately look for and remove any potential causes of any noxious stimuli below the spinal cord lesion level, including bladder distension caused by urine retention, fecal impaction, tight straps from an orthosis or urine retention bag, localized pressure, open pressure ulcers, or exercise. The person should be placed in a sitting or semirecumbent position (not supine) and monitored.

(continued)

TABLE 6-11	Situations That Require First Aid and Appropriate Action (continued)	
Situation	**Description**	**Appropriate Action**
Burn, including chemical burn	The severity of the burn depends on the extent of damage to body tissues.	For minor burns, including first-degree burns and second-degree burns limited to an area no larger than 3 inches (7.6 cm) in diameter, cool the burn by holding the burned area under cool (not cold) running water for 10 or 15 minutes or until the pain subsides. If this is impractical, immerse the burn in cool water or cool it with cold compresses. Cooling the burn reduces swelling by conducting heat away from the skin. Do not put ice on the burn. Next, cover the burn with a sterile gauze bandage. Wrap the gauze loosely to avoid putting pressure on burned skin. For major burns (third-degree), call 911 or the facility's emergency number. Until an emergency unit arrives, do not remove burned clothing, but make sure the victim is no longer in contact with smoldering materials or exposed to electricity, smoke, or heat. Do not immerse large, severe burns in cold water as this can cause a drop in body temperature (hypothermia) and deterioration of blood pressure and circulation (shock). Cover the area of the burn. Use a cool, moist, sterile bandage; clean, moist cloth; or moist towels. When possible, elevate the burned body part or parts above heart level. Check for signs of circulation (breathing, coughing, or movement). If there is no breathing or other sign of circulation, begin CPR.
Cardiac arrest/ heart attack	A cardiac arrest occurs due to the cessation of the blood's normal circulation due to the heart's failure to contract effectively. A heart attack occurs when blood flow to the muscle of the heart is impaired.	All healthcare practitioners should be trained and certified to perform CPR and should be recertified every two years. The emergency services should be contacted as quickly as possible (before initiating CPR). If an automated external defibrillator (AED) is available, it should be applied after two CPR cycles. CPR should be continued until medical assistance arrives or the person shows signs of recovery.
Chemical splash in the eye	Several chemicals used in the clinic can be very corrosive.	Immediately flush the eye with water. Use clean, lukewarm tap water for at least 20 minutes, and use whichever of these approaches is quicker: Get into a shower and, while holding the affected eye or eyes open, aim a gentle stream of lukewarm water on the forehead over the affected eye, or direct the stream on the bridge of the nose if both eyes are affected. Hold the affected eye or eyes open. Place the head down and turn it to the side. Or, ask the person to hold the affected eye open under a gently running faucet.
Choking	Occurs when a foreign object gets lodged in the throat or esophagus, blocking the flow of air.	To ensure that the patient is choking, quickly determine whether the individual demonstrates an inability to talk, difficulty breathing, and an inability to cough forcefully, or whether the skin, lips, and nails turn blue or dusky. If choking occurs, first, deliver five back blows between the person's shoulder blades with the heel of your hand. Next, perform five abdominal thrusts (Heimlich maneuver). The Heimlich maneuver is performed by standing behind the person and wrapping your arms around their waist. The person is then tipped slightly forward. Making a fist with one hand, position it slightly above the person's navel, and, while grasping the fist with the other hand, press hard into the abdomen with a quick, upward thrust (as if trying to lift the person). Alternate between five back blows and five abdominal thrusts until the blockage is dislodged. If the person becomes unconscious, attempt to remove the blockage and perform CPR.
Convulsions/ seizures	Occurs as a result of an electrical imbalance in the brain.	The person should be protected from injury due to the potential of violent or excessive extremity movements and to protect the person's modesty or privacy.
Fainting	Occurs when the blood supply to the brain is momentarily inadequate, resulting in a temporary loss of consciousness.	Position the person on his or her back. If the person is breathing, restore blood flow to the brain by raising the person's legs above heart level—about 12 inches (30 cm)—if possible. Loosen belts, collars, or other constrictive clothing. If the person doesn't regain consciousness within one minute, call 911 or your local emergency number. Also, check the person's airway to be sure it's clear. If vomiting occurs, turn the patient on his/her side. Check for signs of circulation (breathing, coughing, or movement). If absent, begin CPR. Call 911 or your local emergency number. Continue CPR until help arrives or the person responds and begins to breathe.

(continued)

TABLE 6-11	Situations That Require First Aid and Appropriate Action (continued)	
Situation	**Description**	**Appropriate Action**
Fractures	Occurs when damage to the bone is sufficient to interrupt its continuity.	The objectives are to protect the fracture site, avoid further injury to it, prevent shock, reduce pain, and prevent wound contamination if the bone ends have penetrated the skin. The clinician should apply support to the site to stabilize it but should not attempt to align the bone ends. Any open fracture site should be covered with a sterile towel or dressing. If a spinal fracture is suspected, the clinician should use extreme caution and be sure to maintain the head and neck in a neutral position.
Cardiac arrest	Occurs when an artery supplying the heart with blood and oxygen becomes partially or completely blocked. A heart attack generally causes chest pain for more than 15 minutes, but it can also have no symptoms at all.	Call 911 or your local emergency medical assistance number. If possible, have the person chew and swallow an aspirin unless they are allergic to aspirin. Begin CPR.
Heat illness	Several heat illnesses exist, including: ▸ Heatstroke is a body temperature of greater than 40.6°C (105.1°F) due to environmental heat exposure with a lack of thermoregulation and inadequate fluid intake. Symptoms include dry skin, rapid, strong pulse, and dizziness. ▸ Heat exhaustion—can be a precursor of heatstroke; the symptoms include heavy sweating, rapid breathing, and a fast, weak pulse. ▸ Heat syncope—fainting as a result of overheating. ▸ Heat edema—swelling of the digits. ▸ Heat cramps—muscle pains or spasms when exercising in hot weather. ▸ Heat rash—skin irritation from excessive sweating. ▸ Heat tetany—usually results from short periods of stress in intense heat. Symptoms may include hyperventilation, respiratory problems, numbness or tingling, or muscle spasms.	Move the person out of the sun and into a shady or air-conditioned space. Call 911 or emergency medical help. Cool the person by covering him or her with damp sheets or by spraying with cool water. Direct air onto the person with a fan or newspaper. Have the person drink cool water or another nonalcoholic beverage without caffeine, if he or she can.
Insulin-related illnesses	Hypoglycemia—occurs when the blood sugar level is too low. Hyperglycemia—occurs when the blood sugar level is too high.	The goal is to restore the person to a normal insulin glucose state and remove, correct, or compensate for the condition's cause. *Hypoglycemia:* if the person is conscious, provide some form of sugar (eg, orange juice), and monitor the individual. *Hyperglycemia:* this is the more serious of the two, as it can lead to a diabetic coma and death. Ideally, an injection of insulin should be given.

REFERENCES

1. American Physical Therapy Association. Guide to Physical Therapist Practice. 3.0. American Physical Therapy Association; 2014.
2. Lewis PS. Cardiovascular assessment. In Ruppert SD, Dolan JT, Kernicki JG, eds. *Dolan's Critical Care Nursing: Clinical Management Through the Nursing Process.* 2nd ed. Philadelphia: FA Davis; 1996:142-163.
3. Davis MP, Walsh D. Cancer pain: How to measure the fifth vital sign. *Cleve Clin J Med.* 2004;71:625-632.
4. Salcido RS. Is pain a vital sign? *Adv Skin Wound Care.* 2003;16:214.
5. Sousa FA. [Pain: The fifth vital sign]. *Rev Lat Am Enfermagem.* 2002;10:446-447.
6. Lynch M. Pain: The fifth vital sign. Comprehensive assessment leads to proper treatment. *Adv Nurse Pract.* 2001;9:28-36.
7. Lynch M. Pain as the fifth vital sign. *J Intraven Nurs.* 2001;24:85-94.
8. Merboth MK, Barnason S. Managing pain: The fifth vital sign. *Nurs Clin North Am.* 2000;35:375-383.
9. Torma L. Pain—the fifth vital sign. *Pulse.* 1999;36:16.
10. Pain as the fifth vital sign. *J Am Optom Assoc.* 1999;70:619-620.
11. Joel LA. The fifth vital sign: Pain. *Am J Nurs.* 1999;99:9.
12. McCaffery M, Pasero CL. Pain ratings: The fifth vital sign. *Am J Nurs.* 1997;97:15-16.
13. Bailey MK. Physical examination procedures to screen for serious disorders of the low back and lower quarter. La Crosse, WI: Orthopaedic Section, APTA, Inc.; 2003.
14. Schmitz TJ. Vital signs. In O'Sullivan SB, Schmitz TJ, eds. *Physical Rehabilitation.* 5th ed. Philadelphia: FA Davis; 2007:81-120.
15. Dalby M, Gjesdal K. [Resting pulse rate as an indicator of health and disease]. *Tidsskrift for den Norske laegeforening: tidsskrift for praktisk medicin, ny raekke.* 2012;132:1348-1351.
16. Zhang D, Wang W, Li F. Association between resting heart rate and coronary artery disease, stroke, sudden death and noncardiovascular diseases: A meta-analysis. *CMAJ.* 2016;188:E384-E392.
17. DeTurk WE, Cahalin LP. Electrocardiography. In DeTurk WE, Cahalin LP, eds. *Cardiovascular and Pulmonary Physical Therapy: An Evidence-based Approach.* New York: McGraw-Hill; 2004:325-359.
18. Boudet G, Chaumoux A. Ability of new heart rate monitors to measure normal and abnormal heart rate. *J Sports Med Phys Fitness.* 2001;41:546-553.
19. Boudet G, Chamoux A. Heart rate monitors and abnormal heart rhythm detection. *Arch Physiol Biochem.* 2000;108:371-379.
20. Shaffer TH, Wolfson MR, Gault JH. Respiratory physiology. In Irwin S, Tecklin JS, eds. *Cardiopulmonary Physical Therapy.* 2nd ed. St Louis: Mosby;1990:217-244.
21. Collins SM, Cocanour B. Anatomy of the cardiopulmonary system. In DeTurk WE, Cahalin LP, eds. *Cardiovascular and Pulmonary Physical Therapy: An Evidence-based Approach.* New York: McGraw-Hill;2004:73-94.
22. Van de Graaff KM, Fox SI. Respiratory system. In Van de Graaff KM, Fox SI, eds. *Concepts of Human Anatomy and Physiology.* New York: WCB/McGraw-Hill; 1999:728-777.
23. Judge RD, Zuidema GD, Fitzgerald FT. Vital signs. In: Judge RD, Zuidema GD, Fitzgerald FT, eds. *Clinical Diagnosis.* 4th ed. Boston: Little, Brown and Company; 1982:49-58.
24. Huber MA, Terezhalmy GT, Moore WS. White coat hypertension. *Quintessence Int.* 2004;35:678-679.
25. Chung I, Lip GY. White coat hypertension: not so benign after all? *J Hum Hypertens.* 2003;17:807-809.
26. Alves LM, Nogueira MS, Veiga EV, de Godoy S, Carnio EC. White coat hypertension and nursing care. *Can J Cardiovasc Nurs.* 2003;13:29-34.
27. O'Sullivan J, Allen J, Murray A. The forgotten Korotkoff phases: How often are phases II and III present, and how do they relate to the other Korotkoff phases? *Am J Hypertens.* 2002;15:264-268.
28. Venet R, Miric D, Pavie A, Lacheheb D. Korotkoff sound: The cavitation hypothesis. *Med Hypotheses.* 2000;55:141-146.
29. Weber F, Anlauf M, Hirche H, Roggenbuck U, Philipp T. Differences in blood pressure values by simultaneous auscultation of Korotkoff sounds inside the cuff and in the antecubital fossa. *J Hum Hypertens.* 1999;13:695-700.
30. Paskalev D, Kircheva A, Krivoshiev S. A centenary of auscultatory blood pressure measurement: A tribute to Nikolai Korotkoff. *Kidney Blood Press Res.* 2005;28:259-263.
31. Perloff D, Grim C, Flack J, Frohlich ED, Hill M, McDonald M, et al. Human blood pressure determination by sphygmomanometry. *Circulation.* 1993;88:2460-2470.
32. Strugo V, Glew FJ, Davis J, Opie LH. Update: Recommendations for human blood pressure determination by sphygmomanometers. *Hypertension.* 1990;16:594.
33. Higgins JR, Walker SP, Brennecke SP. Re: Which Korotkoff sound should be used for diastolic blood pressure in pregnancy? *Aust N Z J Obstet Gynaecol.* 1998;38:480-481.
34. Likeman RK. Re: Which Korotkoff sound should be used for diastolic blood pressure in pregnancy? *Aust N Z J Obstet Gynaecol.* 1998;38:479-480.
35. Franx A, Evers IM, van der Pant KA, van der Post JA, Bruinse HW, Visser GH. The fourth sound of Korotkoff in pregnancy: A myth. *Eur J Obstet Gynecol Reprod Biol.* 1998;76:53-59.
36. Kelly G. Body temperature variability (Part 1): A review of the history of body temperature and its variability due to site selection, biological rhythms, fitness, and aging. *Altern Med Rev.* 2006;11:278-293.
37. Editors of Nursing. Take care with tympanic temperature readings. *Nursing.* 2007;37:52-53.
38. Sener S, Karcioglu O, Eken C, Yaylaci S, Ozsarac M. Agreement between axillary, tympanic, and mid-forehead body temperature measurements in adult emergency department patients. *Eur J Emerg Med.* 2011;19:252-256.
39. Pursell E, While A, Coomber B. Tympanic thermometry—normal temperature and reliability. *Paediatr Nurs.* 2009;21:40-43.
40. Barton SJ, Gaffney R, Chase T, Rayens MK, Piyabanditkul L. Pediatric temperature measurement and child/parent/nurse preference using three temperature measurement instruments. *J Pediatr Nur.* 2003;18:314-320.
41. Rush M, Wetherall A. Temperature measurement: Practice guidelines. *Paediatr Nurs.* 2003;15:25-28.
42. Denegar CR, Donley PB. Impairment due to pain: Managing pain during the rehabilitation process. In Voight ML, Hoogenboom BJ, Prentice WE, eds. *Musculoskeletal Interventions: Techniques for Therapeutic Exercise.* New York: McGraw-Hill; 2007:99-110.
43. Dray A. Inflammatory mediators of pain. *Br J Anaesth.* 1995;75:125-131.
44. Wiener SL. *Differential Diagnosis of Acute pain by Body Region.* New York: McGraw-Hill; 1993:1-4.
45. Adams RD, Victor M. *Principles of Neurology.* 5th ed. New York: McGraw-Hill, Health Professions Division; 1993.
46. Chusid JG. *Correlative Neuroanatomy & Functional Neurology.* 19th ed. Norwalk, CT: Appleton-Century-Crofts; 1985:144-148.
47. Judge RD, Zuidema GD, Fitzgerald FT. Musculoskeletal system. In: Judge RD, Zuidema GD, Fitzgerald FT, eds. *Clinical Diagnosis.* 4th ed. Boston: Little, Brown and Company; 1982:365-403.
48. Walk D, Poliak-Tunis M. Chronic pain management: An overview of taxonomy, conditions commonly encountered, and assessment. *Med Clin North Am.* 2016;100:1-16.
49. Taylor AJ, Kerry R. When chronic pain is not "chronic pain": Lessons from 3 decades of pain. *J Orthop Sports Phys Ther.* 2017;47:515-517.
50. Huskisson EC. Measurement of pain. *Lancet.* 1974;2:127.
51. Halle JS. Neuromusculoskeletal scan examination with selected related topics. In: Flynn TW, ed. *The Thoracic Spine and Rib Cage: Musculoskeletal Evaluation and Treatment.* Boston: Butterworth-Heinemann; 1996:121-146.
52. Melzack R. The McGill Pain Questionnaire: Major properties and scoring methods. *Pain.* 1975;1:277.
53. Melzack R, Torgerson WS. On the language of pain. *Anaesthiology.* 1971;34:50.
54. Kahn-D'Angel L, Unanue-Rose RA. The special care nursery. In Campbell SK, Vander Linden DW, Palisano RJ, eds. *Physical Therapy for Children.* 3rd ed. St. Louis: Saunders; 2006:1053-1097.
55. Michaleff ZA, Kamper SJ, Stinson JN, Hestbaek L, Williams CM, Campbell P, et al. Measuring musculoskeletal pain in infants, children, and adolescents. *J Orthop Sports Phys Ther.* 2017;47:712-730.
56. Hockenberry MJ, Wilson D, Winkelstein ML. *Wong's Essentials of Pediatric Nursing.* 7th ed. St. Louis: Mosby; 2004.
57. Beyer JE, Denyes MJ, Villarruel AM. The creation, validation, and continuing development of the Oucher: a measure of pain intensity in children. *J Pediat Nurs.* 1992;7:335-346.

CHAPTER 7

Bed Mobility, Patient Positioning, and Draping

CHAPTER OBJECTIVES

At the completion of this chapter, the reader will be able to:

1. Understand the importance of bed mobility to prevent secondary complications

2. Describe some of the precautions when positioning a patient

3. Discuss the biomechanical principles behind correct body mechanics

4. Describe some of the challenges facing a clinician while moving a patient or heavy object

5. Describe some of the mechanical devices that can be used during bed mobility tasks

6. List the 12 principles of good body mechanics

7. Demonstrate how to provide bed mobility to a dependent patient

8. Demonstrate how to instruct a patient in bed mobility

9. Describe the importance and the principles behind patient positioning

10. Describe the importance and the principles behind patient draping

OVERVIEW

Bed mobility activities are designed to increase functional independence or increase patient safety. For example, the patient must frequently adjust their position to prevent the development of joint contractures or skin breakdown. Bed mobility may be assisted by equipment, with help from another individual or individuals, or performed as independently as possible by the patient. There are many occasions when a patient needs to be positioned by the clinician. Examples include when a patient has decreased sensation to pressure or when the patient cannot alter their position independently. In those cases, the recumbent patient's body needs to be frequently moved, so the methods

All figures in this chapter are reproduced with permission from Dutton M: Introduction to Physical Therapy and Patient Skills, 2nd ed. New York, NY: McGraw Hill; 2014.

may have to be taught to nursing staff, family members, or caregivers. In contrast, depending on the patient's medical condition, such as after total joint replacement, the patient may need to learn to restrict certain movements that are contraindicated (see Clinical Pearl).

CLINICAL PEARL

Several medical conditions can result in mobility and position restrictions or contraindications. These include:

▶ *Total hip arthroplasty (THA):* the restrictions and contraindications following this surgical technique depend on the approach the surgeon used:

- The posterolateral approach involves avoiding hip flexion of the hip beyond 60°–90°, 0° hip adduction, and 0° of hip internal rotation.

- The lateral or anterolateral approach involves avoiding hip extension, external rotation, and adduction across the midline.

It is important to remember that these range-of-motion restrictions apply to both hip and trunk motion. For example, lifting the knee while sitting is biomechanically the same as leaning forward at the waist—both result in hip flexion beyond 90°.

▶ *Hemiplegia:* rolling from supine to side lying on the hemiplegic side is relatively straightforward, but rolling to lie on the stronger side presents a greater challenge.

▶ *Spinal cord injury (SCI):* the patient's functional ability post-SCI depends on the level and degree of injury (Table 7-1). For example, an SCI at the sixth cervical vertebra (C6) level will typically allow a patient to achieve the performance of bed mobility independently.

Draping or covering a patient can be a natural consequence of positioning or can be performed to expose a particular body part for an assessment or an intervention, such as passive range of motion (PROM).

Before any treatment session, the clinician should review the patient's chart, which often provides information about the level of assistance the patient requires (Table 10-2), and the clinician should plan ahead of time based on the goals in the plan of care (POC). Some of the preparation may require

TABLE 7-1   **Functional Outcome Related to Level of Spinal Cord Injury**

Level of Lesion	Function/Motion	Care Needs	ADLs	Equipment Needs

C1-C3	Limited head/neck movement
	Rotate/flex neck (sternocleidomastoid)
	Extend neck (cervical paraspinals)
	Speech and swallowing (neck accessories)
	Total paralysis of the trunk, upper and lower extremity
		24 hr care needs
		Able to direct care needs
			Ventilator-dependent
			Impaired communication
			Dependent for all care needs
			Mobility:
			   Power wheelchair,
			   Hoyer lift
				Adapted computer
				Bedside/portable ventilator
				Suction machine
				Specialty bed
				Hoyer lift
				Reclining shower chair

C4	Head and neck control (cervical paraspinals)
	Shoulder shrug (upper traps)
	Inspiration (diaphragm)
	Lack of shoulder control (deltoids)
	Paralysis of the trunk, upper extremity (UE), and lower extremity (LE)
	Inability to cough, low respiratory reserve
		24 hr care needs
		Able to direct care needs
			May or may not be ventilator-dependent
			Improved communication
			Assisted cough
			Dependent for all care needs
			Mobility:
			   Power wheelchair,
			   Hoyer lift
				Adapted computer
				Bedside/portable ventilator as needed
				Suction machine
				Specialty bed
				Hoyer lift
				Reclining shower chair

C5	Shoulder control (deltoids)
	Elbow flexion (biceps/elbow flexors)
	Supinate hands (brachialis and brachioradialis)
	Lacks elbow extension and hand pronation
	Paralysis of the trunk and LE
		10 hr personal care needs
		6 hr homemaking assistance
			Setup/equipment: eating, drinking, face wash, and teeth
			Assisted cough
			Dependent for bowel, bladder, and lower body hygiene
			Dependent for bed mobility and transfers
			Mobility:
			   Hoyer lift or stand pivot
			   Power wheelchair w/ hand controls
			   Manual wheelchair
			   Drive motor vehicle w/ hand controls
				Power and manual wheelchairs
				Adaptive splints/braces
				Page turners/computer adaptations

C6	Wrist extension (extensor carpi ulnaris and extensor carpi radialis longus/brevis) Arm across chest (clavicular pectoralis) Lack elbow extension (triceps) Lack wrist flexion Lack hand control Paralysis of the trunk and LE	6 hr personal care needs 4 hr homemaking assistance	Assisted cough Setup for feeding, bathing, and dressing Independent bed mobility (if sufficient spinal rotation—approximately 66°—can be performed), pressure relief, turns, and skin assessment. May be independent for bowel/bladder care	Independent slide board transfer Manual wheelchair Drive with adaptive equipment
C7	Elbow flexion and extension (biceps/triceps) Arm toward the body (sternal pectoralis) Lack finger function Lack trunk stability	6 hr personal care needs 2 hr homemaking assistance	More effective cough Fewer adaptive aids Independent w/ all ADLs May need adaptive aids for bowel care	Manual wheelchair Transfers without adaptive equipment
C8-T1	Increased finger and hand strength Finger flexion (flexor digitorum) Finger extension (extensor communis) Thumb movement (pollicis longus and brevis) Separate fingers (interossei separates)	4 hr personal care needs 2 hr homemaking assistance	Independent w/ or w/o assistive devices Assist w/ complex meal prep and home management	Manual wheelchair

(continued)

TABLE 7-1   Functional Outcome Related to Level of Spinal Cord Injury (continued)

Level of Lesion	Function/Motion	Care Needs	ADLs	Equipment Needs
T2-T6	Normal motor function of head, neck, shoulders, arms, hands, and fingers Increased use of intercostals Increase trunk control (erector spinae)	3 hr personal care needs/ homemaking	Independent in personal care	Manual wheelchair May have limited walking with extensive bracing Drive with hand controls
T7-T12	Added motor function Increased abdominal control Increased trunk stability	2 hr personal care needs/ homemaking	Independent Improved cough Improved balance control	Manual wheelchair May have limited walking with bracing Driving with hand controls
L2-L5	Added motor function in hips and knees L2 Hip flexors (iliopsoas) L3 Knee extensors (quadriceps) L4 Ankle dorsiflexors (tibialis anterior) L5 Long toe extensors (ext hallucis longus)	May need 1 hr personal care/homemaking	Independent	Manual wheelchair May walk a short distance with braces and assistive devices Driving with hand controls
S1-S5	Ankle plantar flexors (gastrocnemius) Various degrees of bowel, bladder, and sexual function Lower level equals greater function	No personal or homemaker needs	Independent	Increased ability to walk with less adaptive/ supportive devices Manual wheelchair for distance

the rearranging of furniture in the patient room, extra staffing, additional equipment (mechanical lift, positioning pad, draw sheet, etc), and consideration as to how to move the patient without compromising any of the leads or tubes connected to the patient (see Chapter 5).

CLINICAL PEARL

As a patient becomes more independent, less control from the clinician is needed.

ERGONOMICS

Ergonomics is concerned with the interactions among people and other elements of a system. From a physical therapy viewpoint, ergonomics is the design or modification of the working environment to fit the worker to prevent soft tissue injuries and musculoskeletal disorders (MSDs). This design and modification applies to the clinical environment as well as to a patient's workplace. Some of the most important ergonomic recommendations for a patient are described in Table 7-2. The impact of posture is discussed in Chapter 11.

BODY MECHANICS

A lifting task is defined as manually grasping an object with two hands and vertically moving the object without mechanical assistance. Body mechanics refers to how the clinician's

body is positioned or aligned during a lifting task. Correct positioning and alignment place the center of mass (COM) of the clinician close to the patient, which increases the efficiency of movements and limits the stress and strain on musculoskeletal structures.

The Occupational Safety and Health Administration (OSHA) requirements are set by statute, standards, and regulations. According to a fact sheet from OSHA, "lifting heavy items is one of the leading causes of injury in the workplace.*" However, OSHA does not have a standard that limits how much a person may lift or carry. The National Institute for Occupational Safety and Health (NIOSH), though, has developed a mathematical model that helps predict the risk of injury based on the weight being lifted and accounts for several job task variables (Table 7-3). According to this model, a Lifting Index (LI) value of 1.0 or less indicates a nominal risk to healthy employees, whereas an LI greater than 1.0 denotes that the task is high-risk for some fraction of the population. Thus, as the LI increases, the level of injury risk increases correspondingly.

Healthcare workers often experience MSDs, total lost workday injury, and illness incidence at a rate exceeding that of workers in construction, mining, and manufacturing.[1] Most of these injuries are the result of lifting and transferring patients.[2] These injuries incur very high direct costs in

---

*Hospital Safety: Safe Patient Handling Programs, Effectiveness—CMS Fact Sheet (OSHA 3729–2013)-https://www.osha.gov/publications/bytype/fact-sheets.

TABLE 7-2   Ergonomic Recommendations

Position/Activity	Plane of Deviation	Potential Problems	Recommendations
Standing	Sagittal	Prolonged standing in extension can result in excessive lumbar lordosis Prolonged standing in flexion can result in stress on the intervertebral disk	Take frequent breaks or regularly change position Cushioned mats Supportive shoes
Mowing/vacuuming	Sagittal	Prolonged flexion of the lumbar spine	Try to keep the trunk erect
Washing dishes	Sagittal	Prolonged hyperextension of the lumbar spine can irritate the facet joints	Elevate one foot on a stool
Personal hygiene (washing face, cleaning teeth)	Sagittal	Prolonged flexion of the lumbar spine	Minimize the amount of lumbar flexion
Sitting	Sagittal	Increased risk of stress on the intervertebral disc	Avoid sitting for longer than 15 minutes at a time
Reaching up	Sagittal	Prolonged hyperextension of the lumbar spine	Use a step ladder or similar stable device
Getting out of bed	Multiple	Rotational stresses to the lower back	If prone or supine, roll onto the side at the edge of the bed, lower the legs over the side, and push the trunk up with the arms
Getting out of a car	Multiple	Rotational stresses to the lower back	Keep the feet together when turning

workers' compensation, medical treatment, and vocational rehabilitation, as well as indirect costs due to lost production, retraining, and sick or administrative time, the latter of which can be at least four times the direct cost.[3,4] A variety of

TABLE 7-3   NIOSH Lifting Equation

RWL = LC (51) x HM x VM x DM x AM x FM x CM

Calculating the RWL using this formula helps determine which of the task's six components contribute most to the risk. Once the RWL is calculated, the Lifting Index (LI) can be determined to provide a relative estimate of the physical stress associated with a manual lifting job. The goal is to design all lifting jobs to accomplish an LI of 1.0 or less

RWL: Recommended Weight Limit—the maximum acceptable weight (load) that nearly all healthy employees could lift throughout an 8-hour shift without increasing the risk of musculoskeletal disorders (MSDs)

LC: Load constant—the weight of the object lifted

M: Multiplier. The multiplier factors have a value between 0 and 1. The lower the multiplier, the higher the risk, and therefore the lower the RWL

H: Horizontal location of the object relative to the body—the distance from the hands on the load to the midpoint between the ankles

V: Vertical location of the object relative to the floor—starting height of the hands from the ground

D: Distance the object is moved vertically

A: Asymmetry angle or twisting requirement—angle of the load in relation to the body

F: Frequency and duration of lifting activity

C: Coupling or quality of the worker's grip on the object—quality of the grasp or handhold based on the type of handles available

individual factors also play an important role. Individuals who are not in good physical condition tend to have more injuries. Previous trauma or certain medical conditions involving bones, joints, muscles, tendons, nerves, and blood vessels may predispose individuals to injuries. Finally, some psychological factors may influence the reporting of injuries, pain thresholds, and even the speed or degree of healing.

CLINICAL PEARL

It is very important to remember that the greater the load, the greater the risk of injury.

The problem of lifting a patient is compounded by the increasing weight of patients to be lifted due to the obesity epidemic in the United States and the rapidly increasing number of older people who require assistance with their activities of daily living.[5]

When working in healthcare, the physical demands involve pushing, pulling, forceful exertion, repetition, stressful positions or postures, and handling equipment; the amount of force involved can be accurately determined.

Before any activities involving lifting, pushing, or pulling, the clinician must decide whether the transfer is to be performed by a team, a mechanical device, or a combination of both.

▶ *Team.* Choose the best body mechanics possible for everyone involved to accomplish the task with minimal effort and safely. The 13 principles of good body mechanics include:

1. Prepare yourself. Stretch and move around before attempting to lift anything.

2. Plan by estimating the load and clearing the path of travel. Take your time.

3. Stand as close to the load as is feasible. Being as close as possible to the person or object to be lifted or carried allows the combined COM to be maintained within the base of support (BOS). When the COM is centered within the BOS and near the body's midline, both balance and good postural alignment are easier to maintain.

4. Use a BOS that is of the appropriate size and shape—stand with the feet apart, with one foot slightly in front of the other, and the toes pointing slightly outward.

5. Try to maintain normal spinal curvature. If the trunk is maintained in good alignment, the muscles only have to maintain this alignment and do not have to work to extend the trunk during the lifting motion. Whenever possible, the spine should be maintained in a neutral position. A simple method to determine pelvic neutral is to perform an anterior pelvic tilt and then a posterior pelvic tilt to find the midpoint between the two [VIDEO 7-1]. Avoid twisting at the trunk, particularly when the trunk is flexed. Instead, pivot at the feet or take several small steps to rotate the whole body.

6. Whenever possible, lifting should be initiated from the squat position. Getting low and close to the patient or object shortens the lever arm and allows the stronger muscles to operate. The squat's depth should permit the clinician to reach the person or object to be lifted, but not so deep that the leg muscles are moved out of their lifting and lowering power position. This type of squat is achieved by flexing the hips and knees rather than flexing the trunk. The other advantage of this position is that it maintains the COM of the body close to the BOS center—a shorter resistance lever arm requires less effort.

7. When possible, push rather than pull an object, as pushing permits a larger BOS and a lower COM and makes it easier to use the larger muscles more efficiently.

8. Keep the combined COM of the clinician, equipment, or patient within the BOS by holding them close.

9. If possible, elevate the surface to waist height. A load close to the height of the COM conserves energy and maintains stability during a lift.

10. Exhale during exertion to minimize any increase in intraabdominal pressure, which can elevate blood pressure.

11. Avoid rotation of the spine (twisting), particularly when the trunk is flexed. Position the feet pointing in the planned direction and move and pivot the feet during the transfer to avoid twisting and reaching.

12. Before lifting, gently engage the core (abdominal) muscles. Contracting these muscles before lifting may reduce the potential for injury.

13. Know your capabilities and limitations to avoid attempting a task if there is any doubt about completing it safely.

▶ *Mechanical device.* A mechanically assisted or "zero-lift" transfer involves transferring an individual who is unable to provide minimal or any assistance.

When moving large pieces of equipment, the clinician should be positioned behind the equipment or patient, facing the direction of movement. This strategy allows the clinician to:

1. Determine a path free from obstruction

2. Use a lifting or pushing motion

3. Use larger muscles and body weight more efficiently during pushing or lifting

In all cases, plan movements and prepare the area to be used before starting. Use proper body mechanics and safety precautions.

CLINICAL PEARL

When in doubt about your ability to lift or carry a patient or object safely, always obtain additional assistance.

BED MOBILITY

Bed mobility activities are an important component of progressively improving a patient's independence and safety within their abilities. Regardless of the patient's level of dependence, the clinician must always use proper body mechanics while also guarding them. If possible, the height of the transfer surfaces should be adjusted to enhance comfort and safety. As with all planned physical exertion, the clinician should assess whether physical or mechanical assistance is required before attempting the activity. Mechanical assistance can include the use of bed rails, a draw sheet, or an overhead bar or frame in cases where the patient cannot safely perform the activity without equipment. Whenever possible, the patient should be encouraged to participate both mentally and physically in the task, as patient involvement fosters independence and boosts problem-solving. The most common bed mobility activities include the patient turning from a supine to a side lying position and returning; moving from a supine to prone position and returning; moving from a lying to a sitting position and returning; and moving in a variety of horizontal directions (upward, downward, side to side) and returning to the center of the bed. More advanced activities include scooting while supine and sitting, and scooting on the edge of the bed. The clinician should always consider the concepts of COM and BOS during mobility activities. These concepts include:

▶ The greater the mass, the greater the stability.

▶ The greater the friction, the greater the stability.

▶ The larger the BOS, the greater the stability.

▶ The lower the COM, the greater the stability.

▶ The more the BOS is widened in the direction of the line of force, the greater the stability.

From a clinical perspective, the concepts just listed can be applied when moving a patient. For example, when pulling

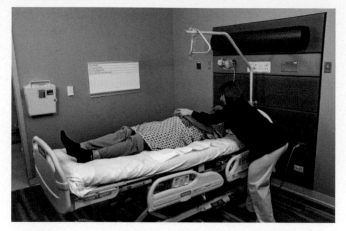

FIGURE 7-1 Folding the patient's arm in preparation for movement.

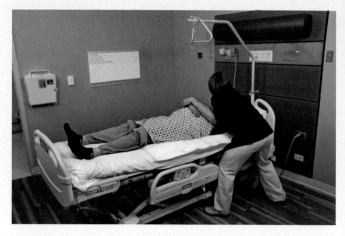

FIGURE 7-3 Moving upper third of patient sideways in bed—initial move.

and sliding a patient, the clinician places his or her COM as close to the patient's COM as possible, widens his or her feet to increase the BOS, and applies the force required to move the patient parallel to the surface of the bed, thereby reducing the energy required. Positioning the patient close to the clinician allows the upper extremity muscles to use short lever arms. This is important because short lever arms can develop greater force than long lever arms, require less energy expenditure, and provide better patient control.

Assisted Mobility

Side-to-Side Movement. With the patient positioned in supine, the clinician folds the patient's arm across the chest (Figure 7-1) and then positions one forearm under the patient's neck, supporting the patient's head, and one forearm under the middle of the patient's back (Figure 7-2). The clinician then gently slides the patient's upper body and head closer to where the clinician is standing (Figures 7-3 and 7-4). Next, the clinician can either place his or her forearms under the patient's lower trunk just distal to the pelvis or use the bed mat (Figure 7-5) before gently sliding that body segment in the same direction as previous (Figure 7-6). Finally, the clinician places his or her forearms under the patient's

thighs and legs (Figure 7-7) and gently slides them toward him or her (Figure 7-8).

Upward Movement. This technique, which normally requires an assistant, is one of the more difficult ones, as it has the most potential for injury to the clinician's shoulders or lower back. If the bed is adjustable, the portion that raises the head and trunk should be flat, and any pillows should be removed from under the patient's head and shoulders. Using the previously mentioned concept that the greater the friction, the greater the stability, the clinician flexes the patient's hips and knees so that only the feet rest flat on the bed. Depending on the patient's level of dependence, their thighs may need to be supported with one or more pillows to maintain the position. The clinician and the assistant stand approximately opposite the patient's mid-chest level, facing toward the patient's head, and with the foot that is farthest from the bed in front of the other foot [VIDEO 7-2]. Using both arms, the lifting team grasps the bed mat, and while keeping close to the patient's chest, the patient is slid upward approximately 6 inches. The technique is repeated until the required position is reached.

Downward Movement. If the bed is adjustable, the portion that raises the head and trunk should be raised. The clinician

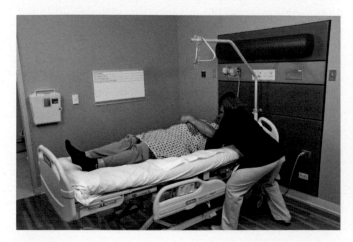

FIGURE 7-2 Clinician positions arms under the patient.

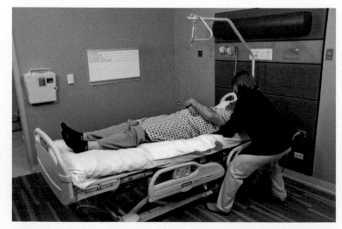

FIGURE 7-4 Moving upper third of patient sideways in bed—end of move.

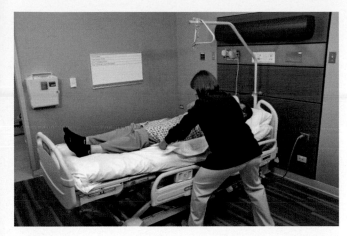

FIGURE 7-5 Moving the middle third of the patient using the bed mat.

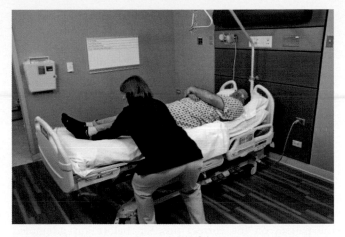

FIGURE 7-7 Moving the lower third of the patient—start position.

and the assistant stand approximately opposite to the patient's waist or hips. Using both arms, the lifting team grasps the bed mat, and while keeping close to the patient's waist, the patient is slid downward. The technique is repeated until the required position is obtained.

Turning from Supine to Side Lying. To turn the patient to the right, the clinician stands on the side of the bed to which the patient is turning, and the patient is positioned close to the edge of the left side of the bed. The right arm is abducted to approximately 45°, and the left lower extremity is crossed over the right lower extremity at the ankle. Using the right hand, the clinician grasps the patient's left hip while holding the patient's left hand against the same hip. The clinician's left hand is used to grasp the patient's left shoulder, and then the patient is rolled into the side lying position.

Turning from Supine to Prone. Moving a patient from supine to prone in a hospital bed does not frequently occur because of modern mattress design. Indeed, given the mattress design, placing a patient prone is likely to be hazardous because of the potential for breathing problems as the face sinks into the mattress. Therefore, the following description is more likely to be used when the patient is on a mat table. The patient is positioned toward one edge of the mat table so that a full rolling movement to the prone position

can occur without the patient coming too near the opposite edge. To roll the patient to the right side of the bed, the patient is first moved to the left side of the bed using the technique described in Side-to-Side Movement. To roll a patient toward the right side of the bed:

► The patient's left lower extremity is crossed over the right lower extremity, with the left ankle resting on top of the right ankle.

► The patient's right upper extremity is abducted, placing the hand under the right hip, palm facing upward against the hip, while the hand and forearm of the left upper extremity are placed across the abdomen.

► The clinician stands on the side of the mat table to which the patient will be turned—in this case, on the patient's right-hand side.

► The clinician's hands are positioned under the patient's left shoulder and lower back to initiate the rolling. When the patient reaches the roll's halfway position, the clinician rotates their hands, positioning them on the patient's anterior surface to control the second half of the roll.

► After the roll is completed, the head is repositioned first, placing it in a comfortable position facing one side

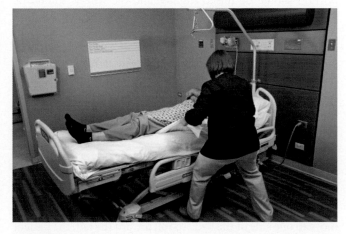

FIGURE 7-6 End of the move using the bed mat.

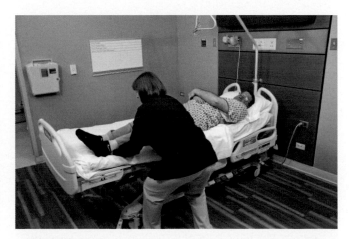

FIGURE 7-8 Moving the lower third of the patient—end position.

(normally toward the side of the roll direction) and ensuring no pressure is being exerted on the patient's eyes, nose, or mouth. Where indicated, a pillow is placed under the trunk and adjusted as necessary (see Prone Position). The upper extremities are placed in a slight abduction position—approximately 20°–30°, and the feet are positioned approximately 6 to 8 inches apart. Generally speaking, rolling a patient from prone to supine is essentially the reverse of rolling the patient from supine to prone.

Independent Mobility

When performing these activities, it is important to instruct the patient on the correct position before any attempted mobility activities. For example, depending on the bed's width, the patient may need to adjust their position by moving forward or backward before attempting to roll. The following techniques may need to be modified based on the patient's size and functional abilities.

Scooting Upward. If the bed is adjustable, the upper portion should be flat, and the wheels should be locked. The patient is positioned in the hooklying position, with the heels close to the buttocks and the upper extremities beside the trunk. The patient is asked to elevate the pelvis using the lower extremities, elevate the upper trunk by simultaneously pressing into the bed with the elbows and the back of the head, and then move toward the head of the bed while pressing down with the lower extremities and depressing the shoulders. The lower and upper extremities are then repositioned before successive movements are attempted. Several other methods can be used to increase patient independence with moving up the bed. These methods are shown in [VIDEOS 7-3 through 7-5].

Before discharge from the hospital, the clinician must review any of the bed mobility skills previously taught to the patient [VIDEO 7-6]. In addition to those previously described, the following should also be reviewed as appropriate.

Video Description

In Video 7-6, several bed mobility skills are reviewed with the patient. These include:

▶ *Hooklying.* Hooklying, which is the supine position with the hips and knees flexed so that the feet are flat on the bed, is a basic bed mobility position from which other skills are derived.

▶ *Bridging.* From the hooklying position, the patient lifts the hips and lower back off the bed. This skill can provide pressure relief while also allowing items such as bedpans and bed linens to be placed underneath the patient.

▶ *Scooting in supine.* This skill, which is a precursor for such skills as rolling and getting out of bed, allows the patient to move up, down, and sideways in the bed. Scooting is made easier by lowering the part of the bed to which the patient is moving. For example, if the

patient moves up the bed, it is easier when the bed's head is lowered.

▶ *Rolling.* This skill can be used to relieve pressure on body tissues and help with air exchange in the lungs. From a functional perspective, the skill allows objects such as linens, slings, and bedpans to be placed under the supine patient. The patient can use head rotation, trunk rotation, and motions of the upper and lower extremities to assist with rolling. The two main types of rolling are a segmental roll, in which the patient moves the shoulder and upper trunk to the side first, followed by the pelvis and lower extremities, and the log roll where the patient moves the whole body at once.

▶ *Supine to sitting.* The sitting position in bed can either occur with the legs extended (long sitting) or with the hips and knees flexed (short sitting). Long sitting is useful for positional adjustments, or when a patient has undergone a total hip arthroplasty and is not permitted to flex the hip beyond 60°. Short sitting is typically used to sit on the side of the bed before standing. To move from supine to sitting requires upper extremity strength in patients with mobility limitations.

▶ *Sitting to supine.* This skill is essentially the reverse of supine to sitting, and the patient uses an upper extremity to control the descent of the trunk into the side lying position before lifting both lower extremities onto the bed.

Side-to-Side Movement. Side-to-side movements are best performed with the patient supine. The patient is asked to assume the hooklying position, have one upper extremity next to the trunk, and the other upper extremity abducted approximately 6 inches from the trunk. The patient is asked to perform a bridge and then move the trunk toward the abducted upper extremity side before lowering the trunk (see Video 7-6). The lower and upper extremities are then repositioned to either move again or for comfort. The activity is practiced so that the patient can move to both the right and the left side.

Scooting Downward. If the bed is adjustable, the upper portion should be raised slightly, and the wheels should be locked. The patient is positioned in the hooklying position with the heels approximately 12 inches distal to the buttocks and the upper extremities positioned next to the trunk. The patient is asked to elevate the pelvis using the lower extremities and to elevate the upper trunk by simultaneously pushing into the bed with the elbows and the back of the head before moving down by pulling with the lower extremities (concentric knee flexion) while simultaneously pushing up with the shoulders and pulling down with the elbows (concentric shoulder extension) or forearms (see Video 7-6). The lower and upper extremities are then repositioned for successive movements.

Rolling from Supine to Sidelying. The patient is asked to move to one side of the bed. To roll toward the left, the patient simultaneously reaches across the chest with the right upper extremity and lifts the right lower extremity diagonally over the left lower extremity, then uses a combination of neck flexors and the abdominal muscles to roll onto the side, or uses the right hand to grasp the edge of the bed/bed rail to pull themselves into the side lying position (see Video 7-6). Once in the side lying position, the BOS can be increased by flexing the lower extremities and reaching back with the right upper extremity. The activity is practiced so that the patient can move into right and left side lying. Alternatively, the patient can perform a log roll by moving the whole body simultaneously. This technique is used frequently following back surgery, as it avoids twisting the spine.

Assuming Sitting. Moving directly from supine to sitting places extreme amounts of torque through the patient's spine. The better techniques do not overstress the patient's spine.

▶ *Supine to long sitting:* providing that the patient has enough strength, the long sitting position can be accomplished using a sit-up from a position propped up on the elbows (see Video 7-6). When minimal assistance is necessary, a trapeze bar can be used while the clinician assists by placing an arm behind the patient's back. In those situations where a trapeze bar is not available, the clinician's forearm can be used.

▶ *Supine to sitting:* if the patient is independent, the patient flexes the hips and knees to 60°–90° and then moves the lower legs over the edge of the bed while using the upper extremities to push down on the table and raise the trunk (see Video 7-6). When minimal assistance is necessary, the clinician grasps the patient's lower extremities and lowers them over the edge of the bed, and helps lift the upper trunk as necessary.

Video Description

VIDEOS 7-7, 7-8, 7-9, and 7-10 show a series of methods to teach a patient how to perform supine-to-sit and sit-to-supine skills based on patient ability. Notice how the clinician always tries to get the patient to do as much of the work as possible, thereby enhancing independence. The clinician also frequently asks the patient whether or not the instructions have been understood. Comprehension is particularly important in Video 7-10 when the postsurgical precautions limit the patient's ability to transfer. Again, the clinician reviews these precautions with the patient, a process that must occur as frequently as necessary.

Scooting in Sitting. Perhaps the most important scoot in sitting is the sideways scoot, which can be used for a patient who is about to return to lying supine in bed. To perform a sideways scoot on the edge of the bed, the patient abducts the arm on the side to which he or she is moving, thus creating a space for the patient's hips to move to. The patient is then asked to push down with both hands into the bed using a fisted hand (less stressful to the wrist than using an open palm with the wrist extended), to depress the shoulders, and to raise the hips off the bed and over to the new position (see

Video 10-6). This technique is repeated until the desired position is achieved. One of two techniques can be used to scoot backward or forward in a sitting position, based on the patient's upper extremity strength:

▶ *Good upper extremity strength:* the patient is asked to lean the trunk slightly forward with the hands by the hips and to press down into the bed. Suppose the bed is at such a height that the patient's feet can touch the floor. In that case, this technique can be assisted by bringing the feet back toward the bed and pushing down on the feet while simultaneously pushing down with the upper extremities before the patient lifts the torso up and then either forward or backward.

▶ *Poor upper extremity strength:* the patient is asked to scoot forward or backward by weight shifting to one side and then moving the opposite hip forward or backward and then repeating this maneuver on the other side until the desired position is achieved.

PATIENT POSITIONING

Immobility can be viewed as a limitation in the purposeful, independent, physical movement of the body or one or both lower extremities. During immobility, bodyweight produces pressure on the skin; subcutaneous tissue; bone; and the circulatory, neural, and lymphatic systems (see Chapter 8). Under normal circumstances, if the bodyweight occurs for long enough, pain and sensory receptors, triggered by localized ischemia, activate and produce a motor response to change positions. If a change in position is not triggered, skin breakdown can occur within 1 to 2 hours. Initially, the skin remains intact, but a nonblanchable erythema appears over the pressure site, which should serve as an early warning sign. Shear and friction forces, together with moisture and chemical irritants, can quickly exacerbate the process. Therefore, to prevent skin breakdown from occurring, it is necessary to move any patient with limited mobility regularly. Frequent patient repositioning (at least every two hours when lying, and every 10 minutes when sitting) is required for conditions including loss of or decreased sensory awareness, paralysis or inability to move independently, bowel and/or bladder incontinence, decreased skin strength, poor nutrition, severe weight loss (cachexia), impaired circulation, an inability to express or communicate discomfort, and a predisposition to contracture development (Table 7-4). In addition to patient positioning, it is also necessary to inspect the patient's skin, especially over bony prominences (Table 7-5), before and immediately after the treatment session. It is also important to remove or reduce folds or wrinkles in the linen beneath the patient to avoid increased skin pressure.

CLINICAL PEARL

Deep venous thrombosis (DVT) and its sequela, pulmonary embolism, are the leading causes of preventable in-hospital mortality in the United States.[6] The Virchow triad,

TABLE 7-4	Soft Tissue Contracture Sites Associated with Prolonged Positioning
Position	**Contracture Sites**
Supine	Shoulder internal rotators, extensors, and adductors Forearm, elbow, wrist, and fingers (depending on the upper extremity position used) Hip and knee flexors Hip external rotators Ankle plantar flexors
Prone	Neck rotators, left or right Shoulder internal/external rotators, extensors, and adductors Forearm, elbow, wrist, and fingers (depending on the upper extremity position used) Ankle plantar flexors
Sidelying	Shoulder adductors and internal rotators Forearm, elbow, wrist, and fingers (depending on the upper extremity position used) Hip adductors and internal rotators Hip and knee flexors
Sitting	Shoulder adductors, internal rotators, and extensors Forearm, elbow, wrist, and fingers (depending on the upper extremity position used) Hip adductors and internal rotators Hip and knee flexors

as first formulated (ie, venous stasis, vessel wall injury, hypercoagulable state), is still the primary mechanism for DVT.[6] Hypercoagulable states include:

► *Genetic:* includes antithrombin C deficiency, protein C deficiency, and protein S deficiency.

► *Acquired:* includes postoperative, postpartum, prolonged bed rest or immobilization, severe trauma, cancer, congestive heart failure, obesity, advanced age, and prior thromboembolism.

No single physical finding or combination of symptoms and signs is sufficiently accurate to establish a DVT diagnosis.[6] The following is a list outlining the most sensitive and specific physical findings in DVT[6-9]:

► Edema, principally unilateral

► If present, tenderness is usually confined to the calf muscles or throughout the thigh's deep veins. Pain and/

or tenderness away from these areas is not consistent with venous thrombosis and usually indicates another diagnosis.

► Venous distention and prominence of the subcutaneous veins.

► Fever: patients may have a fever, usually low grade.

It is important to note that the Homan sign—discomfort in the calf muscles on forced dorsiflexion of the foot with the knee straight—which has been a time-honored sign of DVT, is found in more than 50% of patients without DVT and is present in less than one-third of patients with confirmed DVT, making it very nonspecific.

Prophylactic treatment of DVT includes staying active and mobile whenever possible, medication (heparin, warfarin, aspirin, and dextran), and the use of mechanical modalities such as external pneumatic compression devices and compression stockings.

When appropriate, the clinician should introduce themselves to the patient and explain the purpose of the planned treatment, including how and why the patient is to be positioned. Whenever possible, the patient should be encouraged to be an active participant. To prevent patient injury, the patient's body and extremities should always be fully supported on the mat or table with no partial portion of the body or extremities projecting beyond the surface. The most effective way to position a patient is to position the proximal components (the center of the patient's mass) first. For example, if the pelvis is positioned correctly, the head and extremity positions often occur naturally.

CLINICAL PEARL

Factors to avoid when positioning a patient include:

► Compromising the patient's airway.

► Excessive, prolonged pressure on soft tissues, circulatory, and neurologic structures.

► Poor spinal alignment.

► Positioning the patient's extremities beyond or below the support surface. Extremities that project beyond the support surface are at increased risk for injury, whereas

TABLE 7-5	Bony Prominences Associated with Pressure Ulcers		
Supine	**Prone**	**Sidelying**	**Seated**
Occiput	Forehead	Ears	Spine of scapula
Spine of scapula	The anterior portion of the acromion process	The lateral portion of the acromion process	Vertebral spinous processes
The inferior angle of the scapula	Anterior head of the humerus	The lateral head of the humerus	Ischial tuberosities
Vertebral spinous processes	Sternum	Lateral epicondyle of humerus	
Medial epicondyle of humerus	Anterior superior iliac spine	Greater trochanter	
Posterior iliac crest	Patella	Head of the fibula	
Sacrum	Dorsum of foot	Lateral malleolus	
Coccyx		Medial malleolus	

extremities positioned below the support surface are prone to edema formation.

- Clothing or linen folds beneath the patient, which can produce skin breakdown.
- Excessive and prolonged pressure over bony prominences.
- Friction or shear forces. These can occur if the patient is dragged. A shear force is an applied force that tends to cause an opposite, but parallel, sliding motion of an object's planes.
- Positioning a patient in a way that minimizes interaction with the environment.

The first time a patient is placed in a new position, it is recommended that the skin be checked after 5–10 minutes, and frequently after that, to determine tolerance for the new position.

CLINICAL PEARL

- When inspecting a patient's skin, red areas indicate pressure areas, whereas pale (or blanched) areas may indicate severe, precarious pressure. A red or blanched area that does not return to a normal appearance within an hour must be monitored, and the use of the position that caused the problem should be avoided in the future.
- Subjective complaints of numbness or tingling are indicators of excessive pressure, as is localized edema or swelling.
- The use of supportive devices may cause perspiration buildup, which may lead to skin maceration.

The goals of proper positioning are to:

- Support, stabilize, and provide proper alignment of the axial and appendicular skeletal segments to promote the efficient function of the body systems.
- Provide correct positioning for the administration of effective, efficient, and safe treatment procedures.
- Make the patient as comfortable as possible. However, it is worth remembering that the patient's position of comfort may be the position that could lead to the development of a soft tissue contracture—a limitation of joint motion caused by adaptive shortening in the soft tissue structures, including ligaments, tendons, joint capsule, and muscles. Generally speaking, flexed positions are positions of comfort—for example, hip flexion, knee flexion, and elbow flexion, all common sites for contractures.
- Position the patient based on current medical status. For example, it is worth remembering that a patient with an impaired cardiopulmonary system will not tolerate prolonged positions and will and require frequent monitoring.
- Prevent the development of secondary impairments such as deformities, edema, venous thrombosis, and/or pressure sores. Extra care must be taken with patients who are older, mentally incompetent, paralyzed, or agitated.

CLINICAL PEARL

An immobile patient cannot use their muscles to pump fluid throughout the body toward the heart. Therefore, any extremity positioned below the heart level (dependent position) is at increased risk for edema formation. Similarly, a lack of muscle contraction can produce venous stasis, which increases the risk of the formation of a blood clot or thrombus.

- Provide the patient access to stimulation from the environment.

CLINICAL PEARL

A patient who is being turned or positioned must be lifted rather than dragged across the sheets to prevent skin breakdown.

The clinician must consider what is to be required and what the challenges will be before attempting to reposition a patient, including clinician positioning for optimal body mechanics, appropriate adjustment of the bed height, control of the patient throughout the task, the application of appropriate contact with the patient, and communication with the rest of the rehabilitation team (eg, establishing that any lifting will follow a "1, 2, 3" count). Depending on the patient's environment, the clinician may also have to consider any lines, leads, and tubes attached to the patient. Where possible, it is advisable to include the nursing team in such scenarios. Also, the clinician should assemble the necessary devices that are to be used to support or stabilize the patient. Such devices include pillows, rolled towels, or commercially available devices (eg, bolsters, foam wedges). If a sensitive area must be relieved of pressure, the limb segment can be supported by a pillow or roll just proximal and just distal to the sensitive area. Suppose this type of "bridging" position is used. In that case, the pressure is typically increased, and the circulation is decreased in the adjacent areas, meaning that the time spent in this position must be limited.

CLINICAL PEARL

When attempting to position a patient, the clinician should have several alternatives that can be used based on the patient's condition and ability. For example, a patient with congestive heart failure or chronic obstructive pulmonary disease (COPD) will not tolerate lying flat in a supine position. The clinician should always consider the following factors when positioning a patient:

- Patient safety
- Patient comfort
- Whether the position provides sufficient access to the treatment area

A restraint, which can be pharmacologic or physical, is a means by which a patient can be prevented from harming themselves or others. A pharmacologic restraint is a medication given to control behavior, whereas a physical restraint is prescribed to protect the patient from rolling or falling and to prevent injury. These devices are recommended for short-term use only and should not be used to hinder or restrain a patient for several hours. In fact, the Joint Commission (JC) standards require that a licensed independent practitioner must order restraint or seclusion when applied for behavioral health reasons. The practitioner must conduct an in-person (face-to-face) evaluation of a patient in restraint seclusion at least every 24 hours and at least one hour after initiation.[10] An exception to this would be the use of protective positioning for the patient who:

► Is comatose
► Is mentally or physically incapable of maintaining a safe position
► Is experiencing spasticity
► Has extensive paralysis

CLINICAL PEARL

Physical or pharmacologic restraints, or seclusion, cannot be used without the patient's voluntary consent and the physician's ongoing order. Any patient who is restrained must be monitored at least every 2 hours. Rules, regulations, and guidelines related to the use of restraint and seclusion have been developed and are enforced by various state, local, and federal agencies and by accreditation organizations, including the Department of Public Health (DPH), the Centers for Medicare and Medicaid Services (CMS), and the JC.

Several methods can be used to position/reposition a patient.

Supine Position. The patient is positioned with the shoulders parallel to the hips and the spine straight (Figure 7-9).

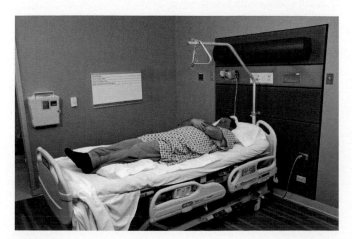

FIGURE 7-9 The supine position.

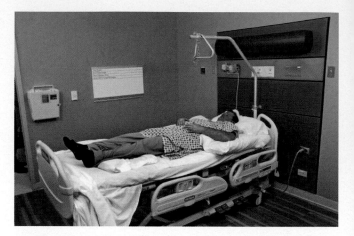

FIGURE 7-10 Using supports for the upper extremities.

The upper extremities may be elevated on pillows by the patient's side or folded on the chest (Figure 7-10) to help prevent edema. The hands should be positioned in an open position to prevent contractures. The hips should be positioned in neutral flexion and/or extension or slightly flexed. A rolled towel can be used to maintain the hips in a neutral position. A small pillow or a cervical roll can be placed under the patient's head while avoiding excessive neck and upper back flexion or scapula abduction (rounded shoulders). A small pillow may also be placed behind the knees to relieve strain on the lower back and prevent knee hyperextension. However, because this position encourages hip and knee flexion that may contribute to lower extremity contractures of the iliopsoas and hamstring muscles, this position should not be maintained for a prolonged period. To relieve pressure on the heel (calcaneus), one of two methods can be used:

► A pillow can be placed under both legs (see Figure 7-9).
► A small, rolled towel can be placed under the patient's ankles while avoiding knee hyperextension.

CLINICAL PEARL

The areas of greatest pressure in the supine position are:
► The occipital tuberosity of the skull
► The spine and inferior angle of the scapula
► The spinous processes of the vertebrae
► The posterior iliac crests
► The sacrum
► The posterior calcaneus

If the patient's hip is positioned in external rotation, the fibular head, the greater trochanter of the hip, and the ankle's lateral malleolus should be regularly monitored.

Prone Position. The patient is positioned with the shoulders parallel to the hips and the spine straight. A small pillow or towel roll is placed under the patient's head, or the head is

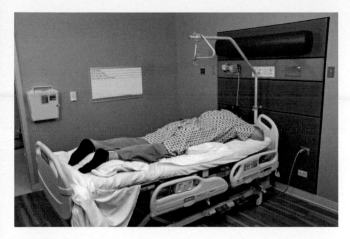

FIGURE 7-11 Prone position with the upper extremities in a T-position.

positioned to the left or right. The patient's upper extremities can be positioned in one of three ways:

► In a T-position with the arms overhead alongside the head (Figure 7-11). Placing the arms overhead increases the lumbar lordosis (see later).

► Along the sides of the patient (Figure 7-12). A folded towel should be placed under each anterior shoulder area to adduct the scapula, reduce the stress on the interscapular muscles, and protect the humeral head.

► With the hands under the head. It is worth remembering that if the upper extremities are positioned above shoulder height, there is an increased propensity for neurovascular compromise. Therefore, this position should only be used when the patient has intact sensation in the arms and when frequent testing for numbness or tingling can be performed.

CLINICAL PEARL

The areas of greatest pressure in the prone position are:
► The forehead
► The lateral ear

► The tip of the acromion process
► The anterior head of the humerus
► The sternum
► The anterior superior iliac spine (ASIS)
► The patella
► The tibial crest
► The dorsum of the foot

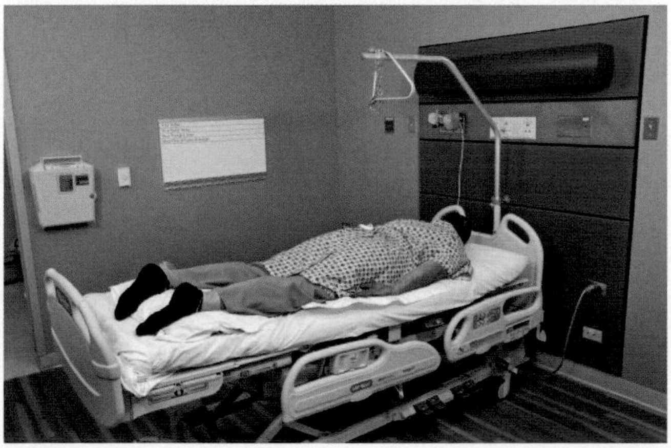

The amount of lordosis and kyphosis of the spine can be controlled using padding. For example, a pillow placed under the patient's lower abdomen will reduce lumbar lordosis (see Figure 7-11), whereas a pillow placed under the middle or upper chest or positioned lengthwise from the pelvis to the thorax can be used to maintain the lordosis. To avoid positioning the patient's ankles in plantar flexion, the patient's feet can be positioned over the end of the bed, or a pillow can be used under the anterior portion of the patient's ankles to relieve stress on the hamstring muscles (see Figure 7-11). The latter position should not be maintained for a prolonged period, as it promotes knee flexion, which can contribute to the development of a knee flexor (hamstrings) contracture.

Side Lying Position. The patient is initially positioned in the center of the bed, with the head, trunk, and pelvis aligned, and both of the lower extremities flexed at the hip and knee. The head is supported by a pillow (Figure 7-13). The uppermost lower extremity is supported on one or two pillows and positioned slightly forward compared to the lowermost extremity to avoid excessive pull on the lower trunk. It is the lowermost lower extremity that provides stability to the patient's pelvis and lower trunk. The upper trunk can be rotated forward or backward:

► If the patient is rotated backward, a pillow is placed behind the patient, and the uppermost upper extremity is extended and supported by that pillow (see Figure 7-13).

► If the patient is rotated forward, a pillow is placed in front of the patient, and the uppermost upper extremity is flexed and supported by that pillow.

FIGURE 7-12 Prone position with the upper extremities along the sides of the patient.

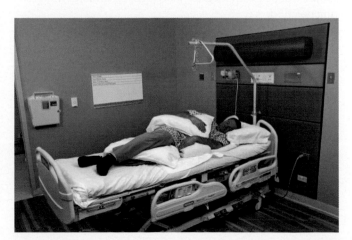

FIGURE 7-13 Side lying position.

141

CLINICAL PEARL

The areas of greatest pressure in the side lying position are:

► The lateral ear
► Lateral ribs
► The lateral acromion process
► The lateral and/or medial epicondyles of the humerus, depending on which upper extremity
► The epicondyles of the humerus
► The greater trochanter of the femur
► The lateral or medial condyle of the femur, depending on which lower extremity is uppermost or closest to the bed
► The lateral or medial malleolus, depending on which lower extremity is uppermost or closest to the bed

Sitting Position. The seated patient must be positioned in a chair with adequate support and stability for the trunk and lower extremities. The patient's upper extremities can be supported on pillows, the chair armrests, a lapboard, or a pillow in the patient's lap. It is important to remember that the patient should not be left unguarded in the sitting position when they cannot maintain the position safely.

CLINICAL PEARL

The areas of greatest pressure in the sitting position are:

► The ischial tuberosities
► The posterior areas of the thigh
► The sacrum
► The spinous processes of the vertebrae (if the patient is leaning against the chair back)
► The medial epicondyle of the humerus (if the elbow rests on a hard surface)

In general, a patient who cannot alter their body position should not be positioned for more than 30 minutes in the sitting position.

Preventative Positioning Based on Diagnosis. Certain diagnoses require specific positioning guidelines to avoid secondary complications related to short-term or prolonged positioning (Table 7-6).

CLINICAL PEARL

A cerebrovascular accident (CVA), or stroke, can either increase or decrease muscle tone on one side of the body. An increase in muscle tone can result in contractures of the upper and/or lower extremity, whereas a decrease in muscle tone can make the affected joints more susceptible to distractive forces and edema.

PATIENT DRAPING

When working with patients, including during transport and treatment, attention must be paid to appropriate draping or dress. Draping involves covering the patient with a sheet(s), gown, or towel(s). Draping a patient appropriately during a therapy session is a seemingly simple yet very important component of a patient's care. When moving a patient, planning is required to maintain appropriate draping during the movement.

The purposes of draping are to:

► Maintaining patient modesty. The patient should be draped with clean linen to expose only the areas or body parts to be treated, with the remainder of the patient's body covered to maintain modesty. If possible, the patient can be alerted ahead of time to bring a change of clothes that would naturally expose the area. For example, asking a patient to wear (or bring) shorts allows the clinician free access to the patient's thigh, knee, and lower leg. Also, if a patient has to be transported to another department, draping may be necessary.
► Provide the clinician with the necessary access to specific areas of the body.
► Absorb perspiration, water, and other various lubricants, or prevent the fluids from contacting the patient's clothing.
► Provide warmth and protection and maintain a comfortable body temperature. For example, when patients are not ambulating, standing, or otherwise bearing weight on their feet, socks or slippers should be worn to provide adequate warmth and protection.
► Protect the skin and clothing from becoming soiled or damaged.
► Protect vulnerable skin areas such as wounds, scars, or stumps.

CLINICAL PEARL

Each patient has an individual sense of modesty and dignity, based on their cultural, religious, or personal beliefs. Thus, the clinician should assume that the patient is extremely modest unless the patient indicates otherwise. Also, any individual with a history of psychological trauma (eg, posttraumatic stress disorder) or abuse (physical, sexual, psychological, or any combination of these) may display an intense emotional reaction to bodily exposure, touch, or certain positions.[11-14]

Before draping, all restrictive clothing, splints, or other devices that will interfere with the treatment should be removed.

CLINICAL PEARL

Although hospital gowns worn by patients are designed to ease dressing and access during nursing care, they may not provide effective draping during the required movements and treatment positions used in physical therapy.

TABLE 7-6	Preventative Positioning Based on Diagnosis	
Diagnosis	**Key Positions to Avoid**	**Recommendations**
Hemiplegia	*Upper Extremity* Shoulder adduction and internal rotation Elbow flexion Forearm supination or pronation Wrist, finger, or thumb flexion Finger and thumb adduction	The upper extremity should be positioned in varying amounts of shoulder abduction and external rotation, elbow extension, slight wrist extension, thumb abduction and extension, finger extension, and slight finger abduction.
	Lower Extremity Hip and knee flexion	The lower extremity should be positioned in varying amounts of hip and knee extension, hip abduction and internal rotation, ankle dorsiflexion, and eversion.
	Hip external rotation Ankle plantar flexion	The involved extremity must be exercised several times per day. The normal alignment of the patient's head and trunk should be maintained.
	Ankle inversion	The use of a sling to support the involved upper extremity should be avoided. Care should be taken when positioning the patient in a side lying position on the affected side. For example, the involved shoulder should be positioned slightly forward so that the scapula is protracted.
Recovering and grafted burn areas	Positions of comfort Flexion or adduction of most peripheral joints (if the burn is located on the flexor or adductor surface of the joint)	Prevention is the key—once a contracture has developed, time, perseverance, and uncomfortable exercise will be necessary to return the joint to a normal functional use position.
Osteoarthritis and rheumatoid arthritis	Positions of comfort Immobility	Promote gentle active or passive range of motion exercises Maintain activity levels within tolerance.
Edema	Involved limb maintained in the dependent position	Encourage elevation of the involved limb at a level higher than the heart.
Pulmonary dysfunction	Supine or recumbent positions	Encourage the patient to elevate the head of the bed when lying Prone lying may benefit some patients as it can improve respiratory mechanics by increasing lung volume and decreasing lung secretions. Chronic obstructive pulmonary disease (COPD) can benefit from the tripod position, where the patient sits and leans forward with their outstretched hands on their knees.
Transfemoral amputation	Hip flexion of the residual limb Hip abduction of the residual limb	Sitting should be limited to no more than 40 minutes of each hour. In the standing or lying position, the residual limb should be maintained in extension (prone lying when the patient is recumbent).
Transtibial amputation	Hip and knee flexion Leg crossing	Sitting should be limited to no more than 40 minutes of each hour. In the standing or lying position, the residual limb should be maintained in extension (prone lying is recommended when the patient is recumbent).
Total hip arthroplasty	If a posterolateral surgical approach was used, the following position should be avoided: ▶ Hip flexion beyond 60°–90° ▶ Hip adduction beyond 0° ▶ Hip internal rotation beyond 0° Full side lying position is contraindicated.	Supine positioning with an abduction wedge or pillow between the legs to prevent hip adduction. Specific attention must be given to the sacral area, which is vulnerable to skin breakdown. Adhere to the surgeon's postoperative protocol.
Total knee arthroplasty	Positions of comfort Knee flexion	Discourage positioning of pillows behind the knee when supine or sitting. Encourage gentle active or passive ROM exercises into knee flexion and extension. Adhere to the surgeon's postoperative protocol.

TABLE 7-7	Common Religious, Cultural, and Ethnic Preferences	
Religious, Cultural, or Ethnic Group	**Preference**
African and Caribbean South Asian (Indian subcontinent) Chinese Hindu women Muslim women Some Latino groups	Strong preference for a healthcare provider of the same sex
Asian Chinese Romany Traveller Orthodox Jewish women	Bodily exposure embarrassment
Some Mormons Rastafarian women	Taboos against wearing garments previously worn by others or against taking off garments that should not be removed
Traditional Egyptians Hindus Orthodox Jews Many North Americans Navajo women Children in many cultural or geographical groups Older individuals in some cultural or geographical groups	Restrictions on touching

Data from Mootoo JS. A guide to spiritual and cultural awareness, Nurs Stand. 2005 Jan 5;19(1):2-18.

A patient's cultural, religious, or personal preferences may affect the clinician's ability to appropriately drape the patient to expose the necessary areas of skin or body parts. Therefore, it is important that, before positioning or draping the patient, the clinician determines whether the patient has specific cultural, religious-based, or personal requests or preferences that would affect the draping process. Table 7-7 outlines some of the more common religious, cultural, and ethnic preferences, although it is important to guard against stereotyping.

CLINICAL PEARL

The American Physical Therapy Association (APTA) has issued guidelines stating that physical therapists and physical therapist assistants are to "provide culturally sensitive care distinguished by trust, respect, and an appreciation for individual differences."

If draping becomes necessary, the clinician should inform the patient that clothing may need to be removed and the purpose of such removal, and obtain permission to proceed. The area to be treated must be exposed and be able to move freely so that observation or palpation of the area can occur and the intervention can be performed effectively. It is important to stress that the body areas will be covered except for the area to

be treated, and that the amount of body area exposed and the length of time it is exposed will be kept to a minimum. When possible, the patient should be educated on how to prepare themselves or be provided with an assistant of the same sex, and the clinician should ask permission before reentering the cubicle, to ensure that the patient is appropriately draped. Suppose the patient cannot remove items of clothing independently. In that case, the clinician must communicate clearly how he or she will assist and then proceed with a matter-of-fact and confident approach to help put the patient at ease while observing the patient for any signs of discomfort or embarrassment. If the clinician needs to leave the treatment area for whatever reason during treatment, the patient should be dressed or draped so that the body is not unduly exposed.

CLINICAL PEARL

The American Medical Association (AMA) recommends that a chaperone be available to all patients on request and that this policy be communicated to the patient in a noticeable form. The APTA recommends providing a same-gender chaperone during patient examination and intervention if requested by the patient or deemed necessary by the clinician.

Only clean and previously unused linen and garments should be used for draping. After each treatment session, any soiled linen and garments must be properly disposed of. The clinician must wear gloves if body fluids have soiled the articles. A gown, sheet, or towel can be used to drape the patient's anterior chest and lower extremities while making sure not to restrict joint motion or access to the area to be treated.

CLINICAL PEARL

Hospital gowns, which open at the back, offer little to enhance patient modesty. However, if appropriate, two gowns can be used. By wearing an additional gown backward so that it opens in the front, better overall coverage of the body can be achieved.

When sheets or blankets are used for draping, they should not be tucked in tightly at the foot of the bed, as this can place the ankles into a position of plantar flexion. The correct draping for a supine patient is depicted in Figure 7-14 for an upper extremity treatment. Figure 7-15 demonstrates the correct draping of the lower extremities for a supine patient. Suppose a lower extremity is to be moved for treatment, and there is potential for the patient's perineum (groin) to be exposed. In that case, the area must be covered with a sheet or towel applied high in the groin and under the thigh to ensure that the area is covered fully (Figure 7-16). Different techniques can be used to drape the trunk. For example, if ultrasound is to be applied to the lower back with the patient in prone, the entire trunk is first covered with a sheet (Figure 7-17); then a towel is placed over the sheet (Figure 7-18), after which the sheet is withdrawn a sufficient amount (Figure 7-19) while simultaneously moving the towel over the treatment area (Figure 7-20).

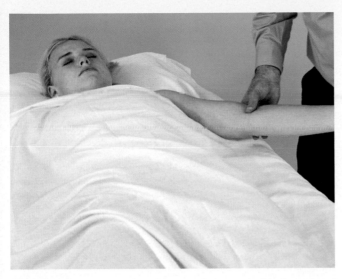

FIGURE 7-14 Correct draping for a supine patient for treatment of the upper extremity.

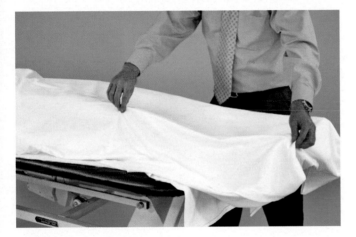

FIGURE 7-15 Correct draping for a supine patient.

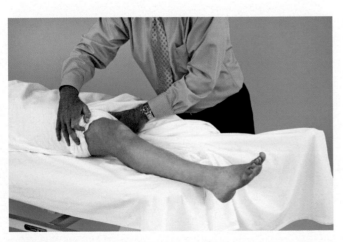

FIGURE 7-16 Correct draping for a supine patient for treatment of the lower extremity.

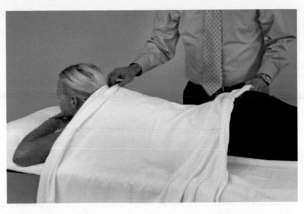

FIGURE 7-17 Draping the entire trunk with a sheet.

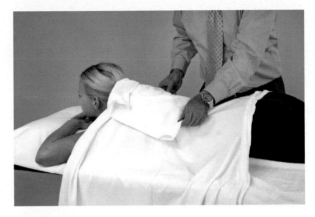

FIGURE 7-18 Towel placed over the sheet.

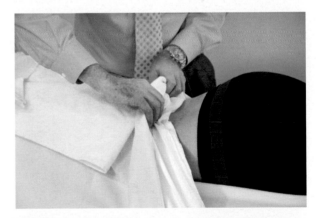

FIGURE 7-19 The sheet is withdrawn.

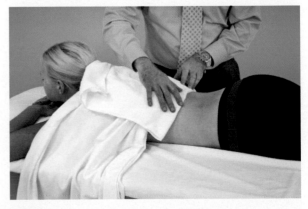

FIGURE 7-20 The towel replaces the sheet.

After the treatment session, the materials used for draping must be placed in the appropriate laundry basket and must not be used with another patient, however clean they may appear. If the treatment procedure has involved the use of lotions or gels, the clinician should provide the patient with a towel to remove any residue.

REFERENCES

1. Bureau of Labor Statistics. Incidence rates for nonfatal occupational injuries and illnesses involving days away from work per 10,000 full-time workers by industry and selected events or exposures leading to injury or illness in 2006. Department: US Department of Labor Washington, DC (2007).
2. White AH. Principles for physical management of work injuries. In: Isernhagen S, ed. *Work Injury.* Gaithersburg, MD: Aspen Publishers; 1988:24-38
3. Grandjean CK, McMullen PC, Miller KP, Howie WO, Ryan K, Myers A, et al. Severe occupational injuries among older workers: Demographic factors, time of injury, place and mechanism of injury, length of stay, and cost data. *Nurs Health Sci.* 2006;8:103-107.
4. Leigh JP, Waehrer G, Miller TR, Keenan C. Costs of occupational injury and illness across industries. *Scand J Work Environ Health.* 2004;30:199-205.
5. Ogden CL, Carroll MD, Curtin LR, McDowell MA, Tabak CJ, Flegal KM. Prevalence of overweight and obesity in the United States, 1999-2004. *JAMA.* 2006;295:1549-1555.
6. Motsch J, Walther A, Bock M, Bottiger BW. Update in the prevention and treatment of deep vein thrombosis and pulmonary embolism. *Curr Opin Anaesthesiol.* 2006;19:52-58.
7. Bounameaux H, Reber-Wasem MA. Superficial thrombophlebitis and deep vein thrombosis: A controversial association. *Arch Interl Med.* 1997;157:1822-1824.
8. Gorman WP, Davis KR, Donnelly R. ABC of arterial and venous disease. Swollen lower limb-1: General assessment and deep vein thrombosis. *BMJ.* 2000;320:1453-1456.
9. Aschwanden M, Labs KH, Engel H, Schwob A, Jeanneret C, Mueller-Brand J, et al. Acute deep vein thrombosis: Early mobilization does not increase the frequency of pulmonary embolism. *Thromb Haemost.* 2001;85:42-46.
10. Guerrero P, Mycyk MB. Physical and chemical restraints (an update). *Emerg Med Clin Nor Am.* 2020;38:437-451.
11. Arias I, Dankwort J, Douglas U, Dutton MA, Stein K. Violence against women: The state of batterer prevention programs. *J Law Med Ethics.* 2002;30:157-165.
12. Bemporad JR, Beresin E, Ratey JJ, O'Driscoll G, Lindem K, Herzog DB. A psychoanalytic study of eating disorders: I. A developmental profile of 67 index cases. *J Am Acad Psych.* 1992;20:509-531.
13. Elton D, Stanley G. Cultural expectations and psychological factors in prolonged disability. *Adv Behav Med.* 1982;2:33-42.
14. Sasano EM, Shepard KF. Sociocultural considerations in physical therapy education. *Phys Ther.* 1973;53:1269-1275.

CHAPTER 8   Mobility

CHAPTER OBJECTIVES

At the completion of this chapter, the reader will be able to:

1. Define the various components of mobility and how they work together to produce functional movements

2. List the different types of physiologic motions

3. Describe the differences among active motions, active-assisted motions, and passive motions

4. Describe the purpose of range of motion (ROM) exercises

5. List the different types of diagonal patterns of motion that can be incorporated therapeutically

6. Interpret the findings of active and passive ROM testing

7. Perform a ROM examination using a goniometer

8. Apply passive range of motion (PROM) techniques to the upper extremity

9. Apply PROM techniques to the lower extremity

OVERVIEW

Normal mobility is necessary for efficient movement. The terms *range of motion (ROM)*, *flexibility*, and *accessory joint motion* are often listed as components of mobility[1]:

▸ ROM. Refers to the distance and direction (eg, flexion, extension, abduction, adduction, internal rotation, and external rotation) a joint can move.

▸ Flexibility. Refers to the passive extensibility of connective tissue that provides the ability for a joint or series of joints to move through a full, nonrestricted, injury-free, and pain-free ROM.

▸ Accessory joint motion. The amount of glide that occurs at the joint surfaces, termed *joint play*.

Physiologic motions are joint and soft tissue movements that can be produced actively or passively. Active motions can

be produced by the patient alone, whereas passive motions are those motions that require assistance to complete. Active assisted motions are those that are a combination of active and passive motions.

CLINICAL PEARL

For a joint to function completely, both the osteokinematic and arthrokinematic motions have to occur normally.

▸ Osteokinematic motion: movements that can be performed voluntarily, eg, how the humerus moves during flexion of the shoulder.

▸ Arthrokinematic motion: the motion(s) of the bone surfaces within the joint, eg, how the convex head of the humerus moves within the concave glenoid cavity of the scapula.

As osteokinematic and arthrokinematic motions are proportional to each other, such that one cannot occur completely without the other, it follows that if an active motion is decreased compared to the same joint on the other side of the body, one or both of these motions may be at fault.

RANGE OF MOTION

ROM exercises are designed to move the joint and soft tissues through the available physiologic ranges of motion.

CLINICAL PEARL

ROM exercises aim to provide sensory stimulation and prevent the adverse effects of immobility (see Chapter 7). These adverse effects include the development of:

▸ Adaptive muscle-tendon shortening

▸ Joint contractures

▸ Deep vein thrombosis (DVT)

▸ Pneumonia and/or aspiration

▸ Urinary tract infection (UTI)

▸ Pressure ulcers

All figures in this chapter are reproduced with permission from Dutton M: Introduction to Physical Therapy and Patient Skills, 2nd ed. New York, NY: McGraw Hill; 2014.

TABLE 8-1	Some of the Benefits of Active Range of Motion (AROM) Exercises

Maintaining the elasticity, strength, and contractile endurance of the muscle

Enhancing local blood circulation

Providing increased sensory awareness

Possible improvements in cardiopulmonary functions if performed at the correct intensity

Possible prevention of thrombus formation

Enhancing bone strength if performed in weight bearing

▶ *Active range of motion (AROM):* performed by the patient independently. AROM exercises are used when the patient can voluntarily contract, control, and coordinate a movement when such a movement is not contraindicated. Contraindications to AROM include a healing fracture site, a healing surgical site, severe and acute soft tissue trauma, and cardiopulmonary dysfunction. The presence of several conditions requires caution with AROM exercises. These include acute rheumatoid arthritis, significant pain or joint swelling, or if the symptoms are intensified with the exercise. The benefits of AROM exercises are outlined in Table 8-1.

▶ *Active assisted range of motion (AAROM):* performed when the patient needs assistance with movement from an external force because of weakness, pain, or muscle tone changes. The assistance may be applied mechanically, manually, or by gravity, while the patient performs a voluntary muscle contraction to the extent he or she can. AAROM exercises are used in the presence of muscular weakness, fatigue, or pain.

▶ *Passive range of motion (PROM):* usually performed when the patient is unable or not permitted to move the body segment actively, and the clinician or family member moves the body segment. PROM exercises are typically used where there is paralysis, when the patient is comatose, in the presence of a healing fracture, or if significant pain is elicited during an active muscle contraction. One of the primary goals of PROM is to counteract the detrimental effects of immobilization. However, it is important to remember that PROM exercises cannot prevent muscle atrophy.

Diagonal Patterns of Motion

Diagonal patterns of motion, which can be performed using PROM, AAROM, or AROM, or with more advanced techniques using resistance, were first incorporated with the techniques of proprioceptive neuromuscular facilitation (PNF), which were based on the theory that the muscles of the body function around three planes of movement in a three-dimensional fashion, with each movement associated with an antagonistic motion. These motions and their antagonists are as follows:

▶ Flexion or extension

▶ Adduction or abduction in the extremities and lateral movement in the trunk

▶ Internal or external rotation

Combinations of these movements work together in spiral and diagonal patterns. The patterns, which integrate sports and daily living motions, are based on an infant's developmental sequence, such as rolling, crawling, and walking. The advantages of diagonal patterns include:

▶ All of the movements involve a combination of motions.

▶ Rotation is incorporated with all movements.

▶ Many of the movements involve the crossing of the midline of the body.

▶ The movements are more functional than movements performed in a planar direction.

There are two fundamental diagonal patterns for the lower extremity (Table 8-2) and for the upper extremity and scapula (Table 8-3), which are referred to as the diagonal 1 (D1) and diagonal 2 (D2) patterns.

These patterns are subdivided into D1 and D2 patterns that move into flexion (D1 flexion and D2 flexion) and D1 and D2 patterns that move into extension (D1 extension and D2 extension). Based on whether the upper extremity or

TABLE 8-2	Lower Extremity Proprioceptive Neuromuscular Facilitation Patterns
Start Position for D1 Pattern	
D1 Extension	**D1 Flexion**
Hip flexed, adducted, and externally rotated	Hip extended, abducted, and internally rotated
Knee flexed	Knee extended
Tibia internally rotated	Tibia externally rotated
Ankle and foot dorsiflexed and inverted	Ankle and foot plantarflexed and everted
Toes extended	Toes flexed
Movement into hip extension, abduction, and internal rotation; ankle plantarflexion; foot eversion; toe flexion	Movement into hip flexion, adduction, and external rotation; ankle dorsiflexion; foot inversion; toe extension
Start Position for D2 Pattern	
D2 Flexion	**D2 Extension**
Hip extended, adducted, and externally rotated	Hip flexed, abducted, and internally rotated
Knee extended	Knee flexed
Tibia externally rotated	Tibia internally rotated
Ankle and foot plantarflexed and inverted	Ankle and foot dorsiflexed and everted
Toes flexed	Toes extended
Movement into hip flexion, abduction, and internal rotation; ankle dorsiflexion; foot eversion; toe extension	Movement into hip extension, adduction, and external rotation; ankle plantarflexion; foot inversion; toe flexion

D1, diagonal 1; D2, diagonal 2.

TABLE 8-3	Upper Extremity and Scapular Proprioceptive Neuromuscular Facilitation Patterns
Start Position for D1 Pattern	
D1 Flexion	**D1 Extension**
Scapula depressed and adducted	Scapula elevated and abducted
Shoulder extended, abducted, and internally rotated	Shoulder flexed, adducted, and externally rotated
Elbow extended	Elbow extended
Forearm pronated	Forearm supinated
Wrist extended and ulnarly deviated	Wrist flexed and radially deviated
Fingers abducted and extended	Fingers adducted and flexed
Thumb extended and abducted	Thumb flexed and adducted
Movement into shoulder flexion, adduction, and internal rotation; scapular elevation and abduction; forearm supination; wrist flexion and radial deviation; finger flexion	Movement into shoulder extension, abduction, and internal rotation; scapular depression and adduction; forearm pronation; wrist extension and ulnar deviation; finger extension
Start Position for D2 Pattern	
D2 Extension	**D2 Flexion**
Scapula elevated and adducted	Scapula depressed and abducted
Shoulder flexed, abducted, and externally rotated	Shoulder extended, adducted, and internally rotated
Elbow extended	Elbow extended
Forearm supinated	Forearm pronated
Wrist extended and radially deviated	Wrist flexed and ulnarly deviated
Fingers extended and abducted	Fingers adducted and flexed
Thumb extended and adducted	Thumb flexed and abducted
Movement into shoulder extension, adduction, and internal rotation; scapular depression and abduction; forearm pronation; wrist flexion and ulnar deviation; finger flexion	Movement into shoulder flexion, abduction, and external rotation; scapular elevation and adduction; forearm supination; wrist extension and radial deviation; finger extension

D1, diagonal 1; D2, diagonal 2.

lower extremity is being used, the terminology can be expanded to D1 flexion lower extremity, D1 flexion upper extremity, and so on. The patterns are named according to the position of the pattern's proximal joint (ie, the shoulder or the hip) at the end position of the pattern. Thus, the pattern is initiated with the proximal joint positioned opposite to its end position. For example, to initiate a D1 flexion diagonal of the upper extremity, which involves flexion, abduction, and external rotation, the shoulder is positioned in the upper extremity's D1 extension position (extension, abduction, and internal rotation).

CLINICAL PEARL

Although it would appear that the use of diagonal patterns for ROM exercises is more efficient than ranging a joint through its anatomic planes because these patterns employ several planes simultaneously, they do not produce as much ROM to the muscles and joints as when the anatomic planes are used.

When performing PNF patterns involving patient contribution (active or resisted motions), the clinician's hand placement is designed to provide a tactile contact and stimulus to the major muscles involved in producing the desired movement, so the hands of the clinician are placed over the muscle or muscles that are to contract while avoiding contact with the muscle or muscles that are to relax during the exercise. When performing the diagonal patterns without patient contribution (passive motion), hand placement is not critical.

Before prescribing any of the ROM exercises, the clinician must determine the purpose of the exercise, the amount of support necessary for the patient, whether stabilization is necessary, the patient's ability to perform the exercise, and the effect of gravity.

Purpose. The most common purpose for ROM exercises is to enhance the patient's functional capacity by maintaining or improving joint motion and range. AROM can affect strength, endurance, and coordination, whereas the benefits of PROM are limited to maintaining or improving joint motion range and assisting in the maintenance of local circulation.

Support Necessary. Support is used to relieve stress on a joint or body segment by controlling the weight of the extremity or body part or compensating for the loss of muscle strength.

Stabilization. Stabilization, which is used to avoid, limit, or prevent movement, is typically used to protect the site of a healing fracture or extensive tissue trauma, and during the acute healing stage.

The Ability of the Patient. Whenever possible, the patient must be allowed to perform at a challenging level without being detrimental to the healing process. To make such a determination, the clinician must be aware of the strengths and weaknesses of the musculoskeletal, neuromuscular, and cardiopulmonary systems of the patient. The clinician must also have a working knowledge of the various stages of healing and such biomechanical concepts as stress, force, torque, levers, and axes of motion.

Effect of Gravity. Gravity can affect an exercise based on the angle at which the exercise is performed:

▶ An active exercise performed perpendicular to the ground is working against gravity if the exercise is directed away from the ground, eg, elbow flexion performed in the sitting or standing position.

▶ An active exercise performed perpendicular to the ground is working with gravity if the exercise is directed toward the ground, eg, elbow extension performed in the sitting or standing position.

▶ An active exercise performed parallel to the ground negates the effect of gravity if the limb is supported, eg, elbow flexion performed on a mat table with the humerus and forearm supported by the table.

INTERPRETATION OF ACTIVE AND PASSIVE RANGE OF MOTION

Both active and passive motions can provide the clinician with valuable information.

Active Range of Motion of the Extremities. During the history, the physical therapist will have deduced the general motions that aggravate or provoke the pain, and other procedures, including the ROM examination, are used to confirm the exact directions of motion that elicit the symptoms. The normal AROM for each of the joints is depicted in Table 8-4.

AROM testing gives the clinician information about the following:

▶ The quantity of available physiologic motion

▶ The presence of muscle substitutions

▶ The willingness of the patient to move

▶ The integrity of the contractile and inert tissues

▶ The quality of motion

▶ Any symptom reproduction

▶ The pattern of motion restriction (eg, capsular or noncapsular)

Capsular and Noncapsular Patterns of Restriction. Cyriax[1] introduced the terms *capsular* and *noncapsular* when describing joint restriction patterns (Table 8-5). A capsular pattern of restriction is a limitation of pain and movement in a joint-specific ratio, usually present with arthritis or following prolonged immobilization.[2] It is worth remembering that a consistent capsular pattern for a particular joint might not exist and that these patterns are based on empirical findings and tradition, rather than on research.[3,4] Significant degeneration of the articular cartilage presents with crepitus (joint noise) on movement when compression of the joint surfaces is maintained.

According to Cyriax, a noncapsular pattern of restriction is a limitation in a joint in any pattern other than a capsular one and may indicate the presence of a joint derangement, a restriction of one part of the joint capsule, or an extra-articular lesion that obstructs joint motion.[2]

Although abnormal motion is typically described as being reduced, abnormal motion may also be excessive. Excessive motion is often missed and is erroneously classified as normal motion. To help determine whether the motion is normal or excessive, PROM, in the form of passive overpressure, and the end-feel are initially assessed by the physical therapist (see next section).

CLINICAL PEARL

Apprehension from the patient during AROM that limits a movement at near or full range suggests instability, whereas apprehension in the early part of the range suggests anxiety caused by pain.

Full and pain-free AROM suggests normalcy for that movement, although it is important to remember that normal *range* of motion is not synonymous with normal motion.[5] Normal motion implies that the control of motion must also be present. This control is a factor of muscle flexibility, joint stability, and central neurophysiologic mechanisms. These factors are highly specific in the body.[6] Also, loss of motion at one joint may not prevent a functional task's performance, although it may result in the task being performed abnormally. For example, the act of walking can still be accomplished in the presence of a knee joint that has been fused into extension.

Repeated movements can give the clinician some valuable insight into the patient's condition[7]:

▶ Symptoms of a postural dysfunction remain unchanged with repeated motions.

▶ Pain from a dysfunction syndrome is increased with tissue loading but ceases at rest.

▶ Repeated motions can indicate the irritability of the condition.

▶ Repeated motions can indicate to the clinician the direction of motion to be used as part of the intervention. For example, if pain increases during repeated motion in a particular direction, exercising in that direction is not indicated. However, if the pain only worsens in part of the range, repeated motion exercises can be used within the range that is pain-free or does not worsen the symptoms.

TABLE 8-4	Active Ranges of Joint Motions			
Joint	**Action**	**Available Degrees of Motion**	**Expected Range**	**Possible Substitutions**
Shoulder	Flexion	0–180	120° of pure GH flexion 150° with GI I, AC, SC, and ST contribution 180° if lumbar hyperextension permitted	Lumbar hyperextension Scapular tipping NB: maintain slight elbow flexion so that long head of triceps does not restrict motion
	Extension	0–40	40°	Lumbar flexion
	Abduction	0–180	90° of pure GH abduction 150° with GH, AC, SC, and ST contribution 180° if lumbar side bending is allowed	Lumbar side bending Excessive scapular upward rotation can contribute to movement
	Internal/external rotation	Internal: 0–70 External: 0–90	70° internal rotation; 90° external rotation	The amount of motion available is influenced by abduction in the frontal plane and whether the measurement is performed in the scapular or frontal planes
	Horizontal adduction	Varies	45°	Trunk rotation
Elbow	Flexion	0–150	150°	Position of forearm (supination/pronation) can affect results
	Extension	Varies according to gender	Males: 0° Females: 10–15°	Towel roll may need to be placed posterior to elbow to allow hyperextension to occur
Forearm	Pronation	80–90	80–90°	Wrist flexion and/or ulnar deviation, abduction and IR of the shoulder, and/or contralateral trunk side bending
	Supination	80–90	80–90°	Wrist extension and/or radial deviation, adduction and ER of the shoulder, and ipsilateral trunk side bending
Wrist	Flexion	0–75	Varies according to generalized hypermobility	Excessive radial or ulnar deviation
	Extension	0–75	75°	Excessive radial or ulnar deviation
	Radial deviation	0–20	20°	MCP abduction or adduction
	Ulnar deviation	0–30	30°	MCP abduction or adduction
Hip	Flexion	0–120	Typically decreases with age	Lumbar spine flexion
	Extension	0–30	Typically decreases with age	Lumbar spine extension
	Abduction	0–45	45°	Hip external rotation, knee flexion/internal rotation, or lateral pelvic tilt
	Adduction	0–30	30°	Hip internal rotation or lateral pelvic tilt
	Internal rotation	0–45	45° (can be decreased in elderly population secondary to osteoarthritis)	Thigh adduction
	External rotation	0–45	45°	Thigh abduction
Knee	Flexion	0–150	135° (depends on the degree of musculature)	May be decreased with adaptive shortening of the rectus femoris

(continued)

TABLE 8-4	Active Ranges of Joint Motions (continued)			
Joint	Action	Available Degrees of Motion	Expected Range	Possible Substitutions
Ankle	Plantarflexion	0–50	30–50°	None
	Dorsiflexion	0–20	10° with the knee extended 20° with the knee flexed	Affected by the degree of gastrocnemius adaptive shortening
Subtalar	Inversion	0–20	20°	None
	Eversion	0–10	10°	None

GH: glenohumeral; AC: acromioclavicular; SC: sternoclavicular; ST: scapulothoracic.

TABLE 8-5	Capsular Patterns of Restriction
Joint	Limitation of Motion (Passive Angular Motion)
Glenohumeral	External rotation > abduction > internal rotation (3:2:1)
Acromioclavicular	No true capsular pattern; possible loss of horizontal adduction and pain (and sometimes slight loss of end range) with each motion
Sternoclavicular	See acromioclavicular joint
Humeroulnar	Flexion > extension (±4:1)
Humeroradial	No true capsular pattern; possible equal limitation of pronation and supination
Superior radioulnar	No true capsular pattern; possible equal limitation of pronation and supination with pain at end ranges
Inferior radioulnar	No true capsular pattern; possible equal limitation of pronation and supination with pain at end ranges
Wrist (carpus)	Flexion = extension
Radiocarpal	See wrist (carpus)
Carpometacarpal	See wrist (carpus)
Midcarpal	See wrist (carpus)
Carpometacarpal 1	Retroposition
Carpometacarpals 2–5	Fan > fold
Metacarpophalangeal 2–5	Flexion > extension (±2:1)
Interphalangeal Proximal (PIP) Distal (DIP)	Flexion > extension (±2:1) Flexion > extension (±2:1)
Hip	Internal rotation > flexion > abduction = extension > other motions
Tibiofemoral	Flexion > extension (±5:1)
Superior tibiofibular	No capsular pattern; pain at the end range of translatory movements
Talocrural	Plantar flexion > dorsiflexion
Talocalcaneal (subtalar)	Varus > valgus
Midtarsal	Inversion (plantar flexion, adduction, supination)
Talonavicular calcaneocuboid	> Dorsiflexion
Metatarsophalangeal 1	Extension > flexion (±2:1)
Metatarsophalangeals 2–5	Flexion ≥ extension
Interphalangeals 2–5 Proximal Distal	Flexion ≥ extension Flexion ≥ extension

Data from Cyriax J. *Textbook of Orthopaedic Medicine, Diagnosis of Soft Tissue Lesions*, 8th ed. London, Bailliere Tindall; 1982.

- Pain increased after the repeated motions may indicate a retriggering of the inflammatory response, and repeated motions in the opposite direction should be explored.

CLINICAL PEARL

It must be remembered that for the full joint motion to occur, multijoint muscles (the muscles that cross two or more joints such as the hamstrings, gastrocnemius, and long flexor and extensors of the hands and feet) must not be lengthened simultaneously over the joints they cross so that they do not prevent full joint motion from occurring. For example, if the clinician performs PROM of ankle dorsiflexion, if the knee is maintained in full extension, the gastrocnemius will prevent full dorsiflexion from occurring. Instead, the clinician should ensure that the knee is flexed.

Active Range of Motion of the Spine. The human zygapophysial joints are capable of only two major motions: gliding upward and gliding downward. If these movements occur in the same direction, flexion or extension of the spine occurs, whereas if the movements occur in opposite directions, side flexion occurs.

Under normal circumstances, an equal amount of gliding occurs at each zygapophysial joint with these motions.

- During flexion, both zygapophysial joints glide superiorly.
- During extension, both zygapophysial joints glide inferiorly.
- During side flexion, the joint on the motion direction side is gliding inferiorly, while the other joint is gliding superiorly. For example, during right side flexion, the right joint is gliding inferiorly, while the left joint is gliding superiorly.

CLINICAL PEARL

Active motion induced by a muscle determines the so-called physiologic ROM,[8] whereas a passive movement causes stretching of the noncontractile elements, such as the ligaments, and determines the anatomic ROM.

Passive Range of Motion of the Extremities. Passive motions are movements performed without the assistance of the patient. Passive movements are performed in the joint's anatomic ROM and normally demonstrate slightly greater ROM than active motion—the barrier to active motion should occur earlier in the range than the barrier to passive motion.

If the patient can complete AROM easily without pain, PROM exercises are usually unnecessary. Cyriax[2] introduced the concept of the end-feel, which is the quality of resistance that occurs at the end range of a joint. The end-feel can indicate the cause of the motion restriction (Tables 8-6 and 8-7).

TABLE 8-6	Normal End-Feels	
Type	**Cause**	**Characteristics and Examples**
Bony	Produced by bone-to-bone approximation	Abrupt and unyielding; it gives the impression that further forcing will break something *Examples:* Normal: elbow extension Abnormal: cervical rotation (may indicate osteophyte)
Elastic	Produced by the muscle-tendon unit; may occur with adaptive shortening	Stretches with elastic recoil and exhibits constant-length phenomenon; further forcing feels as if it will snap something *Examples:* Normal: wrist flexion with finger flexion, the straight-leg raise, and ankle dorsiflexion with the knee extended Abnormal: decreased dorsiflexion of the ankle with the knee flexed
Soft-tissue approximation	Produced by contact of two muscle bulks on either side of a flexing joint where joint range exceeds other restraints	Very forgiving end feel that gives the impression that further normal motion is possible if enough force could be applied *Examples:* Normal: knee flexion and elbow flexion in extremely muscular subjects Abnormal: elbow flexion with obese subject
Capsular	Produced by capsule or ligaments	Various degrees of stretch without elasticity; stretchability is dependent on the thickness of the tissue Strong capsular or extracapsular ligaments produce hard capsular end-feel, whereas a thin capsule produces a softer one The impression given to the clinician is that if further force is applied, something will tear *Examples:* Normal: wrist flexion (soft), elbow flexion in supination (medium), and knee extension (hard) Abnormal: the inappropriate stretchability for a specific joint; if too hard, may indicate hypomobility due to arthrosis; if too soft, hypermobility

Data from Meadows JTS. *Manual Therapy: Biomechanical Assessment and Treatment, Advanced Technique.* Calgary: Swodeam Consulting; 1995.

MOBILITY

TABLE 8-7	Abnormal End-Feels	
Type	**Causes**	**Characteristics and Examples**
Springy	Produced by articular surface rebounding from intra-articular meniscus or disk; the impression is that if forced further, something will collapse	Rebound sensation as if pushing off from a rubber pad *Examples:* Normal: axial compression of the cervical spine Abnormal: knee flexion or extension with displaced meniscus
Boggy	Produced by viscous fluid (blood) within joint	"Squishy" sensation as joint is moved toward its end range; further forcing feels as if it will burst joint *Examples:* Normal: none Abnormal: hemarthrosis at the knee
Spasm	Produced by reflex and reactive muscle contraction in response to irritation of nociceptor, predominantly in articular structures and muscle; forcing it further feels as if nothing will give	Abrupt and "twangy" end to the movement that is unyielding while the structure is being threatened but disappears when threat is removed (kicks back) With joint inflammation, it occurs early in range, especially toward the closed-packed position, to prevent further stress With irritable joint hypermobility, it occurs at the end of what should be the normal range, as it prevents excessive motion from further stimulating the nociceptor Spasm in grade II muscle tears becomes apparent as muscle is passively lengthened and is accompanied by a painful weakness of that muscle *Note:* Muscle guarding is not a true end-feel, as it involves co-contraction *Examples:* Normal: none Abnormal: significant traumatic arthritis, recent traumatic hypermobility, and grade II muscle tears
Empty	Produced solely by pain; frequently caused by serious and severe pathologic changes that do not affect joint or muscle and so do not produce spasm; demonstration of this end-feel is, except for acute subdeltoid bursitis, de facto evidence of serious pathology; further forcing will simply increase pain to unacceptable levels	Limitation of motion has no tissue resistance component, and resistance is from the patient being unable to tolerate further motion due to severe pain; it is not the same feeling as voluntary guarding, but rather it feels as if the patient is both resisting and trying to allow movement simultaneously *Examples:* Normal: none Abnormal: acute subdeltoid bursitis and sign of the buttock
Facilitation	Not truly an end-feel, as facilitated hypertonicity does not restrict motion; it can, however, be perceived near end range	Light resistance as from constant light muscle contraction throughout the latter half of range that does not prevent the end of the range from being reached; resistance is unaffected by the rate of movement *Examples:* Normal: none Abnormal: spinal facilitation at any level

Data from Meadows JTS. *Manual Therapy: Biomechanical Assessment and Treatment,* Advanced Technique. Calgary: Swodeam Consulting; 1995.

The physical therapist will often plan the intervention, and its intensity, on the type of tissue resistance to movement, demonstrated by the end-feel, and on the acuteness of the condition (Table 8-8),[2] as this information may indicate whether the resistance is caused by pain, muscle, capsule ligament, disturbed mechanics of the joint, or a combination.

Both the passive and active ranges of motion can be measured using a goniometer, which has been shown to have a satisfactory level of intraobserver reliability.[8-13] Visual observation using experienced clinicians is equal to measurements by goniometry.[14]

The recording of ROM varies. The American Medical Association (AMA) recommends recording the ROM based on the neutral position of the joint being zero, with the degrees of motion increasing in the direction the joint moves from the zero starting point.[15] A plus sign (+) indicates joint

TABLE 8-8	Abnormal Barriers to Motion and Recommended Manual Techniques	
Barrier	**End-Feel**	**Technique**
Pain	Empty	None
Pain	Spasm	None
Pain	Capsular	Oscillations (I, IV)
Joint adhesions	Early capsular	Passive articular motion stretch (I–V)
Muscle adhesions	Early elastic	Passive physiologic motion stretch
Hypertonicity	Facilitation	Muscle energy (hold/relax, etc)
Bone	Bony	None

hyperextension, and a minus sign (–) indicates an extension lag. The method of recording chosen is not important, provided the clinician chooses a recognized method and documents it consistently with the same patient.

RANGE OF MOTION TECHNIQUES

As previously discussed, ROM can be assessed to provide the clinician with information, but it can also be used therapeutically when a patient cannot independently maintain their mobility, whether globally or at a specific joint. The measurement of ROM is described in the Goniometry section later in the chapter.

When describing a ROM, it is necessary to have a starting position as the reference position. This starting position is referred to as the anatomic reference position. The anatomic reference position for the human body is described as the erect standing position with the feet just slightly separated and the arms hanging by the side, the elbows straight, and the palms of the hand facing forward (Figure 8-1). Movements of the body segments occur in three dimensions along imaginary planes and around various axes of the body.

Planes of the Body. There are three traditional planes of the body, corresponding to the three dimensions of space: sagittal, frontal, and transverse (Figure 8-2).

Axes of the Body. Three reference axes describe human motion: frontal, sagittal, and longitudinal (Figure 8-3). The axis around which the movement takes place is always perpendicular to the plane in which it occurs.

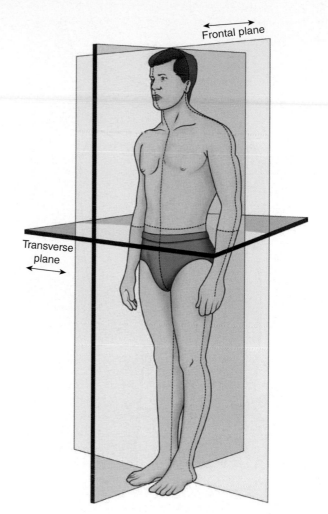

FIGURE 8-2 Planes of the body.

Range of Motion—Upper Extremity

It is assumed that the patient is in the supine position for all of the following techniques unless otherwise stated.

Glenohumeral Joint

Flexion and Extension. Glenohumeral flexion/extension occurs in the sagittal plane (Figure 8-2) around the frontal axis (Figure 8-3).

Pure glenohumeral motion can be assessed by stabilizing the scapula, significantly limiting motion at the glenohumeral joint to approximately 90°. In the following example, the scapular is not stabilized.

Hand Placement. The clinician uses one hand to grasp the patient's wrist while using the other hand to grasp the patient's elbow (Figure 8-4).

Technique. The clinician lifts the patient upper extremity through the available ROM (Figure 8-4) and then returns to the start position. Shoulder extension beyond the body's midline can be accomplished by lowering the arm below the table or bed.

Normal End-feel. The normal end-feel for glenohumeral flexion is firm, resulting from tension in the posterior joint capsule, the posterior band of the coracohumeral ligament, teres major, teres minor, and infraspinatus muscles. If the

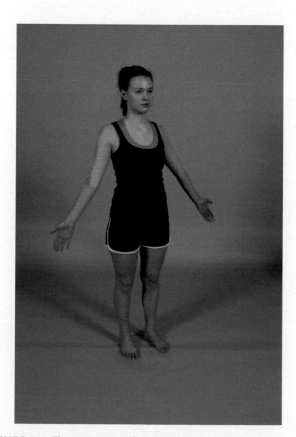

FIGURE 8-1 The anatomic reference position.

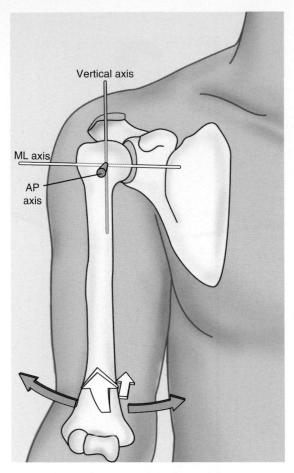

FIGURE 8-3 Axes of the body.

scapular is stabilized, the end-feel for glenohumeral flexion is also firm but results from tension in the latissimus dorsi muscle and the costosternal fibers of the pectoralis major muscle. The normal end-feel for glenohumeral extension is firm because of the tension in the anterior band of the coracohumeral ligament and the anterior joint capsule. For shoulder complex extension, the end-feel is also firm due to the tension in the clavicular fibers of the pectoralis major muscle and the serratus anterior muscle.

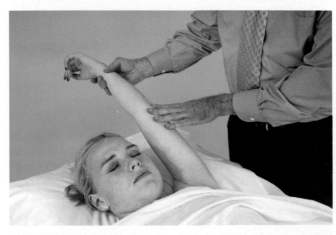

FIGURE 8-4 Shoulder flexion.

CLINICAL PEARL

When performing flexion and extension ROM exercises at the shoulder, it is important to remember the two joint muscles:

▶ *Biceps brachii.* The arm, which is initially positioned with the elbow extended and the forearm pronated, should be lowered below the bed or table level until maximal tension is felt to stretch the long head of the biceps brachii.

▶ *Triceps brachii (long head).* Stretching of this muscle can be achieved by first flexing the shoulder to its point of available motion and then flexing the elbow maximally until the point of maximal tension.

Abduction and Adduction. Motion occurs in the frontal plane (Figure 8-2) around an anterior-posterior (A-P) axis (Figure 8-3).

Hand Placement. The clinician uses one hand to grasp the patient's wrist and the other hand to grasp the patient's elbow (Figure 8-5). The patient's elbow may be extended or flexed.

Technique. The clinician moves the extremity away from the patient's trunk and returns to the start position while avoiding shoulder flexion by maintaining the arm horizontal to the floor (Figure 8-5). If the elbow is extended, the clinician must move his or her feet and step toward the patient's head (Figure 8-5). To avoid the humeral head's impingement on the acromion process, it is important to externally rotate the humerus during this technique. The technique may be modified to prevent excessive elevation of the scapula by using one hand to stabilize the scapula over its superior border.

Normal End-feel. The end-feel for pure glenohumeral abduction is usually firm because of the tension in the middle

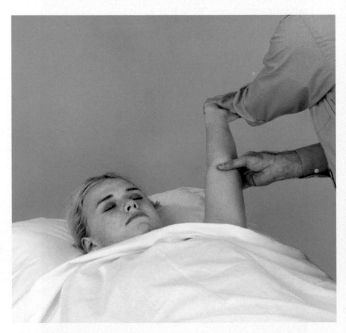

FIGURE 8-5 Shoulder abduction.

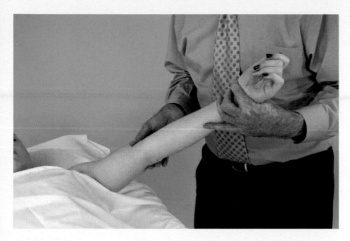

FIGURE 8-6 Horizontal shoulder abduction and adduction.

and inferior bands of the glenohumeral ligament, the inferior joint capsule, and latissimus dorsi and pectoralis major muscles. For shoulder abduction, the end-feel is also firm because of tension in the middle and inferior portion of the trapezius muscle and the rhomboid major and minor muscles.

Horizontal Abduction and Adduction

Hand Placement. Using one hand, the clinician grasps the patient's wrist while using the other hand to grasp the patient's elbow (Figure 8-6). The patient's elbow can be flexed or extended.

Technique. The technique begins with the patient's shoulder abducted to 90° and parallel to the floor. The clinician lifts the patient's arm up and across the upper chest and then returns the arm to the start position. If possible, the patient's arm is lowered below the bed's height or table to achieve full horizontal abduction.

External Rotation. With the patient in the reference position, external rotation of the shoulder occurs in the transverse plane (Figure 8-2) around a longitudinal axis (Figure 8-3).

Hand Placement. Using one hand, the clinician grasps the patient's elbow while grasping the patient's wrist with the other hand (Figure 8-7). The patient's arm is typically positioned in 90° of abduction and 90° of elbow flexion. However,

if this is not possible, the patient's arm can be positioned by the side with the elbow extended or flexed.

Technique. The clinician moves the patient's forearm backward toward the floor so that the humerus externally rotates to a point when the forearm is horizontal to the floor (Figure 8-7) or at the point when the shoulder girdle is felt to move into retraction and is then returned to the start position. Suppose the technique requires the arm to be by the patient's side and the elbow extended. In that case, the clinician uses one hand to grasp the humerus just above the epicondyles and the other hand to grasp the forearm of the wrist, and then rotates or rolls the entire upper extremity in an outward direction. Alternatively, suppose the technique requires the arm to be by the patient's side and the elbow flexed. In that case, the clinician uses one hand to grasp the patient's elbow and the other hand to grasp the distal end of the forearm, and the forearm is moved away from the chest without abducting the shoulder.

Normal End-feel. Using the first technique, the end-feel is firm because of tension in the three bands of the glenohumeral ligament, the coracohumeral ligament, the anterior joint capsule, and the latissimus dorsi, pectoralis major, subscapularis, and teres major muscles. The end-feel for pure glenohumeral external rotation is also firm because of tension in the pectoralis minor and serratus anterior muscles.

Internal Rotation. With the patient in the reference position, external rotation of the shoulder occurs in the transverse plane (Figure 8-2) around a longitudinal axis (Figure 8-3).

Hand Placement. Using one hand, the clinician grasps the patient's elbow while grasping the patient's wrist with the other hand (Figure 8-8). The patient's arm is typically positioned in 90° of abduction and 90° of elbow flexion. However, if this is not possible, the patient's arm can be positioned differently (see below).

Technique. The clinician moves the patient's forearm forward toward the floor so that the humerus internally rotates to a point when the acromion process rises toward the ceiling, signifying that the humeral head is being blocked by the acromion (Figure 8-8), and the shoulder is beginning to move

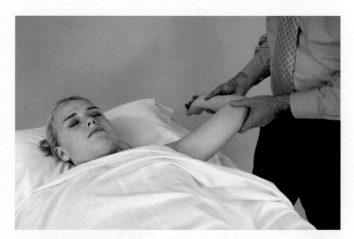

FIGURE 8-7 Shoulder external rotation.

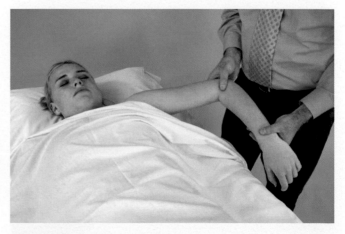

FIGURE 8-8 Shoulder internal rotation.

into protraction and is then returned to the start position. Suppose the technique requires the arm to be by the patient's side and the elbow extended. In that case, the clinician uses one hand to grasp the humerus, just above the epicondyles, and the other hand to grasp the forearm of the wrist, and then rotates or rolls the entire upper extremity in an inward direction. It is not advised to use the technique where the patient's arm is by the side, and the elbow is flexed, as the patient's body blocks the motion of internal rotation, thereby preventing the attainment of complete ROM.

Normal End-feel. Using the first technique, the end-feel is firm because of tension in the middle and inferior portions of the trapezius muscle and the rhomboid major and minor muscles. The end-feel for pure glenohumeral internal rotation is also firm because of tension in the posterior joint capsule and the teres minor and infraspinatus muscles.

Elbow Joint

Flexion and Extension. Motion occurs in the sagittal plane (Figure 8-2) around the frontal axis (Figure 8-3).

Hand Placement. Using one hand, the clinician grasps the distal forearm and hand of the patient while using the other hand to support and stabilize the distal end of the patient's humerus.

Technique. While preventing any shoulder motion, the clinician flexes and extends the patient's elbow with the patient's forearm positioned in neutral (Figure 8-9), then with the patient's forearm positioned in pronation (Figure 8-10), and finally with the patient's forearm positioned in supination (Figure 8-11).

Normal End-feel. The end-feel for elbow flexion is normally one of soft tissue approximation due to compression of the anterior forearm's muscle bulk with that of the anterior upper arm. However, in a very slight individual with a small muscle bulk, the end-feel may be either:

▶ Hard because of the contact between the coronoid process of the ulna and the coronoid fossa of the humerus and contact between the head of the radius and the radial fossa of the humerus.

▶ Firm because of the tension in the posterior joint capsule and the triceps brachii muscle.

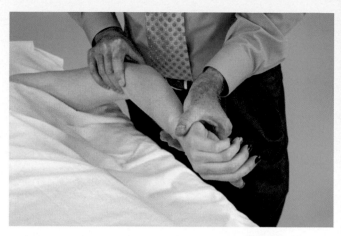

FIGURE 8-10 Approaching the end range of elbow extension and pronation.

The end-feel for elbow extension is typically hard because of contact between the ulna's olecranon process and the olecranon fossa of the humerus. On occasion, the end-feel can be firm because of tension in the anterior joint capsule, the collateral ligaments, and the bulk of the biceps brachii and brachialis muscles.

Forearm Pronation and Supination. With the patient in the anatomic reference position, motion occurs in the transverse plane (Figure 8-2) around a longitudinal axis (Figure 8-3).

Hand Placement. The clinician uses one hand to grasp the patient's distal forearm and the patient's hand while using the other hand to support and stabilize the patient's humerus.

Technique. The technique can be performed with the patient's elbow flexed or extended. While ensuring that no motion occurs at the shoulder, the clinician pronates (Figure 8-10) and supinates (Figure 8-11) the patient's forearm.

Normal End-feel. The normal end-feel for forearm pronation is either hard because of contact between the ulna and the radius or firm because of tension in the posterior (dorsal) radioulnar ligament of the distal (inferior) radioulnar joint, the supinator and biceps brachii muscles, and the interosseous membrane. The normal end-feel for forearm

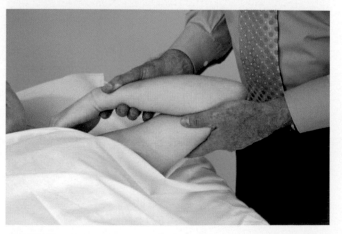

FIGURE 8-9 Elbow flexion.

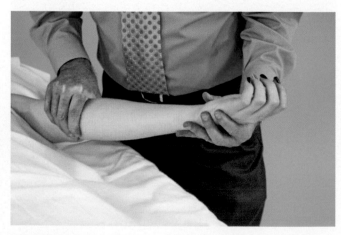

FIGURE 8-11 The end range of elbow extension and supination.

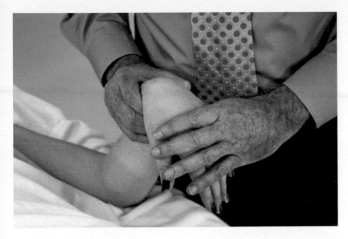

FIGURE 8-12 Wrist flexion.

supination is firm due to tension in the anterior radioulnar ligament of the distal radioulnar joint, interosseous membrane, and the pronator teres and pronator quadratus muscles.

Wrist Joint

Flexion and Extension. Motion occurs in the sagittal plane (Figure 8-2) around a frontal axis (Figure 8-3).

Hand Placement. Using one hand, the clinician grasps the patient's hand over the posterior and anterior surfaces while using the other hand to support and stabilize the forearm.

Technique. The technique can be performed with the patient's elbow flexed or extended. While allowing the patient's fingers to relax, the clinician moves the patient's palm toward the forearm (flexion) (Figure 8-12) and then the posterior aspect of the hand toward the forearm (extension) (Figure 8-13). The technique can then be repeated with the patient's fingers fully flexed in a closed fist position.

Normal End-feel. The end-feel for wrist flexion is firm because of tension in the posterior (dorsal) radiocarpal ligament and the posterior (dorsal) joint capsule. The end-feel for wrist extension is usually firm because of the tension in the anterior (palmar) radiocarpal ligament and the anterior (palmar) joint capsule, but it can be hard due to contact between the radius and the carpal bones.

CLINICAL PEARL

While performing ROM exercises at the wrist, it is important to remember those muscles/tendons that cross multiple joints:

▶ *Extensor digitorum.* This technique can be performed with the patient's elbow flexed or extended. While placing one hand over the posterior aspect of all of the fingers and the patient's hand, the clinician uses the other hand to support and stabilize the forearm. The clinician then sequentially flexes the distal interphalangeal (DIP), proximal interphalangeal (PIP), and metacarpophalangeal (MCP) joints and then gently flexes the wrist.

▶ *Flexor digitorum superficialis and profundus.* This technique can be performed with the patient's elbow flexed or extended. The clinician places one hand over the anterior surface of all of the patient's fingers while using the other hand to support and stabilize the forearm. The clinician then sequentially extends the DIP, PIP, and MCP joints and then gently extends the wrist to the point of maximal tension.

Radial and Ulnar Deviation Motion occurs in the frontal plane (Figure 8-2) around a sagittal axis (Figure 8-3).

Hand Placement. While maintaining the patient's wrist in neutral flexion-extension, the clinician uses one hand to grasp the patient's hand over the posterior and anterior surfaces while using the other hand to support and stabilize the forearm.

Technique. While avoiding any wrist flexion-extension, the clinician moves the patient's hand in a radial (Figure 8-14) and ulnar (Figure 8-15) direction.

Normal End-feel. The end-feel for radial deviation is typically hard because of contact between the radial styloid process and the scaphoid. However, if there is tension in the ulnar collateral ligament, the ulnar carpal ligament, and the ulnar portion of the joint capsule, the end-feel may be firm. The end-feel for ulnar deviation is firm because of tension in the radial collateral ligament and the radial portion of the joint capsule.

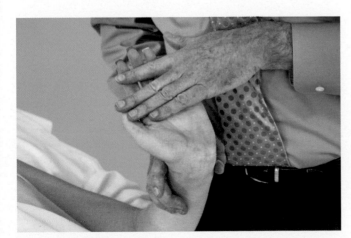

FIGURE 8-13 Wrist extension.

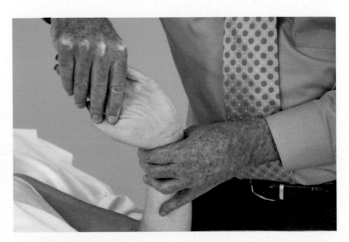

FIGURE 8-14 Radial deviation.

MOBILITY

159

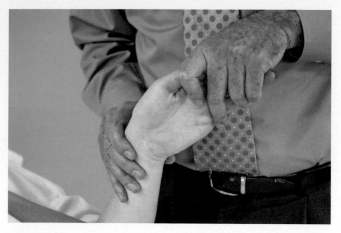

FIGURE 8-15 Ulnar deviation.

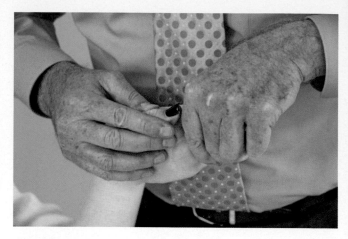

FIGURE 8-17 MCP flexion of the thumb.

Hand and Thumb Joints

Metacarpophalangeal (MCP) Flexion and Extension. Motion occurs in the sagittal plane (Figure 8-2) around a frontal (Figure 8-3) axis.

Hand Placement. Using the thumb and index finger of one hand, the clinician grasps the posterior and anterior surfaces of a metacarpal just proximal to the metacarpal head while using the thumb and index finger of the other hand to grasp the posterior and anterior surfaces of a proximal phalanx (Figure 8-16).

Technique. While stabilizing the metacarpal with one hand, the other hand moves the phalanx upward and downward (Figure 8-16). The technique is repeated for each MCP of the fingers on each hand.

Normal End-feel. The end-feel for MCP flexion can vary from hard, because of contact between the palmar aspect of the proximal phalanx and metacarpal, to firm, because of tension in the posterior joint capsule and the collateral ligaments. The end-feel for MCP extension is firm due to tension in the anterior (palmar) joint capsule and anterior (palmar) fibrocartilaginous plate.

Metacarpophalangeal (MCP) Joint of the Thumb Flexion and Extension. Motion occurs in the frontal plane (Figure 8-2) around an A-P axis (Figure 8-3) when the patient is in the anatomic reference position.

Hand Placement. Using one hand, the clinician stabilizes the first metacarpal to prevent wrist motion and flexion and opposition of the thumb's carpometacarpal (CMC) joint while using the other hand to move the thumb at the MCP joint.

Technique. Once correct stabilization is attained, the clinician moves the thumb around the MCP joint into flexion, toward the palm (Figure 8-17), and then into extension (Figure 8-18), away from the hand.

Normal End-feel. The end-feel for MCP flexion of the thumb is either hard because of contact between the anterior aspect of the proximal phalanx and the first metacarpal or firm because of tension in the posterior joint capsule, the extensor policies brevis muscle, and the collateral ligaments. The end-feel for MCP extension of the thumb is firm, resulting from tension in the anterior joint capsule, anterior (palmar) fibrocartilaginous plate, and the flexor pollicis brevis muscle.

Metacarpophalangeal (MCP) Abduction. Motion occurs in the frontal plane (Figure 8-2) around an A-P axis (Figure 8-3).

Hand Placement. The clinician uses one hand to grasp and stabilize the PIP joints of the first, second, and third fingers while using the other hand to grasp the forefinger.

Technique. While maintaining the MCP and interphalangeal (IP) joint in extension, the clinician gently moves the fourth finger away from the third finger. The clinician then

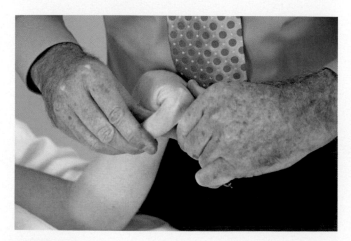

FIGURE 8-16 MCP flexion of the index finger.

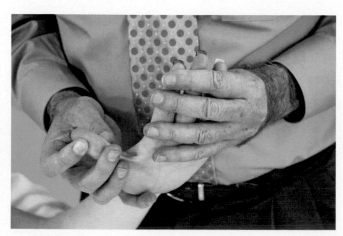

FIGURE 8-18 MCP extension of the thumb.

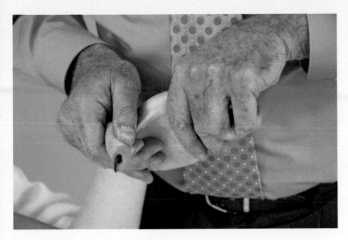

FIGURE 8-19 Thumb abduction.

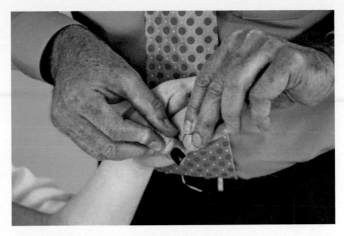

FIGURE 8-20 Thumb opposition.

stabilizes the first and second fingers and moves the third finger away from the second finger. Next, the second finger can be moved to the left and right without stabilizing any of the other fingers.

Normal End-feel. The normal end-feel for MCP abduction is firm because of tension in the collateral ligaments of the MCP joints, the anterior (palmar) interossei muscles, and the fascia of the web space between the fingers.

Thumb (CMC) Abduction and Adduction. Motion occurs in the sagittal plane (Figure 8-2) around a frontal axis (Figure 8-3) when the patient is in the anatomic reference position.

Hand Placement. Using the fingers and thumb of one hand, the clinician grasps the patient's thumb while using the other hand to stabilize the second metacarpal.

Technique. The clinician lifts the thumb away from the palm so that it is perpendicular to the palm while maintaining the MCP and IP joint in extension (Figure 8-19). The thumb is then returned to the palm parallel to the second metatarsal.

Normal End-feel. The end-feel for CMC joint abduction is firm because of tension in the fascia and skin of the web space between the thumb and index finger and tension in the adductor pollicis and first posterior interossei muscles.

Thumb (CMC) Extension and Flexion. Motion occurs in the frontal plane (Figure 8-2) around an A-P axis (Figure 8-3) when the patient is in the anatomic reference position.

Hand Placement. Using the fingers and thumb of one hand, the clinician grasps the patient's thumb while using the other hand to stabilize the second metacarpal.

Technique. The clinician moves the thumb away from the index finger and horizontal to the palm, thereby widening the webspace to its maximum. The thumb is then returned so that it rests next to the side of the second metacarpal.

Normal End-feel. The end-feel for CMC joint flexion can be either soft because of contact between the muscle bulk of the thenar eminence in the palm or firm because of tension in the posterior joint capsule and the extensor pollicis brevis and abductor pollicis brevis muscles. The end-feel for CMC joint extension is firm due to tension in the anterior joint capsule and the adductor pollicis, flexor pollicis brevis, opponens pollicis, and the first posterior interossei muscles.

Thumb Opposition. This motion is a combination of flexion, abduction, and medial-axial rotation that occurs in multiple planes and axes.

Hand Placement. The clinician uses the thumb and index finger of one hand to grasp the patient's thumb while using the other hand to grasp the fifth metacarpal and finger.

Technique. The clinician rolls the patient's thumb toward the fifth finger while maintaining the MCP and IP joint in extension (Figure 8-20), and then returns the thumb to the full extension position.

Normal End-feel. The end-feel can be soft because of contact between the muscle bulk of the thenar eminence and the palm, or firm because of tension in the joint capsule, extensor pollicis brevis muscle, and transverse metacarpal ligament (when moving the fifth finger).

Interphalangeal (IP) Joint of the Thumb Flexion and Extension. Motion occurs in the frontal plane (Figure 8-2) around an A-P axis (Figure 8-3) when the patient is in the anatomic reference position.

Hand Placement. The clinician uses one hand to stabilize the proximal phalanx to prevent flexion or extension of the MCP joint and the other hand to flex the thumb about the IP joint.

Technique. Using the tip of the index finger and the thumb of one hand, the clinician flexes the tip of the thumb around the IP joint into flexion (Figure 8-21) and extension.

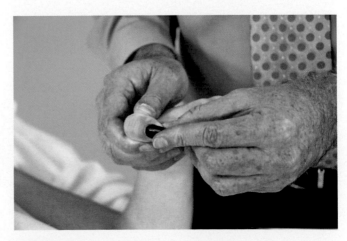

FIGURE 8-21 Flexion of the thumb interphalangeal joint. **161**

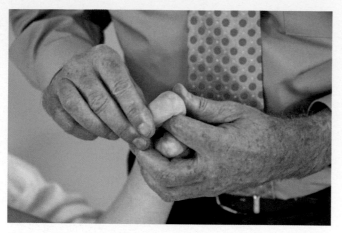

FIGURE 8-22 PIP flexion.

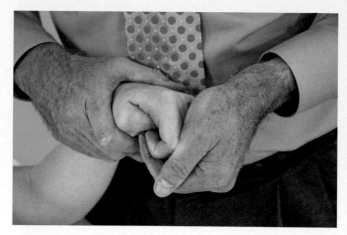

FIGURE 8-24 Combined flexion of the PIP and DIP joints.

Normal End-feel. The normal end-feel for IP flexion is firm because of tension in the collateral ligaments and the posterior joint capsule. The normal end-feel for IP extension is firm because of tension in the anterior joint capsule and the anterior (palmar) fibrocartilaginous plate.

Finger Joints

Flexion and Extension of the Proximal Interphalangeal (PIP) and Distal Interphalangeal (DIP) Joints.
Motion occurs in the sagittal plane (Figure 8-2) around a frontal axis (Figure 8-3).

Hand Placement. Using the thumb and index finger of one hand, the clinician grasps the more proximal phalanx while using the other hand's thumb and index finger to grasp the more distal phalanx. The same technique is used for the PIP (Figure 8-22) and the DIP (Figure 8-23) joints.

Technique. While stabilizing the more proximal phalanx, the clinician moves the more distal phalanx in an upward (extension) and downward (flexion) direction. The technique is repeated for each articulation on each hand, including the thumb. Depending on the intent, the PIP and DIP joints can be flexed (Figure 8-24) and extended as a unit.

Normal End-feel. The end-feel for PIP flexion can be either hard because of contact between the anterior aspect of the middle phalanx and the proximal phalanx, or soft because of soft tissue compression between the anterior aspect of the middle and proximal phalanges. The end-feel for PIP extension is firm due to tension in the anterior (palmar) joint capsule and anterior (palmar) fibrocartilaginous plate. The end-feel for DIP flexion is firm because of tension in the posterior (dorsal) joint capsule, the contralateral ligaments, and the oblique retinacular ligament. The end-feel for DIP extension is firm due to tension in the anterior (palmar) joint capsule and the anterior (palmar) fibrocartilaginous plate.

Diagonal Patterns of the Upper Extremity

Diagonal patterns of motion, incorporating the PNF patterns, can be performed using AROM, AAROM, or PROM as part of a regime, although it must always be remembered that because these patterns employ several planes simultaneously, they do not produce the same amount of ROM to the muscles and joints as when the anatomic planes are used. However, there are times when these more functional movements are appropriate, particularly when a patient can participate. As described in the Diagonal Patterns of Motion section earlier, four major patterns of motions are commonly used, two for the upper extremities (D1 and D2 flexion and extension), and two for the lower extremities (D1 and D2 flexion and extension). Perhaps the major benefit of using PNF patterns instead of the standard anatomic ROM exercises, particularly for the immobile patient, is that they induce some degree of spinal rotation. When used as a method of applying ROM to a patient, hand placement is not as critical. The two patterns for the upper extremities are depicted in Figures 8-25 through 8-28 and **VIDEOS 8-1** and **8-2**.

Video Description

While the PNF techniques are typically performed using a rigid set of hand positions by the clinician and precise movements of the patient's upper or lower extremities, there are occasions when these techniques can be modified based on any ROM restriction found with the patient. If you look closely at Video 8-1, you will notice that the clinician introduces the correct direction of forearm rotation toward the end of the technique to illustrate that there are occasions when the technique's components may have to be modified.

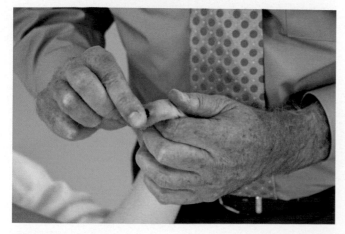

FIGURE 8-23 DIP flexion.

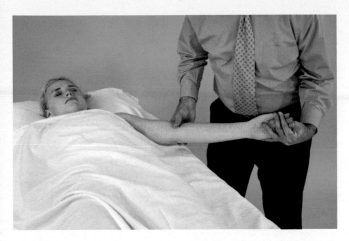

FIGURE 8-25 Upper extremity D1 extension.

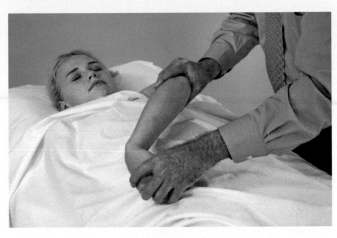

FIGURE 8-27 Upper extremity D2 flexion.

Range of Motion—Lower Extremity

It is assumed that the patient is in the supine position for all of the following techniques unless otherwise stated.

Hip Joint

Hip Flexion. Motion occurs in the sagittal plane (Figure 8-2) around a frontal axis (Figure 8-3).

The ROM exercises for the hip can incorporate motion at the knee and the pelvis. Although the knee motion is more obvious, it is important to remember that hip flexion can induce posterior pelvic rotation, and hip extension can induce anterior pelvic rotation. Based on the ROM exercise's desired outcome, the clinician may determine that the end ranges of hip motion that induce pelvic motion may be necessary.

Hand Placement. The clinician uses one hand to grasp the patient's ankle and the other hand to support the patient's knee.

Technique. The clinician moves the patient's lower extremity into a combination of hip and knee flexion (Figure 8-29) to the appropriate end-feel. Ankle dorsiflexion can also be included. The clinician may also decide to omit the knee flexion and perform hip flexion with knee extension, also known as a straight leg raise (Figure 8-30). This particular maneuver serves to lengthen the posterior thigh's multijoint muscles (the hamstrings) across both the knee and the hip.

The straight leg maneuver can be performed in neutral hip rotation, adduction, and abduction or performed with varying amounts of these motions. For example, the clinician may decide to perform the straight leg raise with the hip in internal rotation and adduction to stretch a specific structure or group of structures.

Normal End-feel. The normal end-feel for hip flexion is usually soft tissue approximation because of contact between the muscle bulk of the anterior thigh and the lower abdomen.

Hip Extension. Motion occurs in the sagittal plane (Figure 8-2) around a frontal axis (Figure 8-3).

The patient is positioned prone.

Hand Placement. The clinician uses one hand to grasp the patient's knee while using the other hand to stabilize the patient's pelvis.

Technique. The clinician raises the patient's thigh from the bed to when the pelvis is felt to begin to rotate anteriorly.

This technique can also be performed with the patient side lying, with the lower extremity being treated uppermost. As before, the clinician uses one hand to monitor the pelvis while using the other hand and arm to support the patient's lower extremity. A modification to the side lying technique can be used to apply tension to the tensor fasciae latae by using a combination of hip extension and hip adduction while stabilizing the pelvis.

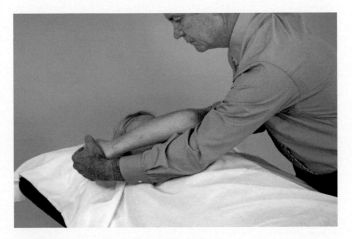

FIGURE 8-26 Upper extremity D1 flexion.

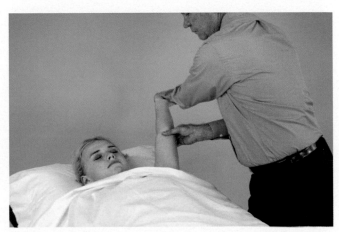

FIGURE 8-28 Upper extremity D2 extension.

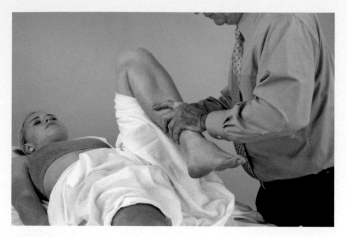

FIGURE 8-29 Hip and knee flexion.

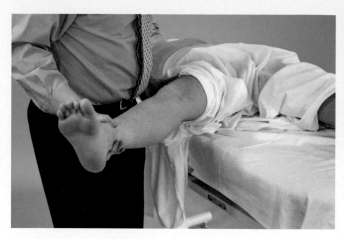

FIGURE 8-31 Hip abduction.

Normal End-feel. The end-feel is firm due to tension in the anterior joint capsule, iliofemoral ligament, and, to a lesser degree, the ischiofemoral and pubofemoral ligaments.

Hip Abduction and Adduction. Motion occurs in a frontal plane (Figure 8-2) around an A-P axis (Figure 8-3).

Hand Placement. The clinician uses one hand to grasp the patient's foot and ankle and the other hand to support the patient's knee or stabilize the pelvis to prevent rotation and lateral tilting.

Technique. The clinician moves the patient's lower extremity so that the hip is abducted (Figure 8-31) and then adducted (Figure 8-32). To ensure that the hip abduction occurs beyond the midline, the patient's contralateral lower extremity may need to be elevated or positioned in hip abduction.

Normal End-feel. The end-feel for abduction is firm because of tension in the inferior-medial joint capsule, pubofemoral ligament, ischiofemoral ligament, and the inferior band of the iliofemoral ligament. Also, depending on the degree of adaptive shortening, the adductor magnus, adductor longus, adductor brevis, pectineus, and gracilis muscles may contribute to the firmness of the end-feel. The end-feel for adduction is firm because of tension in the superior-lateral joint capsule and the iliofemoral ligament's superior band. Also, depending on the degree of adaptive shortening, the gluteus medius and

minimus and the tensor fascia latae muscles may contribute to the end-feel's firmness.

Hip External and Internal Rotation. Motion occurs in a transverse plane (Figure 8-2) around a longitudinal axis (Figure 8-3) when the subject is in the anatomic reference position.

Hand Placement. The clinician uses one hand to grasp the patient's foot and ankle and the other hand to support the patient's knee. The patient's hip and knee are positioned at approximately 90°.

Technique. The clinician moves the patient's foot toward the midline for external rotation of the hip (Figure 8-33) and away from the midline for internal rotation of the hip (Figure 8-34).

Normal End-feel. The end-feel for internal rotation is firm because of tension in the posterior joint capsule and the ischiofemoral ligament and muscle tension from the external rotators of the hip (piriformis, obturator internis and externus, gemelli superior and inferior, quadratus femoris, and the posterior fibers of the gluteus medius and gluteus maximus). The end-feel for external rotation is also firm due to tension in the anterior joint capsule, iliofemoral ligament, and pubofemoral ligament. Also, tension from the hip's internal rotators (the anterior portion of the gluteus medius, the gluteus

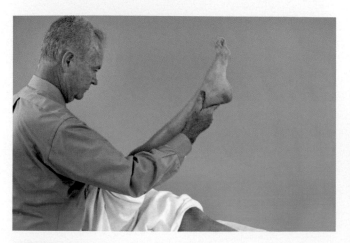

FIGURE 8-30 Hip flexion and knee extension.

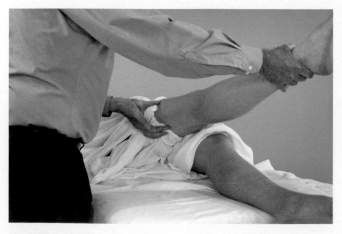

FIGURE 8-32 Hip adduction.

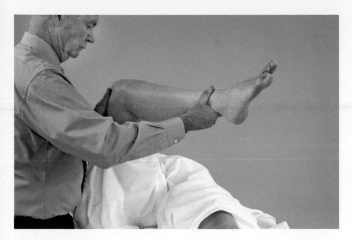

FIGURE 8-33 Hip external rotation.

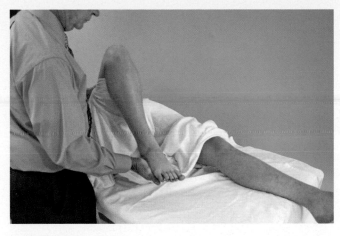

FIGURE 8-35 Knee flexion.

minimus, the adductor magnus and longus, and the pectineus muscles) may enhance the firmness of the end-feel.

Knee Joint

Knee Flexion and Extension. Motion occurs in the sagittal plane (Figure 8-2) around a frontal axis (Figure 8-3).

Hand Placement. The clinician uses one hand to grasp the patient's foot and ankle and the other hand to support the patient's knee.

Technique. The patient's knee is flexed (Figure 8-35) to the appropriate end-feel. This technique can be modified by positioning the patient prone (with a pillow under the hips to maintain pelvic neutral) to stretch the two joint muscles of the hip and knee, especially the rectus femoris. The clinician uses one hand to grasp the patient's ankle and the other hand to monitor the patient's pelvis. The clinician flexes the patient's knee to where anterior pelvic rotation motion is felt to occur.

Normal End-feel. The end-feel for knee flexion is normally one of soft tissue approximation because of contact between the posterior calf and thigh muscle bulk or between the heel and the buttocks. However, if there is a significant adaptive shortening of the rectus femoris muscle, the end-feel is firm because of tension in this muscle. The end-feel for knee extension is firm because of tension in the posterior joint capsule,

the oblique and arcuate popliteal ligaments, collateral ligaments, and the anterior and posterior cruciate ligaments.

Ankle Joint

Dorsiflexion and plantarflexion motions occur in the sagittal plane (Figure 8-2) around a frontal axis (Figure 8-2). The motions of inversion and eversion consist of a combination of motions:

▶ *Inversion:* a combination of supination, adduction, and plantarflexion occurring in varying degrees throughout the various joints of the ankle and foot.

▶ *Eversion:* a combination of pronation, abduction, and dorsiflexion occurring in varying degrees throughout the various joints of the ankle and foot.

Dorsiflexion

Hand Placement. Using one hand, the clinician stabilizes the patient's lower leg while using the other hand on the sole of the patient's foot.

Technique. The clinician uses the hand on the sole of the patient's foot to dorsiflex the ankle (Figure 8-36).

Normal End-feel. The end-feel is firm because of tension in the joint capsules, the calcaneofibular ligament, the anterior and posterior talofibular ligament, the posterior calcaneal ligaments, the anterior, posterior, lateral, and interosseous

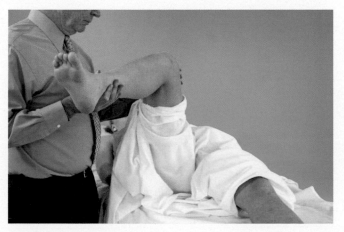

FIGURE 8-34 Hip internal rotation.

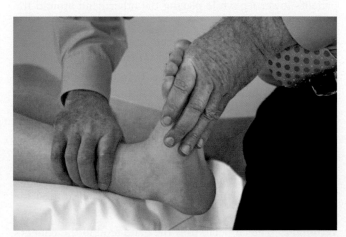

FIGURE 8-36 Ankle dorsiflexion.

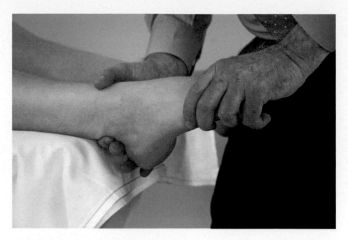

FIGURE 8-37 Ankle plantarflexion.

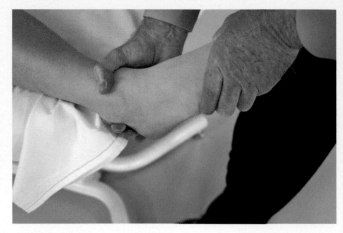

FIGURE 8-38 Ankle inversion.

talocalcaneal ligaments, the posterior talonavicular ligament, the posterior calcaneocuboid ligament, the lateral band of the bifurcate ligament, the transverse metatarsal ligament, and various anterior and posterior and interosseous ligaments of the smaller joints of the foot. Also, tension from the fibularis longus and brevis muscles can enhance the end-feel's firmness.

Plantarflexion

Hand Placement. Using one hand, the clinician stabilizes the patient's lower leg while placing the other hand on the posterior aspect of the patient's foot.

Technique. The clinician uses the hand on the posterior aspect of the patient's foot to plantarflex the ankle (Figure 8-37).

Normal End-feel. The end-feel can be either hard because of contact between the calcaneus and the floor of the sinus tarsi or firm because of tension in the joint capsules, the deltoid ligament, the plantar calcaneonavicular and calcaneocuboid ligaments, the medial talocalcaneal ligament, the medial band of the bifurcate ligament, the transverse metatarsal ligament, the posterior talonavicular ligament and, various posterior, anterior and interosseous ligaments of the smaller joints of the foot. Also, tension from the tibialis posterior muscle can also enhance the firmness of the end-feel.

Inversion

Hand Placement. Using one hand, the clinician stabilizes the patient's lower leg while placing the other hand around the patient's foot.

Technique. The clinician uses the hand around the patient's foot to apply motion into inversion (Figure 8-38).

Normal End-feel. The end-feel is firm because of tension in the lateral joint capsule, the calcaneofibular ligament, the anterior and posterior talofibular ligaments, and the lateral, posterior, anterior, and interosseous talocalcaneal ligaments.

Eversion

Hand Placement. Using one hand, the clinician stabilizes the patient's lower leg while placing the other hand around the patient's foot.

Technique. The clinician uses the hand around the patient's foot to apply motion into eversion (Figure 8-39).

Normal End-feel. The end-feel is either hard because of contact between the calcaneus and the floor of the sinus tarsi or firm because of tension in the deltoid ligament, the medial talocalcaneal ligament, and the tibialis posterior muscle.

Toe Joints

Flexion and extension of the toe joints occur in the sagittal plane (Figure 8-2) around a frontal axis (Figure 8-3).

Metatarsophalangeal (MTP) Flexion

Hand Placement. Using one hand, the clinician stabilizes the patient's foot while using the other hand to grasp the patient's toes.

Technique. The clinician moves the toes into flexion around the MTP joint (Figure 8-40). This technique can be performed at each of the MTP joints for more specificity.

Normal End-feel. The end-feel is firm because of tension in the posterior joint capsule and the collateral ligaments, in addition to tension in the extensor digitorum brevis muscle.

Metatarsophalangeal (MTP) Extension

Hand Placement. Using one hand, the clinician stabilizes the patient's foot while using the other hand to grasp the patient's toes.

Technique. The clinician moves the toes into extension around the MTP joint (Figure 8-41). The technique can be performed at each of the MTP joints for more specificity.

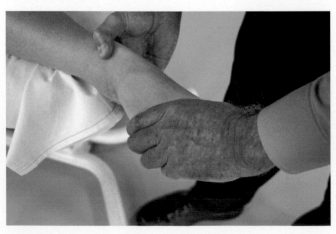

FIGURE 8-39 Ankle eversion.

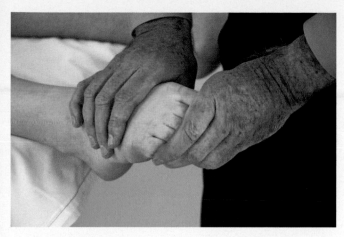

FIGURE 8-40 MTP flexion.

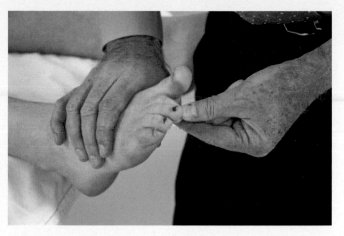

FIGURE 8-42 Interphalangeal joint flexion.

Normal End-feel. The end-feel is firm because of tension in the plantar joint capsule, the plantar fibrocartilaginous plate, flexor hallucis brevis, flexor digitorum brevis, and flexor digiti minimi muscles.

Interphalangeal (IP) Flexion and Extension

Hand Placement. Using one hand, the clinician stabilizes the patient's foot while using the other hand to grasp the patient's toes.

Technique. The clinician moves each toe into flexion (Figure 8-42) and extension (Figure 8-43). The technique is repeated with the great toe into flexion (Figure 8-44) and extension (Figure 8-45).

Diagonal Patterns of the Lower Extremity

As with the upper extremity, diagonal patterns of motion, incorporating the PNF patterns, can be performed using AROM, AAROM, or PROM as part of a regime (VIDEOS 8-3 and 8-4). The diagonal patterns of the lower extremity have a greater potential for inducing motion at the lumbar and thoracic spine, particularly at the extremes of range. The clinician must determine whether ROM into these regions is desired or not and place limits on the ROM accordingly. As stated earlier, although it would appear that the use of diagonal patterns is a more efficient method of applying ROM to a series of joints rather than ranging a series of individual joints,

these PNF patterns do not produce the same amount of ROM to the muscles and joints as when the individual joints are moved through their various ranges of motion. When used as a method of applying ROM to a patient, hand placement is not as critical. The two patterns for the lower extremities are depicted in Figures 8-46 through 8-49.

Combined Ranges of Motion

When performing PROM exercises, the clinician may apply combined motions simultaneously (VIDEO 8-5). For example, when performing ROM to the lower extremities, the clinician may use a technique that incorporates ankle dorsiflexion, knee flexion, and hip flexion. Also, the clinician may decide to superimpose hip internal rotation and hip external rotation onto the technique.

Video Description

In Video 8-5, the clinician demonstrates a combined technique of hip flexion, knee flexion, and dorsiflexion for the lower extremity. Notice how the clinician adds internal rotation and external rotation of the hip to the technique. Also, note how the clinician uses his larger trunk muscles to perform the ROM technique rather than just his arm muscles.

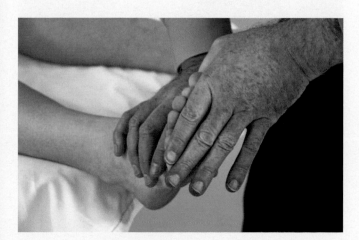

FIGURE 8-41 MTP extension.

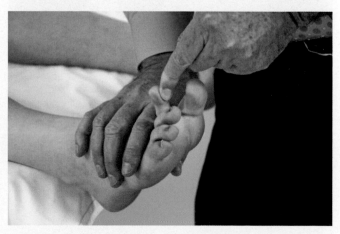

FIGURE 8-43 Interphalangeal joint extension.

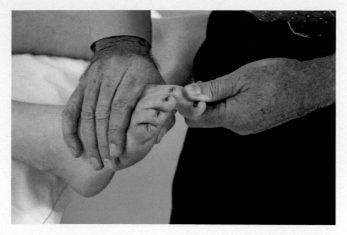

FIGURE 8-44 Great toe flexion.

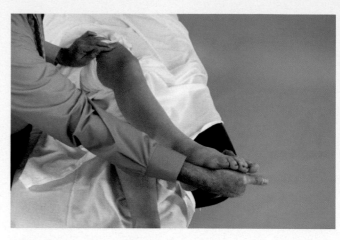

FIGURE 8-47 Lower extremity D1 flexion.

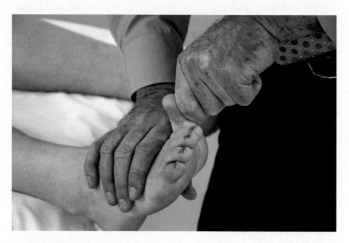

FIGURE 8-45 Great toe extension.

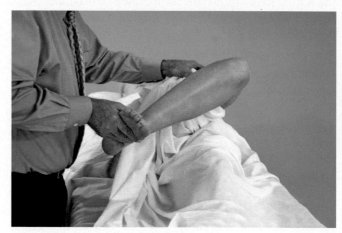

FIGURE 8-48 Lower extremity D2 flexion.

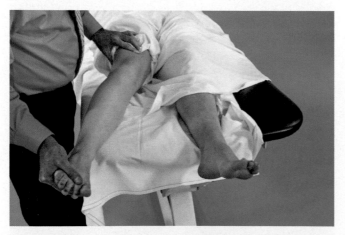

FIGURE 8-46 Lower extremity D1 extension.

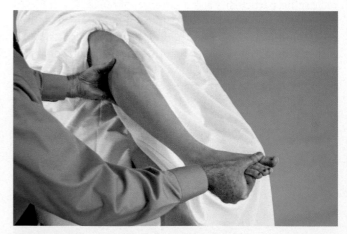

FIGURE 8-49 Lower extremity D2 extension.

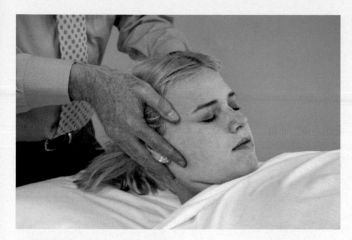

FIGURE 8-50 Cervical flexion.

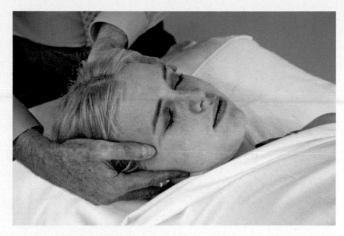

FIGURE 8-52 Cervical side bending to the right.

Range of Motion—The Spine

Cervical Spine

Hand Placement. Standing at the foot of the bed, the clinician uses both hands to support the patient's head.

Technique. While supporting the patient's head, the clinician moves the patient's head and cervical spine into flexion (Figure 8-50), rotation to the right (Figure 8-51) and left, and side flexion to the right (Figure 8-52) and left.

Wherever possible, cervical spine motion should be assessed with AROM in either the sitting or standing position (VIDEO 8-6) so that the effect of the compression of the head on the ROM can be noted.

Video Description

In Video 8-6, the patient demonstrates AROM of the cervical spine. To the trained eye, this patient demonstrates a loss of ROM in one direction. Can you spot it?

Lumbar Spine Although PROM can be applied to the lumbar spine, achieving end ranges of motion is very difficult. Whenever possible, AROM of the lumbar spine in the sitting or standing position (VIDEO 8-7) should be assessed so that the effect of the trunk's compression on the ROM can be noted.

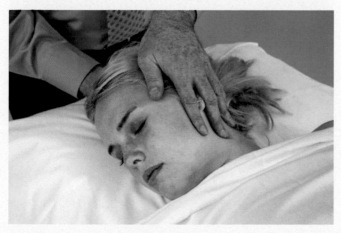

FIGURE 8-51 Cervical rotation to the right.

Video Description

In Video 8-7, the patient performs AROM of the lumbar spine. What do you consider the cause of the apparent decrease in lumbar flexion?

GONIOMETRY

The term *goniometry* is derived from two Greek words, *gonia*, meaning angle, and *metron*, meaning measure. Thus, a goniometer is an instrument used to measure angles. In physical therapy, goniometry is used to measure the total amount of available motion at a specific joint. Goniometry can be used to measure both active and passive ROM.

Goniometers are produced in various sizes and shapes and are usually constructed of either plastic or metal (Figure 8-53). The two most common types of instruments used to measure joint angles are the bubble inclinometer and the traditional goniometer.

▶ *Bubble goniometer* (Figure 8-54). The bubble goniometer, which has a 360° rotating dial and scale with fluid indicator, can be used for flexion and extension; abduction and adduction; and rotation in the neck, shoulder, elbow, wrist, hip, knee, ankle, and spine.

▶ *Traditional goniometer.* The traditional goniometer, which can be used for flexion and extension; abduction and adduction; and rotation in the shoulder, elbow, wrist, hip, knee, and ankle, consists of three parts:

■ *A body.* The body of the goniometer is designed like a protractor and may form a full or half circle. A measuring scale is located around the body. The scale can extend either from 0° to 180° and 180° to 0° for the half-circle models, or from 0° to 360° and from 360° to 0° on the full-circle models. The intervals on the scales can vary from 1° to 10°.

■ *A stationary arm.* The stationary arm is structurally a part of the body and cannot move independently of the body.

■ *A moving arm.* The moving arm is attached to the fulcrum in the center of the body by a rivet or

169

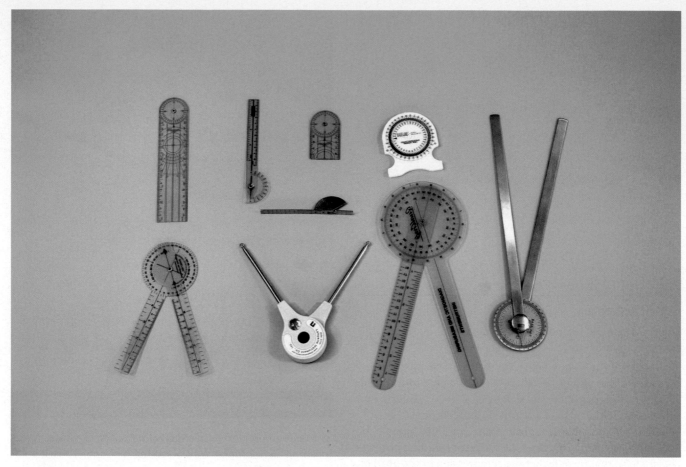

FIGURE 8-53 The various types of goniometers.

screw-like device that allows the moving arm to move freely on the device's body. In some instruments, the screw-like device can be tightened to fix the moving arm in a certain position or loosened to permit free movement.

The correct selection of which goniometer device to use depends on the joint angle to be measured. The length of arms varies among instruments and can range 3–18 inches.

Extendable goniometers (Figure 8-55) allow varying ranges 9½–26 inches. The longer-armed goniometers or the bubble inclinometer are recommended when the landmarks are farther apart, such as when measuring hip, knee, elbow, and shoulder movements. In the smaller joints such as the wrist, hand, foot, and ankle, a traditional goniometer with a shorter arm is used.

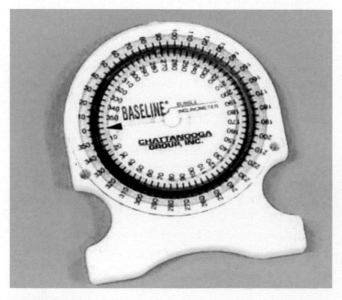

FIGURE 8-54 Bubble goniometer.

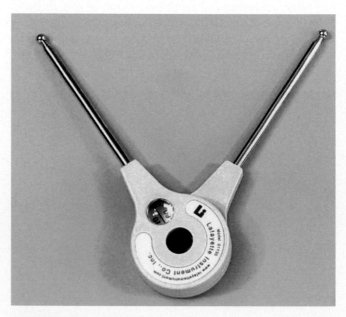

FIGURE 8-55 Extendable goniometer.

The general procedure for measuring ROM involves the following:

1. The patient is positioned in the recommended testing position close to the edge of the treatment table or bed and should be correctly draped. While stabilizing the proximal joint component, the clinician gently moves the distal joint component through the available ROM until the end-feel is determined (see Range of Motion Examination). An estimate is made of the available ROM, and the distal joint component is returned to the starting position. For brevity, the following descriptions of goniometric measurements do not include the PROM assessment, but the reader should consider it as read.

2. The clinician palpates the relevant bony landmarks and aligns the goniometer.

3. A record is made of the starting measurement. The goniometer is then removed, and the patient moves the joint through the available ROM. Once the joint has been moved through the available ROM, the goniometer is replaced and realigned, and the measurement is read and recorded.

The standard testing procedures for each of the upper and lower extremity joints are outlined in Tables 8-9 and 8-10.

TABLE 8-9	Goniometric Techniques for the Upper Extremity			
Joint	**Motion**	**Fulcrum**	**Proximal Arm**	**Distal Arm**
Shoulder	Flexion	Acromion process	Midaxillary line of the thorax	Lateral midline of the humerus using the lateral epicondyle of the humerus for reference
	Extension	Acromion process	Midaxillary line of the thorax	Lateral midline of the humerus using the lateral epicondyle of the humerus for reference
	Abduction	Anterior aspect of the acromion process	Parallel to the midline of the anterior aspect of the sternum	Medial midline of the humerus
	Adduction	Anterior aspect of the acromion process	Parallel to the midline of the anterior aspect of the sternum	Medial midline of the humerus
	Internal rotation	Olecranon process	Parallel or perpendicular to the floor	Ulna using the olecranon process and ulnar styloid for reference
	External rotation	Olecranon process	Parallel or perpendicular to the floor	Ulna using the olecranon process and ulnar styloid for reference
Elbow	Flexion	Lateral epicondyle of the humerus	Lateral midline of the humerus using the center of the acromion process for reference	Lateral midline of the radius using the radial head and radial styloid process for reference
	Extension	Lateral epicondyle of the humerus	Lateral midline of the humerus using the center of the acromion process for reference	Lateral midline of the radius using the radial head and radial styloid process for reference
Forearm	Pronation	Lateral to the ulnar styloid process	Parallel to the anterior midline of the humerus	Dorsal aspect of the forearm, just proximal to the styloid process of the radius and ulna
	Supination	Medial to the ulnar styloid process	Parallel to the anterior midline of the humerus	Ventral aspect of the forearm, just proximal to the styloid process of the radius and ulna
Wrist	Flexion	Lateral aspect of the wrists over the triquetrum	Lateral midline of the ulna using the olecranon and ulnar styloid process for reference	Lateral midline of the fifth metacarpal
	Extension	Lateral aspect of the wrists over the triquetrum	Lateral midline of the ulna using the olecranon and ulnar styloid process for reference	Lateral midline of the fifth metacarpal

(continued)

TABLE 8-9   Goniometric Techniques for the Upper Extremity (continued)

Joint	Motion	Fulcrum	Proximal Arm	Distal Arm
	Radial deviation	Over the middle of the posterior aspect of the wrist over the capitate	Posterior midline of the forearm using the lateral epicondyle of the humerus for reference	Posterior midline of the third metacarpal
	Ulnar deviation	Over the middle of the posterior aspect of the wrist over the capitate	Posterior midline of the forearm using the lateral epicondyle of the humerus for reference	Posterior midline of the third metacarpal
Thumb	Carpometacarpal flexion	Over the anterior aspect of the first carpometacarpal joint	Anterior midline of the radius using the anterior surface of the radial head and radial styloid process for reference	Anterior midline of the first metacarpal
	Carpometacarpal extension	Over the anterior aspect of the first carpometacarpal joint	Anterior midline of the radius using the anterior surface of the radial head and radial styloid process for reference	Anterior midline of the first metacarpal
	Carpometacarpal abduction	Over the lateral aspect of the radial styloid process	Lateral midline of the second metacarpal using the center of the second metacarpal or phalangeal joint for reference	Lateral midline of the first metacarpal using the center of the first metacarpal or phalangeal joint for reference
	Carpometacarpal adduction	Over the lateral aspect of the radial styloid process	Lateral midline of the second metacarpal using the center of the second metacarpal or phalangeal joint for reference	Lateral midline of the first metacarpal using the center of the first metacarpal or phalangeal joint for reference
Fingers	Metacarpophalangeal flexion	Over the posterior aspect of the metacarpophalangeal joint	Over the posterior midline of the metacarpal	Over the posterior midline of the proximal phalanx
	Metacarpophalangeal extension	Over the posterior aspect of the metacarpophalangeal joint	Over the posterior midline of the metacarpal	Over the posterior midline of the proximal phalanx
	Metacarpophalangeal abduction	Over the posterior aspect of the metacarpophalangeal joint	Over the posterior midline of the metacarpal	Over the posterior midline of the proximal phalanx
	Metacarpophalangeal adduction	Over the posterior aspect of the metacarpophalangeal joint	Over the posterior midline of the metacarpal	Over the posterior midline of the proximal phalanx
	Proximal interphalangeal flexion	Over the posterior aspect of the proximal interphalangeal joint	Over the posterior midline of the proximal phalanx	Over the posterior midline of the middle phalanx
	Proximal interphalangeal extension	Over the posterior aspect of the proximal interphalangeal joint	Over the posterior midline of the proximal phalanx	Over the posterior midline of the middle phalanx
	Distal interphalangeal flexion	Over the posterior aspect of the proximal interphalangeal joint	Over the posterior midline of the middle phalanx	Over the posterior midline of the distal phalanx
	Distal interphalangeal extension	Over the posterior aspect of the proximal interphalangeal joint	Over the posterior midline of the middle phalanx	Over the posterior midline of the distal phalanx

TABLE 8-10	Goniometric Techniques for the Lower Extremity			
Joint	**Motion**	**Fulcrum**	**Proximal Arm**	**Distal Arm**
Hip	Flexion	Over the lateral aspect of the hip joint using the greater trochanter of the femur for reference	Lateral midline of the pelvis	Lateral midline of the femur using the lateral epicondyle for reference
	Extension	Over the lateral aspect of the hip joint using the greater trochanter of the femur for reference	Lateral midline of the pelvis	Lateral midline of the femur using the lateral epicondyle for reference
	Abduction	Over the anterior superior iliac spine (ASIS) of the extremity being measured	Aligned with an imaginary horizontal line extending from one ASIS to the other ASIS	Anterior midline of the femur using the midline of the patella for reference
	Adduction	Over the anterior superior iliac spine (ASIS) of the extremity being measured	Aligned with an imaginary horizontal line extending from one ASIS to the other ASIS	Anterior midline of the femur using the midline of the patella for reference
	Internal rotation	Anterior aspect of the patella	Perpendicular to the floor or parallel to the supporting surface	Anterior midline of the lower leg using the crest of the tibia and a point midway between the two malleoli for reference
	External rotation	Anterior aspect of the patella	Perpendicular to the floor or parallel to the supporting surface	Anterior midline of the lower leg using the crest of the tibia and a point midway between the two malleoli for reference
Knee	Flexion	Lateral epicondyle of the femur	Lateral midline of the femur using the greater trochanter for reference	Lateral midline of the fibula using the lateral malleolus and fibular head for reference
	Extension	Lateral epicondyle of the femur	Lateral midline of the femur using the greater trochanter for reference	Lateral midline of the fibula using the lateral malleolus and fibular head for reference
Ankle	Dorsiflexion	Lateral aspect of the lateral malleolus	Lateral midline of the fibula using the head of the fibula for reference	Parallel to the lateral aspect of the fifth metatarsal
	Plantarflexion	Lateral aspect of the lateral malleolus	Lateral midline of the fibula using the head of the fibula for reference	Parallel to the lateral aspect of the fifth metatarsal
	Inversion	Anterior aspect of the ankle midway between the malleoli	Anterior midline of the lower leg using the tibial tuberosity for reference	Anterior midline of the second metatarsal
	Eversion	Anterior aspect of the ankle midway between the malleoli	Anterior midline of the lower leg using the tibial tuberosity for reference	Anterior midline of the second metatarsal
Subtalar	Inversion	Posterior aspect of the ankle midway between the malleoli	Posterior midline of the lower leg	Posterior midline of the calcaneus
	Eversion	Posterior aspect of the ankle midway between the malleoli	Posterior midline of the lower leg	Posterior midline of the calcaneus

The following sections describe how to measure joint ROM for the major joints of the upper extremity.

Shoulder Complex

Shoulder motion occurs at the glenohumeral, scapulothoracic, acromioclavicular, and sternoclavicular joints. There must also be available motion in the cervical and upper thoracic spine for full shoulder motion to occur. For the following measurements, the patient is positioned supine with both hips and knees flexed and the feet is placed on the bed to flatten the lumbar spine unless otherwise stated.

Shoulder Flexion. When measuring glenohumeral flexion, allowing the motion to occur at the other joints provides a more functional reading. However, if the clinician requires a pure glenohumeral motion measurement, the other joints must be manually blocked. This is best achieved by stabilizing the scapula to prevent it from elevating, upwardly rotating, and posteriorly tilting. In the following description, the scapula is not stabilized; instead, the thorax is stabilized to prevent extension of the spine.

Upper Extremity Position. The glenohumeral joint is initially positioned in 0° of abduction, adduction, and rotation, and the forearm is positioned in 0° of supination and pronation so that the palm faces the body.

Goniometer Placement. The fulcrum is centered close to the acromion process. The proximal arm is aligned with the midaxillary line of the thorax. The distal arm is aligned with the lateral midline of the humerus, using the lateral epicondyle of the humerus as a landmark.

Technique. The shoulder is moved passively or actively to the end range of available shoulder flexion (Figure 8-56), and a measurement is made (Figure 8-57).

Shoulder Extension. The patient is positioned prone.

Upper Extremity Position. The glenohumeral joint is positioned in 0° of abduction and rotation, the elbow is positioned in slight flexion, and the forearm is positioned in 0° of supination and pronation. If a measurement of pure glenohumeral extension is required, the scapula must be stabilized to prevent elevation and anterior tilting.

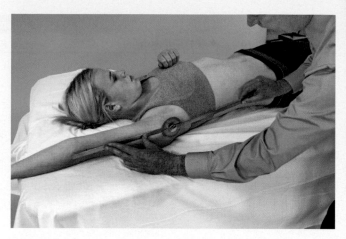

FIGURE 8-57 Goniometric measurement of shoulder flexion.

Goniometer Placement. The fulcrum is centered close to the acromion process. The proximal arm is aligned with the thorax's midaxillary line, and the distal arm is aligned with the lateral midline of the humerus using the lateral epicondyle of the humerus as a landmark.

Technique. The shoulder is moved passively or actively to the end range of available shoulder extension (Figure 8-58). The clinician can measure AROM (Figure 8-59) or PROM, or both if a comparison is made.

Shoulder Abduction. Although measured here with the patient positioned supine, shoulder abduction can be measured with the patient in sitting or prone, which has the advantage of allowing free movement of the scapula.

Upper Extremity Position. The glenohumeral joint is positioned in 0° of flexion and extension and full external rotation. The palm faces anteriorly to prevent the greater tubercle of the humerus from impacting the upper portion of the glenoid fossa or acromion process. Pure glenohumeral abduction can be measured by stabilizing the scapula to prevent its upward rotation and elevation.

Goniometer Placement. The fulcrum is centered close to the anterior aspect of the acromion process, the proximal arm is aligned so that it is parallel to the midline of the anterior aspect of the sternum, and the distal arm is aligned with the medial midline of the humerus using the medial epicondyle

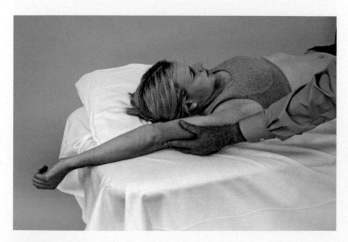

FIGURE 8-56 Passive shoulder flexion.

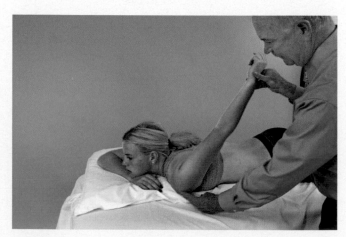

FIGURE 8-58 Passive shoulder extension.

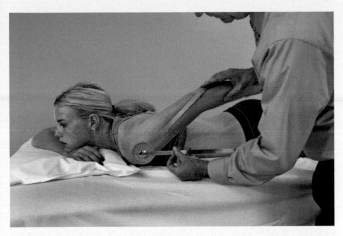

FIGURE 8-59 Goniometric measurement of shoulder extension.

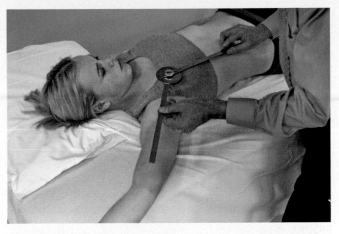

FIGURE 8-61 Goniometric measurement of shoulder abduction.

as a landmark. Suppose shoulder abduction is measured with the patient in the seated position. In that case, the fulcrum is centered close to the posterior aspect of the acromion process. The proximal arm is aligned parallel to the vertebral column's spinous processes, and the distal arm is aligned with the lateral midline of the humerus, using the lateral epicondyle as a landmark.

Technique. The shoulder is moved passively or actively to the end range of available shoulder abduction (Figure 8-60), and a goniometric measurement of AROM (Figure 8-61) or PROM is made for a comparison

CLINICAL PEARL

Shoulder adduction is not typically measured, as it represents the patient's arm by the side. The further motion toward the patient's midline is considered horizontal adduction.

Shoulder Internal Rotation

Upper Extremity Position. The patient is positioned prone. The glenohumeral joint is positioned in 90° of shoulder abduction with the forearm perpendicular to the supporting surface and at 0° of supination/pronation so that the palm faces the feet. If necessary, a rolled-up towel can be placed

under the humerus so that it is positioned level with the acromion process.

Goniometer Placement. The fulcrum is centered over the olecranon process. The proximal arm is aligned so that it is either parallel to or perpendicular to the floor. The distal arm is aligned with the ulna, using the olecranon process and ulnar styloid as landmarks.

Technique. The shoulder is moved passively or actively to the end range of shoulder internal rotation (Figure 8-62), and a measurement is taken (Figure 8-63).

Shoulder External Rotation. The patient position is the same as for internal rotation of the shoulder.

Goniometer Placement. The goniometer alignment is the same as for shoulder internal rotation.

Technique. The shoulder is moved passively or actively to the end range of shoulder external rotation (Figure 8-64), and a measurement is taken (Figure 8-65).

Alternatively, shoulder internal rotation can be measured with the patient in supine (Figure 8-66), as can shoulder external rotation (Figure 8-67), using the start position for the goniometer as depicted in Figure 8-68.

Elbow/Forearm Complex

For the following measurements, the patient is positioned supine with both hips and knees flexed and the feet placed

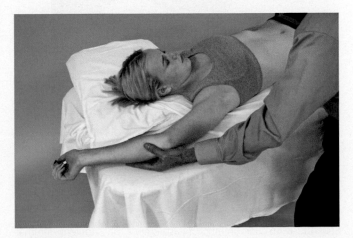

FIGURE 8-60 Passive shoulder abduction.

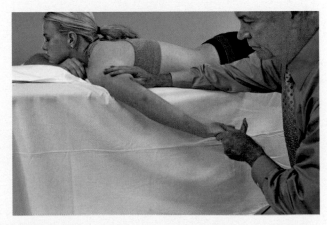

FIGURE 8-62 Passive shoulder internal rotation.

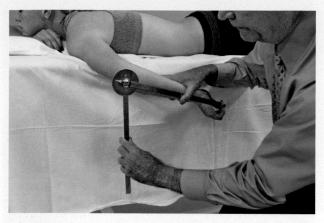

FIGURE 8-63 Goniometric measurement of shoulder internal rotation.

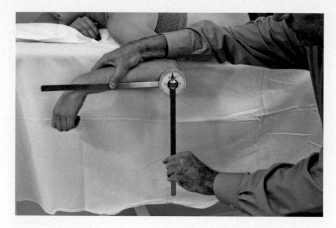

FIGURE 8-65 Goniometric measurement of shoulder external rotation.

on the bed to flatten the lumbar spine unless otherwise stated.

Flexion/Extension. A pad can be placed under the distal end of the humerus to allow for elbow extension.

Upper Extremity Position. The glenohumeral joint is positioned in 0° of flexion, extension, and abduction so that the arm is close to the side of the body.

Goniometer Placement. The goniometer placement is the same for flexion and extension. The fulcrum is centered over the lateral epicondyle of the humerus, the proximal arm is aligned with the lateral midline of the humerus (using the acromion process as a landmark), and the distal arm is aligned with the lateral midline of the radius, using the styloid process as a landmark.

Technique. To measure elbow flexion, the elbow is passively or actively flexed to the end of the available range, and a measurement is taken (Figure 8-69). The upper extremity is positioned correctly to measure elbow extension, and a measurement is taken (Figure 8-70).

Forearm Pronation. This measurement can also be performed with the patient seated.

Upper Extremity Position. The glenohumeral joint is positioned in 0° of flexion, extension, abduction, and rotation so that the upper arm is close to the side of the body, and the elbow is flexed to 90° with the forearm midway between supination and pronation.

Goniometer Placement. The fulcrum is centered lateral to the ulnar styloid process, the proximal arm is aligned parallel to the anterior midline of the humerus, and the distal arm is aligned across the posterior aspect of the forearm, just proximal to the styloid processes of the radius and ulna (Figure 8-71).

Technique. The forearm is pronated passively or actively to the end of the available ROM (Figure 8-72), and a measurement is taken (Figure 8-73).

Forearm Supination. The patient is positioned as for the forearm pronation measurement.

Goniometer Placement. The fulcrum is aligned medial to the ulnar styloid process. The proximal arm is aligned parallel to the anterior midline of the humerus. The distal arm is

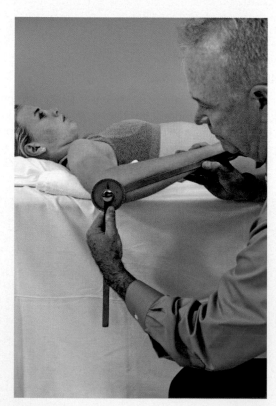

FIGURE 8-66 Goniometric measurement of shoulder internal rotation with the patient in supine.

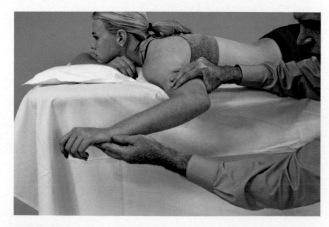

FIGURE 8-64 Passive shoulder external rotation.

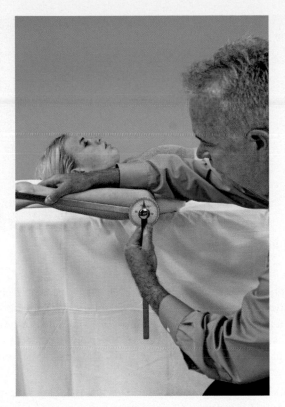

FIGURE 8-67 Goniometric measurement of shoulder external rotation with the patient in supine.

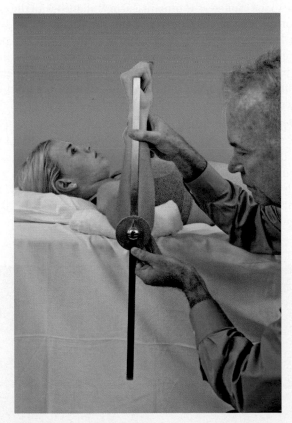

FIGURE 8-68 Start position for the goniometer to measure internal and external rotation with the patient in supine.

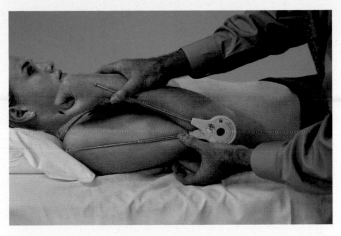

FIGURE 8-69 Goniometric measurement of elbow flexion.

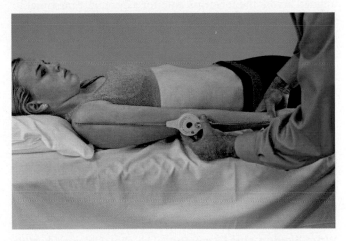

FIGURE 8-70 Goniometric measurement of elbow extension.

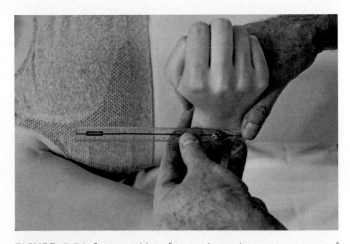

FIGURE 8-71 Start position for goniometric measurement of forearm supination/pronation.

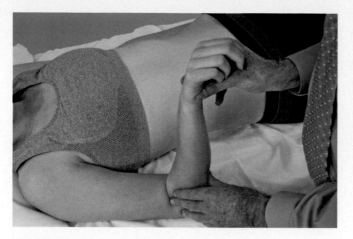

FIGURE 8-72 Passive forearm pronation.

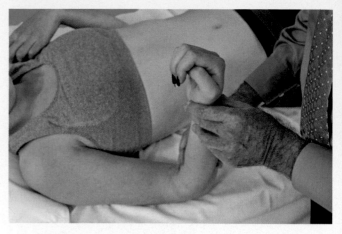

FIGURE 8-74 Passive forearm supination.

aligned across the forearm's anterior aspect, just proximal to the styloid process (Figure 8-71).

Technique. The forearm is moved passively or actively to the end of the available ROM (Figure 8-74), and a measurement is taken (Figure 8-75).

An alternative technique to measure forearm supination and pronation involves having the patient hold a pen or pencil in a close-fisted hand. The goniometer can then be aligned using the end of the pen as a landmark (Figure 8-76).

Wrist Joints

For the following measurements, the patient is seated next to a supporting surface to support the forearm, but the hand is free to move.

Wrist Flexion and Extension. The clinician should stabilize the forearm to prevent supination or pronation.

Goniometer Placement. The goniometer placement is the same for wrist flexion and wrist extension. The fulcrum is centered over the lateral aspect of the wrist, close to the triquetrum. The proximal arm is aligned with the ulna's lateral midline, using the olecranon process as a landmark, and the distal arm is aligned with the lateral midline of the fifth metacarpal. The patient's palm is moved downward for wrist flexion and upward for wrist extension while avoiding extension of the fingers.

Technique. To measure wrist flexion, the wrist is actively or passively flexed to the end of the available ROM (Figure 8-77), and a measurement is taken (Figure 8-78). To measure wrist extension, the wrist is actively or passively extended to the end of the available ROM (Figure 8-79), and a measurement is taken (Figure 8-80).

Radial Deviation and Ulnar Deviation. The patient is positioned as for wrist flexion/extension.

Goniometer Placement. The goniometer placement is the same for radial deviation and ulnar deviation. The fulcrum is centered over the middle of the posterior aspect of the wrist close to the capitate, the proximal arm is aligned with the posterior midline of the forearm, using the lateral epicondyles as a landmark, and the distal arm is aligned with the posterior midline of the third metacarpal. For radial deviation, the patient's hand moves toward the patient's body, whereas for ulnar deviation, the patient's hand moves away from the patient's body.

Technique. To measure radial deviation, the wrist is passively or actively moved to the end of the available ROM for radial deviation (Figure 8-81), and a measurement is taken (Figure 8-82). To measure ulnar deviation, the wrist is passively or actively moved to the end of the available ROM for ulnar deviation (Figure 8-83), and a measurement is taken (Figure 8-84).

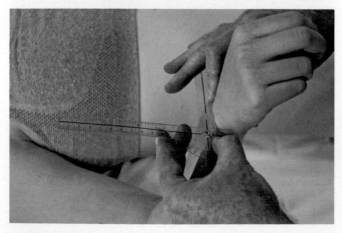

FIGURE 8-73 Goniometric measurement of forearm pronation.

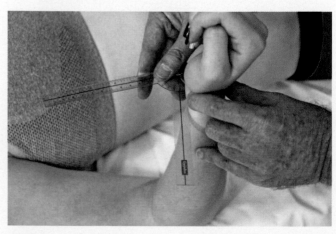

FIGURE 8-75 Goniometric measurement of forearm supination.

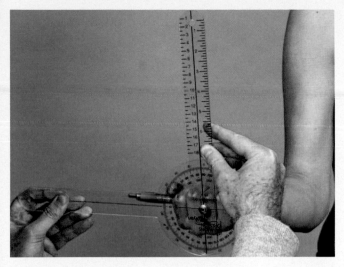

FIGURE 8-76 Alternative method for measuring forearm supination/pronation.

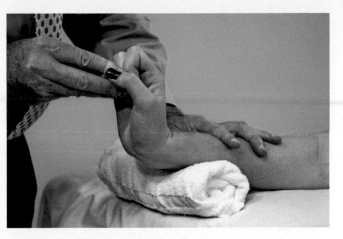

FIGURE 8-79 Passive wrist extension—less motion occurs if the fingers are extended.

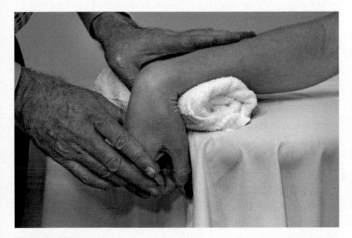

FIGURE 8-77 Passive wrist flexion—more motion occurs if the fingers are extended.

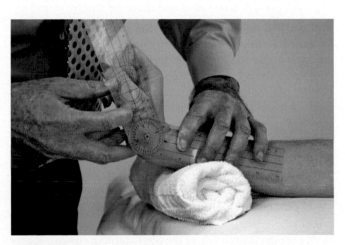

FIGURE 8-80 Goniometric measurement of wrist extension.

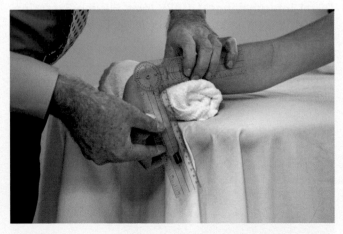

FIGURE 8-78 Goniometric measurement of wrist flexion.

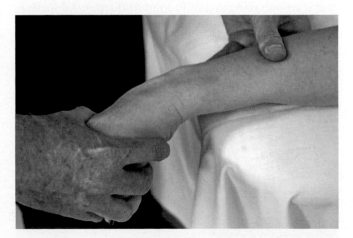

FIGURE 8-81 Passive radial deviation.

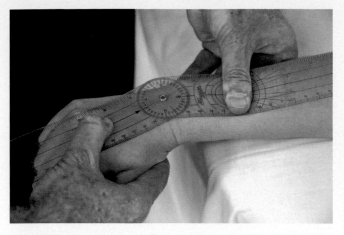

FIGURE 8-82 Goniometric measurement of radial deviation.

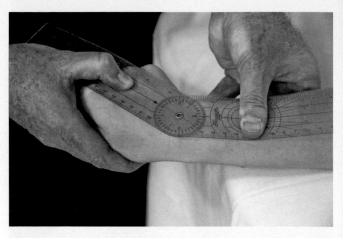

FIGURE 8-84 Goniometric measurement of ulnar deviation.

Finger Joints

The patient's position for these joints is typically in sitting, with the forearm supported and midway between pronation and supination, the wrist positioned in 0° of flexion and extension, and neutral radial and ulnar deviation.

Metacarpophalangeal (MCP) Joint Flexion/Extension. While performing these measurements, the clinician must ensure that the MCP joint is maintained in a neutral position relative to abduction and adduction and to avoid too much motion occurring at the proximal interphalangeal and distal interphalangeal joints. The same technique is used for all of the MCP joints of the fingers.

Goniometer Placement. The goniometer placement is the same for MCP flexion and MCP extension. The fulcrum is centered over the posterior aspect of the MCP joint. The proximal arm is aligned over the posterior midline of the metacarpal. The distal arm is aligned over the posterior midline of the proximal phalanx. For the index finger, the fulcrum is centered over the thumb side of the MCP joint, the proximal arm is aligned with the radial styloid, and the distal arm is aligned over the thumb side of the phalanx (Figure 8-85).

Technique. A measurement is taken for MCP flexion (Figure 8-86) and MCP extension (Figure 8-87).

Metacarpophalangeal (MCP) Joint Abduction/Adduction. The same technique is used for all of the MCP joints of the fingers.

Goniometer Placement. The goniometer placement is the same for MCP joint abduction and MCP joint adduction. The fulcrum is centered over the posterior aspect of the MCP joint. The proximal arm is aligned over the posterior midline of the metacarpal. The distal arm is aligned over the posterior midline of the proximal phalanx (Figure 8-88).

Technique. A measurement is taken for MCP abduction (Figure 8-89) and MCP abduction (Figure 8-90).

Proximal Interphalangeal (PIP) Joint Flexion/Extension. The clinician attempts to stabilize the proximal phalanx to prevent motion at the wrist and MCP joint.

Goniometer Placement. The goniometer placement is the same for PIP joint flexion and PIP joint extension. The fulcrum is centered over the posterior aspect of the PIP joint. The proximal arm is aligned over the posterior midline of the proximal phalanx. The distal arm is aligned over the posterior midline of the middle phalanx. The same technique is used for each of the PIP joints of the fingers. It is questionable whether measurement of PIP joint extension is possible, as any loss of PIP extension is technically a measurement of PIP flexion.

Technique. A measurement is taken for PIP joint flexion (Figure 8-91).

Distal Interphalangeal (DIP) Joint Flexion/Extension. The MCP joint is positioned in 0° of flexion, extension,

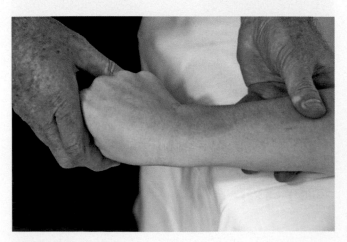

FIGURE 8-83 Passive ulnar deviation.

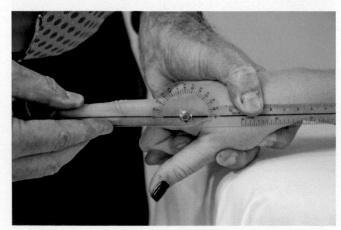

FIGURE 8-85 Goniometer placement for MCP flexion/extension.

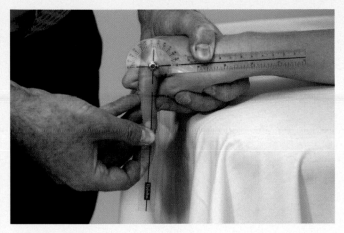

FIGURE 8-86 Goniometric measurement for MCP flexion of the index finger.

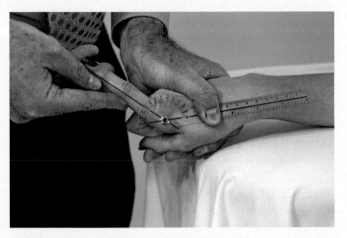

FIGURE 8-87 Goniometric measurement for MCP extension of the index finger.

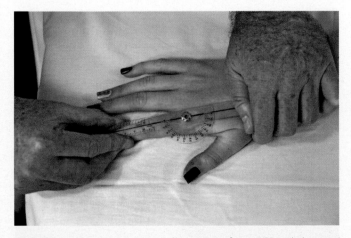

FIGURE 8-88 Goniometer placement for MCP abduction/adduction.

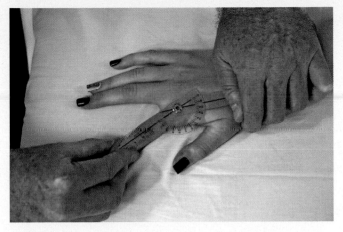

FIGURE 8-89 Goniometric measurement for MCP abduction.

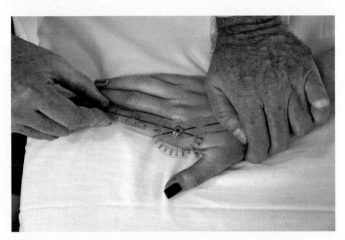

FIGURE 8-90 Goniometric measurement for MCP adduction.

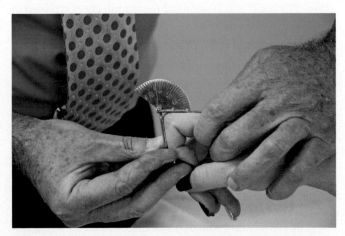

FIGURE 8-91 Goniometric measurement for PIP joint flexion.

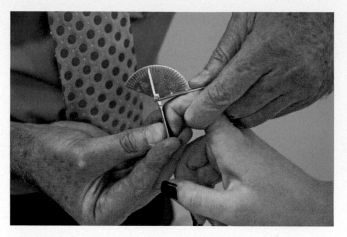

FIGURE 8-92 Goniometric measurement for DIP joint flexion.

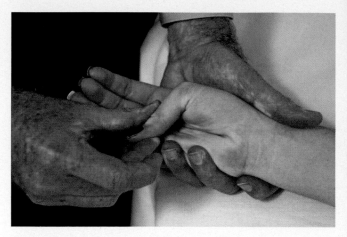

FIGURE 8-93 Passive thumb CMC joint flexion.

abduction, and adduction, with the PIP joint positioned in approximately 70° to 90° of flexion. The clinician attempts to stabilize the middle phalanx to prevent further flexion or extension of the wrist, MCP joints, and PIP joints.

Goniometer Placement. The goniometer placement is the same for DIP joint flexion and DIP joint extension. The fulcrum is centered over the posterior aspect of the PIP joint. The proximal arm is aligned over the posterior midline of the middle phalanx. The distal arm is aligned over the posterior midline of the distal phalanx. The same technique is used for each of the DIP joints of the fingers. As with PIP joint extension, it is questionable whether measurement of DIP joint extension is possible, as any loss of DIP extension is technically a measurement of DIP flexion.

Technique. A measurement is taken for DIP joint flexion (Figure 8-92).

Thumb Joints

The patient position for these joints is typically seated, with the forearm supported in supination, the wrist positioned in 0° of flexion and extension, and neutral radial and ulnar deviation. The MCP and IP joints of the thumb are positioned in 0° of flexion and extension.

Carpometacarpal (CMC) Flexion and Extension

Goniometer Placement. The fulcrum is centered over the first CMC joint's anterior aspect. The proximal arm is aligned parallel to the anterior midline of the radius, and the distal arm is aligned with the anterior midline of the first metacarpal. CMC flexion occurs when the thumb moves toward the palm, and CMC extension occurs when the thumb moves away from the palm.

Technique. The CMC joint is passively or actively moved into the available ROM for flexion (Figure 8-93), and a measurement is taken (Figure 8-94). The CMC joint is passively or actively moved into the available ROM for extension (Figure 8-95), and a measurement is taken (Figure 8-96).

Carpometacarpal (CMC) Abduction and Adduction.
The patient positioning is the same as for CMC flexion and extension.

Goniometer Placement. The goniometer placement is the same for CMC abduction and CMC adduction. The fulcrum

is centered midway between the posterior aspect of the first and second carpometacarpal joints. The proximal arm is aligned parallel to the anterior midline of the radius, and the distal arm is aligned with the lateral midline of the first metacarpal. CMC abduction occurs when the thumb moves away from the hand, whereas CMC adduction occurs when it moves toward the hand.

Technique. The CMC joint is passively or actively moved into the available ROM for abduction (Figure 8-97), and a measurement is taken (Figure 8-98).

Thumb Opposition. The patient positioning is the same as for CMC flexion and extension.

Goniometer Placement. The ruler component of a goniometer is typically used to measure the amount of thumb opposition by calculating the distance between the tip of the thumb and the tip of the fifth digit.

Technique. The thumb and little finger are actively or passively moved together in the direction of opposition (Figure 8-99), and a measurement is taken (Figure 8-100). In most cases, the thumb and little fingertips will be able to touch, so Figure 8-100 demonstrates a case where this is not possible.

Metacarpophalangeal (MCP) Joint of the Thumb Flexion and Extension. The patient positioning is the same as for CMC flexion and extension.

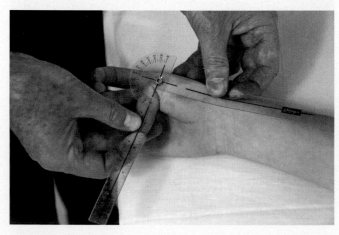

FIGURE 8-94 Goniometric measurement of thumb CMC joint flexion.

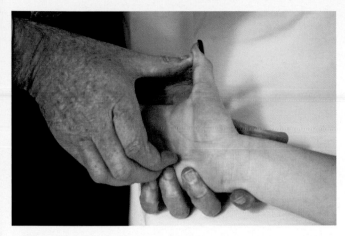

FIGURE 8-95 Passive thumb CMC joint extension.

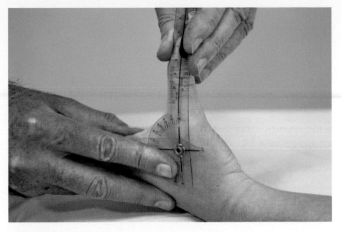

FIGURE 8-98 Goniometric measurement of thumb CMC joint abduction.

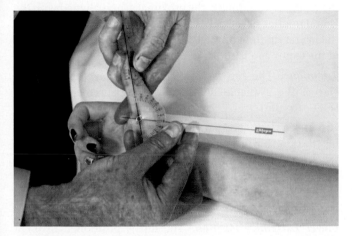

FIGURE 8-96 Goniometric measurement of thumb CMC joint extension.

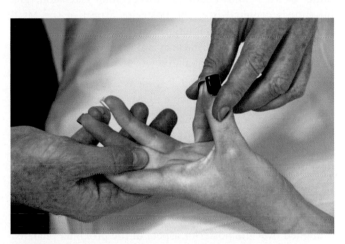

FIGURE 8-99 Passive opposition of thumb and little finger.

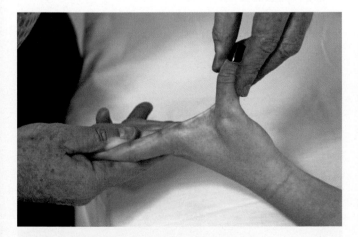

FIGURE 8-97 Passive thumb CMC joint abduction.

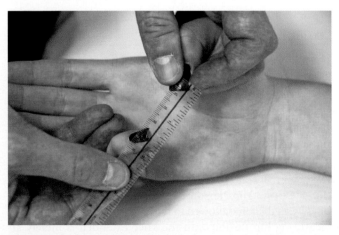

FIGURE 8-100 Goniometric measurement of active thumb opposition.

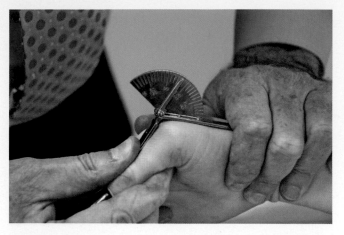

FIGURE 8-101 Goniometric measurement of thumb MCP flexion.

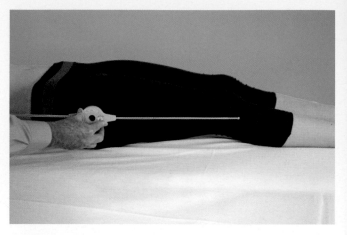

FIGURE 8-102 Goniometer position for hip flexion.

Goniometer Placement. The goniometer placement is the same for MCP joint flexion and MCP joint extension. The fulcrum is centered over the posterior aspect of the MCP joint. The proximal arm is aligned over the posterior midline of the metacarpal. The distal arm is aligned with the posterior midline of the proximal phalanx.

Technique. The thumb's MCP joint is actively or passively flexed to the end of the available ROM, and a measurement is taken (Figure 8-101).

Interphalangeal (IP) Joint of the Thumb Flexion and Extension. The patient positioning is the same as for CMC flexion and extension.

Goniometer Placement. The goniometer placement is the same for IP flexion and IP extension. The fulcrum is centered over the posterior surface of the IP joint. The proximal arm is aligned over the posterior aspect of the proximal phalanx. The distal arm is aligned with the posterior midline of the distal phalanx.

Technique. The thumb's IP joint is actively or passively flexed to the end of the available ROM, and a measurement is taken.

Lower Extremity

The following sections describe in detail how to measure joint ROM for the major joints of the lower extremity.

Hip Joint

The patient is positioned in supine to measure hip flexion, hip abduction, and hip adduction, seated to measure hip internal rotation and external rotation, and prone to measure hip extension.

Hip Flexion. Hip flexion can be measured in one of two ways, with the knee allowed to flex, or with the knee extended. Measuring hip flexion with the knee extended is merely an indication of the length of the patient's hamstrings rather than a true measurement of hip joint motion. Hip flexion with the knee flexed is described here.

Lower Extremity Position. The hip is positioned in 0° of abduction, abduction, and rotation, with the knee motion unrestricted.

Goniometer Placement. The fulcrum is centered over the lateral aspect of the hip joint using the greater trochanter of the femur as a landmark, the proximal arm is aligned with the lateral midline of the pelvis, and the distal arm is aligned with the lateral midline of the femur, using the lateral epicondyle of the femur as a landmark (Figure 8-102).

Technique. The hip is actively or passively flexed to the end of the available ROM, and a measurement is taken (Figure 8-103).

Hip Extension. The patient is positioned in prone. As with hip flexion, hip extension can be measured in one of two ways, with the knee allowed to flex, or with the knee extended. Measuring hip extension with the knee flexed can be misleading due to tension from the rectus femoris muscle, which can restrict motion.

Lower Extremity Position. The hip is positioned in 0° of abduction, abduction, and rotation, with the knee motion unrestricted.

Goniometer Placement. The goniometer placement and alignment is the same as for hip flexion, except that the patient is positioned in prone (Figure 8-104).

Technique. The hip is actively or passively extended to the end of the available ROM, and a measurement is taken (Figure 8-105).

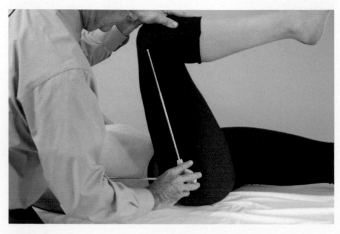

FIGURE 8-103 Goniometric measurement of hip flexion.

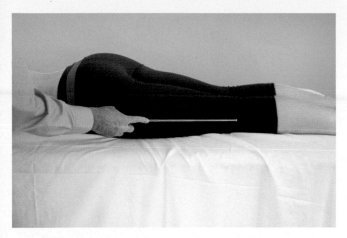

FIGURE 8-104 Goniometer position for hip extension.

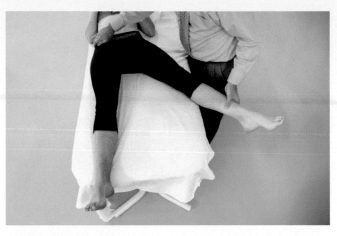

FIGURE 8-106 Passive hip abduction while monitoring contralateral ASIS.

Hip Abduction/Adduction

Lower Extremity Position. The patient is positioned in prone. The lower extremity is kept as straight as possible. It is worth remembering that, in order for full hip adduction to take place, the contralateral hip must be abducted to allow the hip being measured to complete its full ROM.

Goniometer Placement. The goniometer placement for hip abduction and hip adduction is the same. The fulcrum is centered over the anterior superior iliac spine (ASIS) of the extremity being measured, the proximal arm is aligned with an imaginary horizontal line extending from one ASIS to the other ASIS, and the distal arm is aligned with the anterior midline of the femur using the midline of the patella as a landmark.

Technique. The hip is actively or passively abducted to the end of the available ROM (Figure 8-106), and a measurement is taken (Figure 8-107). To measure hip adduction, the hip is actively or passively adducted to the end of the available ROM (Figure 8-108), and a measurement is taken (Figure 8-109).

Hip Internal Rotation/External Rotation. The patient is seated on a supporting surface, with the knee flexed over the edge.

Lower Extremity Position. The hip is in 0° of abduction and adduction and 90° of flexion. If necessary, a towel roll

is placed under the distal end of the femur to maintain the femur in a horizontal plane.

Goniometer Placement. The goniometer placement for hip internal rotation and hip external rotation is the same. The fulcrum is centered over the anterior aspect of the patella, the proximal arm is aligned so that it is perpendicular to the floor all parallel to the supporting surface, and the distal arm is aligned with the anterior midline of the lower leg, using the tibial crest and a point midway between the two malleoli as reference points.

Technique. The hip is actively or passively internally rotated to the end of the available ROM (Figure 8-110), and a measurement is taken (Figure 8-111). To measure external rotation of the hip, the hip is actively or passively externally rotated to the end of the available ROM (Figure 8-112), and a measurement is taken (Figure 8-113).

Tibiofemoral Joint

To assess tibiofemoral joint flexion and extension, the patient is typically positioned in prone. However, in the presence of significant adaptive shortening of the rectus femoris muscle, knee flexion can be measured with the patient in supine.

Tibiofemoral Joint Flexion/Extension. During these measurements, it is important to stabilize the femur to prevent rotation, flexion, or extension of the hip.

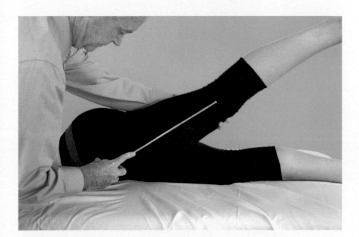

FIGURE 8-105 Goniometric measurement of hip extension.

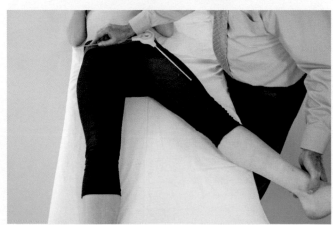

FIGURE 8-107 Goniometric measurement of hip abduction.

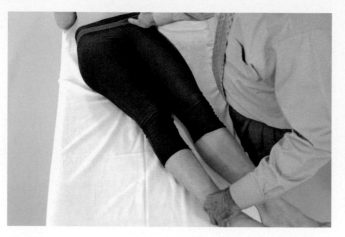

FIGURE 8-108 Passive hip adduction while monitoring contralateral ASIS.

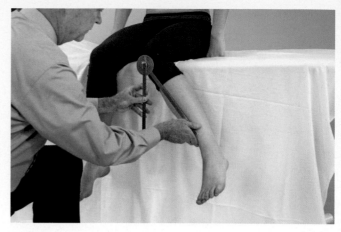

FIGURE 8-111 Goniometric measurement of hip internal rotation.

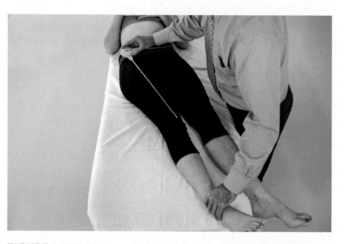

FIGURE 8-109 Goniometric measurement of hip adduction.

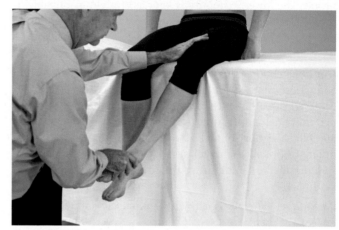

FIGURE 8-112 Passive hip external rotation.

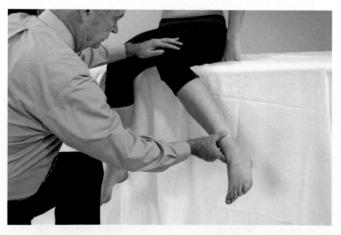

FIGURE 8-110 Passive hip internal rotation.

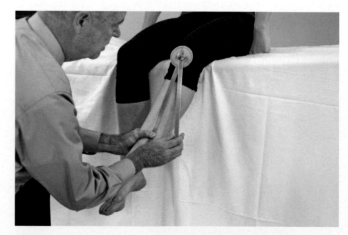

FIGURE 8-113 Goniometric measurement of hip external rotation.

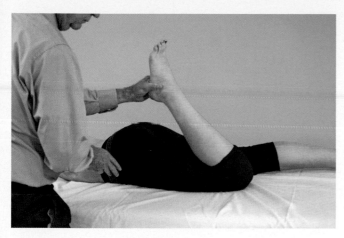

FIGURE 8-114 Passive knee flexion.

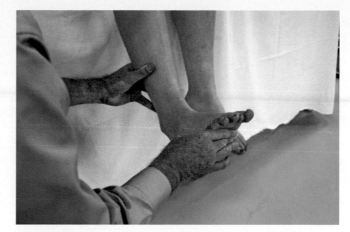

FIGURE 8-116 Passive ankle dorsiflexion.

Lower Extremity Position. The hip is positioned in 0° of abduction, adduction, flexion, extension, and rotation.

Goniometer Placement. The goniometer placement for tibiofemoral flexion and tibiofemoral extension is the same. The fulcrum is centered over the lateral epicondyle of the femur, the proximal arm is aligned with the lateral midline of the femur, using the greater trochanter at a landmark, and the distal arm is aligned with the lateral midline of the fibula, using the lateral malleolus as a landmark.

Technique. The knee is actively or passively flexed to the end of the available ROM (Figure 8-114), and a measurement is taken (Figure 8-115). This measurement can also be taken with the patient in supine.

Ankle Joint

The ankle joint can be assessed with the patient in sitting, prone, or supine. For a more accurate measurement of ankle motion, the patient's knee should be flexed to at least 30° to remove any influence from the gastrocnemius complex.

Dorsiflexion and Plantarflexion. The patient is positioned in sitting or supine.

Goniometer Placement. The goniometer placement is the same for dorsiflexion and plantarflexion. The fulcrum is centered over the lateral aspect of the lateral malleolus, the

proximal arm is aligned with the lateral midline of the fibula, using the head of the fibula as a landmark, and the distal arm is aligned parallel to the lateral aspect of the fifth metatarsal, or parallel to the inferior aspect of the calcaneus.

Technique. The ankle is actively or passively dorsiflexed to the end of the available ROM (Figure 8-116), and a measurement is taken (Figure 8-117). To measure ankle plantarflexion, the ankle is actively or passively plantarflexed to the end of the available ROM (Figure 8-118), and a measurement is taken (Figure 8-119).

Subtalar Joint Inversion and Eversion. The patient is positioned in prone.

Goniometer Placement. The goniometer placement is the same for inversion and eversion. The fulcrum is centered over the posterior aspect of the ankle, midway between the malleoli, the proximal arm is aligned with the posterior midline of the lower leg, and the distal arm is aligned with the posterior midline of the calcaneus.

Technique. The ankle is actively or passively inverted to the end of the available ROM (Figure 8-120), and a measurement is taken (Figure 8-121). For ankle eversion, the ankle is actively or passively everted to the end of the available ROM (Figure 8-122), and a measurement is taken (Figure 8-123).

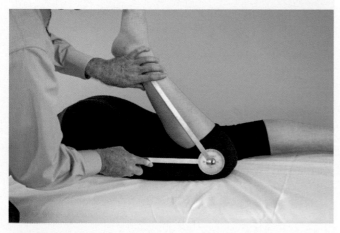

FIGURE 8-115 Goniometric measurement of knee flexion with the patient prone.

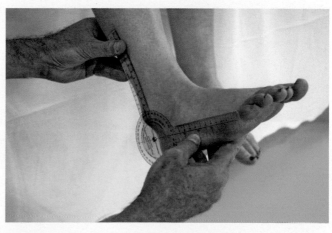

FIGURE 8-117 Goniometric measurement of ankle dorsiflexion.

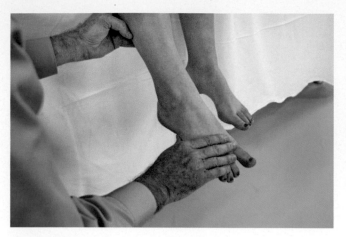

FIGURE 8-118 Passive ankle plantarflexion.

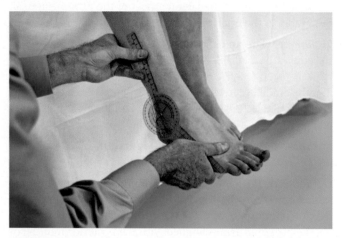

FIGURE 8-119 Goniometric measurement of ankle plantarflexion.

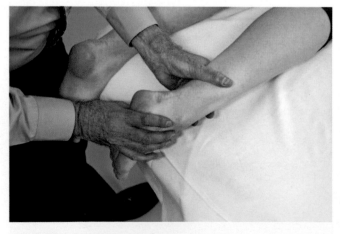

FIGURE 8-120 Passive subtalar joint inversion.

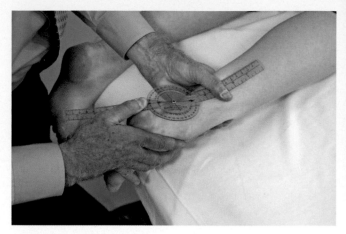

FIGURE 8-121 Goniometric measurement of subtalar joint inversion.

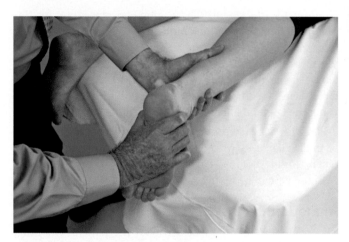

FIGURE 8-122 Passive subtalar joint eversion.

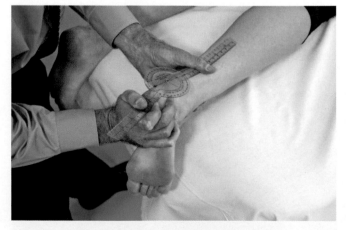

FIGURE 8-123 Goniometric measurement of subtalar joint eversion.

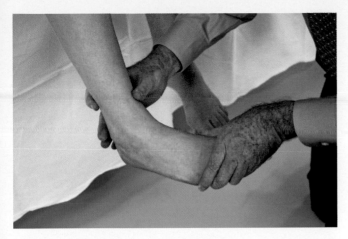

FIGURE 8-124 Passive tarsal joint inversion.

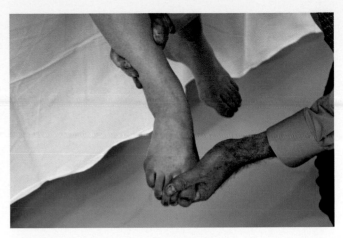

FIGURE 8-126 Passive tarsal joint eversion.

Tarsal Joint Inversion and Eversion. The patient is positioned in sitting.

Goniometer Placement. The goniometer placement is the same for inversion and eversion. The fulcrum is centered over the anterior aspect of the ankle midway between the malleoli, the proximal arm is aligned with the anterior midline of the lower leg, using the tibial crest for reference, and the distal arm is aligned with the anterior midline of the second metatarsal.

Technique. The tarsal joints are actively or passively inverted to the end of the available ROM (Figure 8-124), and a measurement is taken (Figure 8-125). For tarsal joint eversion, the tarsal joints are actively or passively everted to the end of the available ROM (Figure 8-126), and a measurement is taken (Figure 8-127).

Toe Joints

Metatarsophalangeal (MTP) Joint Flexion and Extension. The patient is positioned in sitting or supine with the MTP and IP joints positioned in 0° of flexion and extension.

Goniometer Placement. The goniometer placement is the same for MTP joint flexion and MTP joint extension. The fulcrum is aligned over the posterior aspect of the MTP joint, the proximal arm is aligned over the posterior midline of the metatarsal, and the distal arm is aligned over the posterior midline of the proximal phalanx.

Technique. The MTP joint is actively or passively flexed to the end of the available ROM (Figure 8-128), and a measurement is taken (Figure 8-129). To measure MTP joint extension, the MTP joint is actively or passively extended to the end of the available ROM (Figure 8-130), and a measurement is taken (Figure 8-131).

CLINICAL PEARL

Although motions such as abduction of the great toe (Figure 8-132), flexion/extension of the individual PIP joints, and flexion/extension of the individual distal DIP joint can theoretically be measured, one has to question the usefulness of these measurements. A more practical approach is to perform a visual assessment of combined PIP and DIP joint flexion/extension and great toe abduction (if the patient is able to perform such an action).

The Spine

Goniometric measurement of spinal motion brings its own set of challenges. Over the years, various methods have been put forward that have incorporated the use of a tape measure, the use of standard goniometers, and the use of specialized goniometers, such as the bubble goniometer. Most of the problems have

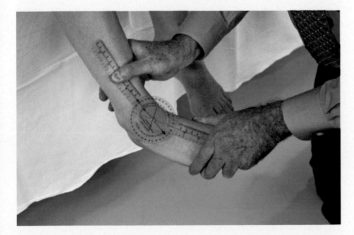

FIGURE 8-125 Goniometric measurement of tarsal joint inversion.

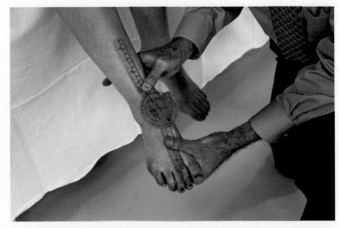

FIGURE 8-127 Goniometric measurement of tarsal joint eversion.

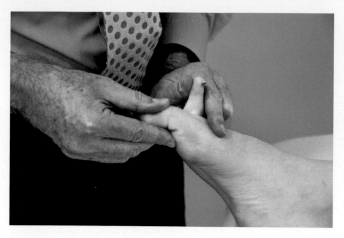

FIGURE 8-128 Passive MTP joint flexion of the great toe.

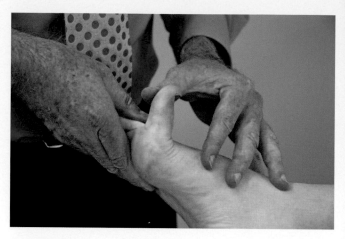

FIGURE 8-130 Passive MTP joint extension of the great toe.

stemmed from determining the best appropriate landmarks, the wide variations in body types, and whether such measurements have sufficient interrater and intrarater reliability.

Whichever method is chosen, it is important to remember that, as with other joints in the body, the ROM in the spine may vary according to a number of factors, including structural alterations, the individual's age, neck girth and length, body habitus, diurnal changes,[16] neurologic disease, or other factors unrelated to the disability for which the exam is being performed. Without taking body size into account, measurements may underestimate or overestimate ROM.[17]

Cervical Spine

Cervical Rotation

Traditional Goniometer Method. The fulcrum is centered over the center of the superior aspect of the head, the proximal arm is aligned parallel to an imaginary line between the two acromion processes, and the distal arm is aligned with the tip of the nose.

Tape Measure Method. A tape measure can be used to measure the distance between the tip of the chin and the acromion process.

Bubble Goniometer Method. The dual inclinometer method, using two bubble goniometers, is the approach recommended in the AMA's *Guides to the Evaluation of Permanent*

Impairment,[15] and is often considered the clinical standard for assessing cervical ROM in the clinic.[18,19] This method requires accurate identification of anatomic landmarks (Table 8-11). Both inter- and intrarater reliability studies have shown the inclinometry method to be reliable.[20-23] Others dispute this conclusion and contend that the inclinometer method is flawed and should not be used in clinical settings.[24,25] The normal ROM using this method is 80° or greater from the neutral position for active motion. To measure cervical rotation using a bubble goniometer, the patient is positioned in prone, and the goniometer is aligned over the crown of the head in the transverse plane (Figure 8-133). The goniometer is zeroed out and the patient is asked to rotate the head to the right (Figure 8-134), and then to the left (Figure 8-135). These measurements can also be taken with the patient seated.

CLINICAL PEARL

Using the bubble goniometer method, the full arc of passive cervical rotation range depends on the age of the patient[8]:

▶ 20–29: 183° ± 11
▶ 30–49: 172° ± 13
▶ ≥50: 155° ± 15

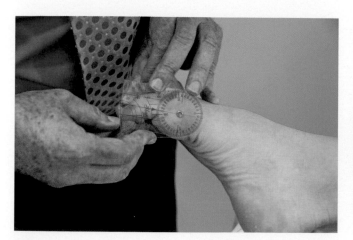

FIGURE 8-129 Goniometric measurement of flexion of the great toe.

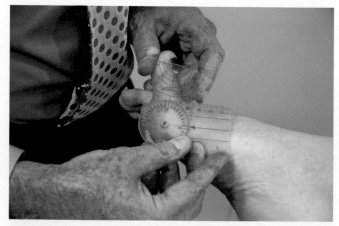

FIGURE 8-131 Goniometric measurement of extension of the great toe.

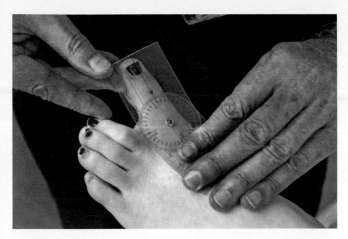

FIGURE 8-132 Goniometric measurement of great toe abduction.

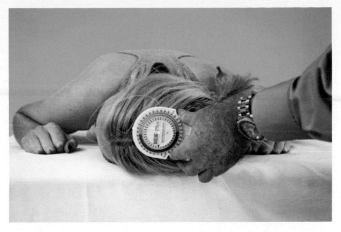

FIGURE 8-134 Goniometric measurement for right cervical rotation.

TABLE 8-11	The American Medical Association Inclinometer Technique for Measuring Cervical ROM
Range	**Method**
Flexion	Two inclinometers are used, which are aligned in the sagittal plane. The center of the first inclinometer is placed over the T1 spinous process. The center of the second one is placed on top of the head, parallel to a line drawn from the eye's corner to the ear, where the temple of eyeglasses would sit. The patient is asked to flex the neck, and both inclinometer angles are recorded. The cervical flexion angle is calculated by subtracting the T1 from the calvarium inclinometer angle.
Extension	Two inclinometers can be used, which are aligned as for measuring cervical flexion. The patient is asked to extend the neck, and both inclinometer angles are recorded. The cervical extension angle is calculated by subtracting the T1 from the calvarium inclinometer angle.
Rotation	The patient is positioned supine. One inclinometer is used, and it is aligned in the transverse plane. The base of the inclinometer is placed over the forehead. The patient is asked to rotate the neck, and the inclinometer angle is recorded. The test is repeated on the other side.
Side bending	Two inclinometers are used, which are aligned in the frontal plane. The center of the first inclinometer is placed over the T1 spinous process. The center of the second one is placed on top of the head, over the calvarium. The patient is asked to side bend the neck, and both inclinometer angles are recorded. The cervical side-bending angle is calculated by subtracting the T1 from the calvarium inclinometer angle.

ROM: range of motion
Data from American Medical Association. *Guides to the Evaluation of Permanent Impairment.* 5th ed. Chicago IL: American Medical Association; 2001.

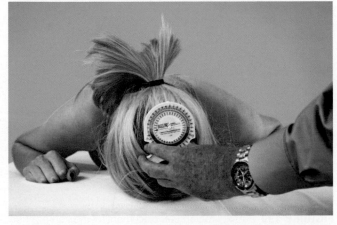

FIGURE 8-133 Bubble goniometer placement for cervical rotation.

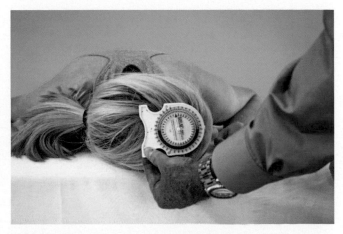

FIGURE 8-135 Goniometric measurement for left cervical rotation.

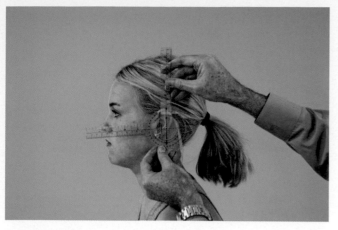

FIGURE 8-136 Goniometer placement for the start position for cervical flexion.

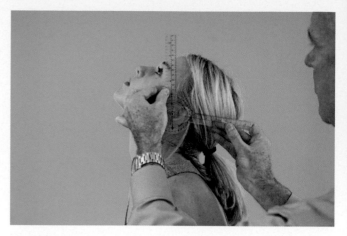

FIGURE 8-138 Goniometric measurement of cervical extension.

Cervical Flexion and Extension

Traditional Goniometer Method. The fulcrum is centered over the external auditory meatus, the proximal arm is aligned so that it is either perpendicular or parallel to the ground, and the distal arm is aligned with the base of the skull or with the end of the eye brow (the tip of the nose can also be used) (Figure 8-136). The patient is then asked to flex the cervical spine (Figure 8-137) and to extend the cervical spine (Figure 8-138).

Tape Measure Method. A tape measure can be used to measure the distance between the tip of the chin and the sternal notch, while making sure that the patient's mouth remains closed.

Bubble Goniometer Method. See Table 8-11. The normal ROM for cervical flexion using this technique is 60° or greater from the neutral position, and 75° or greater from the neutral position for active motion.[8] Two inclinometers are used, which are aligned in the sagittal plane. The center of the first inclinometer is placed over the T1 spinous process. The center of the second one is placed on top of the head (calvaria), parallel to a line drawn from the corner of the eye to the ear, where the temple of eyeglasses would sit, and both inclinometer angles are recorded. From the start position (Figure 8-139), the patient is asked to flex the cervical spine (Figure 8-140) and both inclinometer angles are recorded,

and then to extend the cervical spine (Figure 8-141). Again, both inclinometer angles are recorded. The cervical flexion and extension angles are calculated by subtracting the T1 angles from the calvarian inclinometer angles. For example: 45 degrees (reading at calvaria) − 5 degrees (reading at T1) = 40 degrees of flexion.

CLINICAL PEARL

Using the bubble goniometer method, the full arc of passive flexion/extension range depends on the age of the patient[8]:

▶ 20–29: 151° ± 17

▶ 30–49: 141° ± 35

▶ ≥50: 129° ± 14

Cervical Side Bending. When measuring cervical side bending, the clinician should stabilize the shoulder girdle to prevent lateral flexion of the thoracic and lumbar spine.

Traditional Goniometer Method. The fulcrum is centered over the spinous process of the C7 vertebra, the proximal arm is aligned with the spinous processes of the thoracic vertebra so that the arm is perpendicular to the ground, and the distal

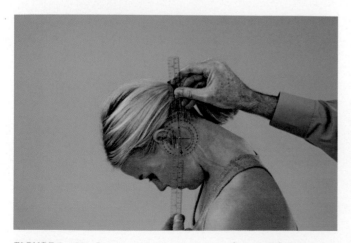

FIGURE 8-137 Goniometric measurement of cervical flexion.

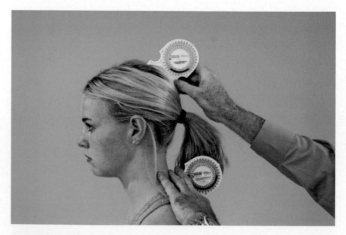

FIGURE 8-139 Bubble goniometer placement for the start position for cervical flexion.

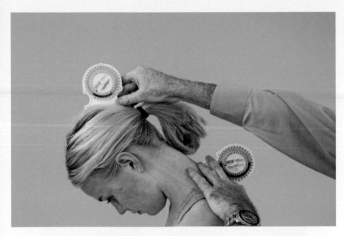

FIGURE 8-140 Goniometric measurement of cervical flexion.

arm is aligned with the posterior midline of the head, using the occipital protuberance as a landmark.

Tape Measure Method. A tape measure can be used to measure the distance between the mastoid process and the acromion process.

Bubble Goniometer Method. See Table 8-11. The normal range of cervical side bending using this method is 45° or greater from the neutral position for active motion. The center of the first inclinometer is placed over the T1 spinous process. The center of the second one is placed on top of the head, over the calvaria, and both inclinometer angles are recorded. From the start position (Figure 8-142), the patient is asked to side bend the cervical spine to the left (Figure 8-143), and then to the right (Figure 8-144). As before, the inclinometer angles for each motion are recorded. The cervical side-bending angle is calculated by subtracting the T1 from the calvarian inclinometer angle.

CLINICAL PEARL

Using the bubble goniometer method, the full arc of passive right/left cervical side bending range depends on the age of the patient[8]:

► 20–29: 101° ± 11
► 30–49: 93° ± 13
► ≥50: 80° ± 17

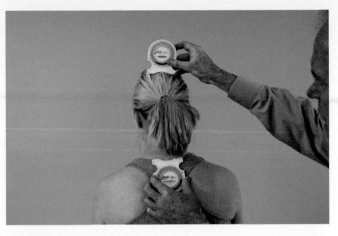

FIGURE 8-142 Bubble goniometer placement for the start position for cervical side bending.

Thoracic Spine

Oftentimes, thoracic spine motion is measured simultaneously with lumbar spine motion using a variety of methods, none of which are really satisfactory. To objectively measure thoracic motion and differentiate thoracic spine motion from lumbar spine motion, the bubble goniometer techniques by the AMA are recommended.[15]

Flexion. To measure thoracic flexion, two inclinometers are used and are aligned in the sagittal plane. The center of the first inclinometer is placed over the T1 spinous process. The center of the second one is placed over the T12 or L1 spinous process (Figure 8-145). The patient is asked to slump forward, as though trying to place the forehead on the knees (Figure 8-146), and both inclinometer angles are recorded. The thoracic flexion angle is calculated by subtracting the T12 from the T1 inclinometer angle. The patient should be able to flex approximately 50° from the neutral position.[26,27] The clinician observes for any paravertebral fullness during flexion, which might alter the measurement. The thoracic spine during flexion should curve forward in a smooth and even manner, and there should be no evidence of segmental rotation or side bending. To decrease pelvic and hip movements, McKenzie advocates examining thoracic flexion with the patient seated.[28]

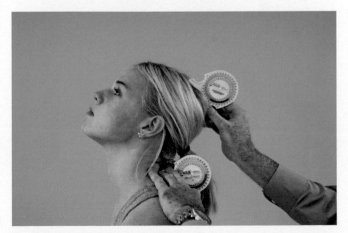

FIGURE 8-141 Goniometric measurement of cervical extension.

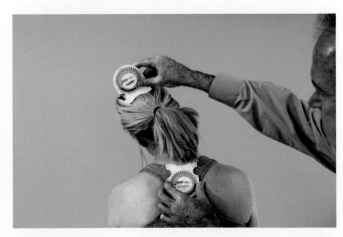

FIGURE 8-143 Goniometric measurement of cervical side bending to the left.

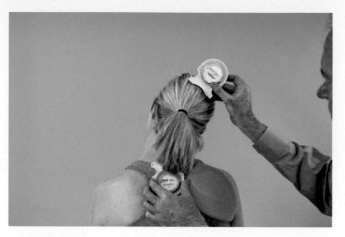

FIGURE 8-144 Goniometric measurement of cervical side bending to the right.

Extension. Clinical guidelines for measurements of thoracic extension recommend that ROM be defined with reference to the magnitude of the kyphosis measured in standing. However, to date, the relationship between the magnitude of the thoracic kyphosis and the amount of thoracic extension movement has not been reported.[29] Thoracic extension may be measured using the same technique and inclinometer positions as described for flexion (Figure 8-147). The thoracic extension angle is calculated by subtracting the T12 or L1 from the T1 inclinometer angle. The patient should be able to extend approximately 15–20° from the neutral position.[27] Alternatively, thoracic extension can be measured using a tape

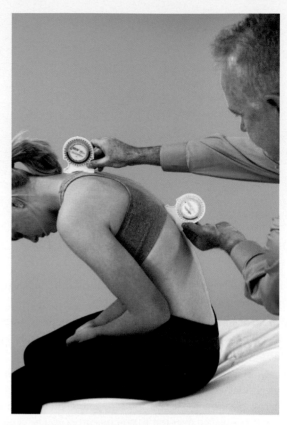

FIGURE 8-146 Goniometric measurement of thoracic flexion.

measure. The distance between two points (the C7 and T12 spinous processes) is measured. A 2.5-cm difference between neutral and extension measurements is considered normal.[30,31] During thoracic extension, the thoracic curve should curve

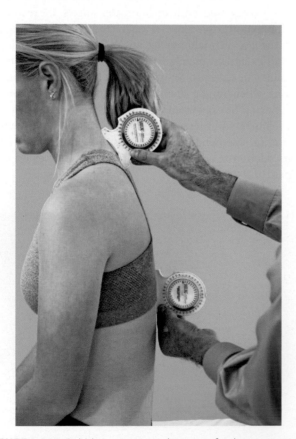

FIGURE 8-145 Bubble goniometer placement for the start position of thoracic flexion and extension.

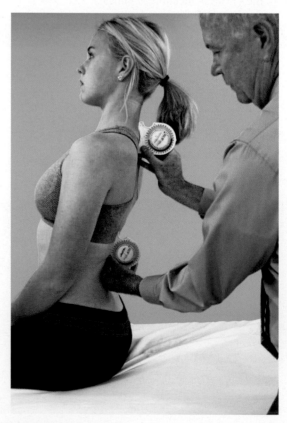

FIGURE 8-147 Goniometric measurement of thoracic extension.

backward or straighten. As with flexion, there should be no evidence of segmental rotation or side bending.

Rotation. Rotation is a primary movement of the thoracic spine and a key component of functional activities. Thoracic rotation can be measured objectively using a tape measure or two bubble goniometers.

Tape Measure Method. Pavelka[32] devised a simple objective clinical method to measure thoracolumbar rotation using a tape measure that can be used to detect asymmetries in rotation. The tape is placed over the L5 spinous process and over the jugular notch on the superior aspect of the manubrium. A measurement is taken before and after full trunk rotation. The measurements from each side are then compared.

Bubble Goniometer Method. The patient is positioned in sitting, and is then asked to flex forward as close to horizontal as possible. One bubble goniometer is positioned at the T1 level and the other at the T12 level, both in the frontal plane. Both goniometers are zeroed out, and then the patient is instructed to rotate the trunk to one side. The clinician records both the T1 and the T12 inclinations and subtracts the T12 from the T1 inclination to arrive at the thoracic rotation angle. The technique is then repeated to the opposite side. The patient should be able to rotate 30° or greater from the neutral position.[33,34] Active thoracic rotation of less than 20° can result in an impairment of function during activities of daily living involving the thoracic spine.[30]

Side Bending. Side bending can be measured objectively using a tape measure,[35] or using two bubble goniometers.

Tape Measure Method. Two ink marks are placed on the skin of the lateral trunk. The upper mark is made at a point where a horizontal line through the xiphisternum crosses the frontal line. The lower mark is made at the highest point on the iliac crest. The distance between the two marks is measured in centimeters, with the patient standing erect, and again after full ipsilateral side bending. The second measurement is subtracted from the first, and the remainder is taken as an index of lateral spinal mobility.

Bubble Goniometer Method. The patient is positioned in standing, and one goniometer is placed flat against the T1 spinous process and the other flat against the T12/L1 spinous process (Figure 8-148). Both goniometers are zeroed out, and then the patient is asked to side bend the thoracic spine to the left side (Figure 8-149) and then to the right side (Figure 8-150). The T1 inclination angle is subtracted from the T12/L1 inclination angle to arrive at the thoracic side bending angle. The patient should be able to side bend 20-40° from the neutral position.

Lumbar Spine

Lumbar spine motion can be measured using a variety of methods.

Flexion and Extension. Flexion and extension can be measured using two bubble goniometers or a tape measure.

Tape Measure Method. Using the modified Schober technique, the patient is positioned in relaxed standing. A point is drawn with the skin marker at the spinal intersection of a line joining S1. Additional marks are made 10 cm above and 5 cm below S1 (Figure 8-151). The patient is then asked to bend

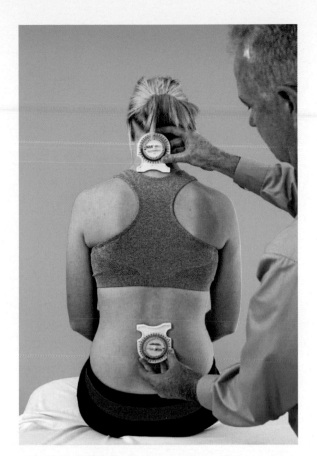

FIGURE 8-148 Bubble goniometer placement for the start position of thoracic side bending.

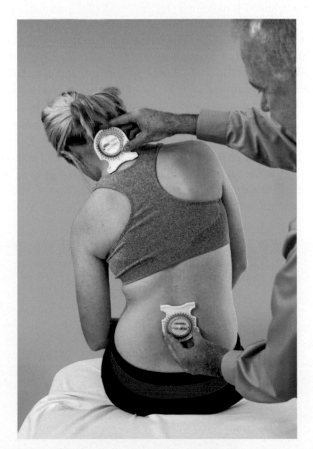

FIGURE 8-149 Goniometric measurement of thoracic side bending to the left.

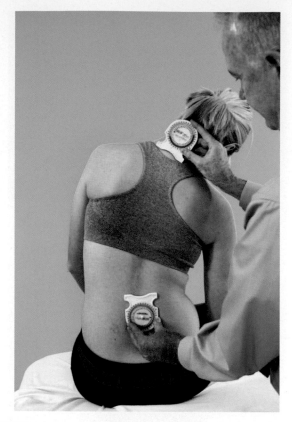

FIGURE 8-150 Goniometric measurement of thoracic side bending to the right.

forward and the distance between the marks 10 cm above and 5 cm below S1 is measured (Figure 8-152). Despite this method's simplicity, Reynolds[36] found this measurement of motion to have good reliability, with Pearson correlation coefficients of 0.59 for lumbar flexion and 0.75 for extension. In another study by Fitzgerald and colleagues,[37] the Pearson correlation coefficient was found to be 1.0 for lumbar flexion and 0.88 for lumbar extension in a study of young, healthy subjects.

Bubble Goniometer Method. The patient is positioned in standing with the lumbar spine in a neutral position. The clinician places one bubble goniometer over the T12/L1 spinous process in the sagittal plane, and the other goniometer at the level of the sacrum, also in the sagittal plane (Figure 8-153). Both goniometers are zeroed out, and the patient is then

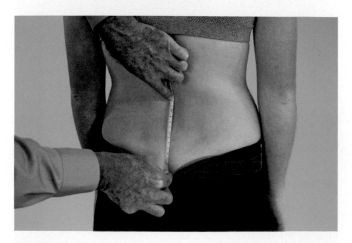

FIGURE 8-151 Start position for the modified Schober technique.

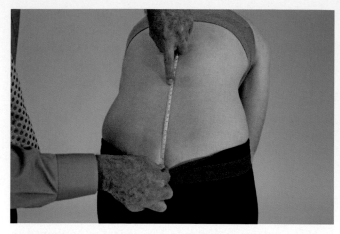

FIGURE 8-152 End position for the modified Schober technique.

asked to flex the trunk forward (Figure 8-154). The clinician notes the inclinations of both goniometers and subtracts the sacral inclination from the T12/L1 inclination to obtain the lumbar flexion angle. The patient is then asked to extend the trunk (Figure 8-155). The clinician subtracts the sacral inclination from the T12/L1 inclination to obtain the lumbar extension angle. The normal ROMs for flexion and extension vary according to patient age and gender[38] (Table 8-12).

Side Bending. Side bending can be measured with the patient standing with the feet together using a standard goniometer, a tape measure, or two bubble goniometers.

Standard Goniometer Method. The fulcrum is centered over the posterior aspect of the spinous process of S1, the proximal arm is aligned so that it is perpendicular to the ground, and

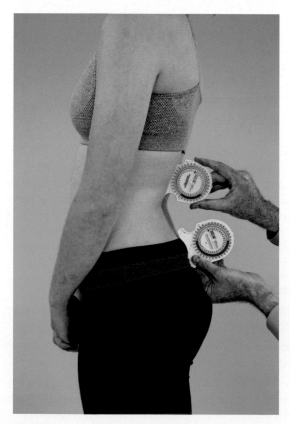

FIGURE 8-153 Bubble goniometer placement for the start position of lumbar spine flexion and extension.

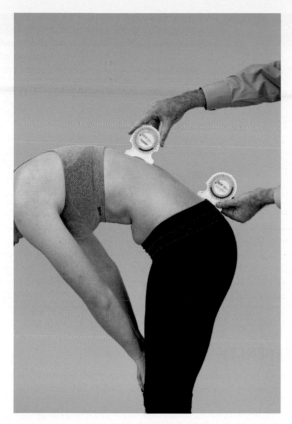

FIGURE 8-154 Goniometric measurement for lumbar spine flexion.

TABLE 8-12	Normal Ranges of Motion for Lumbar Spine Flexion and Extension Based on Patient Age and Gender		
Gender	**Age Range**	**Normal Range of Flexion in Degrees**	**Normal Range of Extension in Degrees**
Male	15–30 years old	66	38
	31–60 years old	58	35
	>61 years old	49	33
Female	15–30 years old	67	42
	31–60 years old	60	40
	>61 years old	44	36

Data from Loebl WY. Measurement of spinal posture and range of spinal movement. *Ann Phys Med*. 1967;9(3):103-110.

the distal arm is aligned with the posterior aspect of the spinous process of C7.

Tape Measure Method. A tape measure is used to measure the distance between the tip of the middle finger and the floor.

Bubble Goniometer Method. The clinician places one goniometer flat at the T12/L1 spinous process in the frontal plane and the other goniometer at the superior aspect of the sacrum, also in the frontal plane (Figure 8-156). Both goniometers are zeroed out, and then the patient is asked to side bend the trunk to the right side (Figure 8-157) and the inclination is recorded from both goniometers. The clinician subtracts the sacral inclination from the T12/L1 inclination to obtain the lumbar side bending angle. The technique is then repeated to the left side (Figure 8-158). The normal ranges of motion for flexion and extension vary according to patient age and gender (Table 8-13).[36,38]

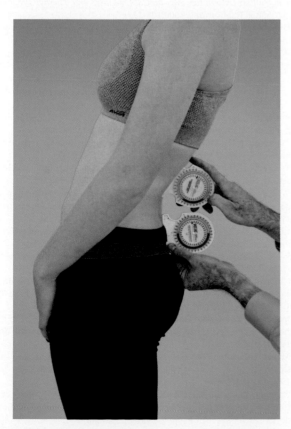

FIGURE 8-155 Goniometric measurement for lumbar spine extension.

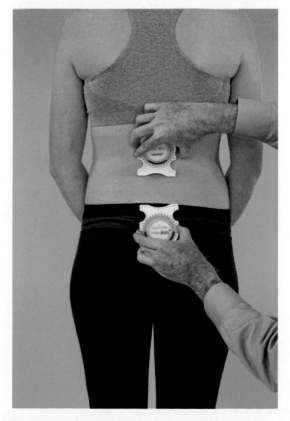

FIGURE 8-156 Bubble goniometer placement for the start position of lumbar spine side bending.

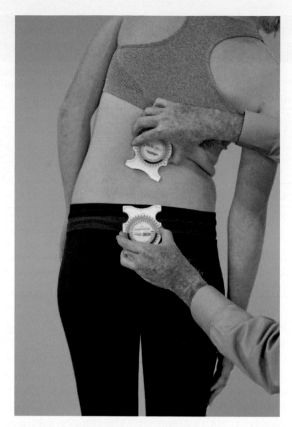

FIGURE 8-157 Goniometric measurement of lumbar spine side bending to the right.

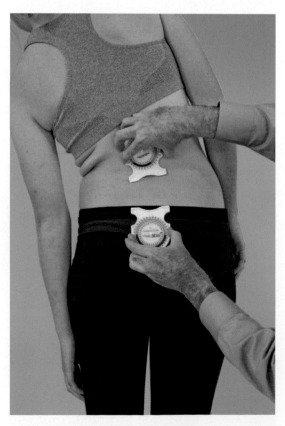

FIGURE 8-158 Goniometric measurement of lumbar spine side bending to the left.

TABLE 8-13	Normal Ranges of Motion for Lumbar Side Bending Based on Gender and Age	
Gender	**Age Range**	**Normal Range of Flexion in Degrees**
Male	20–29 years old	38 ± 5.8
	31–60 years old	29 ± 6.5
	>61 years old	19 ± 4.8
Female	15–30 years old	35 ± 6.4
	31–60 years old	30 ± 5.8
	>61 years old	23 ± 5.4

Data from Fitzgerald GK, Wynveen KJ, Rheault W, et al. Objective assessment with establishment of normal values for lumbar spinal range of motion. *Phys Ther.* 1983;63(11):1776-1781 and Einkauf DK, Gohdes ML, Jensen GM, et al. Changes in spinal mobility with increasing age in women. *Phys Ther.* 1987 Mar;67(3):370-375.

REFERENCES

1. Dutton M. Improving mobility. In: Dutton M, ed. *Dutton's Orthopaedic: Examination, Evaluation and Intervention,* 4th ed. New York: McGraw-Hill; 2016:521-556.
2. Cyriax J. *Textbook of Orthopaedic Medicine, Diagnosis of Soft Tissue Lesions,* 8th ed. London: Bailliere Tindall; 1982.
3. Hayes KW. An examination of Cyriax's passive motion tests with patients having osteoarthritis of the knee. *Phys Ther.* 1994;74:697.
4. Rothstein JM. Cyriax reexamined. *Phys Ther.* 1994;74:1073.
5. Farfan HF. The scientific basis of manipulative procedures. Clinics in Rheumatic Diseases. 1980;6:159-177.
6. Harris ML. Flexibility. *Phys Ther.* 1969;49:591-601.
7. McKenzie R, May S. Physical examination. In: McKenzie R, May S, eds. *The Human Extremities: Mechanical Diagnosis and Therapy.* Waikanae, NZ: Spinal Publications; 2000:105-121.
8. Dvorak J, Antinnes JA, Panjabi M, et al. Age and gender related normal motion of the cervical spine. *Spine.* 1992;17:S393-S398.
9. White DJ. Musculoskeletal examination. In: O'Sullivan SB, Schmitz TJ, eds. *Physical Rehabilitation,* 5th ed. Philadelphia: FA Davis; 2007:159-192.
10. Petersen CM, Hayes KW. Construct validity of Cyriax's selective tension examination: Association of end-feels with pain ath the knee and shoulder. *J Orthop Sports Phys Ther.* 2000;30:512-527.
11. Boone DC, Azen SP, Lin C-M, Spence C, Baron C, Lee L. Reliability of goniometric measurements. *Phys Ther.* 1978;58:1355-1360.
12. Mayerson NH, Milano RA. Goniometric measurement reliability in physical medicine. *Arch Phys Med Rehab.* 1984;65:92-94.
13. Riddle DL, Rothstein JM, Lamb RL. Goniometric reliability in a clinical setting: Shoulder measurements. *Phys Ther.* 1987;67:668-673.
14. Williams JG, Callaghan M. Comparison of visual estimation and goniometry in determination of a shoulder joint angle. *Physiotherapy.* 1990;76:655-657.
15. Cocchiarella L, Andersson GBJ, eds. *Guides to the Evaluation of Permanent Impairment,* 5th ed. Chicago: American Medical Association; 2001.
16. Wing P, Tsang I, Gagnon F. Diurnal changes in the profile shape and range of motion of the back. *Spine.* 1992;17:761-766.
17. Chibnall JT, Duckro PN, Baumer K. The influence of body size on linear measurements used to reflect cervical range of motion. *Phys Ther.* 1994;74:1134-1137.
18. Mayer TG, Kondraske G, Beals SB, Gatchel RJ. Spinal range of motion. Accuracy and sources of error with inclinometric measurement. *Spine.* 1997;22:1976-1984.
19. Mayer T, Brady S, Bovasso E, Pope P, Gatchel RJ. Noninvasive measurement of cervical tri-planar motion in normal subjects. *Spine.* 1993;18:2191-2195.
20. Capuano-Pucci D, Rheault W, Aukai J, Bracke M, Day R, Pastrick M. Intratester and intertester reliability of the cervical range of motion device. *Arch Phys Med Rehabil.* 1991;72:338-340.

21. Ordway NR, Seymour R, Donelson RG, Hojnowski L, Lee E, Edwards WT. Cervical sagittal range-of-motion analysis using three methods. Cervical range-of-motion device, 3space, and radiography. *Spine*. 1997;22:501-508.

22. Nilsson N, Christensen HW, Hartvigsen J. The interexaminer reliability of measuring passive cervical range of motion, revisited. *J Manipulative Physiol Ther*. 1996;19:302-305.

23. Nilsson N. Measuring passive cervical motion: A study of reliability. *J Manipulative Physiol Ther*. 1995;18:293-397.

24. Youdas JW, Carey JR, Garrett TR. Reliability of measurements of cervical spine range of motion: Comparison of three methods. *Phys Ther*. 1991;71:98-104.

25. Chen SP, Samo DG, Chen EH, Crampton AR, Conrad KM, Egan L, et al. Reliability of three lumbar sagittal motion measurement methods: Surface inclinometers. *J Occup Environ Med*. 1997;39:217-223.

26. Raou RJP. *Recherches sur la mobilité vertebrale en fonction des types rachidiens*. Paris: Thèse; 1952.

27. Lawrence DJ, Bakkum B. Chiropractic management of thoracic spine pain of mechanical origin. In: Giles LGF, Singer KP, eds. *Clinical Anatomy and Management of Thoracic Pain*. Oxford: Butterworth-Heinemann; 2000:244-256.

28. McKenzie RA. *The Cervical and Thoracic Spine: Mechanical Diagnosis and Therapy*. Waikanae, NZ: Spinal Publications; 1990.

29. Edmondston SJ, Waller R, Vallin P, Holthe A, Noebauer A, King E. Thoracic spine extension mobility in young adults: Influence of subject position and spinal curvature. *J Orthop Sports Phys Ther*. 2011;41: 266-273.

30. Evans RC. *Illustrated Essentials in Orthopedic Physical Assessment*. St. Louis: Mosby-Year Book; 1994.

31. Magee DJ. *Orthopedic Physical Assessment*. Philadelphia: WB Saunders; 1997.

32. Pavelka K, Von. Rotationsmessung der wirbelsaule. *A Rheumaforschg*. 1970;29:366.

33. Gonon JP, Dimnet J, Carret JP, et al. Utilité de l'analyse cinématique de radiographies dynamiques dans le diagnostic de certaines affections de la colonne lombaire. In: Simon L, Rabourdin JP, eds. *Lombalgies et médecine de rééducation*. Paris: Masson; 1983:27-38.

34. White AA. An analysis of the mechanics of the thoracic spine in man. *Acta Orthopaedica Scandinavica*. 1969;127(Suppl):8-92.

35. Moll JMH, Wright V. Measurement of spinal movement. In: Jayson MIV, ed. *The Lumbar Spine and Back Pain*. New York: Grune and Stratton; 1981: 93-112.

36. Reynolds PM. Measurement of spinal mobility: A comparison of three methods. *Rheumatol Rehabil*. 1975;14:180-185.

37. Fitzgerald GK, Wynveen KJ, Rheault W, Rothschild B. Objective assessment with establishment of normal values for lumbar spinal range of motion. *Phys Ther*. 1983;63:1776-1781.

38. Loebl WY. Measurement of spinal posture and range of spinal movement. *Ann Phys Med*. 1967;9:103-110.

Manual Muscle Testing

CHAPTER 9

CHAPTER OBJECTIVES

At the completion of this chapter, the reader will be able to:

1. Understand the importance of manual muscle testing

2. Perform a gross muscle screening of a patient's strength

3. Perform specific manual muscle tests to the shoulder

4. Perform specific manual muscle tests to the elbow

5. Perform specific manual muscle tests to the wrist and forearm

6. Perform specific manual muscle tests to the hand

7. Perform specific manual muscle tests to the hip

8. Perform specific manual muscle tests to the knee

9. Perform specific manual muscle tests to the leg and foot

10. Perform specific manual muscle tests of the trunk

11. Describe the strengths and weaknesses of the various grading systems used with manual muscle testing

12. Interpret the different results that can be obtained from a manual muscle test

OVERVIEW

Movement of the body or any of its parts involves considerable activity from the nervous and musculoskeletal systems. The nervous system provides cognition, perception, and sensory integration and is primarily involved in controlling movement, while the nervous and musculoskeletal systems provide the power behind the movement. If a functional limitation is highlighted during the patient's physical examination, the physical therapist determines the cause of the functional and/or participation restrictions. If the cause is poor muscle performance, a progression of exercises to enhance muscle performance is added to the plan of care (POC). Muscle performance can be assessed by measuring

All figures in this chapter are reproduced with permission from Dutton M: Introduction to Physical Therapy and Patient Skills, 2nd ed. New York, NY: McGraw Hill; 2014.

several parameters: strength, endurance, and power. This chapter provides an overview of how the strength component of muscle performance can be assessed. The improvement of muscle strength is an integral component of most rehabilitation programs. Strength may be defined as the amount of force that an individual may exert in a single maximum muscular contraction against a specific resistance or the ability to produce torque at a joint.[1] Manual muscle testing, performed grossly or specifically, is a simple way to assess the ability of a muscle, or a group of muscles, to perform a single maximum muscular contraction in an isometric fashion.

CLINICAL PEARL

The three main types of muscle contraction are[2]:

► Isometric. Isometric exercises provide a static contraction with a variable and accommodating resistance without producing any appreciable muscle-length change.

► Concentric. A concentric contraction produces a shortening of the muscle such that the origin and insertion of the muscle move closer together. A muscle performs a concentric contraction when it lifts a load/weight that is less than the maximum tetanic tension it can generate.

► Eccentric. An eccentric contraction occurs when a muscle slowly lengthens as it gives in to an external force greater than the contractile force it is exerting. In reality, the muscle does not lengthen but merely returns from its shortened position to its normal resting length.

GROSS MUSCLE SCREENING

Muscle testing requires that the patient be able to control the tension developed in the muscles voluntarily. A patient with a central nervous system (CNS) disorder who demonstrates spasticity is not an appropriate candidate for muscle testing.

A gross muscle screening is performed on a patient when a quick assessment of the patient's general muscle strength is required. If any weakness is found during the gross muscle screening test, a specific muscle test is then performed. It is important to remember that the gross muscle screening does not detail the determination of strength; it only provides the clinician with information about whether a region of the body is either normal or weak. An example of when a gross muscle screening would be used is when the clinician is preparing the patient to get out of a wheelchair and to ambulate using a standard walker—the clinician needs to determine whether the patient has sufficient strength to weight bear through the lower extremities and to weight bear through the upper extremities. Regardless of the type of muscle testing used, the procedure is innately subjective and depends on the subject's ability to exert a maximal contraction. This ability can be negatively affected by such factors as pain, poor comprehension, motivation, cooperation, fatigue, and fear.

The gross muscle testing procedures for the body's main regions are described in Table 9-1. As mentioned, one of the more common gross muscle testing procedures is the one performed by the clinician before gait training with an assisted device when the clinician is not sure of the patient's capabilities. In this scenario, the clinician must efficiently assess the strength of the major muscle groups used when using an assistive device. The muscle groups tested include the shoulder abductors (Figure 9-1), the shoulder flexors (Figure 9-2), the shoulder extensors (Figure 9-3), the elbow flexors (Figure 9-4), the elbow extensors (Figure 9-5), the wrist extensors (Figure 9-6), the wrist flexors (Figure 9-7), the hip flexors (Figure 9-8), the knee extensors (Figure 9-9), the knee flexors and hip extensors (the hamstrings) (Figure 9-10), the hip abductors (Figure 9-11), the ankle dorsiflexors (Figure 9-12), and the ankle plantarflexors (Figure 9-13). Any detected weakness during these tests should prompt the clinician to specifically test the individual muscles involved in the weakened group.

SPECIFIC MUSCLE TESTING

Specific muscle testing, called manual muscle testing (MMT), is a procedure for assessing the voluntary function and strength of individual muscles and muscle groups based on the ability of specific muscles to effectively perform against various levels of gravity and manual resistance forces.

CLINICAL PEARL

Maximum muscular strength is the maximum amount of tension or force that a muscle or muscle group can voluntarily exert in one maximal effort when the type of muscle contraction, limb velocity, and joint angle are specified.

MMT is typically used when the gross muscle screening shows specific muscle weakness or to measure improvements in strength. From a physiologic viewpoint, MMT measures the capability of the musculotendinous units to generate motion.[3]
Several factors can influence the results from MMT:

▶ The length of the muscle at the time of the contraction. The amount of tension a muscle produces depends on its length as it contracts. Each muscle has its optimal length to produce optimal tension—for some muscles, the lengthened position is more favorable than the shortened position. Generally speaking, as a muscle continues to lengthen, it eventually reaches a point of passive insufficiency, where it is not capable of generating its maximum force output.

▶ Whether the muscle acts on one joint or multiple joints. As a one-joint muscle shortens, or as the distal and proximal attachments of a two-joint muscle approach each other during a concentric contraction, the tension diminishes.

▶ The type of muscle contraction. Physiologically, a muscle can generate its greatest tension during an eccentric contraction, less tension when contracting isometrically, and even less tension when contracting concentrically.[4]

▶ The speed of contraction. The faster a muscle produces a concentric contraction, the less ability the muscle has to generate tension—as velocity increases, tension decreases.

▶ The length of the moment arm. As a muscle moves through its range of motion, the torque generated varies with the moment arm's length (distance from the axis of rotation). For example, as the elbow moves from full extension into flexion, the moment arm increases, reaching its maximum at approximately 90° of flexion, and then decreases throughout the remainder of the range of motion.

▶ Whether the muscle is working against gravity or with gravity. The force of gravity has the greatest leverage and, therefore, can produce the greatest toll on the body segment when the segment is horizontal.

Strength values using MMT have traditionally been used between similar muscle groups on opposite extremities or antagonistic ratios. This information is then used to determine whether a patient is fully rehabilitated. An agonist muscle contracts to produce the desired movement. From a rehabilitation viewpoint, knowledge of a specific muscle's synergists and antagonists is very important:

▶ *Synergist.* Synergist muscles are muscle groups that work together with the agonist to produce a desired movement.[5] In essence, a synergist muscle can be viewed as a muscle's helper muscle, as the force generated by the synergists works in the same direction. Synergist muscles may need to be strengthened so that they can assist the agonist muscle.

▶ *Antagonists.* The antagonist muscle can oppose the desired movement. Antagonists allow movement by relaxing and lengthening gradually to ensure that the desired motion occurs and does so in a coordinated and controlled fashion. Care must be taken to ensure that the antagonist muscles are not adaptively shortened and monitor whether the antagonist muscles are not overpowering the agonist muscle.

The synergists and antagonist muscles are provided for each of the specific muscle tests to assist the clinician.

To accurately perform a specific muscle test, the clinician must know the following:

▶ The origin and insertion of the muscle being tested.
▶ The function of the muscle being tested. Muscles rarely perform a single action; instead, they form groups of actions that overlap with the functions of other muscles.

TABLE 9-1	Gross Muscle Screening	
Patient Position	**Tested Muscle Group**	**Procedure**
Supine	Hip flexors	The patient is instructed to raise both legs off the supporting surface simultaneously while keeping both legs straight. The position is held for 10 seconds. The hip flexors can also be tested in the sitting position.
	Hip abductors	The patient is instructed to abduct the legs to each side and hold the position while the clinician attempts to bring the legs together.
	Hip adductors	The patient is instructed to keep the legs together while the clinician attempts to separate the legs.
	Hip extensors	The patient is instructed to flex the hips and knees while keeping the soles of the feet on the supporting surface and raising the pelvis from the sitting surface. This position is held for 10 seconds.
	Shoulder flexors and scapular upward rotators	The patient is instructed to flex the shoulder to 90° with the elbow straight and hold the position while the clinician attempts to push the arms into extension.
	Shoulder extensors and scapular downward rotators	The patient is instructed to flex the shoulder to 90° with the elbow straight and hold the position while the clinician attempts to push the arms into flexion.
	Shoulder horizontal abductors	The patient is instructed to flex the shoulder to 90° with the elbow straight and to hold the position while the clinician attempts to push the arms together into horizontal adduction.
	Shoulder adductors	The patient is instructed to bring their hands together in front of the chest while keeping the elbows straight and holding this position. The clinician attempts to separate the arms into horizontal abduction.
	Neck and trunk flexors	The patient is instructed to hold both arms straight in front of their body and then raise the head and shoulders from the supporting surface and hold this position.
Supine or sitting	Shoulder abductors	The patient is instructed to abduct the shoulder to the side up to shoulder level with the elbows straight. The clinician attempts to push the arms down to the patient's sides into shoulder adduction.
	Shoulder adductors	The patient is instructed to abduct the shoulder to the side up to shoulder level with the elbows straight. The clinician attempts to push the arms over the patient's head into shoulder abduction.
	Shoulder internal rotators	The patient is instructed to hold the arms at the sides, flex the elbows to approximately 90°, and place the forearms in neutral. The clinician attempts to push the arms outward into external rotation of the shoulder.
	Shoulder external rotators	The patient is instructed to hold the arms at the sides, flex the elbows to approximately 90°, and place the forearms in neutral. The clinician attempts to push the arms inward into internal rotation of the shoulder.
	Elbow flexors	The patient is instructed to hold the arms at the sides, flex the elbows to approximately 90°, and place the forearms in neutral. The clinician attempts to push the forearms toward the supporting surface into elbow extension.
	Elbow extensors	The patient is instructed to hold the arms at the sides, flex the elbows to approximately 90°, and place the forearms in neutral. The clinician attempts to push the forearms toward the shoulders into elbow flexion.
	Forearm supinators	The patient is instructed to hold the arms at the sides, flex the elbows to approximately 90°, and place the forearms in neutral. The clinician attempts to turn the palms toward the body into pronation.
	Forearm pronators	The patient is instructed to hold the arms at the sides, flex the elbows to approximately 90°, and place the forearms in neutral. The clinician attempts to turn the palms away from the body into supination.
	Wrist flexors	The patient is instructed to hold the arms at the sides, flex the elbows to approximately 90°, and place the forearms in neutral. The clinician attempts to push the palms upward into wrist extension.

(continued)

| TABLE 9-1 | Gross Muscle Screening (continued) |

Patient Position	Tested Muscle Group	Procedure
	Wrist extensors	The patient is instructed to hold the arms at the sides, flex the elbows to approximately 90°, and place the forearms in neutral. The clinician attempts to push the hand down into wrist flexion.
	Finger flexors	The patient is instructed to hold the arms at the sides, flex the elbows to approximately 90°, and place the forearms in neutral. The clinician places his or her index and middle fingers into the patient's hand, and the patient is asked to squeeze the fingers. The clinician then attempts to pull the fingers out.
	Finger extensors	The patient is instructed to hold the arms at the sides, flex the elbows to approximately 90°, and place the forearms in neutral. The patient is asked to straighten the fingers, and then the clinician attempts to push the fingers into flexion.
	Anterior interossei	The patient is instructed to hold the arms at the sides, flex the elbows to approximately 90°, and place the forearms in neutral. The patient is asked to adduct the fingers, and then the clinician attempts to pull the fingers into abduction.
	Posterior interossei	The patient is instructed to hold the arms at the sides, flex the elbows to approximately 90°, and place the forearms in neutral. The patient is asked to abduct the fingers, and then the clinician attempts to push the fingers into adduction.
	Opponens pollicis	The patient is instructed to hold the arms at the sides, flex the elbows to approximately 90°, and place the forearms in neutral. The clinician places his or her index finger between the patient's thumb and each finger one at a time while asking the patient to pinch the finger.
Sitting	Latissimus dorsi and triceps	The patient is instructed to place both hands on the supporting surface next to the hips, keeping the elbows straight and the shoulder shrugged. The patient is then asked to depress the scapular by lifting the buttocks off the supporting surface.
	Upper trapezius and levator scapulae	The patient is instructed to shrug the shoulders toward the ears and to hold the position. The clinician attempts to push the shoulders down into depression.
	Internal rotators of the hip and evertors of the feet	The patient is instructed to evert the foot and to hold the position while the clinician pushes on the lateral border of each foot into inversion and external rotation of the hip.
	External rotators of the hip and invertors of the feet	The patient is instructed to invert the foot and to hold the position while the clinician pushes on the medial border of each foot into eversion and internal rotation of the hip.
Prone	Rhomboids, middle trapezius, and posterior deltoid	The patient is instructed to flex the elbows level with the shoulders, then pinch or adduct the scapulae together, and then raise the arms from the supporting surface. The clinician attempts to push the arms downward.
	Elbow and shoulder extensors	The patient is instructed to raise the arm off the supporting surface while keeping the arms at the sides and the elbows straight. The clinician attempts to push the arms downward.
	Extensors of the hips, back, neck, and shoulders	The patient is instructed to keep the arms at the sides and to raise the head, shoulders, arms, and legs off the supporting surface simultaneously by arching the back. The position is held for 10 seconds.
Prone or sitting	Hamstrings	The patient is instructed to flex the knees to about 90°. The clinician attempts to pull the knees into extension.
	Quadriceps	The patient is instructed to flex the knees to about 90°. The clinician attempts to push the knees into flexion.
Standing	Gastrocnemius/soleus	The patient is instructed to stand on one leg with one finger on the supporting surface for balance. The patient is then asked to rise up on tiptoes and to repeat 10 times. The other leg is then tested.
	Dorsiflexors	The patient is instructed to walk on the heel for 10 steps.
	Hip and knee extensors	The patient is instructed to do five partial deep-knee bends.

MANUAL MUSCLE TESTING

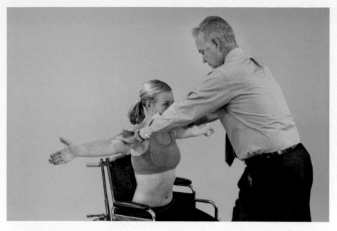

FIGURE 9-1 Gross muscle testing of the shoulder abductors.

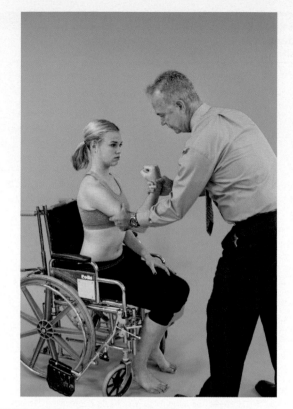

FIGURE 9-4 Gross muscle testing of the elbow flexors.

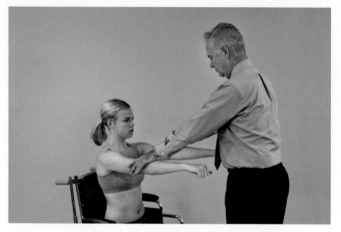

FIGURE 9-2 Gross muscle testing of the shoulder flexors.

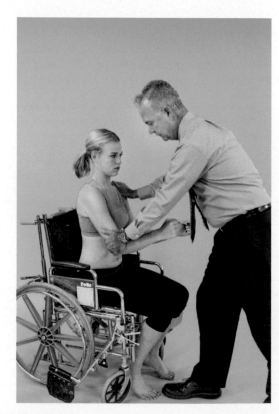

FIGURE 9-3 Gross muscle testing of the shoulder extensors.

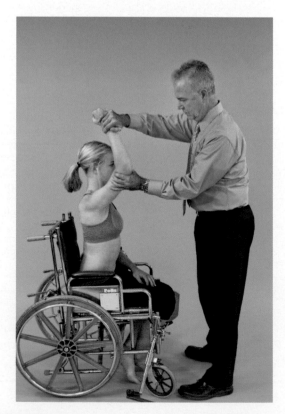

FIGURE 9-5 Gross muscle testing of the elbow extensors.

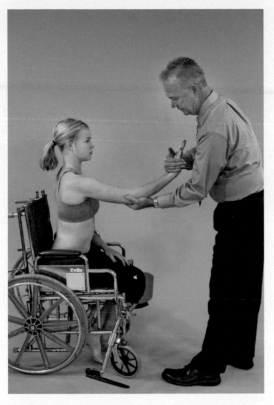

FIGURE 9-6 Gross muscle testing of the wrist extensors.

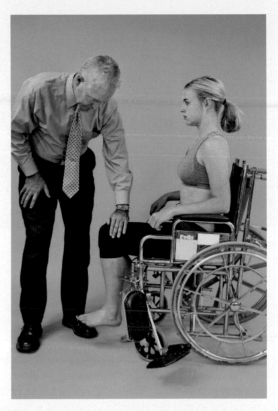

FIGURE 9-8 Gross muscle testing of the hip flexors.

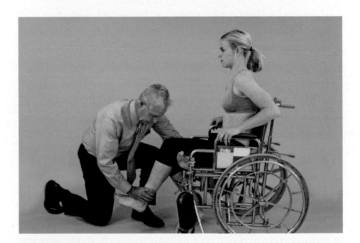

FIGURE 9-9 Gross muscle testing of the knee extensors.

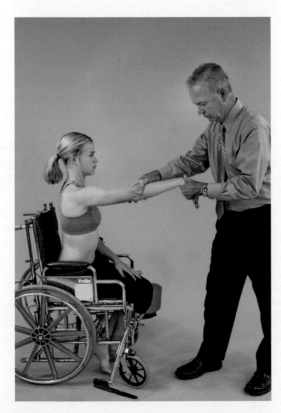

FIGURE 9-7 Gross muscle testing of the wrist flexors.

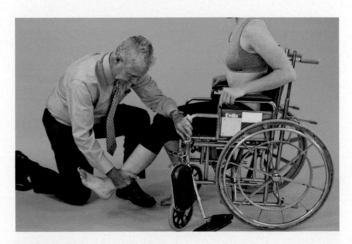

FIGURE 9-10 Gross muscle testing of the knee flexors and hip extensors.

205

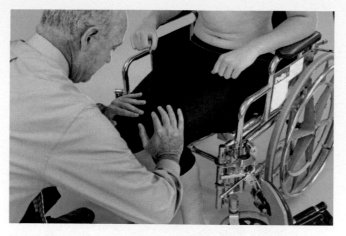

FIGURE 9-11 Gross muscle testing of the hip abductors.

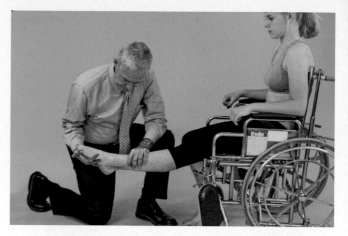

FIGURE 9-13 Gross muscle testing of the ankle plantarflexors.

For that reason, if a component of a muscle's function is lost, other muscles that have duplicate functions can compensate for that loss.

► How to eliminate substitute or trick motions. This is best accomplished by using standardized testing positions. Where appropriate, these motions are included in each test procedure so that the clinician is aware of what to avoid.

► How to skillfully apply resistance. Pressure should be applied slowly, very gently, and gradually before progressing to the maximum resistance tolerable.

► The standard positions for each muscle test, based on the effects of gravity. Typically the patient is positioned in either an antigravity or a gravity-eliminated position.

► The standard methods of grading muscle strength. Several grading methods have been described (Table 9-2).

It should be noted that there is considerable variability in the amount of resistance that normal muscles can hold against. The application of resistance throughout the arc of motion (referred to as a *make* test or *active resistance* test), in addition to resistance applied at only one point in the arc of motion (referred to as a *break* test) can help in judging the strength of a muscle.[6]

The main purposes of specific muscle testing are as follows:

► To help determine a diagnosis. For example, specific muscle testing can aid in precisely localizing a lesion in the peripheral nervous system.

► To establish a baseline for muscle reeducation and exercise.

► To determine a patient's need for supportive apparatus (orthosis, an assistive device for ambulation, or splints).

► To help determine a patient's progress.

CLINICAL PEARL

MMT is less sensitive in detecting strength deficits in stronger muscles compared to weaker muscles.[6]

As mentioned, several scales have been devised to assess muscle strength, including numerical, descriptive, and fractional (Table 9-2). The patient is positioned in an antigravity position for grades 3–5 and in a gravity-eliminated position for grades 0–2. If the muscle strength is less than grade 3, then the methods advocated in muscle testing manuals must be used.[6] For the testing methods and positions described in this chapter, it is assumed that the patient has a grade of 3–5. Alternative gravity-eliminated/minimized positions will also be provided.

Many problems exist with the grading systems. The grading systems for MMT produce ordinal data with unequal rankings between grades. For example, a muscle grade of 4 is not equivalent to 75% of the strength represented by a grade 5; it is a natural grade determined by the effect of gravity, manual resistance, the patient's age, and so forth. In general, the grades 5 (normal) and 4 (good) typically encompass a large range of a muscle's strength—although a score of 5 does not mean that the muscle is normal in every circumstance (eg, when at the onset of fatigue or in a state of exhaustion)—whereas the grades of 3 (fair), 2 (poor), and 1 (trace) include a much narrower range.[6] As a result, scores of 4 or 5 require some subjectivity, which can increase the variability between testers, whereas the precise definitions for 0–3 scores produce

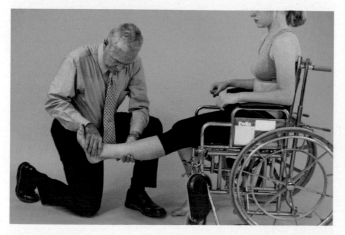

FIGURE 9-12 Gross muscle testing of the ankle dorsiflexors.

TABLE 9-2	Manual Muscle Grading		
Numerical	Descriptive	Fractional	Description
10	Normal	5/5	Ability to complete test movement and/or hold test position against gravity and maximum (strong) pressure
9	Good +	4+/5	Ability to complete test movement and/or hold test position against gravity and slightly less than maximum (moderate to strong) pressure
8	Good	4/5	Ability to complete test movement and/or hold test position against gravity and moderate pressure
7	Good –	4–/5	Ability to complete test movement and/or hold test position against gravity and slightly less than moderate (slight to moderate) pressure
6	Fair +	3+/5	Ability to complete test movement and/or hold test position against gravity and minimal (slight) pressure
5	Fair	3/5	Ability to complete test movement and/or hold test position against gravity but cannot hold if even slight pressure is applied
4	Fair –	3–/5	Ability to complete at least 1/2 of test movement against gravity. Cannot complete full test movement against gravity. NOTE: Kendall and colleagues[a] refer to this as a very gradual release from the antigravity test position
3	Poor +	2+/5	Ability to initiate test movement against gravity, but completes less than 1/2 of test movement range, OR ability to complete test movement in a gravity-lessened position against resistance throughout the range, OR ability to complete test movement and hold test position in a gravity-lessened position against pressure
2	Poor	2/5	Ability to complete test movement in gravity-lessened position with friction reduced. No movement against gravity
1	Poor –	2–/5	Ability to initiate or complete partial test movement in a gravity-lessened position with friction reduced; unable to complete the full range of test movement.
T	Trace	1/5	Feeble but palpable muscle contraction or prominent tendon during muscle contraction with no visible motion of the part
0	Zero	0/5	No palpable muscle contraction

[a]Data from Kendall FP, McCreary EK, Provance PG. *Muscles: Testing and Function*. Baltimore, MD: Williams & Wilkins; 1993.

little tester-to-tester variability. Some of the confusion arises from the descriptions of maximal, moderate, minimal, or considerable, which removes much of the objectivity from the tests. It has been advocated by some to add + or – to the scales. The – is used to describe that the test range is not complete, but the motion is over one-half the standard test range of motion (eg, a grade of 2– with a patient who achieves more than one-half of the standard range, with gravity eliminated). The + is used to describe the test range of less than one-half of the test range (eg, a grade of 2+ with a patient who achieves less than one-half of the standard range, in the anti-gravity position).

CLINICAL PEARL

If the clinician is having difficulty differentiating between a grade 4 and a grade 5, the eccentric "break" method of muscle testing may be used. This procedure starts as an isometric contraction, but then the clinician applies sufficient force to cause an eccentric contraction or a "break" in the patient's isometric contraction.

CLINICAL PEARL

Studies have demonstrated that reliability in MMT is dependent on the specific muscle being examined. For example, Florence and colleagues[7] found high reliability in the proximal muscles as opposed to the distal muscles, and Barr and colleagues[8] found the upper-body muscles to be more reliably tested than the lower-body ones.[9]

To be a valid test, strength testing must elicit a maximum contraction of the muscle being tested. The following strategies ensure that this occurs:

1. *Comparing the passive range of motion to the active range of motion.* To achieve a grade of 3–5, the muscle must move through the entire available range. One of the most common mistakes is to overgrade or undergrade a muscle by assessing a muscle in a patient who cannot achieve the full available range of motion.

2. *Placing the joint which the muscle to be tested crosses in, or close to, its open packed position.* This strategy helps

protect the joint from excessive compressive forces and the surrounding inert structures from excessive tension. The body area or segment to be evaluated is exposed, and the subject is properly draped. It is important to remember that the position used is dependent on the overall condition and comfort of the patient.

3. *Placing the muscle to be tested in a shortened position.* This puts the muscle in an ineffective physiologic position and has the effect of increasing motor neuron activity. Three basic factors must be considered with specific muscle testing: (1) the weight of the limb or distal segment with a minimal effect of gravity on the moving segment; (2) the weight of the limb plus the effects of gravity on the limb or segment; and (3) the weight of the limb or segment plus the effects of gravity plus manual resistance.

4. *Using standardized positions.* If the muscle to be tested is not isolated, the clinician is merely testing a muscle group rather than an individual muscle. Initially, the standardized gravity-minimized positions may be necessary to avoid the weight of the moving body segment on the force measurement. For example, to test the strength of the hip abductors, the patient is positioned supine so that the muscle action pulls in a horizontal plane relative to the ground.[6]

5. *Stabilizing the appropriate parts of the body.* When performing a specific muscle test, the emphasis is placed on correct stabilization of the body part on which the muscle originates and careful avoidance of substitution by other muscle groups to enhance accuracy. Substitutions by other muscle groups during testing indicate the presence of weakness. It does not, however, tell the clinician the cause of the weakness.

6. *Apply force at the appropriate location.* The force is typically applied distally on the segment to where the muscle insertion occurs, except when a longer lever is needed. The application of force is usually made at the end of the range with one-joint muscles and midrange with two-joint muscles. Resistance is always applied at right angles to the long axis of the segment. The clinician applies the force in a direction opposite to the torque (the rotary force around an axis, which is a combination of the force along the longitudinal axis of the segment on which the muscle attaches and another force that is at right angles to the axis of motion) exerted by the muscle being tested.

7. *Consider the patient's age, size, strength, occupation, and neuromuscular condition.* It is important to remember that the standardized positions apply to the adult population and may need to be adjusted for the aged or younger subjects. Also, the clinician should know his or her limitations.

8. *For grades 3–5, ask the patient to perform an eccentric muscle contraction.* This can be accomplished by using the command, "Don't let me move you." Because the tension at each cross-bridge and the number of active cross-bridges are greater during an eccentric contraction, the maximum eccentric muscle tension developed is greater with an eccentric contraction than with a concentric one.

9. *Breaking the contraction.* It is important to break the patient's muscle contraction to ensure that the patient is making a maximal effort and that the muscle's full power is being tested. Although force values determined with make and break tests are highly correlated, break tests usually result in greater force values than make tests,[10,11] so they should not be used interchangeably.

10. *Holding the contraction for at least 5 seconds.* Weakness resulting from nerve palsy has a distinct fatigability. The muscle demonstrates poor endurance because it usually can only sustain a maximum muscle contraction for about 2 to 3 seconds before complete failure occurs. This strategy is based on the theories behind muscle recruitment, wherein a normal muscle, while performing a maximum contraction, uses only a portion of its motor units, keeping the remainder in reserve to help maintain the contraction. With its fewer functioning motor units, a palsied muscle has very few, if any, motor units in reserve. If a muscle appears to be weaker than normal, further investigation is required, as follows:

    a. The test is repeated three times. Muscle weakness resulting from disuse will be consistently weak and should not become weaker with several repeated contractions.

    b. Another muscle that shares the same innervation is tested. Knowledge of both spinal and peripheral nerve innervation will aid the clinician in determining which muscle to select.

11. *Comparing findings with uninvolved side.* One study found no statistically significant difference in force between the dominant and nondominant lower extremities but did find the difference between the dominant and nondominant upper extremities.[12] Sapega[13] states that a difference in muscle force between sides of greater than 20% probably indicates an abnormality, whereas a difference of 10% to 20% possibly indicates abnormality.

As always, these tests cannot be evaluated in isolation but have to be integrated into a total clinical profile before drawing any conclusion about the patient's condition. Many factors can influence the results from MMT, including:

► Age
► Type of contraction (isometric, concentric, or eccentric)
► Muscle size
► Speed of contraction
► Training effect
► Joint position
► Fatigue
► Nutrition status
► Level of motivation
► Pain
► Body type
► Limb dominance

Although the grading of muscle strength has its role in the clinic, and the ability to isolate the various muscles is very important in determining the source of nerve palsy, specific grading of individual muscles does not give the clinician much information on the ability of the structure to perform functional tasks. Also, isometric muscle force measurements are specific to a point or small range in the joint range excursion and, thus, cannot be used to predict dynamic force capabilities.[17-19]

More recently, the use of quantitative muscle testing (QMT) has been recommended to assess strength, as it produces interval data that describe force production. QMT methods include:

▸ *The use of handheld dynamometers.* Although more costly and time-consuming than manual muscle testing, handheld dynamometry can improve objectivity and sensitivity. Patients are typically asked to push against the dynamometer in a maximal isometric contraction (make test) or hold a position until the clinician overpowers the muscle producing an eccentric contraction (break test).[6] Normative force values for particular muscle groups by patient age and gender have been reported, with some authors including regression equations that take into account body weight and height.[20]

▸ *The use of an isokinetic dynamometer.* This is a stationary, electromechanical device that controls the moving body segment's velocity by resisting and measuring the patient's effort so that the body segment cannot accelerate beyond a preset angular velocity.[6] Isokinetic dynamometers measure torque and range of motion as a function of time and can analyze the ratio between the eccentric contraction and concentric contraction of a muscle at various positions and speeds.[26] This ratio is aptly named the *eccentric/concentric ratio.*[27] The ratio is calculated by dividing the eccentric strength value by the concentric strength value. Various authors[28,29] have demonstrated that the upper limit of this ratio is 2.0 and that lower ratios indicate pathology.[27,30] Alternatively, the same recommendations for manual muscle testing advocated by Sapega[13] can be used: a difference in muscle force between sides of greater than 20% probably indicates an abnormality, while the

difference of 10% to 20% possibly indicates abnormality. To ensure the validity of isokinetic dynamometry measurements, calibration of equipment is necessary and should be performed each day of testing at the same speed and damp setting to be used during the testing.[31]

One of the major criticisms of MMT is the overestimation of strength when a muscle is weak as identified by QMT, compared to the same muscle being graded as normal by MMT, such that a theoretical percentage score based on MMT is likely to overestimate the strength of a patient.[9] Studies that compare the reliability of MMT and QMT often conclude that MMT may be consistent and reliable, but it is unable to detect subtle differences in strength.[32,33] Thus, although MMT results are more consistent, the variation produced by QMT can appreciate differences in strength undetectable in MMT.[9] For example, Beasley[2] showed that 50% of the knee extensor strength needed to be lost before MMT was able to identify weakness.

MUSCLE TESTING OF THE SHOULDER COMPLEX

Several significant muscles control motion at the shoulder and provide dynamic stabilization. Rarely does a single muscle act in isolation at the shoulder. For simplicity, the muscles acting at the shoulder may be described in terms of their functional roles: scapular rotators, humeral propellers, humeral positioners, and shoulder protectors (Table 9-3).[34]

TABLE 9-3	Muscles of the Shoulder Complex
Scapular rotators Trapezius Serratus anterior Levator scapulae Rhomboid major Rhomboid minor	
Humeral propellers Latissimus dorsi Teres major Pectoralis major Pectoralis minor	
Humeral positioners Deltoid	
Shoulder protectors Rotator cuff (supraspinatus, infraspinatus, teres minor, and subscapularis) Long head of the biceps brachii	

209

Scapular Rotators

The scapular rotators comprise the trapezius, serratus anterior, levator scapulae, rhomboid major, and rhomboid minor.[34] As a group, these muscles are involved with motions at the scapulothoracic articulation, and their proper function is vital to the normal biomechanics of the whole shoulder complex. The scapular muscles can contract isometrically, concentrically, or eccentrically, depending on the desired movement and whether it involves acceleration or deceleration. To varying degrees, the serratus anterior and all parts of the trapezius cooperate during the scapula's upward rotation.

Trapezius. The trapezius muscle (Figure 9-14) originates from the medial third of the superior nuchal line, the external occipital protuberance, the ligamentum nuchae, the apices of the seventh cervical vertebra, all the thoracic spinous processes, and the supraspinous ligaments of the cervical and thoracic vertebrae. According to anatomy and function, this muscle is traditionally divided into middle, upper, and lower parts (see Figure 9-14).

► The upper fibers descend to attach to the lateral third of the posterior border of the clavicle.

► The middle fibers of the trapezius run horizontally to the medial acromial margin and the superior lip of the spine of the scapula.

► The inferior fibers ascend to attach to an aponeurosis, gliding over a smooth triangular surface at the medial end of the scapular spine to a tubercle at the lateral scapular apex.

The nerve supply to the trapezius is from the spinal accessory (cranial nerve [CN] XI) and the anterior ramus of C2-4.

Upper Trapezius. The upper portion of the trapezius originates from the external occipital protuberance, medial one-third of the superior nuchal line, the ligamentum nuchae, and the seventh cervical vertebra's spinous process (see Figure 9-14). It inserts on the lateral one-third of the clavicle and acromion processes of the scapula. It has been suggested that the upper fibers of this muscle have a different motor supply than the middle and lower portions.[35,36] Recent clinical and anatomic evidence seem to suggest that the spinal accessory nerve (CN XI) provides the most important and consistent motor supply to all portions of the trapezius muscle and that although the C2-4 branches of the cervical plexus are present, no particular elements of innervation within the trapezius have been determined.[37]

One of the functions of the upper trapezius is to produce shoulder girdle elevation on a fixed cervical spine. For the trapezius to perform this action, the anterior neck flexors must stabilize the cervical spine to prevent the simultaneous occipital extension from occurring. Failure to prevent this occipital extension would allow the head to translate anteriorly, resulting in a decrease in the length, and therefore the efficiency, of the trapezius,[38] and an increase in the cervical lordosis. The synergist muscles for the upper trapezius include the rhomboid major and minor, the middle trapezius, the levator scapulae, and the serratus anterior. The antagonists for the upper trapezius include the lower trapezius, pectoralis minor, subclavius, pectoralis major

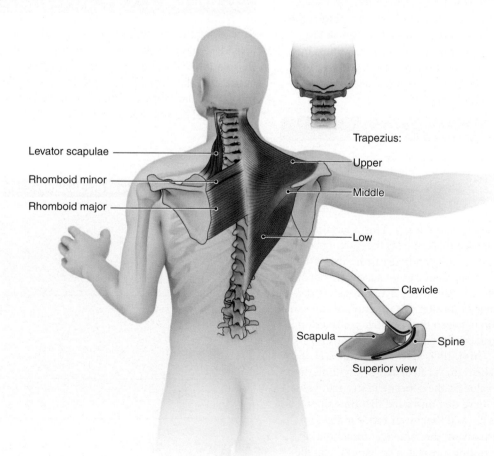

Levator scapulae
Rhomboid minor
Rhomboid major

Trapezius:
Upper
Middle
Low
Clavicle
Scapula
Spine
Superior view

FIGURE 9-14 Trapezius muscle.

(sternal portion), serratus anterior, and latissimus dorsi. An upper trapezius weakness results in a decrease in the ability to approximate the acromial end of the scapula and the occiput, difficulty raising the head from a prone position, and difficulty with abduction and flexion of the humerus above shoulder level.[39] Adaptive shortening of the muscle results in elevation of the shoulder girdle. This muscle is a common location for trigger points.

To specifically test this muscle, the patient is seated with the arm relaxed at the sides. The patient is asked to raise the shoulder as high as possible and extend and rotate the occiput toward the elevated shoulder (Figure 9-15). The clinician stabilizes the top of the patient's shoulders with one hand and applies resistance against the head in the direction of cervical flexion anterolaterally (see Figure 9-15). The command given to the patient is, "Don't let me separate your head and shoulder." Substitution or trick motions can include abduction and upward rotation of the scapula (serratus anterior), elevation and downward rotation of the scapula (rhomboid major and minor), anterior tilting of the scapula (pectoralis minor), and elevation of the first and second ribs (scalenus muscle group).

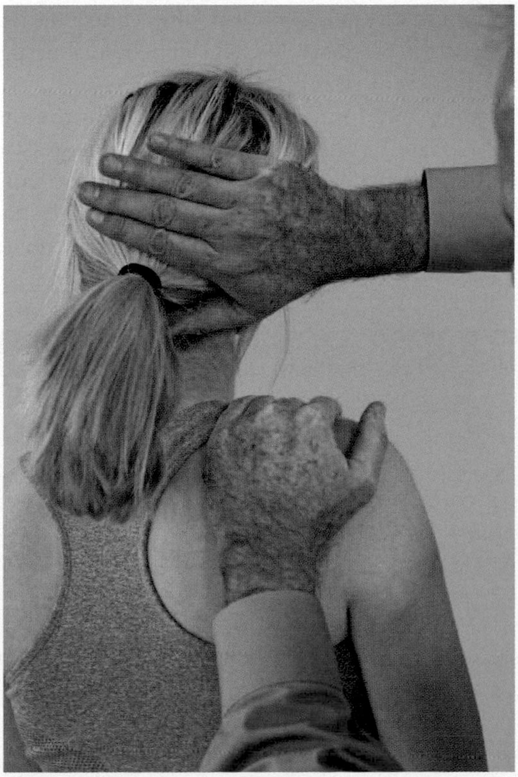

The gravity minimized/eliminated position for this muscle is with the patient positioned supine or prone with the upper limb and shoulder supported.

Middle Trapezius. The middle portion of the trapezius originates from the spinous processes of the first through fifth thoracic vertebrae and inserts on the medial margin of the acromion and the superior lip of the scapular spine (see Figure 9-14), forming the cervicothoracic part of the muscle. Working alone, this muscle produces scapular adduction (retraction). The middle trapezius synergists include the rhomboid major and minor, the upper and lower trapezius, the levator scapulae, and the serratus anterior (depending on its action). The middle trapezius antagonists include the lower trapezius (depending on its action), serratus anterior, pectoralis minor, and pectoralis major (sternal portion).

To test this muscle specifically, the patient is positioned prone with the shoulder abducted to 90°, the elbow extended, and the upper extremity externally rotated so that the thumb points toward the ceiling (Figure 9-16). The clinician applies pressure against the forearm in a downward direction toward the table. The command given to the patient is, "Don't let me push your arm down while keeping your elbow straight and your thumb pointing upward." Substitution or trick motions can include trunk rotation, horizontal abduction of the shoulder (posterior deltoid) elevation and downward rotation of the scapula (rhomboid major and minor), depression and downward rotation of the scapula (lower trapezius), synergistic contraction of the upper and lower fibers of the trapezius muscle, and synergistic contraction of the lower trapezius and the rhomboids. The gravity-minimized/eliminated position for this muscle is with the patient positioned in sitting with the upper limb supported on a friction-free surface in a position of 90° of abduction and 90° of elbow flexion.

Lower Trapezius. The lower fibers of this muscle originate from the spinous processes of the sixth through twelfth thoracic vertebrae (see Figure 9-14) and insert at the tubercle of the apex of the spine of the scapula. Working alone, the lower trapezius muscle stabilizes the scapula against lateral displacement (abduction) produced by the serratus anterior and stabilizes the scapula against scapular elevation produced by the levator scapulae. The lower trapezius synergists include

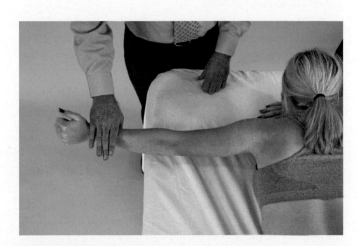

FIGURE 9-15 Test position for the upper portion of the trapezius.

FIGURE 9-16 Test position for the middle trapezius.

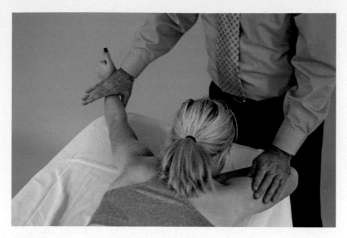

FIGURE 9-17 Test position for the lower trapezius.

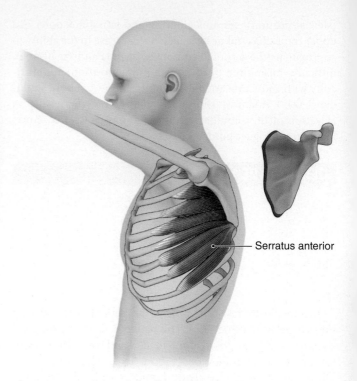

— Serratus anterior

FIGURE 9-18 Serratus anterior muscle.

the rhomboid major and minor, the middle and upper trapezius, the pectoralis minor, and the latissimus dorsi. The lower trapezius antagonists include the upper trapezius, levator scapulae, rhomboid major and minor, and serratus anterior.

To test this muscle specifically, the patient is positioned in prone with the arm placed diagonally overhead, and the shoulder is externally rotated (Figure 9-17). The clinician applies pressure against the forearm downward toward the table. The command given to the patient is, "Don't let me push your arm down while keeping your arm diagonally upward and your thumb facing upward." Substitution or trick motions can include assistance from the posterior deltoid, latissimus dorsi, or pectoralis major. The gravity-minimized/eliminated position for this muscle is with the patient positioned in prone with the arms by the sides and the upper extremity supported by the clinician. The patient is asked to depress and adduct the scapula through the full range of motion.

Serratus Anterior. The muscular digitations of the serratus anterior (Figure 9-18) originate from the upper 8–10 ribs and fascia over the intercostals. The muscle is composed of three functional components[41,42]:

► The upper component originates from the first and second ribs and inserts on the scapula's superior angle.

► The middle component arises from the second, third, and fourth ribs and inserts along the anterior aspect of the medial scapular border.

► The lower component is the largest and most powerful, originating from the fifth through ninth ribs. It runs anterior to the scapula and inserts on the medial border of the scapula.

The serratus anterior is activated with all shoulder movements, but especially during shoulder flexion and abduction.[42] Working in synergy with the upper and lower trapezius, as part of a force couple, the main function of the serratus anterior is to protract and upwardly rotate the scapula,[43,44] while providing a strong, mobile base of support to position the glenoid optimally for maximum efficiency of the upper extremity.[45] Its lower fibers draw the lower angle of the scapula forward to rotate the scapula upward while maintaining the scapula on the thorax during arm elevation.[46] This moves the coracoacromial arch out of the path of the advancing greater tuberosity and opposes the excessive elevation of the scapula by the levator scapulae and trapezius muscles.[47] Without upward rotation and protraction of the scapula by the serratus anterior, full glenohumeral (G-H) elevation is not possible. In fact, in patients with complete paralysis of the serratus anterior, Gregg and colleagues[45] reported that abduction is limited to 110°.

Dysfunction of serratus anterior muscle causes winging of the scapula if the patient attempts to elevate the arm.[48,49] Scapulothoracic dysfunctions can also contribute to G-H instability, as the scapula's normal stable base is destabilized during abduction or flexion.[49-51]

The serratus anterior muscle is innervated by the long thoracic nerve (C5–7).* The serratus anterior synergists include the upper and lower trapezius, pectoralis minor, latissimus dorsi, and subclavius. The antagonists for the serratus anterior include the middle trapezius, levator scapulae, and rhomboids.

CLINICAL PEARL

Paralysis or weakness of the serratus anterior muscle results in disruption of normal shoulder kinesiology. The disability may be slight with partial paralysis or profound with complete paralysis. As a rule, persons with complete or marked paralysis of the serratus anterior cannot elevate the arms above 110° of abduction.[40]

To specifically test this muscle, the patient is positioned supine, standing, or sitting.

---

*Two mnemonics can be used for this muscle: SALT (serratus anterior—long thoracic) and "C5, 6, 7 raise your arms to heaven"

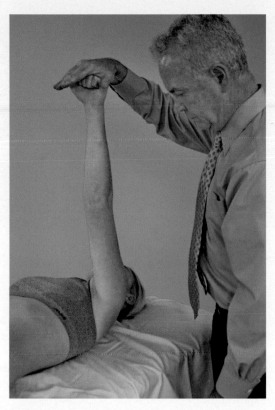

FIGURE 9-19 Test position for the serratus anterior—patient supine.

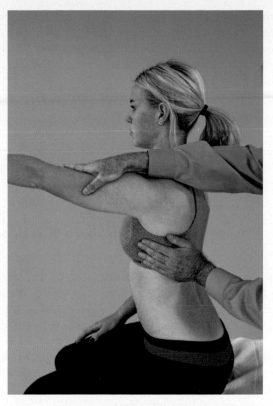

FIGURE 9-20 Test position for the serratus anterior—patient sitting.

▶ *Supine:* the patient is asked to flex the shoulder to 90° with slight abduction and with the elbow in extension. From this position, the patient moves the arm upward toward the ceiling by abducting the scapula. The clinician applies resistance by grasping around the forearm and elbow and applying a downward and inward pressure toward the table (Figure 9-19). The command given to the patient is, "Try to lift your arm higher by moving your shoulder forward while I push down on it."

▶ *Standing:* the patient places a hand against the wall with the shoulder in forward flexion to 80–90° and the elbows locked in extension. While monitoring the inferior angle of the scapula for any winging, the command given to the patient is, "Push against the wall."

▶ *Sitting:* this test focuses on the upward rotation action of the serratus in the abducted position. The patient is asked to move the humerus into approximately 120° to 130° of flexion. Using one hand, the clinician wraps the thumb and index finger around the scapula's inferior aspect, and the other hand is placed on the anterior aspect of the arm (Figure 9-20). The command given to the patient is, "Keep your arm still while I try and push it down," as the clinician pushes downwardly on the arm while applying a resistive force with the other hand into internal rotation of the inferior angle of the scapula.

Substitution or trick motions typically occur in sitting and can include flexion or rotation of the vertebrae.

The gravity-minimized/eliminated position for this muscle is with the patient positioned in sitting with the upper limb resting on a table, with the shoulder positioned in 90° of flexion, and the elbow extended.

Levator Scapulae. The levator scapulae muscle (see Figure 9-14) originates by tendinous strips from the transverse processes of the atlas, axis, and C3 and C4 vertebrae and descends diagonally to insert on the superomedial angle of the scapula.

The levator scapulae can act on either the cervical spine or the scapula. If it acts on the cervical spine, it can produce extension, side bending, and rotation of the cervical spine to the same side.[52] When acting on the scapula during upper extremity flexion or abduction, the levator scapulae muscle acts as an antagonist to the lower trapezius muscle and provides eccentric control of upward scapular rotation in the higher ranges of motion.[53]

Both the trapezius and levator scapulae muscles are activated with increased upper extremity loads.[38,42,54]

The levator scapulae muscle is innervated by the posterior (dorsal) scapular nerve (C3–5). The synergists for the levator scapulae include all portions of the trapezius and the rhomboid major and minor. The levator scapulae's antagonists include the lower trapezius, pectoralis minor, pectoralis major (lower portion), subclavius, serratus anterior, and latissimus dorsi.

To test this muscle specifically, the patient is positioned in sitting with the arms relaxed at the sides. The patient is asked to raise the shoulder as high as possible while the clinician generates resistance downward on top of the shoulder (see Figure 9-15). The command given to the patient is, "Don't let me push your shoulder down." It is worth remembering that it is difficult to differentiate the levator scapulae's strength from that of the upper trapezius. For this reason, the levator scapulae strength is often assessed together with the rhomboids or with the upper trapezius.

213

Rhomboid Major and Minor. The rhomboid muscles help control scapular positioning, particularly with horizontal flexion and extension of the shoulder complex.[53] Based on anatomy and function, the rhomboids are divided into major and minor portions.

▶ The rhomboid major muscle (see Figure 9-14) originates from the second to fifth thoracic spinous processes and the overlying supraspinous ligaments. The fibers descend to insert on the medial scapular border between the root of the scapular spine and the inferior angle of the scapula.

▶ The rhomboid minor muscle (see Figure 9-14) originates from the lower ligamentum nuchae and the seventh cervical and first thoracic spinous processes and attaches to the medial border of the scapula at the root of the spine of the scapula.

The rhomboid muscles are innervated by the posterior (dorsal) scapular nerve (C4–5). Working together, the rhomboid muscles adduct and elevate the scapula, and downwardly rotate the scapula. The rhomboid major muscle helps stabilize the scapula against the rib cage. The synergists for both of the rhomboids include all portions of the trapezius muscle and the levator scapulae. The antagonists for the rhomboids include the lower trapezius, pectoralis major and minor, serratus anterior, and latissimus dorsi.

To test this muscle specifically, the patient is positioned in prone with the head turned toward the tested side, the elbow flexed, and the ipsilateral humerus abducted, slightly extended, and externally rotated (Figure 9-21a). The clinician applies pressure with one hand against the patient's arm in the direction of abducting the scapula and externally rotating the inferior angle, while the other hand is placed against the patient's shoulder in the direction of depression (see Figure 9-21a). The command given to the patient is, "Don't let me push your arm down." Substitution or trick motions can include assistance from the wrist extensors, middle trapezius, posterior deltoid, latissimus dorsi, teres major, and levator scapulae. An alternative test can be performed with the patient positioned in prone with the upper extremity positioned in 90° of abduction and internally rotated so that the

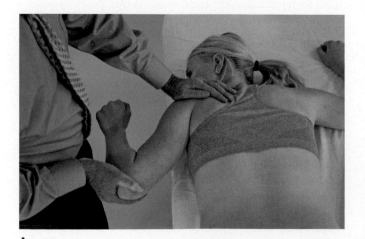

A

FIGURE 9-21A Test position for the rhomboids (and levator scapulae).

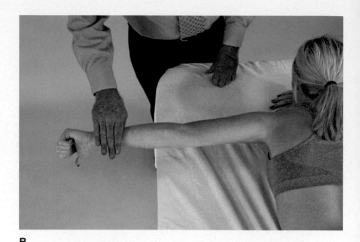

B

FIGURE 9-21B Alternate test position for the rhomboids.

thumb is pointing down (Figure 9-21b). The patient is asked to raise the arm toward the ceiling and to hold the position while the clinician applies a downward force to the patient's forearm. The gravity-minimized/eliminated position for this muscle is with the patient sitting with the hand resting on the lumbar spine.

Humeral Propellers

The mass of the shoulder's internal rotators (subscapularis, anterior deltoid, pectoralis major, latissimus dorsi, and teres major) is much greater than that of the external rotators (infraspinatus, teres minor, and posterior deltoid).[40] This fact explains why the shoulder internal rotators produce about 1.75 times greater isometric torque than the external rotators.[55] Peak torques of the internal rotators also exceed the external rotators when measured isokinetically, under both concentric and eccentric conditions.[40,56]

Latissimus Dorsi. The latissimus dorsi muscle (Figure 9-22) originates from the spinous processes of the last six thoracic vertebrae, the lower three or four ribs, the lumbar and sacral spinous processes through the thoracolumbar fascia, the posterior third of the external lip of the iliac crest, and a slip from the inferior scapular angle. The scapular slip allows the latissimus dorsi to act at the scapulothoracic articulation. The latissimus dorsi inserts on the intertubercular sulcus of the humerus. The latissimus dorsi functions as an extensor, adductor, and powerful internal rotator of the shoulder and assists in scapular depression, retraction, and downward rotation.[57] It is innervated by the thoracodorsal nerve (C6–8). The synergists for the latissimus dorsi include the teres major, anterior and posterior deltoid, triceps brachii, erector spinae, subscapularis, and pectoralis major. The antagonists for the latissimus dorsi include the middle trapezius, supraspinatus, infraspinatus, teres minor, anterior and posterior deltoid, coracobrachialis, biceps brachii, and pectoralis major (clavicular portion).

To test this muscle specifically, the patient is positioned in prone with the shoulder internally rotated and adducted and the palm facing upward (Figure 9-23). The patient is asked to extend the shoulder while keeping the elbow straight.

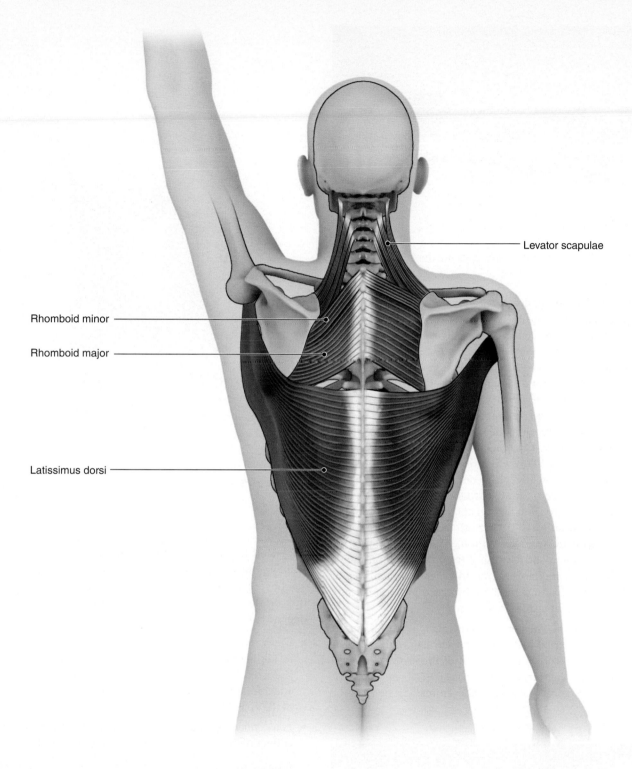

Rhomboid minor

Rhomboid major

Latissimus dorsi

Levator scapulae

FIGURE 9-22 Latissimus dorsi.

The command given to the patient is, "While keeping your palm facing the ceiling, don't let me push your arm down." The clinician stabilizes the thorax, and resistance is given proximal to the elbow joint using a force that combines shoulder abduction and minimal flexion (see Figure 9-23). Substitution or trick motions can include scapular adduction with no shoulder motion, anterior tipping, and abduction of the scapula, assistance from the teres major, posterior deltoid, or pectoralis major (sternal head). The gravity-minimized/eliminated position for this muscle is with the patient positioned in side lying, with the upper limb supported in 90° of shoulder flexion and internal rotation, and with the elbow flexed.

Teres Major. The teres major (see Figure 9-22) originates from the inferior third of the lateral border of the scapula, just superior to the inferior angle. The teres major tendon inserts on the medial lip of the intertubercular groove of the humerus. The teres major functions to complement the actions of the latissimus dorsi in that it extends, adducts, and internally rotates the G-H joint. It is innervated by the lower subscapular nerve (C5, C6). The synergists for the teres major

215

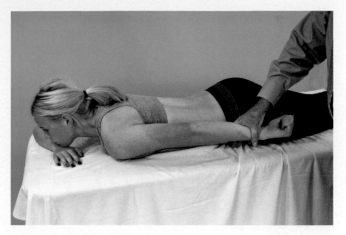

FIGURE 9-23 Test position for the latissimus dorsi.

include the latissimus dorsi, anterior and posterior deltoid, triceps brachii (long head), pectoralis major, and subscapularis. The antagonists for the teres major are numerous and include the middle deltoid, supraspinatus, infraspinatus, teres minor, coracobrachialis, biceps brachii, anterior and posterior deltoid, and pectoralis major (clavicular portion).

To test this muscle specifically, the patient is positioned in prone with the upper extremity extended, abducted, and medially rotated and with the back of the hand resting on the small of the back. The clinician places a hand against the arm proximal to the elbow (Figure 9-24), and the command given to the patient is, "Keeping your hand against your back, don't let me move your arm toward the table," while the clinician generates a force into flexion and abduction of the upper extremity. Substitution or trick motions can include scapular adduction without shoulder motion, external rotation of the glenohumeral joint, and assistance from the latissimus dorsi, pectoralis major, and teres minor. In general, the teres major muscle is not tested in a gravity-eliminated position because it will only contract against resistance.

Pectoralis Major. The pectoralis major (Figure 9-25) originates from the sternal half of the clavicle, half of the anterior surface of the sternum, to the level of the sixth or seventh costal cartilage, the sternal end of the sixth rib, and the aponeurosis of the obliquus externus abdominis. The fibers of the

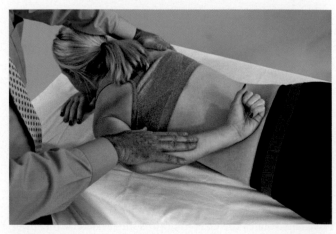

FIGURE 9-24 Test position for the teres major.

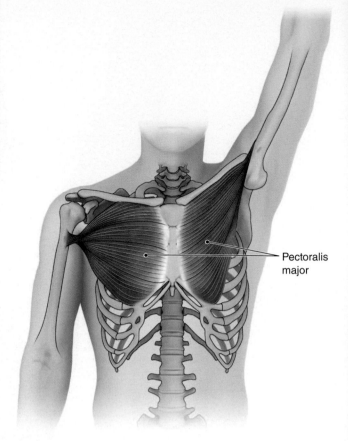

FIGURE 9-25 Pectoralis major muscle.

pectoralis major converge to form a tendon that inserts on the lateral lip of the intertubercular sulcus of the humerus. Although this muscle does not insert on the scapula, it does act on the scapulothoracic articulation through its insertion on the humerus. The function of the pectoralis muscle depends on which fibers are activated:

▶ *Upper fibers (clavicular head)*—internal rotation, horizontal adduction, flexion, abduction (once the humerus is abducted 90°, the upper fibers assist in further abduction), and adduction (with the humerus below 90° of abduction) of the G-H joint

▶ *Lower fibers (sternal head)*—internal rotation, horizontal adduction, extension, and adduction of the G-H joint

From a functional perspective, this muscle is important with crutch walking or ambulation within the parallel bars. The pectoralis major is innervated by the medial (lower fibers) and lateral (upper fibers) pectoral nerves (C8–T1 and C5–7, respectively). The synergists for the clavicular portion include the pectoralis major (sternal portion), subscapularis, latissimus dorsi, teres major, anterior and middle deltoid, coracobrachialis, pectoralis minor, serratus anterior, and biceps brachii. The antagonists for the clavicular portion include the latissimus dorsi, teres major, middle and posterior deltoid, infraspinatus, triceps brachii (long head), teres minor, and supraspinatus. The synergists for the sternal portion include the pectoralis major (clavicular portion), posterior deltoid, latissimus dorsi, teres major, triceps brachii (long head), and pectoralis minor. The antagonists for the sternal portion include the supraspinatus, deltoid, trapezius, serratus anterior, levator scapulae, and rhomboids.

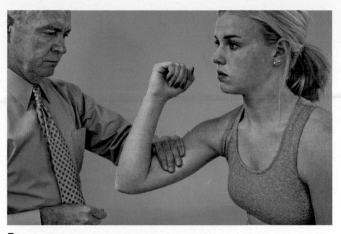

B

FIGURE 9-26B Test position for the coracobrachialis.

CLINICAL PEARL

The pectoralis major and latissimus dorsi muscles are referred to as *humeral propeller* muscles as they demonstrate a positive correlation both between peak torque and pitching velocity and during the propulsive phase of the swim stroke.

To specifically test this muscle, the patient is positioned supine. The patient's arm position depends on which portion of the muscle is being tested:

▶ *The clavicular portion (upper fibers):* the patient's arm is positioned in 60–90° of shoulder abduction, and the elbow is slightly flexed. The patient is then asked to adduct the shoulder horizontally as the clinician applies resistance at the forearm (or proximal to the elbow if the elbow flexors are weak) in a downward and outward direction (Figure 9-26). The coracobrachialis, a synergist of the upper fibers, can also be assessed (Figure 9-26a).

▶ *The sternal portion (lower fibers):* the patient's arm is positioned in 120° of shoulder abduction with the elbow slightly flexed. The patient is asked to move the arm down and inward across the body as the clinician applies resistance at the elbow in an up and outward direction (Figure 9-27).

Substitution or trick motions can include trunk rotation and assistance from the anterior deltoid, coracobrachialis, and biceps brachii. The gravity-minimized/eliminated position for this muscle is with the patient positioned in sitting with the shoulder positioned in neutral rotation and 90° of abduction, the elbow flexed to 90°, and the upper limb supported.

Pectoralis Minor. The pectoralis minor (Figure 9-28) originates from the outer surface of the upper margins of the third to fifth ribs near their cartilage. The fibers of the pectoralis minor ascend laterally, converging into a tendon that inserts on the coracoid process of the scapula.

Working alone, this muscle depresses the shoulder, downwardly rotates the scapula, and protracts the scapula.

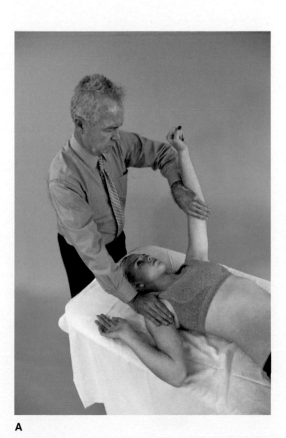

A

FIGURE 9-26A Test position for the pectoralis major—upper fibers.

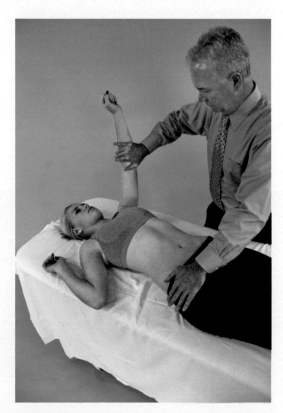

FIGURE 9-27 Test position for the pectoralis major—lower fibers.

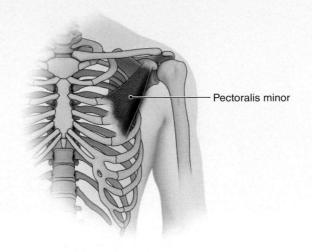

FIGURE 9-28 Pectoralis minor muscle.

This muscle can also assist with rib elevation during forced inspiration. The pectoralis minor muscle is innervated by the medial pectoral nerve (C6–8). The pectoralis minor is prone to adaptive shortening, particularly if the patient commonly adopts a rounded shoulder posture, which in turn can result in impingement on the cords of the brachial plexus or the axillary vessels. The synergists to this muscle include the pectoralis major, lower trapezius, serratus anterior, latissimus dorsi, levator scapulae, rhomboid major and minor, and middle trapezius. The antagonists of this muscle are the trapezius, levator scapulae, latissimus dorsi, serratus anterior, and rhomboid major and minor.

To specifically test this muscle, the patient is positioned supine with the arms at the sides, and the patient is asked to lift the shoulder girdle from the table (without using force from the elbow or hand) and to hold the position while the clinician applies resistance against the anterior aspect of the shoulder (Figure 9-29) in a downward direction toward the table. Substitution or trick motions can include flexion of the wrist or fingers, giving the appearance of anterior tipping of the scapula. The gravity-minimized/eliminated position for this muscle is with the patient positioned in sitting with the hand resting on the small of the back.

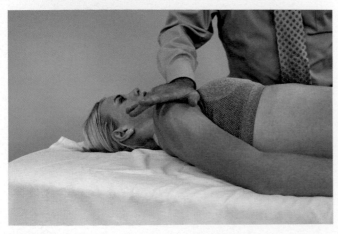

FIGURE 9-29 Test position for pectoralis minor.

Humeral Positioners

Deltoid. The deltoid muscle originates from the lateral third of the clavicle, the superior surface of the acromion, and the scapular spine (Figure 9-30). It inserts into the deltoid tuberosity of the humerus. The deltoid can be described as three separate muscles—anterior, middle, and posterior—all of which function as humeral positioners, positioning the humerus in space.[34]

Working alone, the three separate muscles of the deltoid can produce shoulder horizontal adduction, shoulder flexion, internal rotation of the shoulder, and shoulder scaption (arm elevated in the scapular plane). Working in a combined fashion, the deltoid can produce shoulder abduction. The deltoid muscle is innervated by the axillary nerve (C5-6). The synergists and antagonists of this muscle depend on which of the three portions is being used:

► *Anterior deltoid (see Figure 9-30).* The synergists include the middle and posterior deltoid, subscapularis, biceps brachii, pectoralis major, coracobrachialis, and supraspinatus. The antagonists include the triceps brachii (long head), posterior deltoid, latissimus dorsi, teres major, infraspinatus, and teres minor.

► *Middle deltoid (see Figure 9-30).* The synergists are the supraspinatus, posterior deltoid, and anterior deltoid. The antagonists are latissimus dorsi, teres major, coracobrachialis, and triceps brachii (long head).

► *Posterior deltoid (see Figure 9-30).* The synergists are the teres minor, latissimus dorsi, teres major, triceps brachii (long head), and infraspinatus.

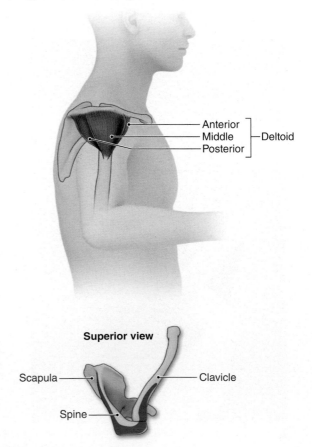

FIGURE 9-30 Deltoid muscle.

To specifically test this muscle, the patient's arm position used depends on which portion of the muscle is being tested:

▶ *Anterior deltoid.* The patient is positioned in sitting or supine with the shoulder abducted in minimal flexion and external rotation. The command given to the patient is, "Place your arm diagonally outward from your body and hold it against my resistance." While stabilizing the patient's shoulder with one hand, the clinician uses the other hand to apply resistance to the anterior and medial aspect of the arm proximal to the elbow in the direction of abduction and minimal extension (Figure 9-31). Substitution or trick motions can include elevating the shoulder and leaning backward; assistance from the biceps brachii, coracobrachialis, or pectoralis major (clavicular head); or moving the scapula. The gravity-minimized/eliminated position for this muscle is with the patient positioned in side lying with the upper extremity supported and the shoulder positioned in neutral, and the elbow flexed.

▶ *Middle deltoid.* The patient is positioned in sitting with the arm abducted to 90°, and the elbow flexed to approximately 90°. The patient is asked to hold this position while the clinician applies resistance just proximal to the elbow in a downward direction (Figure 9-32). Substitution or trick motions can include trunk flexion to the opposite side or assistance from the biceps brachii, supraspinatus, or serratus anterior. The gravity-minimized/eliminated position for this muscle is with the patient positioned supine with the upper extremity supported, and the elbow flexed to 90°.

▶ *Posterior deltoid.* The patient positioned in sitting with the shoulder abducted to approximately 90° and positioned

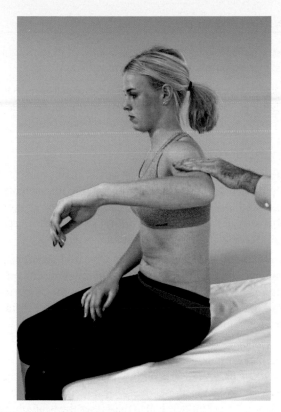

FIGURE 9-32 Test position for the middle deltoid.

in minimal shoulder extension and internal rotation. The patient is asked to push the arms back toward the clinician as the clinician uses one hand to stabilize the shoulder and the other hand to apply resistance to the posterolateral aspect of the arm, proximal to the elbow, in the direction of shoulder abduction and slight flexion (Figure 9-33). Substitution or trick motions can include assistance from the long head of the triceps or adduction of the scapula without horizontally abducting the shoulder. The gravity-minimized/eliminated position for this muscle is with the patient positioned in sitting with the upper extremity supported on a table and the shoulder and elbow flexed to 90°.

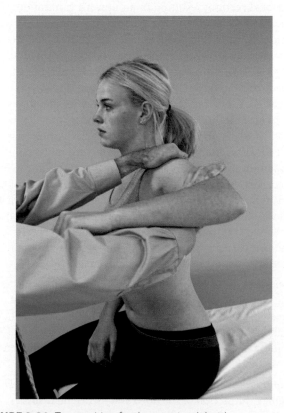

FIGURE 9-31 Test position for the anterior deltoid.

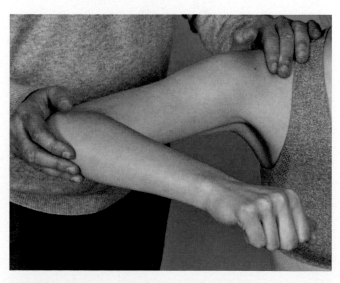

FIGURE 9-33 Test position for the posterior deltoid.

Shoulder Protectors

Rotator Cuff (RC). The RC muscles consist of the supraspinatus, infraspinatus, teres minor, and subscapularis:

▶ *Supraspinatus (Figure 9-34).* The supraspinatus muscle originates above the scapular spine, in the supraspinatus fossa, and inserts on the greater tuberosity of the humerus. Working alone, the supraspinatus abducts or elevates the G-H joint.

▶ *Infraspinatus (Figure 9-35).* The infraspinatus muscle originates below the scapular spine, in the infraspinatus fossa, and inserts on the posterior aspect of the greater tuberosity of the humerus. Working alone, the infraspinatus externally rotates the G-H joint.

▶ *Teres minor (see Figure 9-35).* The teres minor muscle originates on the lateral scapula border and inserts on the inferior aspect of the greater tuberosity of the humerus. Working alone, the teres minor muscle externally rotates the G-H joint.

▶ *Subscapularis (Figure 9-36).* The subscapularis muscle originates on the scapula's anterior surface, sitting directly over the ribs, and inserts on the lesser tuberosity of the humerus. Working alone, the subscapularis is an internal rotator of the shoulder. It also depresses the head of the humerus, allowing it to move freely in the G-H joint during elevation of the arm. Internal rotation of the shoulder dominates over external rotation secondary to the greater muscle mass of the subscapularis.

The RC muscles are referred to as the protectors of the shoulder because, in addition to working individually to move the humerus, they have an important role in the function of the shoulder and serve the following roles[34]:

▶ *Assist in the rotation of the shoulder and arm.* At the G-H joint, elevation through abduction of the arm requires that the greater tuberosity of the humerus pass under the coracoacromial arch. For this to occur, the humerus must externally rotate, and the acromion must elevate.[58] External rotation of the humerus is produced actively by a contraction of the infraspinatus and teres minor and joint capsule twisting. A force couple exists in the transverse plane between the subscapularis anteriorly and the infraspinatus and teres minor posteriorly in which co-contraction of the infraspinatus, teres minor, and subscapularis muscles both depresses and compresses the humeral head during overhead movements.

CLINICAL PEARL

The importance of the external rotation during humeral elevation can be demonstrated clinically. Suppose the humerus is held in full internal rotation. In that case, only about 60° of G-H abduction is passively possible before the greater tuberosity impinges against the coracoacromial arch and blocks further abduction. This helps explain why individuals with marked internal rotation contractures cannot abduct fully but can elevate the arm in the sagittal plane.

In the frontal plane, there is another force couple between the deltoid and the inferior RC muscles (infraspinatus, subscapularis, and teres minor). With the arm fully adducted, contraction of the deltoid produces a vertical force in a superior direction, resulting in an upward translation of the humeral head relative to the glenoid. Co-contraction of the inferior RC muscles produces both a compressive force and a downward translation of the humerus that counterbalances the deltoid's force, thereby stabilizing the humeral head.

Electromyography (EMG) studies have shown that during casual elevation of the arm in normal shoulders, the deltoid and the RC act continuously throughout the motion of abduction, each reaching a peak of activity between 120° and 140° of abduction.[59,60] However, during more rapid and precise movements such as those involved with throwing, a more selective pattern emerges with specific periods of great intensity.[61] Weakening of the RC appears to allow the deltoid to elevate the proximal part of the humerus in the absence of an adequate depressor effect from the RC. A decrease in the subacromial space is created, and impingement of the RC on the anterior aspect of the acromion occurs.[62,63]

▶ *Reinforce the G-H capsule.* The RC muscles, together with the glenohumeral ligament (and the long head of the biceps—often referred to as the fifth RC muscle), enhance stability. For example, firing the RC muscles increases the middle G-H ligament tension when the arm is abducted to 45° and externally rotated.[64]

▶ *Control much of the active arthrokinematics of the G-H joint.* Contraction of the horizontally oriented supraspinatus produces a compression force directly into the

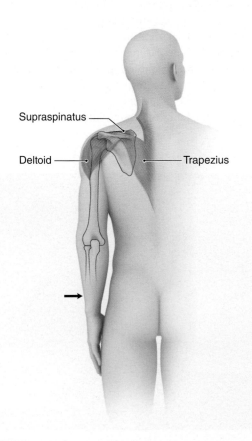

Supraspinatus

Deltoid

Trapezius

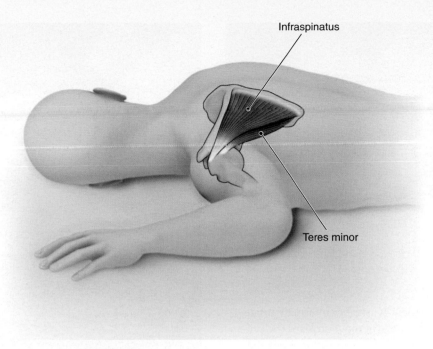

FIGURE 9-35 Infraspinatus and teres minor muscles.

glenoid fossa.[62] This compression force holds the humeral head securely in the glenoid cavity during its superior roll, which provides stability to the joint, and also maintains a mechanically efficient fulcrum for elevation of the arm.[62] In the shoulder's midrange position, when all of the passive restraints are lax, joint stability is achieved almost entirely by the RC. Also, as previously mentioned, without adequate supraspinatus force, the near-vertical line of force of a contracting deltoid tends to jam or impinge the humeral head superiorly against the coracoacromial arch.[40]

The synergists and antagonists of the RC muscles depend on the individual muscles of the group:

▶ *Teres minor.* The synergists are the infraspinatus and the posterior deltoid. The antagonists are the anterior deltoid,

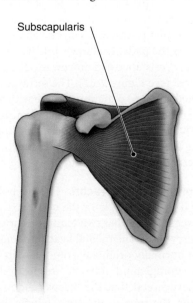

FIGURE 9-36 Subscapularis muscle.

subscapularis, pectoralis major, latissimus dorsi, and teres major.

▶ *Subscapularis.* The synergists are the pectoralis major, anterior deltoid, teres major, and latissimus dorsi. The antagonists are the infraspinatus, posterior deltoid, and teres minor.

▶ *Supraspinatus.* The synergist is the middle deltoid. The antagonists are the teres major, latissimus dorsi, and pectoralis major.

▶ *Infraspinatus.* The synergists are the teres minor and posterior deltoid. The antagonists are the subscapularis, pectoralis major, latissimus dorsi, anterior deltoid, and teres major.

Each of the muscles of the RC can be specifically tested, with the patient setup dependent on which muscle is being tested:

▶ *Teres minor.* The patient is positioned prone with the shoulder abducted to 90° and the arm supported by the table so that the forearm is permitted to move freely (Figure 9-37). The patient is asked to externally rotate the shoulder so that the forearm moves toward the ceiling. The patient is asked to hold this position while the clinician applies resistance at the patient's wrist in a downward direction with one hand while using the other hand to support the patient's elbow (see Figure 9-37). The teres minor can also be tested with the patient in supine with the humerus in external rotation and the elbow held at a right angle. Using one hand, the clinician stabilizes the upper arm while using the other arm to apply pressure in the direction of internal rotation of the humerus (Figure 9-38).

▶ *Subscapularis.* The patient is positioned prone with the shoulder abducted to 90° and the upper arm resting on the table so that the forearm is permitted to move freely

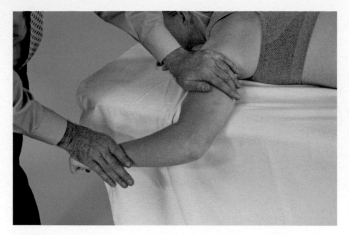

FIGURE 9-37 Test position for the shoulder external rotators—teres minor and infraspinatus–patient prone.

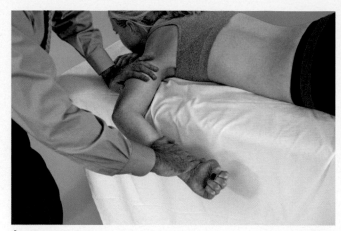

A

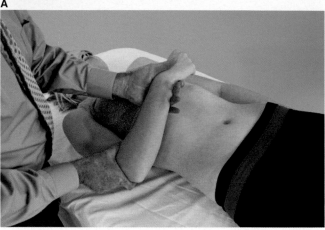

B

FIGURE 9-39 a. Test position for the shoulder internal rotators—subscapularis. b. Alternate test position for the subscapularis.

(Figure 9-39a). The patient is asked to internally rotate the shoulder so that the forearm moves toward the ceiling. The patient is asked to hold the position while the clinician applies resistance at the wrist in a downward direction with one hand while using the other hand to support the patient's arm (see Figure 9-39). The subscapularis can also be tested with the patient in supine with the upper arm at the side and the elbow held at a right angle (Figure 9-39b). Using one hand to stabilize the patient's upper arm, the clinician uses the other hand to apply force against the inner aspect of the patient's wrist and forearm in the direction of external rotation. Substitution or trick motions can include scapular abduction, pronation of the forearm, and assistance from the pectoralis major, teres major, and latissimus dorsi. The gravity-minimized/eliminated position for this muscle is with the patient positioned in prone with the shoulder flexed over the table's edge.

▶ *Supraspinatus.* The patient is positioned in sitting with the arm by the side and the head rotated ipsilaterally and extended. Using one hand, the clinician palpates the supraspinatus; the other hand applies resistance at the elbow into shoulder adduction while the patient is asked to raise the arm into shoulder abduction. This is a difficult

muscle to isolate, as it works in conjunction with the middle deltoid.

▶ *Infraspinatus.* The patient is positioned prone with the shoulder abducted to 90° and the arm supported by the table so that the forearm is permitted to move freely (see Figure 9-37). The patient is asked to rotate the shoulder externally so that the forearm moves toward the ceiling and holds that position. Using one hand, the clinician stabilizes the patient's elbow while using the other hand to apply resistance in a downward direction at the patient's wrist (see Figure 9-37). The infraspinatus can also be tested with the patient in supine with the humerus in external rotation and the elbow held at a right angle. Using one hand, the clinician stabilizes the upper arm while using the other arm to apply pressure in the direction of internal rotation of the humerus (see Figure 9-38).

Long Head of the Biceps Brachii. The biceps brachii muscle is a large fusiform muscle in the upper extremity's anterior compartment, which has two tendinous origins from the scapula (Figure 9-40). The medial head and long head of the biceps (LHB) normally originate from the scapula's coracoid process and supraglenoid tubercle, respectively. However, researchers have noted that the biceps tendon's origin varies, not only in the type of insertion (single, bifurcated, or trifurcated) but also in the specific anatomic location where

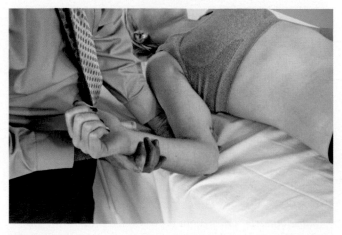

FIGURE 9-38 Test position for the shoulder external rotators–teres minor and infraspinatus—patient supine.

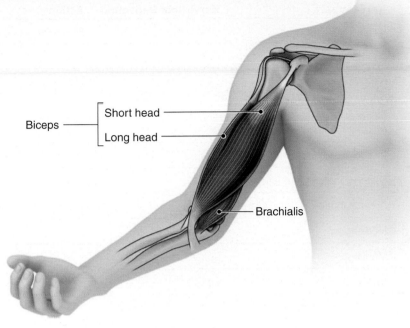

FIGURE 9-40 Biceps brachii and brachialis muscles.

Biceps
— Short head
— Long head

— Brachialis

it inserts.[65,66] The proximal LHB tendon receives some arterial supply from labral branches of the suprascapular artery.[67] As it leaves its origin, the LHB tendon is surrounded by a synovial sheath, which ends at the distal end of the bicipital groove, making the tendon an intra-articular but extra-synovial structure.[65] As the LHB tendon moves between the greater and lesser tuberosities, it is stabilized in position by the tendoligamentous sling made up of the coracohumeral ligament, superior G-H ligament, and fibers from the supraspinatus and subscapularis.[65,68] Once in the bicipital groove, the LHB tendon passes under the transverse humeral ligament, which bridges the groove.[69] After coursing through the groove, the two heads join to form the biceps muscle belly at the deltoid insertion level.[70] The medial tendon is interarticular, lying inside the G-H capsule.[71-73] This tendon is not as common a source of shoulder pain as the long tendon, and it rarely ruptures.[71-73]

The biceps' function as a forearm supinator and secondarily as an elbow flexor is well known (see Muscle Testing of the Elbow).[74] At the shoulder joint, however, the LHB tendon's function is less clear, with most references regarding it as a weak flexor of the shoulder.[75] Cadaveric studies have suggested that the LHB tendon functions as a humeral head depressor (in full external rotation), an anterior stabilizer, a posterior stabilizer, a limiter of external rotation, a lifter of the glenoid labrum, and a humeral head compressor of the shoulder.[76-79] The muscle has also been described as having an important role in decelerating the rapidly moving arm during activities such as forceful overhand throwing.[65] In the anatomic position, the biceps cannot elevate the humerus. If the arm is externally rotated 90°, the long head's tendon aligns with the muscle belly to form a straight line across the humeral head. As the biceps contracts in this position, the humeral head rotates beneath the tendon, resisting external rotation of the humeral head and increasing the anterior

stability of the G-H joint.[80-82] Contraction of the long head of the biceps when the arm is abducted and externally rotated fixes the humeral head snugly against the glenoid cavity, as the resultant force passes obliquely through the center of rotation of the humeral head and at right angles to the glenoid.[80] The humeral head is prevented from moving upward by the biceps tendon's hoodlike action, which exerts a downward force and assists the cuff's depressor function.[83-85] Interestingly, the biceps tendon was wider in cuff-deficient shoulders in one study.[86]

The musculocutaneous nerve innervates the biceps brachii muscle.

CLINICAL PEARL

Several pathological conditions have been associated with the LHB tendon, including LHB tendon degeneration, SLAP lesions, LHB tendon anchor abnormalities, and LHB tendon instability.[69]

The strength of the LHB is assessed in combination with the short head of the biceps (see Elbow Flexors later).

MUSCLE TESTING OF THE ELBOW

A summary of the muscles of the elbow is outlined in Table 9-4.

Elbow Flexors

Anatomic, biomechanic, and electromyographic analyses have demonstrated that the primary elbow flexors are the biceps, brachialis, and brachioradialis (see Table 9-4).[87] The pronator teres, flexor carpi radialis (FCR), flexor carpi ulnaris

TABLE 9-4	Muscles of the Elbow, Forearm, Wrist, and Hand: Their Actions, Nerve Supply, and Nerve Root Derivation		
Muscles	**Nerve Supply**	**Nerve Root Derivation**	**Action**
Triceps	Radial	C7-C8	Elbow extension
Anconeus	Radial	C7-C8, (T1)	
Brachialis	Musculocutaneous	C5-C6, (C7)	Elbow flexion
Biceps brachii	Musculocutaneous	C5-C6	
Brachioradialis	Radial	C5-C6, (C7)	
Biceps brachii	Musculocutaneous	C5-C6	Supination of the forearm
Supinator	Posterior interosseous (radial)	C5-C6	
Pronator quadratus	Anterior interosseous (median)	C8, T1	Pronation of the forearm
Pronator teres	Median	C6-C7	
Flexor carpi radialis	Median	C6-C7	
Extensor carpi radialis longus	Radial	C6-C7	Extension of the wrist
Extensor carpi radialis brevis	Posterior interosseous (radial)	C7-C8	
Extensor carpi ulnaris	Posterior interosseous (radial)	C7-C8	
Flexor carpi radialis	Median	C6-C7	Flexion of the wrist
Flexor carpi ulnaris	Ulnar	C7-C8	
Flexor carpi ulnaris	Ulnar	C7-C8	Ulnar deviation of the wrist
Extensor carpi ulnaris	Posterior interosseous (radial)	C7-C8	
Flexor carpi radialis	Median	C6-C7	Radial deviation of the wrist
Extensor carpi radialis longus	Radial	C6-C7	
Abductor pollicis longus	Posterior interosseous (radial)	C7-C8	
Extensor pollicis brevis	Posterior interosseous (radial)	C7-C8	
Extensor digitorum communis	Posterior interosseous (radial)	C7-C8	Extension of the fingers
Extensor indicis	Posterior interosseous (radial)	C7-C8	
Extensor digiti minimi	Posterior interosseous (radial)	C7-C8	
Flexor digitorum profundus	Lateral: anterior interosseous (median)	C8, T1	Flexion of the fingers (lateral aspect flexes the 2nd and 3rd digits; medial aspect flexes the 4th and 5th digits
	Medial: ulnar	C8, T1	
Flexor digitorum superficialis	Median	C7-C8, T1	Flexion of the fingers

(FCU), and extensor carpi radialis longus (ECRL) muscles are considered to be weak flexors of the elbow.[88] Most elbow flexors, and essentially all the major supinator and pronator muscles, have their distal attachments on the radius.[89] Contraction of these muscles, therefore, pulls the radius proximally against the humeroradial joint.[90,91] The combined efforts of all the elbow flexors can create large amounts of elbow flexion torque. The interosseous membrane transfers a component of this muscle force to the radius and the ulna, thereby dissipating some of the force.[89]

Biceps Brachii. The biceps is a two-headed muscle that spans two joints. The short head of the biceps arises from the tip of the coracoid process of the scapula, whereas the long head arises from the supraglenoid tuberosity of the scapula (see Figure 9-40). The biceps has two insertions: the radial tuberosity and the lacertus fibrosus (see Figure 9-40).

At the elbow, the biceps is the dominant flexor, but it also functions as a forearm supinator.[92] The supination action of the biceps increases the more the elbow is flexed and is maximal at 90°. It diminishes again when the elbow is fully flexed.

No,[93] or limited,[94] biceps muscle activity has been demonstrated during elbow flexion, with the forearm pronated.[88] The biceps, via its long head, also functions as a shoulder flexor (see Muscles of the Shoulder earlier).

The musculocutaneous nerve innervates the biceps brachii muscle.

The synergists of the biceps include the brachialis and brachioradialis, supinator, anterior deltoid, coracobrachialis, pectoralis major (clavicular portion), FCR, FCU, pronator teres, and extensor carpi radialis longus and brevis. The antagonists include the triceps brachii and anconeus, pronator teres, pronator quadratus, posterior deltoid, and latissimus dorsi.

To test this muscle specifically, the patient is positioned in sitting with the elbow flexed to approximately 90° and the forearm in supination. Using one hand to stabilize the patient's shoulder, the clinician uses the other hand to apply resistance over the anterior aspect of the patient's forearm while asking the patient to hold the position of elbow flexion against the resistance (Figure 9-41). As with all elbow flexors, the gravity-minimized/eliminated position is with the patient positioned in sitting with the arm supported on a table at 90° of abduction, the shoulder in neutral rotation, and the elbow extended. When testing any of the elbow flexors, substitution or trick motions can include shoulder extension and assistance from the pronator teres or the wrist and finger extensors and flexors.

Brachialis. The brachialis (see Figure 9-40) originates from the lower two-thirds of the anterior surface of the humerus and inserts on the ulnar tuberosity and coronoid process. The brachialis is the workhorse of the elbow and functions to bend the elbow regardless of the degree of pronation and supination of the forearm.[94] It is the most powerful flexor of the elbow when the forearm is pronated.[95]

The musculocutaneous and radial nerves innervate the brachialis muscle.

The synergists of the brachialis include the biceps brachii, brachioradialis, extensor carpi radialis longus and brevis, pronator teres, FCR, and FCU. The antagonists of this muscle include the triceps brachii and anconeus.

To test this muscle specifically, the patient is positioned in sitting or supine with the elbow flexed and the forearm

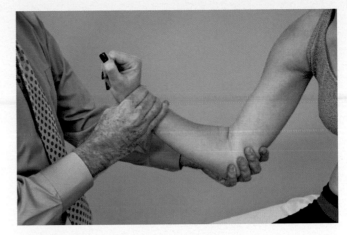

FIGURE 9-42 Test position for the brachialis.

pronated (Figure 9-42). Using one hand to stabilize the patient's elbow, the clinician places the other hand over the posterior surface of the patient's forearm proximal to the wrist and applies a force in the direction of elbow extension while asking the patient to try and prevent the motion (see Figure 9-42).

Brachioradialis. The brachioradialis (Figure 9-43) arises from the proximal two-thirds of the lateral supracondylar ridge of the humerus and the lateral intermuscular septum. It travels down the forearm and inserts on the lateral border of the styloid process on the distal aspect of the radius.

The brachioradialis appears to have several functions, two of which occur with rapid movements of elbow flexion. Initially, it functions as a shunt muscle, overcoming centrifugal forces acting on the elbow and then adding power to increase flexion speed.[92]

The brachioradialis also functions to bring a pronated or supinated forearm back into the neutral position of pronation and supination. In the neutral or pronated position, the muscle acts as a flexor of the elbow, an action that diminishes when the forearm is held in supination.[94,96]

The radial nerve innervates the brachioradialis muscle.

The synergists of the brachioradialis include the biceps brachii, brachialis, supinator, pronator teres, pronator quadratus, FCR, FCU, palmaris longus, and flexor digitorum

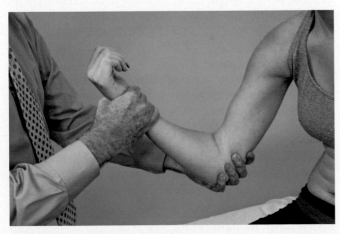

FIGURE 9-41 Test position for the biceps brachii.

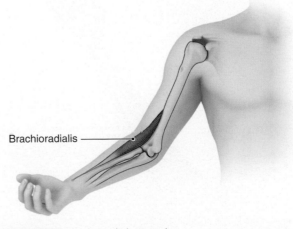

FIGURE 9-43 Brachioradialis muscle.

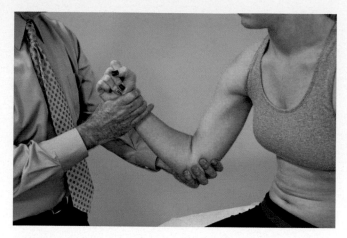

FIGURE 9-44 Test position for the brachioradialis.

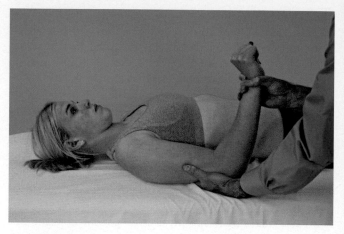

FIGURE 9-46 Test position for the pronator teres

superficialis (FDS). The antagonists include the triceps brachii and anconeus, extensor carpi radialis longus and brevis, extensor carpi ulnaris (ECU), and extensor digitorum communis (EDC).

To test this muscle specifically, the patient is positioned in sitting or supine with the elbow flexed and the forearm placed in a neutral position halfway between supination and pronation (Figure 9-44). Using one hand to stabilize the patient's elbow, the clinician places the other hand proximal to the patient's wrist and applies a force into elbow extension while asking the patient to resist the movement.

Pronator Teres. The pronator teres (Figure 9-45) has two heads of origin: a humeral head and an ulnar head. The humeral head arises from the medial epicondylar ridge of the humerus and common flexor tendon, whereas the ulnar head arises from the medial aspect of the coronoid process of the ulna. The pronator teres inserts on the anterolateral surface of the midpoint of the radius. The muscle functions predominantly to pronate the forearm but can also assist with elbow flexion.[95-97]

The median nerve innervates the pronator teres.

The synergists of this muscle include the biceps brachii, brachioradialis, brachialis, FCR, FCU, palmaris longus, FDS,

and the pronator quadratus. The antagonists of this muscle include the triceps brachii and anconeus, biceps brachii, brachioradialis, and supinator.

To test this muscle specifically, the patient is positioned in sitting or supine with the elbow flexed to approximately 60° and the forearm fully pronated (Figure 9-46). Using one hand, the clinician stabilizes the patient's elbow against the patient's thorax while placing the other hand proximal to the patient's wrist (see Figure 9-46). The patient is asked to maintain the position while the clinician generates a force into forearm supination. Substitution or trick motions can include trunk flexion to the contralateral side and abduction and internal rotation of the shoulder. The gravity-minimized/eliminated position for this muscle is with the patient positioned in sitting with the shoulder supported on a table at 90° of flexion, the elbow flexed to 90°, and the forearm perpendicular to the table.

Extensor Carpi Radialis Longus (ECRL). The ECRL arises from a point superior to the lateral epicondyle of the humerus on the lower third of the supracondylar ridge, just distal to the brachioradialis. It travels down the forearm to insert on the posterior surface of the base of the second metacarpal (Figure 9-47). The muscle functions as a weak flexor of the elbow and provides wrist extension and radial deviation.

The radial nerve innervates the ECRL. The synergists of this muscle include ECU, FCR, EDC, extensor indicis (EI), extensor pollicis longus (EPL), extensor pollicis brevis (EPB), and abductor pollicis longus (APL). The antagonists of this muscle include the ECU, FCU, FCR, palmaris longus, flexor digitorum profundus (FDP), flexor digitorum superficialis (FDS), and flexor pollicis longus (FPL).

To test this muscle specifically, the patient is positioned in sitting or supine with the elbow extended and the forearm just short of full pronation. Using one hand, the clinician supports the patient's forearm, and the patient is asked to extend the wrist in a radial direction (Figure 9-48). Using the other hand, the clinician applies pressure on the posterior aspect of the patient's hand along the second through fourth metacarpal bones in an ulnar direction while asking the patient to prevent the movement (Figure 9-48).

Flexor Carpi Radialis (FCR). The FCR (Figure 9-49) arises from the common flexor tendon on the medial epicondyle of

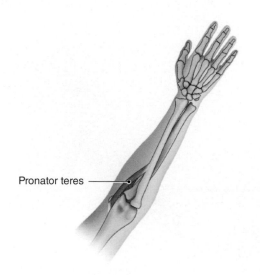

Pronator teres —

FIGURE 9-45 Pronator teres muscle.

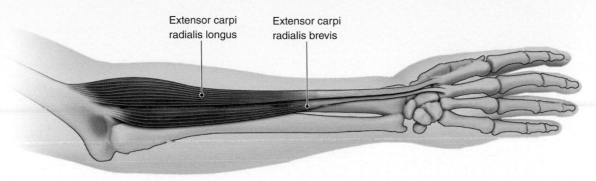

FIGURE 9-47 Extensor carpi radialis longus and brevis.

the humerus and inserts on the base of the second and third metacarpal bones. The FCR not only functions to flex the elbow and wrist but also assists in pronation and radial deviation of the wrist.

The median nerve innervates the FCR. The synergists of this muscle include the FCU, palmaris longus, FDP, FDS, FPL, extensor carpi radialis longus and brevis, EPB, and APL. The antagonists of this muscle include the FCU, ECU, FPL, extensor carpi radialis longus and brevis, EDC, EI, and EPL.

To test this muscle specifically, the patient is positioned in sitting or supine, with the wrist flexed and ulnarly deviated and the forearm in supination. Using one hand, the clinician supports the patient's forearm while using the index and middle finger of the other hand to apply pressure on the thenar eminence in an ulnar and extension direction (Figure 9-50). The patient is asked to prevent this motion.

Flexor Carpi Ulnaris (FCU). The FCU (Figure 9-51) arises from two heads. The humeral head arises from the medial humeral epicondyle as part of the common flexor tendon, while the ulnar head arises from the proximal portion of the subcutaneous border of the ulna. The FCU inserts directly onto the pisiform, the hamate via the pisohamate ligament, and onto the anterior surface of the base of the fifth metacarpal, via the pisometacarpal ligament. The FCU functions to assist with elbow flexion in addition to flexion and ulnar deviation of the wrist.

The ulnar nerve innervates the FCU. The synergists of this muscle include the FCR, palmaris longus, FDP, FDS, FPL,

ECU, biceps brachii, brachialis, pronator teres, brachioradialis, and extensor carpi radialis longus and brevis. The antagonists of this muscle include the triceps brachii and anconeus, ECRL, ECRB, ECU, EDC, EI, extensor digiti minimi (EDM), EPL, EPB, FCR, and APL.

To test this muscle specifically, the patient is positioned supine or sitting with the forearms supported, the wrist flexed, and the fingers relaxed. The patient is asked to flex and ulnarly deviate the wrist. While stabilizing the wrist with one hand, the clinician generates a radial and extension force with the other hand on the medial aspect of the patient's hand (Figure 9-52).

Forearm Pronators

Pronator Teres. See earlier discussion.

Pronator Quadratus. The fibers of the pronator quadratus run perpendicular to the arm's direction, running from the most distal quarter of the anterior ulna to the distal quarter of the anterior radius (Figure 9-53). It is the only muscle that attaches only to the ulna at one end and the radius at the other end.

The pronator quadratus, which is the main pronator of the hand, is innervated by the anterior interosseous branch of the median nerve. The synergists for this muscle include the pronator teres, brachioradialis, and FCR. The antagonists include the biceps brachii, brachioradialis, and supinator.

To test this muscle specifically, the patient is positioned in sitting or supine with the elbow completely flexed and the forearm pronated. Using one hand to stabilize the patient's elbow, the clinician places the other hand proximal to the patient's wrist and applies a force into supination while asking the patient to prevent the movement (Figure 9-54).

Flexor Carpi Radialis. See earlier discussion.

Forearm Supinators

Biceps. See earlier discussion. It is important to remember that the biceps's effectiveness as a supinator is greatest when the elbow is flexed to 90°, placing the biceps tendon at a 90° angle to the radius. In contrast, with the elbow flexed only 30°, much of the rotational efficiency of the biceps is lost.[98]

Supinator. The supinator (Figure 9-55) originates from the lateral epicondyle of the humerus, the lateral collateral ligament (LCL), the annular ligament, the supinator crest, and

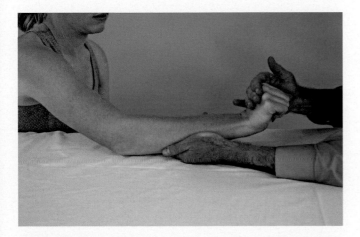

FIGURE 9-48 Test position for the extensor carpi radialis longus and brevis

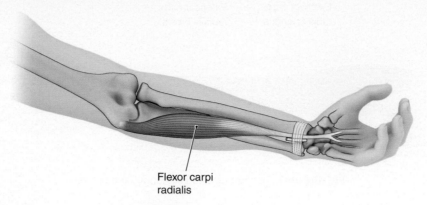

Flexor carpi
radialis

FIGURE 9-49 Flexor carpi radialis muscle.

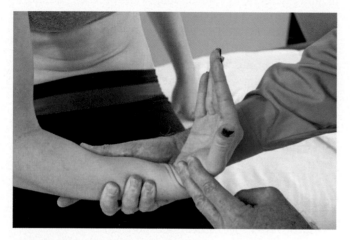

FIGURE 9-50 Test position for the flexor carpi radialis.

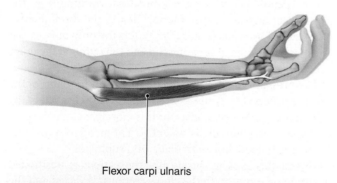

Flexor carpi ulnaris

FIGURE 9-51 Flexor carpi ulnaris muscle.

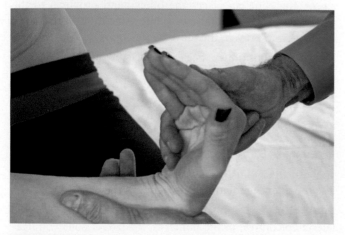

FIGURE 9-52 Test position for the flexor carpi ulnaris.

the ulnar fossa. It inserts on the superior third of the anterior and lateral surface of the radius. The supinator muscle is a relentless forearm supinator, similar to the brachialis during elbow flexion. The supinator functions to supinate the forearm in any elbow position, whereas the previously mentioned ECRL and ECRB work as supinators during fast movements and against resistance.

The nervous system usually recruits the supinator muscle for low-power tasks that require a supination motion only, while the biceps remains relatively inactive—a fine example of the law of parsimony.[87]

The radial nerve innervates the supinator.

CLINICAL PEARL

The muscles about the elbow help provide stability by compressing the joint surfaces through muscular contraction.[99] The flexor and pronator muscles, which originate at the medial epicondyle, provide additional static and dynamic support to the medial elbow,[97] with the FCU and FDS being the most effective in this regard.[100]

The synergists for the supinator include the biceps brachii and the brachioradialis. The antagonists include the pronator teres, pronator quadratus, brachioradialis, and FCR.

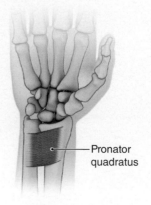

Pronator
quadratus

FIGURE 9-53 Pronator quadratus muscle.

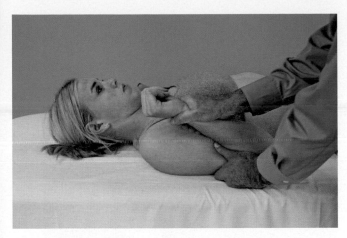

FIGURE 9-54 Test position for the pronator quadratus.

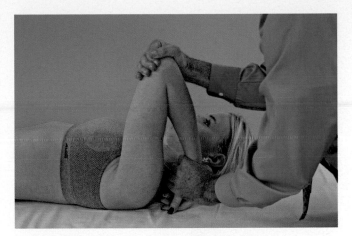

FIGURE 9-56 Test position for the supinator.

To specifically test this muscle, the patient is positioned in standing or sitting. The patient's arm can be positioned in one of two ways:

▶ The shoulder flexed to 90°, the elbow fully flexed, and the forearm fully supinated (Figure 9-56).

▶ The shoulder and elbow extended behind the patient, and the forearm supinated (Figure 9-57).

Using one hand to stabilize the patient's upper arm at the elbow, the clinician places the other hand just proximal to the patient's wrist and applies a force into pronation while asking the patient to prevent the motion.

Elbow Extensors

Two muscles extend the elbow: the triceps and the anconeus (see Table 9-4).

Triceps Brachii. The triceps brachii (Figure 9-58) has three heads of origin. The long head arises from the infraglenoid tuberosity of the scapula, the lateral head from the posterior and lateral surface of the humerus, and the medial head from the lower posterior surface of the humerus. The muscle inserts on the superoposterior surface of the olecranon and deep fascia of the forearm. The triceps has its maximal force in movements that combine both elbow extension and shoulder

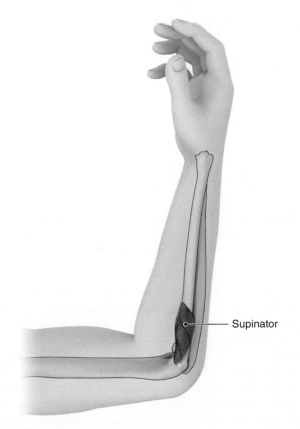

FIGURE 9-55 Supinator muscle.

Supinator

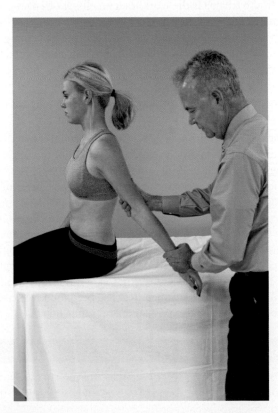

FIGURE 9-57 Alternate test position for the supinator.

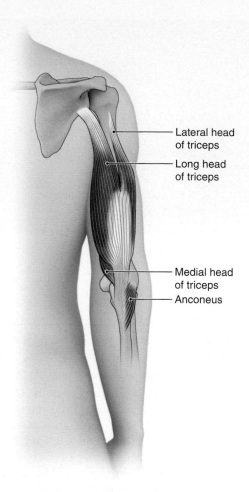

FIGURE 9-58 Triceps brachii and anconeus.

extension. Like the biceps, it is a two-joint muscle. The medial head of the triceps is the workhorse of elbow extension, with the lateral and long heads recruited during heavier loads.[77] During strong contractions of the triceps—for example, a push-up, which involves a combination of elbow extension and shoulder flexion—as the triceps strongly contracts to extend the elbow, the shoulder simultaneously flexes by the action of the anterior deltoid, which overpowers the shoulder extension torque of the long head of the triceps.[98]

Anconeus. The anconeus arises from the lateral epicondyle of the humerus and inserts on the lateral aspect of the olecranon and posterior surface of the ulna (see Figure 9-58). The exact function of the anconeus in humans has yet to be determined, although it appears as a fourth head of the elbow extension mechanism, similar to the quadriceps of the knee.[89] It has been suggested that in addition to assisting with elbow extension, the anconeus functions to stabilize the ulnar head in all positions (except radial deviation) and pull the subanconeus bursa and the joint capsule out of the way during extension, thus avoiding impingement.[97,101] The anconeus has also been found to stabilize the elbow during forearm pronation and supination.[94]

CLINICAL PEARL

Tendinopathy of the anconeus can mimic lateral elbow tendinopathy (tennis elbow), while hypertrophy of the anconeus muscle can compress the ulnar nerve.[102]

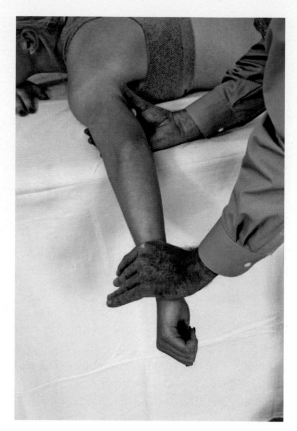

FIGURE 9-59 Test position for the triceps brachii—patient prone.

The radial nerve innervates the triceps brachii and anconeus.

The synergists of the triceps brachii and anconeus include the latissimus dorsi, teres major, and posterior deltoid. The antagonists include the biceps brachii, brachioradialis, brachialis, FCR, FCU, pronator teres, and the extensor carpi radialis longus and brevis.

To specifically test the triceps brachii and anconeus, three different positions can be used:

► *Patient prone.* The patient abducts the shoulder to 90°, extends the elbow fully, and then unlocks it slightly (Figure 9-59).

► *Patient supine.* The patient abducts the shoulder to 90°, extends the elbow fully, and then unlocks it slightly (Figure 9-60).

► *Patient sitting.* The patient abducts the shoulder to 160–180°, extends the elbow fully, and then unlocks it slightly (Figure 9-61). This position is the one used most commonly.

With each of the previous positions, the clinician uses one hand to stabilize the upper arm and places the other hand proximal to the patient's wrist. The patient is asked to hold the arm position while the clinician applies a force into elbow flexion.

Substitution or trick motions can include flexion of the shoulder. The gravity-minimized/eliminated position for this muscle is with the patient positioned in sitting with the shoulder supported in 90° of abduction and internal rotation, and with the elbow flexed and the forearm in neutral.

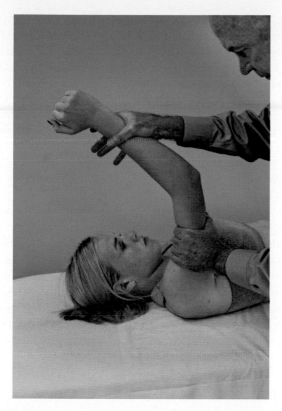

FIGURE 9-60 Test position for the triceps brachii—patient supine.

MUSCLE TESTING OF THE WRIST AND FOREARM

The muscles of the forearm are contained within three major fascial compartments, the anterior forearm, the posterior forearm, and the compartment referred to as the mobile wad (Table 9-5), all of which can be described as the 18 extrinsic muscles that originate in the forearm and insert within the hand.[103] The flexors, located in the anterior compartment, flex the wrist and digits, whereas the extensors, located in the posterior compartment, extend the wrist and the digits.

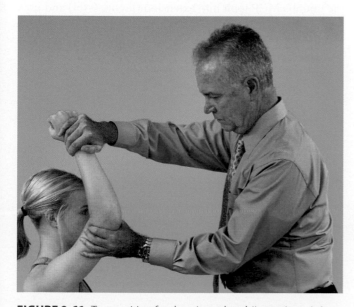

FIGURE 9-61 Test position for the triceps brachii—patient sitting.

TABLE 9-5	Muscle Compartments of the Forearm
Compartment	**Principal Muscles**
Anterior	Pronator teres
	Flexor carpi radialis
	Palmaris longus
	Flexor digitorum superficialis
	Flexor digitorum profundus
	Flexor pollicis longus
	Flexor carpi ulnaris
	Pronator quadratus
Posterior	Abductor pollicis longus
	Extensor pollicis brevis
	Extensor pollicis longus
	Extensor digitorum communis
	Extensor digitorum proprius
	Extensor digiti quinti
	Extensor carpi ulnaris
Mobile wad	Brachioradialis
	Extensor carpi radialis longus
	Extensor carpi radialis brevis

The extrinsic group, whose muscle bellies lie proximal to the wrist, joins with the intrinsic muscles located entirely within the hand. This design provides for a large number of muscles to act on the hand without excessive bulkiness. The extrinsic tendons enhance wrist stability by balancing flexor and extensor forces and compressing the carpals.

The amount of tendon excursion determines the available range of motion at a joint. Calculating the amount of tendon excursion needed to produce a certain number of joint motion degrees involves an appreciation of geometry. A circle's radius equals approximately 1 radian (57.29°). The mathematical radius, which is equivalent to the moment arm, represents the amount of tendon excursion required to move the joint through 1 radian.[104] For example, if a joint's moment arm is 10 mm, the tendon must glide 10 mm to move the joint 60° (approximately 1 radian) or 5 mm to move the joint 30° (½ radian).[105]

Anterior Compartment of the Forearm

Superficial Muscles

Pronator Teres. See earlier discussion.

Flexor Carpi Radialis (FCR). See earlier discussion.

Palmaris Longus. The inconsistent palmaris longus (see Figure 9-49) arises from the medial humeral epicondyle as part of the common flexor tendon and inserts on the transverse carpal ligament and palmar aponeurosis. The function of the palmaris longus is to flex the wrist, and it may play a role in thumb abduction in some people.[106]

The median nerve innervates the palmaris longus. The synergists of this muscle include the FCR, FCU, FDP, FDS, and FPL. The antagonists of this muscle include the ECU, extensor carpi radialis longus and brevis, EDC, EPL, and EI.

To test this muscle specifically, the patient is positioned in sitting or supine with the forearm supinated and is asked to flex the wrist and cup the palm (Figure 9-62). While supporting

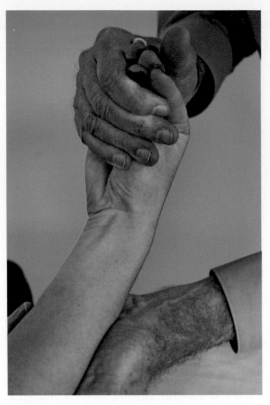

FIGURE 9-62 Test position for the palmaris longus.

the patient's forearm with one hand, the clinician uses the other hand to apply an uncupping and wrist extension force to the thenar and hypothenar eminences of the patient's hand (see Figure 9-62).

Flexor Carpi Ulnaris (FCU). See earlier discussion.

Intermediate Muscle

Flexor Digitorum Superficialis (FDS). The FDS has a three-headed origin (Figure 9-63). The humeral head arises from the medial humeral epicondyle as part of the common flexor tendon. The ulnar head arises from the coronoid process of the ulna. The radial head arises from the oblique line of the radius. The FDS inserts on the middle phalanx of the

medial four digits via a split, "sling" tendon. The FDS serves to flex the proximal and middle interphalangeal joints of the medial four digits and assist with elbow flexion and wrist flexion. The FDS possesses tendons that are capable of relatively independent action at each finger.

The median nerve innervates the FDS. The synergists of this muscle include the FDP, FCR, FCU, palmaris longus, lumbricals, interossei, abductor digiti minimi (ADM), flexor digiti minimi (FDM), and opponens digiti minimi (ODM). The antagonists to this muscle include the extensor carpi radialis longus and brevis, ECU, EDC, EI, lumbricals, and interossei.

To test this muscle specifically, the patient is positioned in sitting or supine with the forearm supported in supination and the metacarpophalangeal (MCP) joint stabilized by the clinician. The patient is asked to bend the middle phalanx of the finger (Figure 9-64) while maintaining the three fingers not being tested in extension and preventing the wrist from flexing excessively (see Figure 9-64). The clinician tests each finger individually by applying an extension force to the anterior aspect of the middle phalanx while asking the patient to resist the movement.

Deep Muscles

Flexor Pollicis Longus (FPL). The FPL has its origin on the anterior surface of the radius, medial border of the coronoid process of the ulna, and the adjacent interosseous membrane. It inserts on the distal phalanx of the thumb (Figure 9-65). The FPL functions to flex the thumb.

The FPL is innervated by the anterior interosseous branch of the median nerve. The synergists of this muscle include the FCR, FCU, palmaris longus, FDP, FDS, flexor pollicis brevis (FPB), abductor pollicis brevis (APB), and adductor pollicis (AP). The antagonists to this muscle include the extensor carpi radialis longus and brevis, ECU, EDC, EI, EPL, EPB, APB, and APL.

To test this muscle specifically, the patient is positioned in sitting or supine with the hand resting on a surface and the forearm in supination. Using one hand, the clinician stabilizes the thumb's MCP joint into extension (Figure 9-66) and uses

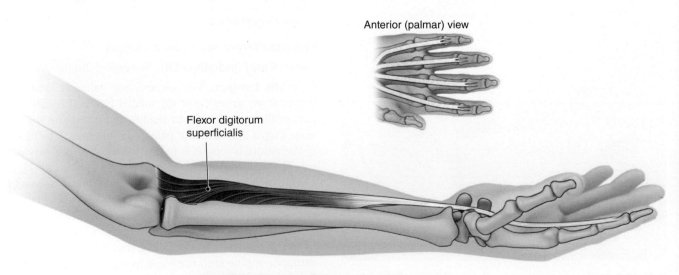

Anterior (palmar) view

Flexor digitorum
superficialis

FIGURE 9-63 Flexor digitorum superficialis muscle.

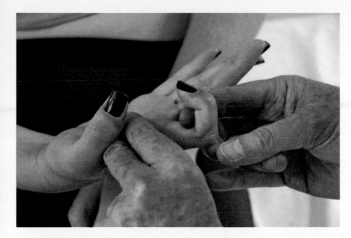

FIGURE 9-64 Test position for the flexor digitorum superficialis.

the other hand to generate an extension force to the anterior aspect of the distal phalanx of the thumb (see Figure 9-66).

Flexor Digitorum Profundus (FDP). The FDP arises from the medial and anterior surfaces of the proximal ulna, the adjacent interosseous membrane, and the forearm's deep fascia (Figure 9-67). The FDP inserts on the base of the distal phalanges of the medial four digits. The FDP functions to flex the distal interphalangeal (DIP) joints after the FDS flexes the second phalanges and assists with flexion of the wrist. The tendons of the FDS and FDP are held against the phalanges by a fibrous sheath. At strategic locations along the sheath, five dense annular pulleys (designated A1, A2, A3, A4, and A5) and three thinner cruciform pulleys (designated C1, C2, and C3) prevent the tendons from bowstringing.[105]

> ### CLINICAL PEARL
>
> Tendinous connections between the FDP and the FPL are a common anatomic anomaly, which has been linked to a condition causing chronic forearm pain, called Linburg syndrome,[107] although the association is by no means conclusive.[108]

The FDP has a dual nerve supply: the medial two heads are supplied by the ulnar nerve, whereas the lateral two heads are supplied by the median nerve's anterior interosseous branch. The synergists of this muscle include the FCR, FCU, palmaris longus, FDS, FPL, lumbricals, interossei, ADM, FDM, and ODM. The antagonists of this muscle include the extensor carpi radialis longus and brevis, ECU, EDC, EI, EPL, lumbricals, and interossei.

To test this muscle specifically, the patient is positioned in sitting or supine with the wrist in a neutral position or

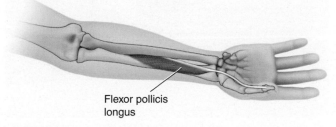

Flexor pollicis longus

FIGURE 9-65 Flexor pollicis longus muscle.

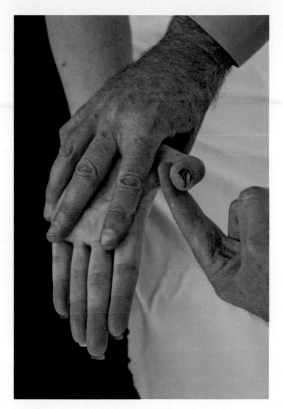

FIGURE 9-66 Test position for flexor pollicis longus.

slightly extended. Using one hand, the clinician stabilizes the proximal and middle phalanges of the finger to be tested. The patient is asked to flex the finger's DIP joint while the clinician applies an extension force to the anterior aspect of the DIP (Figure 9-68).

Pronator Quadratus. See earlier discussion.

Posterior Compartment of the Forearm

Superficial Muscles

Extensor Carpi Radialis Longus (ECRL). See earlier discussion.

Extensor Carpi Radialis Brevis (ECRB). The ECRB arises from the common extensor tendon on the lateral epicondyle of the humerus and the radial collateral ligament (see Figure 9-47). It inserts on the posterior surface of the base of the third metacarpal bone. The muscle stretches across the radial head during pronation, resulting in increased tensile stress when the forearm is pronated, the wrist is flexed, and the elbow is extended. The more medial location of the ECRB compared to the ECRL makes it the primary wrist extensor, but it also has a slight action of radial deviation.

> ### CLINICAL PEARL
>
> The ECRB and ECRL are commonly considered similar muscles, but they differ in many respects.[109] The ECRB, because of its origin on the epicondyle, is not affected by the elbow position, so that all of its action is on the wrist.[110] Taken together, both ECR tendons comprise about 10% of the forearm's muscle mass and 76% of the muscle mass of the extensors of the wrist.[111] The ECRL has longer muscular fibers, mostly at the level of the elbow.

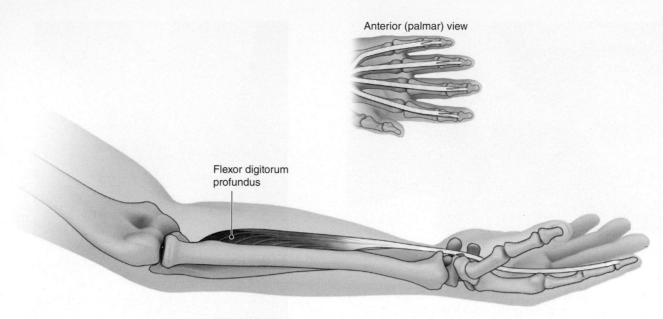

Anterior (palmar) view

Flexor digitorum
profundus

FIGURE 9-67 Flexor digitorum profundus muscle.

The ECRB receives its nerve supply from the posterior interosseous branch of the radial nerve. The synergists and antagonists of this muscle are similar to those of the ECRL except those that cross the elbow.

To test this muscle specifically, the patient is positioned in sitting or supine with the elbow fully flexed (to place the ECRL in a position of mechanical insufficiency) and the forearm just short of full pronation supported by the examiner or the table (Figure 9-69). The patient is asked to extend the wrist in a radial direction and to hold that position while the clinician applies pressure on the posterior aspect of the hand along with the second and third metacarpal bones.

Extensor Digitorum Communis (EDC). The EDC, which consists of the extensor indices, EDM, and extensor digitorum, arises from the lateral humeral epicondyle, part of the common extensor tendon, and inserts on the lateral and posterior aspect of the medial four digits (Figure 9-70). The EDC functions to extend the medial four digits.

The EDC is innervated by the posterior interosseous branch of the radial nerve. The synergists of this muscle include the extensor carpi radialis longus and brevis, ECU,

EI, EPL, lumbricals, and interossei. The antagonists of this muscle include the FCR, FCU, palmaris longus, FDP, FDS, FPL, lumbricals, interossei, ADM, FDM, and ODM.

To specifically test this muscle, the patient is positioned supine or sitting with the forearm pronated. The wrist is positioned in neutral—halfway between flexion and extension—and the MCP and proximal interphalangeal (PIP) joints slightly flexed. The patient is asked to extend the MCP of the finger to be tested and to hold that position. The clinician uses one hand to stabilize the wrist and, using two fingers of the other hand, applies pressure against the posterior surfaces of the patient's proximal phalanges (Figure 9-71).

Extensor Digiti Minimi (EDM). The EDM arises from a muscular slip from the ulnar aspect of the extensor digitorum muscle and inserts on the fifth digit's proximal phalanx. The EDM extends the MCP of the fifth digit and, in conjunction with the lumbricals and interossei, extends the interphalangeal joints of the fifth digit. The EDM also assists in abduction of the fifth digit.

The EDM is innervated by the posterior interosseous branch of the radial nerve.

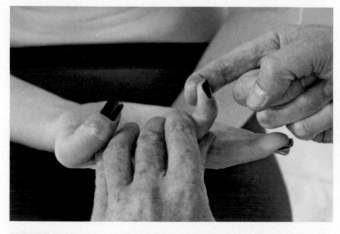

FIGURE 9-68 Test position for flexor digitorum profundus muscle.

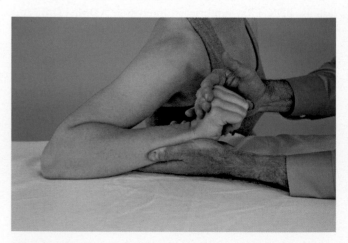

FIGURE 9-69 Test position for the extensor carpi radialis brevis.

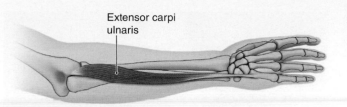

FIGURE 9-72 Extensor carpi ulnaris muscle.

To test this muscle specifically, the patient is positioned supine or sitting with the forearm pronated, the wrist positioned in neutral—halfway between flexion and extension—and the MCP and PIP joints slightly flexed. The patient is asked to extend the MCP of the fifth digit and to hold that position. The clinician uses one hand to stabilize the wrist and, using two fingers of the other hand, applies pressure against the posterior surface of the patient's proximal phalange.

Extensor Carpi Ulnaris (ECU). The ECU arises from the common extensor tendon on the lateral epicondyle of the humerus and the posterior border of the ulna (Figure 9-72). It inserts on the medial side of the base of the fifth metacarpal bone. The ECU is an extensor of the wrist in supination and primarily causes ulnar deviation of the wrist in pronation, working in synergy with the FCU to prevent radial deviation during pronation.[110]

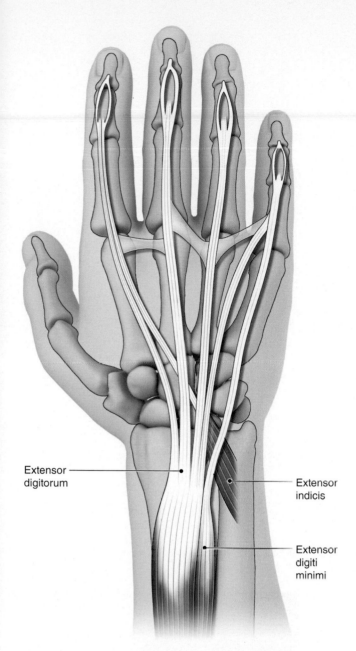

Extensor digitorum

Extensor indicis

Extensor digiti minimi

FIGURE 9-70 Extensor digitorum communis muscle.

CLINICAL PEARL

Extension of the wrist is dependent on three muscles:

► ECRL

► ECRB

► ECU

The ECRL only becomes a wrist extensor after the radial deviation is balanced against the ECU's ulnar forces.

The ECU, the EPL antagonist, has the weakest moment of extension, which becomes zero when the forearm is fully pronated.

Thus, the three wrist extensors have very different moment arms of extension. The ECRB is the most effective extensor of the wrist because it has the greatest tension and the most favorable moment arm.[110]

The ECU is innervated by the posterior interosseous branch of the radial nerve. The synergists for this muscle include the FCU, FPL, extensor carpi radialis longus and brevis, EDC, EI, and EPL. This muscle's antagonists include the FCR, ECRL, ECRB, EPB, APL, FCU, palmaris longus, FDP, FDS, and FPL.

To test this muscle specifically, the patient is positioned sitting or supine with the forearm positioned in complete pronation. The patient is asked to extend the wrist in an ulnar direction and to hold this position. Using one hand to stabilize the patient's forearm, the clinician uses the other hand to apply pressure to the posterior aspect of the patient's hand along the fifth metacarpal bone in a radial direction (Figure 9-73).

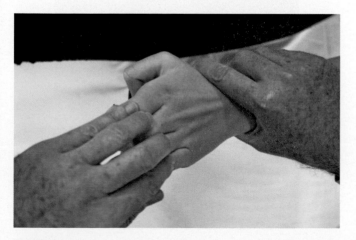

FIGURE 9-71 Test position for the extensor digitorum communis.

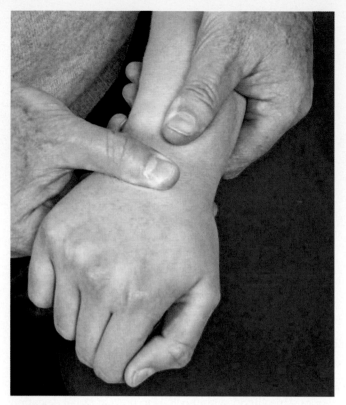

FIGURE 9-73 Test position for the extensor carpi ulnaris.

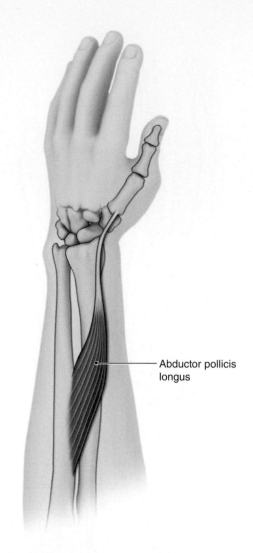

Abductor pollicis longus

FIGURE 9-74 Abductor pollicis longus muscle.

Deep Muscles

Abductor Pollicis Longus (APL). The APL arises from the dorsal surface of the proximal portion of the radius, ulna, and interosseous membrane and inserts on the ventral surface of the base of the first metacarpal (Figure 9-74). The APL functions in abduction, extension, and external rotation of the first metacarpal.

The APL is innervated by the posterior interosseous branch of the radial nerve. The synergists of this muscle include the FCR, extensor carpi radialis longus and brevis, APB, and EPB. The antagonists of this muscle include the FCU, ECU, FPL, FPB, and AP.

To specifically test this muscle, the patient is positioned sitting or supine. The patient is asked to abduct and slightly extend the thumb and to hold that position. Using one hand, the clinician stabilizes the patient's hand and uses the other hand to apply an adduction and flexion force against the lateral aspect of the distal first metacarpal (Figure 9-75).

Extensor Pollicis Brevis (EPB). The EPB arises from the posterior surface of the radius and interosseous membrane, just distal to the APL's origin. It inserts on the posterior surface of the thumb's proximal phalanx via the extensor expansion (Figure 9-76). The EPB functions to extend the proximal phalanx of the thumb.

The EPB is innervated by the posterior interosseous branch of the radial nerve. The synergists of this muscle include the FCR, ECRL, ECRB, APL, and APB. The antagonists of this muscle include the FCU, ECU, FPL, FPB, and AP.

To specifically test this muscle, the patient is positioned sitting or supine with the MCP joint of the thumb extended. Using one hand, the clinician stabilizes the patient's hand

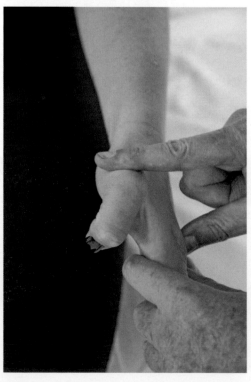

FIGURE 9-75 Test position for the abductor pollicis longus.

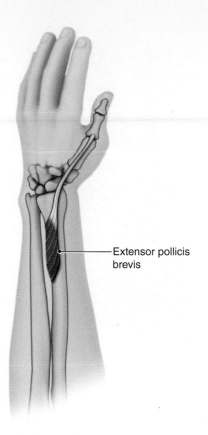

FIGURE 9-76 Extensor pollicis brevis muscle.

while using a finger from the other hand to apply a flexion force against the proximal phalanx of the thumb (Figure 9-77).

Extensor Pollicis Longus (EPL). The EPL arises from the posterior surface of the midportion of the ulna and

interosseous membrane. It inserts on the posterior surface of the thumb's distal phalanx via the extensor expansion (Figure 9-78). The EPL functions to extend the distal phalanx of the thumb and is thus involved in extension of the middle phalanx and the thumb's MCP joint.

The EPL is innervated by the posterior interosseous branch of the radial nerve. The synergists of this muscle include the APB, FPB, AP, ECRL, ECRB, ECU, EDC, EI, and first anterior interosseous. The antagonists of this muscle include the FPL, FPB, APB, FCR, FCU, palmaris longus, FDP, and FDS.

To specifically test this muscle, the patient is positioned in sitting or supine with the thumb extended. The clinician uses one hand to stabilize the patient's hand and uses the other to apply a flexion force to the distal phalanx of the posterior surface of the patient's thumb (Figure 9-79).

Extensor Indicis (EI). The EI arises from the posterior surface of the ulna, distal to the other deep muscles, and inserts on the extensor expansion of the index finger. The EI is involved in extension of the proximal phalanx of the index finger.

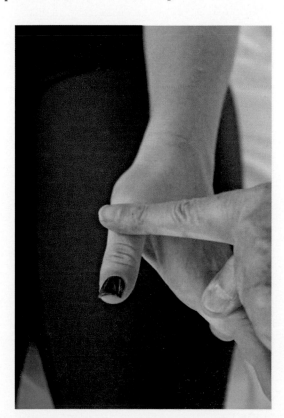

FIGURE 9-77 Test position for the extensor pollicis brevis.

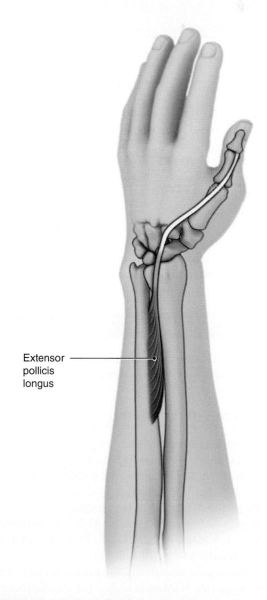

Extensor pollicis longus

FIGURE 9-78 Extensor pollicis longus muscle.

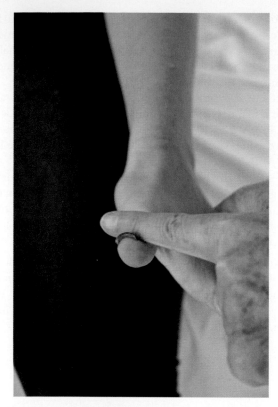

FIGURE 9-79 Test position for the extensor pollicis longus.

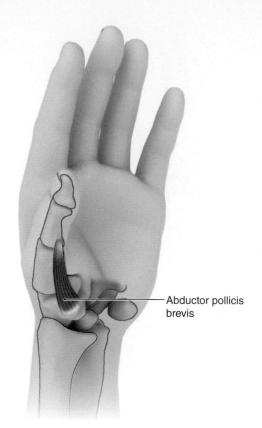

Abductor pollicis brevis

FIGURE 9-80 Abductor pollicis brevis muscle.

The EI is innervated by the posterior interosseous branch of the radial nerve. The synergists of this muscle include the extensor carpi radialis longus and brevis, ECU, EDC, EPL, lumbricals, and interossei. The antagonists of this muscle include the FCR, FCU, palmaris longus, FDP, FDS, FPL, lumbricals, and interossei.

To test this muscle specifically, the patient is positioned in sitting or supine and is asked to extend the index finger. The clinician uses one hand to stabilize the patient's hand and uses the other hand to generate a flexion force to the posterior aspect of the proximal phalanx of the index finger (see Figure 9-71).

MUSCLE TESTING OF THE HAND

The hand muscles originate and insert within the hand and are responsible for fine finger movements.

Short Muscles of the Thumb

Abductor Pollicis Brevis (APB). The APB arises from the flexor retinaculum and the trapezium bone and inserts on the radial aspect of the proximal phalanx of the thumb (Figure 9-80). The APB functions to abduct the first metacarpal and proximal phalanx of the thumb.

The median nerve innervates the APB. The synergists of this muscle include the APL, FPL, and FPB. The antagonists of this muscle include the APL and EPL.

To test this muscle specifically, the patient is positioned in sitting or supine and is asked to abduct the thumb. Using one hand, the clinician stabilizes the patient's wrist and hand and

uses the other hand to generate a downward force against the proximal phalanx of the patient's thumb (Figure 9-81).

Flexor Pollicis Brevis (FPB). The FPB arises from two heads. The superficial head arises from the flexor retinaculum

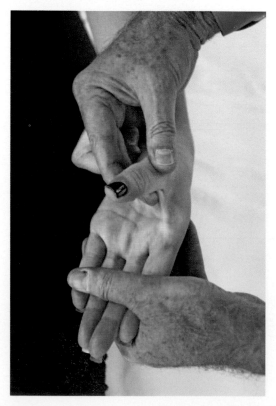

FIGURE 9-81 Test position for the abductor pollicis brevis.

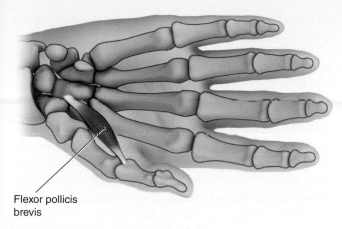

Flexor pollicis
brevis

FIGURE 9-82 Flexor pollicis brevis muscle.

and the trapezium bone, whereas the deep head arises from the floor of the carpal canal (Figure 9-82). The FPB inserts on the base of the proximal phalanx of the thumb. The FPB functions to flex the proximal phalanx of the thumb.

The FPB has dual innervation—the superficial head receives its innervation from the median nerve, whereas the deep head is innervated by the ulnar nerve. The synergists to this muscle include the FPL, APB, and AP. The antagonists of this muscle include the EPL and EPB.

To test this muscle specifically, the patient is positioned in sitting or supine and is asked to flex the thumb. Using one hand, the clinician stabilizes the patient's wrist and hand and uses the other hand to apply an extension force to the anterior surface of the proximal phalanx of the patient's thumb (Figure 9-83).

Opponens Pollicis (OP). The OP arises from the flexor retinaculum and the trapezium bone and inserts along the radial surface of the first metacarpal (Figure 9-84). The OP functions to flex, rotate, and slightly abduct the first metacarpal across the palm to allow for opposition to each of the other digits.

The median nerve innervates the OP. The synergists of this muscle include the FPB and AP. The antagonists include the EPL and EPB.

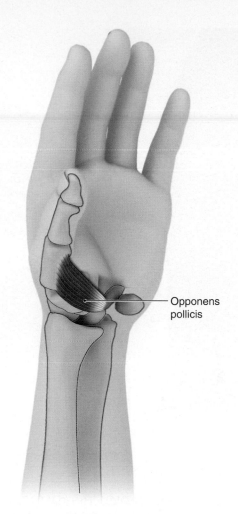

Opponens
pollicis

FIGURE 9-84 Opponens pollicis muscle.

To test this muscle specifically, the patient is positioned in sitting or supine and is asked to touch his or her thumb to the little finger (a combination of flexion, abduction, and slight internal rotation). The clinician uses one hand to stabilize the patient's wrist and hand. The other hand generates pressure to the thumb's metacarpal bone in an adduction and external rotation and extension direction (Figure 9-85).

Adductor Pollicis (AP). The AP arises from two heads. The transverse head originates from the anterior surface of the shaft of the third metacarpal, whereas the oblique head originates from the trapezium, trapezoid, and capitate bones (Figure 9-86) and the base of the second and third metacarpal bone. The AP inserts on the ulnar side of the base of the proximal phalanx of the thumb. The AP functions to adduct the carpometacarpal joint and adducts and assists in flexion of the MCP joints and thumb opposition. The AP may also assist in extending the interphalangeal joint.

The AP is innervated by the deep branch of the ulnar nerve. The synergists of this muscle include the EPL, FPL, FPB, OP, and first anterior interossei. The antagonists include the APB, APL, FPL, and EPB.

To test this muscle specifically, the patient is positioned in sitting or supine and is asked to move the thumb toward the palm. Using one hand, the clinician stabilizes the patient's wrist and hand while using the other to apply an abduction force to the inner aspect of the thumb (Figure 9-87).

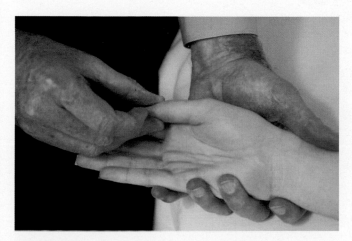

FIGURE 9-83 Test position for the flexor pollicis brevis.

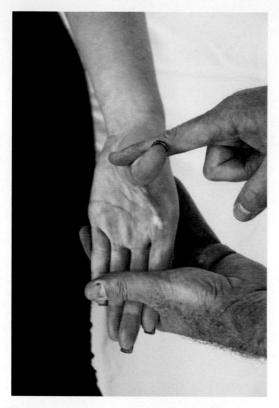

FIGURE 9-85 Test position for the opponens pollicis.

Short Muscles of the Fifth Digit

Abductor Digiti Minimi (ADM). The ADM arises from the pisiform bone and the tendon of the FCU. It inserts on the ulnar aspect of the base of the proximal phalanx of the fifth digit, together with the FDM brevis (Figure 9-88). The ADM functions to abduct the fifth digit.

The ADM is innervated by the deep branch of the ulnar nerve. The synergists for this muscle include the interossei, FDP, FDS, and fourth lumbrical. The antagonists to this muscle include the anterior interossei, EDC, and EDM.

To test this muscle specifically, the patient is positioned sitting or supine and is asked to abduct the little finger. The clinician uses one hand to stabilize the patient's wrist and hand and the other to apply an adduction force against the ulnar aspect of the middle phalanx of the patient's fifth digit (Figure 9-89).

Flexor Digiti Minimi (FDM). The FDM originates from the flexor retinaculum and the hook of the hamate bone (Figure 9-90). It inserts on the ulnar aspect of the base of the proximal phalanx of the fifth digit, together with the ADM. The FDM functions to flex the proximal phalanx of the fifth digit.

CLINICAL PEARL

Deep branches of the ulnar artery and nerve enter the thenar mass and course into the hand's deep region by passing between the ABD and the FDM.

The FDM is innervated by the deep branch of the ulnar nerve. The synergists for this muscle include the opponents digiti minimi (ODM), lumbricals 3 and 4, interossei, FDP, and FDS. The antagonists include the EDC and EDM.

To test this muscle specifically, the patient is positioned sitting or supine and is asked to flex the little finger at the MCP joint while maintaining the interphalangeal joint in extension. Using one hand, the clinician stabilizes the patient's hand while

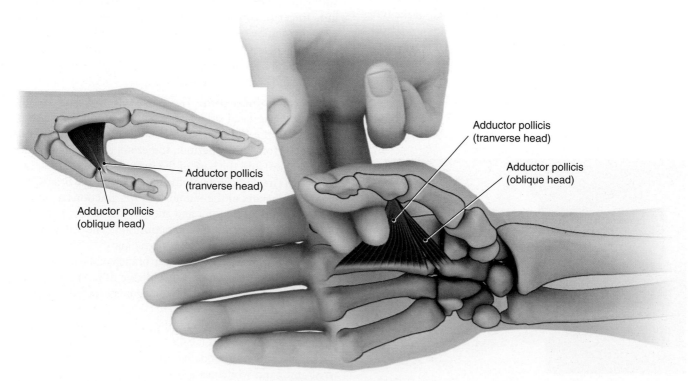

Adductor pollicis (tranverse head)

Adductor pollicis (oblique head)

Adductor pollicis (tranverse head)

Adductor pollicis (oblique head)

FIGURE 9-86 Adductor pollicis.

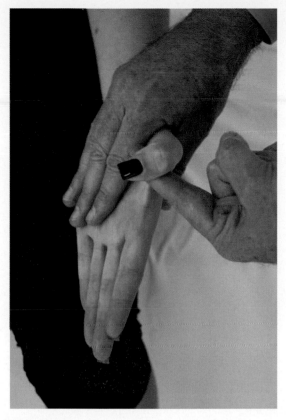

FIGURE 9-87 Test position for the adductor pollicis.

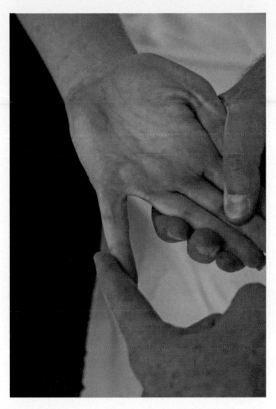

FIGURE 9-89 Test position for the abductor digiti minimi.

using the other to apply an extension force against the flexed proximal phalanx of the patient's fifth digit (Figure 9-91).

Opponens Digiti Minimi (ODM). The ODM arises from the flexor retinaculum and the hook of the hamate bone and inserts on the ulnar border of the shaft of the fifth metacarpal bone (Figure 9-92). The ODM functions to provide a small amount of flexion and external rotation of the fifth digit.

The ODM is innervated by the deep branch of the ulnar nerve. The synergists of this muscle include the FDM, ADM, fourth lumbricals, third and fourth anterior interossei, FDS, and FDP. The antagonists include the EDC, EDM, and ADM.

To test this muscle specifically, the patient is positioned in sitting or supine and is asked to cup the fifth metacarpal toward the thumb. Using one hand, the clinician stabilizes the patient's hand while using the index finger of the other hand to push against the first metacarpal of the fifth digit and apply a downward force (Figure 9-93).

Interosseous Muscles of the Hand

The interossei muscles of the hand are divided by anatomy and function into anterior (palmar) and posterior (dorsal) interossei.

Anterior Interossei. The three anterior (palmar) interossei have various origins and insertions (Figure 9-94). The first interosseus originates from the ulnar surface of the second metacarpal bone and inserts on the ulnar side of the proximal phalanx of the second digit. The second palmar interosseus arises from the radial side of the fourth metacarpal bone and inserts into the radial side of the proximal phalanx of the fourth digit. The third palmar interosseus originates from the radial side of the fifth metacarpal bone and inserts into the radial side of the proximal phalanx of the fifth digit. Each of the anterior interossei functions to adduct the digit to which it is attached toward the middle digit. The anterior interossei also function to extend the distal and then the middle phalanges.

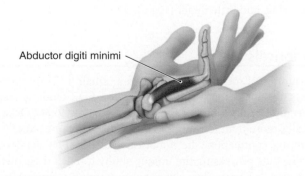

Abductor digiti minimi

FIGURE 9-88 Abductor digiti minimi muscle.

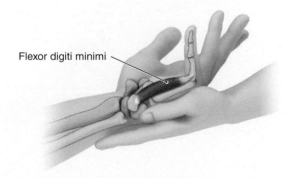

Flexor digiti minimi

FIGURE 9-90 Flexor digiti minimi muscle.

241

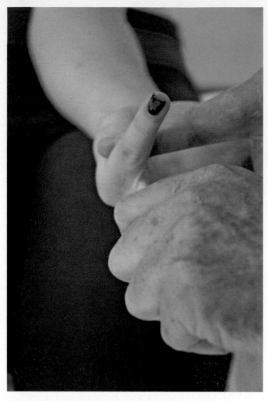

FIGURE 9-91 Test position for the flexor digiti minimi.

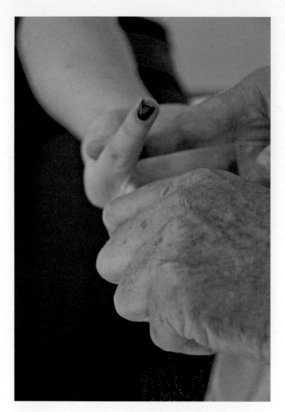

FIGURE 9-93 Test position for the opponens digit minimi.

The anterior interossei are innervated by the deep branch of the ulnar nerve. The synergists to the anterior interossei include the posterior interossei, lumbricals, FDP, FDS, EI, EDC, EDM, ADM, FDM, ODM, and AP. The antagonists to the anterior interossei include the posterior interossei, EDC, EI, EDM, ADM, FDP, FDS, and lumbricals.

To specifically test this muscle group, the patient is positioned sitting or supine with the digits not being tested stabilized and the finger being tested brought toward the midline. One by one, the clinician applies pressure in an abduction direction against the appropriate phalanx of the thumb, index, ring, and little finger (Figure 9-95).

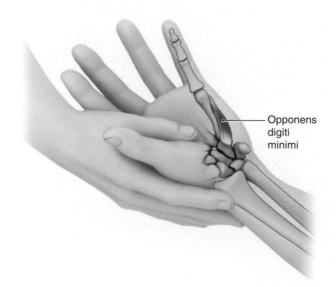

Opponens digiti minimi

FIGURE 9-92 Opponens digiti minimi muscle.

Posterior Interossei. The four posterior (dorsal) interossei have a varied origin and insertion similar to those of their anterior counterparts (see Figure 9-94). The posterior interossei originate via two heads from adjacent sides of the metacarpal bones. The first posterior interosseous muscle inserts into the radial side of the proximal phalanx of the second digit. The second inserts into the radial side of the proximal phalanx of the third digit. The third inserts into the ulnar side of the proximal phalanx of the third digit, and the fourth inserts into the ulnar side of the proximal phalanx of the fourth digit. The posterior interossei abduct the index, middle, and ring fingers from the midline of the hand.

The posterior interossei receive their innervation from the deep branch of the ulnar nerve.

To specifically test this muscle group, the patient is positioned sitting or supine with the digits not being tested stabilized and the finger being tested moved away from the midline. One by one, the clinician applies pressure in the direction of adduction against the appropriate phalanx of the thumb, index, ring, and little finger (Figure 9-96).

Lumbricals

The lumbrical muscles are usually four small intrinsic muscles of the hand that originate from the FDP tendons and insert into the dorsal hood apparatus (see Figure 9-94). Occasionally, more than four lumbricals are found in one hand.[112]

During contraction, the lumbricals pull the FDP tendons distally, thus possessing the unique ability to relax their own antagonist.[113] They perform interphalangeal joint extension with the MCP joint held in extension and assist in MCP flexion.[110]

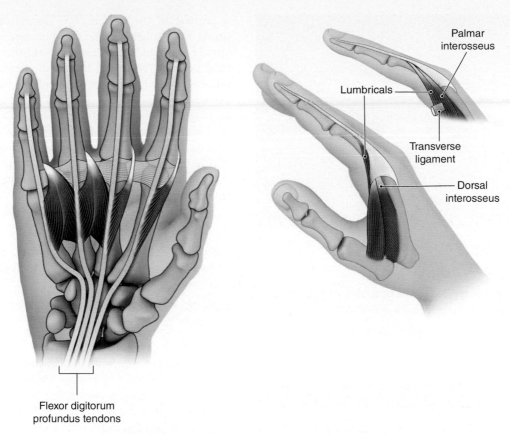

FIGURE 9-94 Lumbricals, anterior and posterior interossei.

The lumbrical muscles also serve an important role in the hand's proprioception, providing feedback about the position and movement of the hand and finger joints.[113]

CLINICAL PEARL

In instances of lumbrical spasm or contracture, attempts to flex the fingers via the FDP result in the transmission of force through the lumbricals into the extensor apparatus, producing extension rather than flexion.[113] A "lumbrical plus" deformity occurs if there is an excessive lumbrical force or an imbalance of opposing forces, which produces an exaggerated lumbrical action (ie, MCP joint flexion and interphalangeal joint extension).[113]

The lumbricals have dual innervation. Lumbricals I and II are innervated typically by the median nerve, whereas the third and fourth lumbricals are innervated by the ulnar nerve. The synergists for the lumbricals include the posterior interossei, FDP, FDS, ADM, FDM, ODM, EDC, extensor indices, and anterior interossei. The antagonists include the EDC, extensor indices, anterior interossei, FDP, and FDS.

To test this muscle group specifically, the patient is positioned in sitting or supine and is asked to place the hand into an intrinsic plus position (Figure 9-97) and hold a piece of paper. Using one hand, the clinician tries to pull a sheet of paper from the patient's grasp. The pressure is thus applied in two distinct phases:

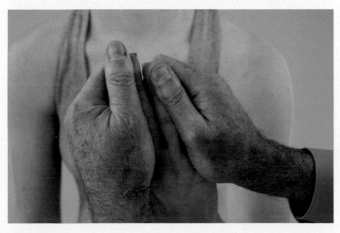

FIGURE 9-95 Test position for the anterior interossei.

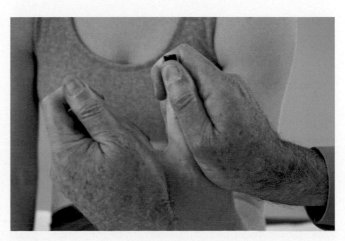

FIGURE 9-96 Test position for the posterior interossei.

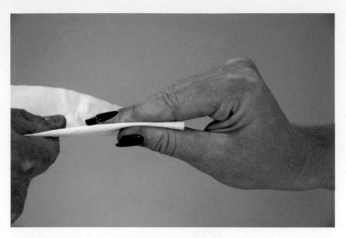

FIGURE 9-97 Test position for the lumbricals.

1. A flexion force is applied to the posterior surfaces of the distal and middle phalanges.
2. An extension force is applied to the anterior surfaces of the proximal phalanges.

MUSCLE TESTING OF THE HIP

The hip joint is surrounded by many muscles that accelerate, decelerate, and stabilize the hip joint. Indeed, 21 muscles cross the hip, providing both triplanar movement and stability between the femur and acetabulum.[114] Consequently, any abnormal performance of the hip muscles may alter the distribution of forces across the joint articular surfaces, potentially causing, or at least predisposing, degenerative changes in the articular cartilage, bone, and surrounding connective tissues.[114]

CLINICAL PEARL

Because the hip joint can move through a wide ROM, a muscle's line of pull may be altered with changing hip position, which makes describing a muscle's action difficult. For example, the gluteus medius orientation allows it to work as an internal rotator with the hip flexed, yet as a weak external rotator with the hip extended.[115] Similarly, the tensor fasciae latae (TFL) is a hip abductor and flexor, depending upon the hip position, while being a weak internal rotator in all positions.[77]

The hip muscles and their respective actions are outlined in Tables 9-6 and 9-7.

Iliopsoas. The iliopsoas muscle, formed by the iliacus and psoas major muscles (Figure 9-98), is the most powerful hip flexor. This muscle also functions as a weak adductor and external rotator of the hip. The iliopsoas attaches to the hip joint capsule, thereby affording it some support. Because the muscle spans both the axial and appendicular components of the skeleton, it also functions as a trunk flexor and affords an important element of vertical stability to the lumbar spine, especially when the hip is in full extension and passive tension

is greatest in the muscle.[114,116] Theoretically, a sufficiently strong and isolated bilateral contraction of any hip flexor muscle will rotate the femur toward the pelvis, the pelvis (and possibly the trunk) toward the femur, or both actions simultaneously.[114] The synergists of this muscle include the sartorius, pectineus, TFL, adductor brevis and longus, adductor magnus (anterior portion), gluteus minimus, rectus femoris, gluteus medius, gluteus maximus, piriformis, biceps femoris (long head), and gracilis. The antagonists of this muscle include the erector spinae, gluteus maximus, adductor magnus (posterior portion), gluteus medius, hamstrings, gluteus minimus, TFL, and sartorius.

To specifically test this muscle, the patient is positioned in supine or sitting:

▶ *Supine.* The patient's lower extremity is positioned in knee extension, slight hip abduction, and flexion of the hip (Figure 9-99).
▶ *Sitting.* With the knee flexed, the patient flexes the hip (Figure 9-100).

With both positions, the clinician applies pressure in the direction of hip extension and abduction while the patient attempts to prevent the motion. Caution should be taken to ensure that the patient does not externally rotate the femur, as this will cause the hip adductors to contract. Substitution or trick motions can include hip abduction and external rotation, hip abduction and internal rotation, or assistance from the rectus femoris. The gravity-minimized/eliminated position for this muscle is with the patient positioned in side lying with the extremity supported on a friction-free surface and the hip positioned in neutral rotation with the knee flexed to 90°.

Gluteus Maximus. The gluteus maximus (Figure 9-101) is the largest and most important hip extensor and external rotator of the hip. The muscle consists of a larger superficial and a deep portion. The inferior gluteal nerve, which innervates the muscle, is located on the deep portion.

The gluteus maximus is usually active only when the hip is flexed, such as during stair climbing or cycling or when hip extension is resisted.[117] The synergists for this muscle include the adductor magnus, gluteus medius, hamstrings, gluteus minimus, TFL, piriformis, sartorius, iliopsoas, adductor brevis and longus, pectineus, and gracilis. The antagonists of this muscle include the iliopsoas; pectineus; TFL; adductor magnus, brevis, and longus; gluteus medius and minimus; sartorius; rectus femoris; gracilis; and piriformis.

To specifically test this muscle, the patient is positioned in prone with the knee flexed to at least 90° (to eliminate hamstring activation), and the hip extended (Figure 9-102). The clinician applies a force over the l femur in the direction of hip flexion while the patient attempts to prevent the motion. Substitution or trick motions can include assistance from the hamstrings or an increase in lumbar lordosis. The gravity-minimized/eliminated position for this muscle is with the patient positioned in side lying with the extremity supported, the hip flexed to 90°, and the knee flexed.

Gluteus Medius. The gluteus medius (Figure 9-103) is critical for balancing the pelvis in the frontal plane during one-leg stance,[118] which accounts for approximately 60% of the

TABLE 9-6	Origin, Insertion, and Innervation of Muscles Acting across the Hip Joint		
Muscle	**Origin**	**Insertion**	**Innervation**
Adductor brevis	External aspect of the body and inferior ramus of the pubis	The line from the greater trochanter of the linea aspera of the femur	Obturator nerve
Adductor longus	In the angle between the pubic crest and the symphysis	The middle third of the linea aspera of the femur	Obturator nerve
Adductor magnus	Inferior ramus of pubis, ramus of ischium, and the inferolateral aspect of the ischial tuberosity	To the linea aspera and adductor tubercle of the femur	Obturator nerve and tibial portion of the sciatic nerve
Biceps femoris	The long head arises from the sacrotuberous ligament and posterior aspect of the ischial tuberosity. The short head does not act across the hip	On the lateral aspect of the head of the fibula, the lateral condyle of the tibial tuberosity, the lateral collateral ligament, and the deep fascia of the leg	The tibial portion of the sciatic nerve, S1
Gemelli (superior and inferior)	Superior–posterior (dorsal) surface of the ischial spine and inferior-upper part of the ischial tuberosity	Superior- and the inferior-medial surface of the greater trochanter	Sacral plexus
Gluteus maximus	Posterior gluteal line of the ilium, iliac crest, aponeurosis of the erector spinae, the posterior (dorsal) surface of the lower part of the sacrum, side of the coccyx, sacrotuberous ligament, and intermuscular fascia	Iliotibial tract of the fasciae latae and gluteal tuberosity of the femur	Inferior gluteal nerve
Gluteus medius	The ilium's outer surface between the iliac crest and the posterior gluteal line, anterior gluteal line, and fascia	The lateral surface of the greater trochanter	Superior gluteal nerve
Gluteus minimus	The ilium's outer surface between the anterior and inferior gluteal lines and the greater sciatic notch margin	On the anterior surface of the greater trochanter	Superior gluteal nerve
Gracilis	The body and inferior ramus of the pubis	The superior medial surface of the proximal tibia, just proximal to the tendon of the semitendinosus	Obturator nerve
Iliacus	Superior two-thirds of the iliac fossa and upper surface of the lateral part of the sacrum	Fibers converge with the tendon of the psoas major to the lesser trochanter	Femoral nerve
Obturator externus	Rami of the pubis, ramus of the ischium, and medial two-thirds of the obturator membrane's outer surface	Trochanteric fossa of the femur	Obturator nerve
Obturator internus	Internal surface of the anterolateral wall of the pelvis and obturator membrane	Medial surface of the greater trochanter	Sacral plexus
Pectineus	Pectineal line	Along a line extending from the lesser trochanter to the linea aspera	Femoral or obturator or accessory obturator nerves
Piriformis	The pelvic surface of the sacrum, the gluteal surface of the ilium, the capsule of the sacroiliac joint, and the sacrotuberous ligament	The upper border of the greater trochanter of the femur	Sacral plexus
Psoas major	Transverse processes of all the lumbar vertebrae bodies and intervertebral disks of the lumbar vertebrae	Lesser trochanter of the femur	Lumbar plexus
Quadratus femoris	Ischial body next to the ischial tuberosity	Quadrate tubercle on femur	Nerve to quadratus femoris
Rectus femoris	Two heads, from the anterior–inferior iliac spine, and a reflected head from the groove above the acetabulum	The upper border of the patella	Femoral nerve

(continued)

TABLE 9-6	Origin, Insertion, and Innervation of Muscles Acting across the Hip Joint (continued)		
Muscle	**Origin**	**Insertion**	**Innervation**
Sartorius	Anterior–superior iliac spine and notch below it	The upper part of the medial surface of the tibia in front of the gracilis	Femoral nerve
Semimembranosus	Ischial tuberosity	The posterior-medial aspect of the medial condyle of the tibia	Tibial nerve
Semitendinosus	Ischial tuberosity	The upper part of the tibia's medial surface behind the attachment of the sartorius and below that of the gracilis	Tibial nerve
Tensor fascia latae	The anterior part of the iliac crest's outer lip and the lateral surface of the anterior superior iliac spine	Iliotibial tract	Superior gluteal nerve

TABLE 9-7	Hip Actions and Muscles If in Anatomic Position	
Hip Action	**Prime Movers**	**Assistant Movers**
Flexors	Iliopsoas Sartorius Tensor fasciae latae Rectus femoris Pectineus Adductor longus	Adductor brevis Gracilis Gluteus minimus (anterior fibers)
Extensors	Gluteus maximus Semitendinosus Semimembranosus Biceps femoris (long head) Adductor magnus (posterior head)	Gluteus medius (middle and posterior fibers) Adductor magnus (anterior head)
Abductors	Gluteus medius (all fibers) Gluteus minimus (all fibers) Tensor fasciae latae	Sartorius Rectus femoris Piriformis
Adductors	Adductor magnus (anterior and posterior heads) Adductor longus Adductor brevis Gracilis Pectineus	Biceps femoris (long head) Gluteus maximus (posterior fibers) Quadratus lumborum Obturator externus
External rotators	Gluteus maximus Gemellus inferior Gemellus superior Obturator internus Quadratus femoris Piriformis (at less than 60° hip flexion)	Gluteus medius (posterior fibers) Gluteus minimus (posterior fibers) Biceps femoris (long head) Sartorius Obturator externus
Internal rotators	No prime movers	Semitendinosus Semimembranosus Gracilis Piriformis (at 90° hip flexion) Gluteus medius (anterior fibers) Adductor longus Adductor brevis Pectineus Adductor magnus (posterior head) Gluteus minimus (anterior fibers) Tensor fasciae latae

Data from Anderson LC, Blake DJ. The anatomy and biomechanics of the hip joint, *J Back Musculoskelet Rehabil* 1994 Jan 1;4(3):145-153 and Neumann DA. Kinesiology of the hip: a focus on muscular actions, *J Orthop Sports Phys Ther* 2010 Feb;40(2):82-94.

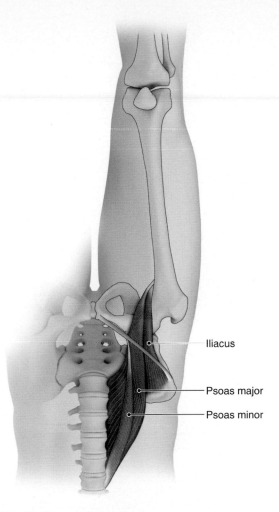

FIGURE 9-98 Iliopsoas muscle.

Iliacus

Psoas major

Psoas minor

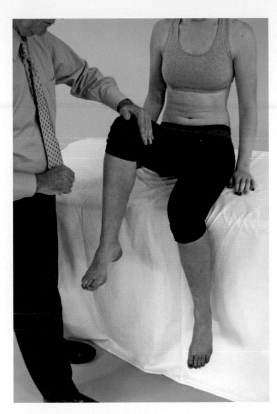

FIGURE 9-100 Test position for iliopsoas—patient sitting.

gait cycle.[119] During one-leg stance, approximately 3 times the body weight is transmitted to the hip joint, with two-thirds of that being generated by the hip abductor mechanism.[119] In addition to its role as a stabilizer, the gluteus medius also functions as a decelerator of hip adduction.

Because of its shape, the gluteus medius is known as the deltoid of the hip. The muscle can be divided into two functional parts: an anterior portion and a posterior portion. The anterior portion works to flex, abduct, and internally rotate the hip. The posterior portion extends and externally rotates the hip. The superior gluteal nerve and the superior and inferior gluteal vessels are located on the deep surface of this muscle. The synergists of this muscle include the gluteus maximus and minimus, TFL, sartorius, iliopsoas, rectus femoris, pectineus, adductor longus and brevis, adductor magnus, gracilis, hamstrings, and piriformis. The antagonists of the muscle include the TFL, sartorius, iliopsoas, rectus femoris, pectineus, adductor longus

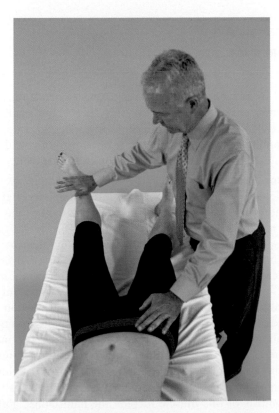

FIGURE 9-99 Test position for iliopsoas—patient supine.

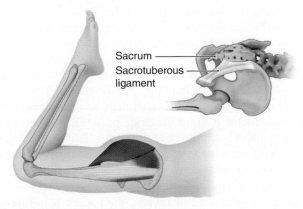

Sacrum
Sacrotuberous ligament

FIGURE 9-101 Gluteus maximus muscle.

247

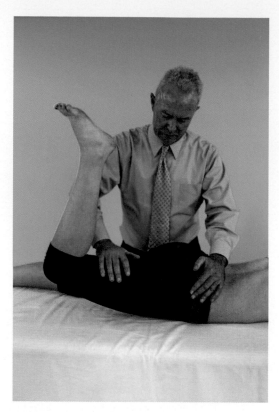

FIGURE 9-102 Test position for gluteus maximus.

and brevis, adductor magnus, gracilis, hamstrings, gluteus maximus, piriformis, and gluteus minimus.

To specifically test this muscle, the patient is positioned in side lying with the tested leg uppermost. The patient's hip is positioned in abduction, slight extension, and external rotation (Figure 9-104). While stabilizing the pelvis with one hand, the clinician applies a force of abduction and minimal flexion to the hip while the patient attempts to prevent the motion. Substitution or trick motions can include assistance from the quadratus lumborum and the lateral abdominals, which can tilt the pelvis laterally, giving the appearance of abduction; assistance from the gluteus maximus (superior fibers); or allowing the patient to roll slightly toward the supine position, which places the TFL in a more favorable position for hip abduction. The gravity-minimized/eliminated position for this muscle is with the patient positioned supine with the extremity on a friction-free surface.

Gluteus Minimus. The gluteus minimus (Figure 9-105) is a rather thin muscle situated between the gluteus medius muscle and the external surface of the ilium. The muscle is the major internal rotator of the femur. It receives assistance from the TFL, semitendinosus, semimembranosus, and gluteus medius.[117] The gluteus minimus also abducts the thigh and helps the gluteus medius with pelvic support. The synergists of this muscle include the gluteus medius, TFL, sartorius, iliopsoas, rectus femoris, pectineus, adductor longus and brevis, adductor magnus (anterior portion), gracilis, hamstrings, gluteus maximus, and piriformis. The antagonists of this muscle include the adductor longus and brevis, adductor magnus, gracilis, sartorius, iliopsoas, hamstrings, gluteus maximus, piriformis, pectineus, and gluteus medius.

To specifically test this muscle, the patient is positioned in side lying with the tested side uppermost. The patient is

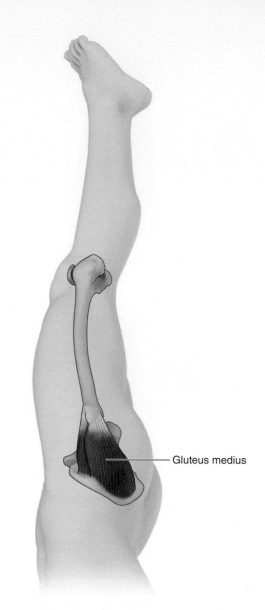

Gluteus medius

FIGURE 9-103 Gluteus medius muscle.

asked to abduct the hip while avoiding any rotation, flexion, or extension of the hip (Figure 9-106). While stabilizing the pelvis with one hand, the clinician applies an adduction and minimal extension force to the lower extemity while the patient attempts to prevent the motion from occurring.

Tensor Fasciae Latae (TFL). The TFL (Figure 9-107) envelops the muscles of the thigh and seldom works alone. In addition to counteracting the backward pull of the gluteus maximus on the iliotibial band (ITB), the TFL also flexes, abducts, and externally rotates the hip. The trochanteric bursa is found deep in this muscle as it passes over the greater trochanter and is a common source of lateral thigh pain.[120] The attachment of the TFL via the ITB to the anterolateral tibia provides a flexion moment in knee flexion and an extension moment in knee extension.[81] The synergists of this muscle include the iliopsoas, sartorius, pectineus, gluteus medius and minimus, gracilis, adductor longus and brevis, adductor magnus (anterior portion), gluteus maximus, piriformis, rectus femoris, and hamstrings. The antagonists of this muscle include the hamstrings, gluteus medius, adductor magnus, adductor longus and brevis,

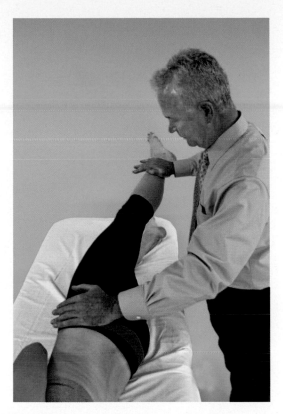

FIGURE 9-104 Test position for gluteus medius.

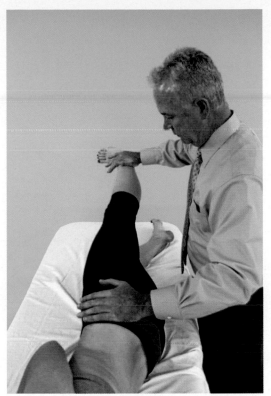

FIGURE 9-106 Test position for gluteus minimus.

pectineus, gracilis, gluteus maximus, piriformis, sartorius, iliopsoas, and piriformis.

To specifically test this muscle, the patient is positioned supine with the knee extended. The patient is asked to abduct, flex, and internally rotate the hip and to hold the position

(Figure 9-108) while the clinician applies resistance in the direction of hip extension and hip abduction (the rotational component is not resisted) on the distal tibia. Substitution or trick motions can include assistance from the hip flexors. The gravity-minimized/eliminated position for this muscle is with the patient positioned in long-sitting with the hips supported on the table, flexed to 45° and in neutral rotation, and the upper extremities supporting the trunk.

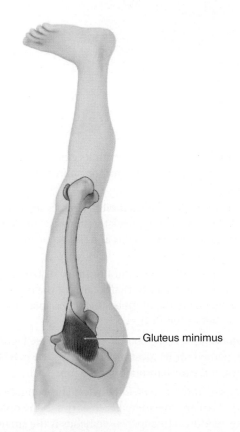

—— Gluteus minimus

FIGURE 9-105 Gluteus minimus muscle.

CLINICAL PEARL

The ITB or iliotibial tract begins as a wide covering of the superior and lateral aspects of the pelvis and thigh in continuity with the fasciae latae (see Figure 9-101). It inserts distal and lateral to the patella at the tubercle of Gerdy on the tibia's lateral condyle. Anteriorly, it attaches to the lateral border of the patella. Posteriorly, it is attached to the tendon of the biceps femoris. Laterally, it blends with an aponeurotic expansion from the vastus lateralis (see Muscles of the Knee).[121] Like the patella tendon, the ITB can be viewed as a ligament or a tendon. Its location adjacent to the center of rotation of the knee allows it to function as an anterolateral stabilizer of the knee in the frontal plane[122] and flex and extend the knee.[123,124] In knee flexion greater than 30°, the ITB becomes a weak knee flexor and an external rotator of the tibia.

During static standing, the primary function of the ITB is to maintain knee and hip extension, providing the thigh muscles an opportunity to rest. While walking or running, the ITB helps maintain the hip flexion and is a major supporter of the knee in squatting from full extension until 30° of flexion.

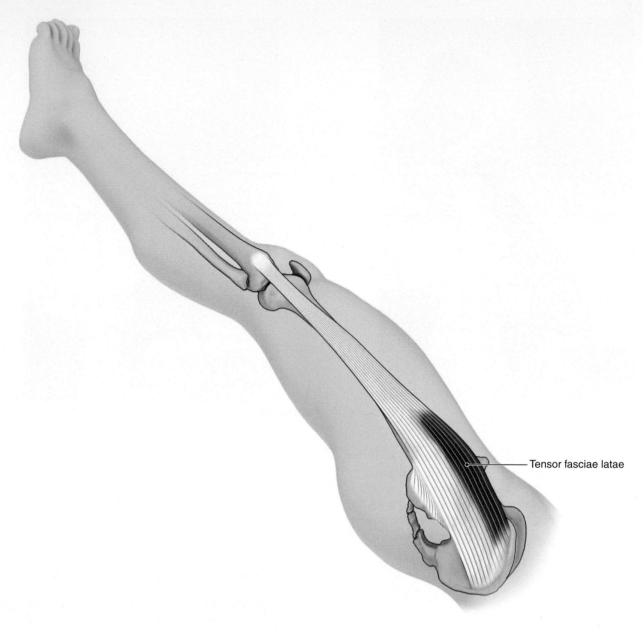

Tensor fasciae latae

FIGURE 9-107 Tensor fasciae latae muscle.

Rectus Femoris. The rectus femoris muscle (Figure 9-109), one of the four quadriceps muscles, is a two-joint muscle that arises from two tendons: one, the anterior or straight, from the anterior inferior iliac spine; the other, the posterior or reflected, from a groove above the brim of the acetabulum. The rectus femoris combines movements of flexion at the hip and extension at the knee. It functions more effectively as a hip flexor when the knee is flexed, such as when a person kicks a ball.[117] The specific test for this muscle is described in the section Muscle Testing of the Knee.

Hip External Rotators. The hip external rotators (Figure 9-110) include the piriformis, quadratus femoris, obturator internus, obturator externus, gemellus superior, and gemellus inferior.

▶ *Piriformis.* The piriformis (see Figure 9-110) is the most superior of the external rotators of the hip. The piriformis is an external rotator of the hip at less than 60° of hip flexion. At 90° of hip flexion, the piriformis reverses its muscle action, becoming an internal rotator and abductor of the hip.[125] The piriformis, with its close association with the sciatic nerve, can be a common source of buttock and leg pain.[126-129]

▶ *Quadratus femoris.* The quadratus femoris muscle (see Figure 9-110) is a flat, quadrilateral muscle located between the inferior gemellus and the superior aspect of the adductor magnus.

▶ *Obturator internus.* The obturator internus (see Figure 9-110) is normally an external rotator of the hip and an internal rotator of the ilium but becomes an abductor of the hip at 90° of hip flexion.[130]

▶ *Obturator externus.* The obturator externus (see Figure 9-110), named for its location external to the pelvis, is an adductor and external rotator of the hip.[131]

▶ *Superior and inferior gemelli muscles.* These muscles (see Figure 9-110) are considered accessories to the obturator internus tendon. The superior gemellus is the smaller of the two.[131]

250

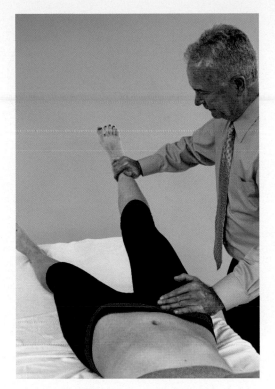

FIGURE 9-108 Test position for tensor fasciae latae.

CLINICAL PEARL

The quadratus femoris and the inferior gemellus share the same innervation (L4–L5).[131] The obturator internus and superior gemellus also share the same innervation (L5–S1).[131]

The external rotators of the hip are tested as a group. The patient is positioned in sitting with the thigh supported on the table and the lower leg over the table's edge. The patient rotates the hip externally such that the foot moves toward the contralateral side (Figure 9-111). Using one hand, the clinician stabilizes the patient's thigh while, with the other hand, generating a force of internal rotation of the hip by applying pressure to the inner aspect of the leg (see Figure 9-111).

CLINICAL PEARL

In a manner generally similar to the infraspinatus and teres minor at the G-H joint, the short external rotators of the hip also like to provide an important element of mechanical stability to the hip articulation.[119] Interestingly, the popular posterior surgical approach to a total hip arthroplasty used by some surgeons necessarily cuts through at least part of the hip's posterior capsule, potentially disrupting several of the short external rotators tendons.[114] Studies have reported a significant reduction in posterior hip dislocation incidence when the surgeon carefully repairs the posterior capsule and external rotator tendons.[114,132,133]

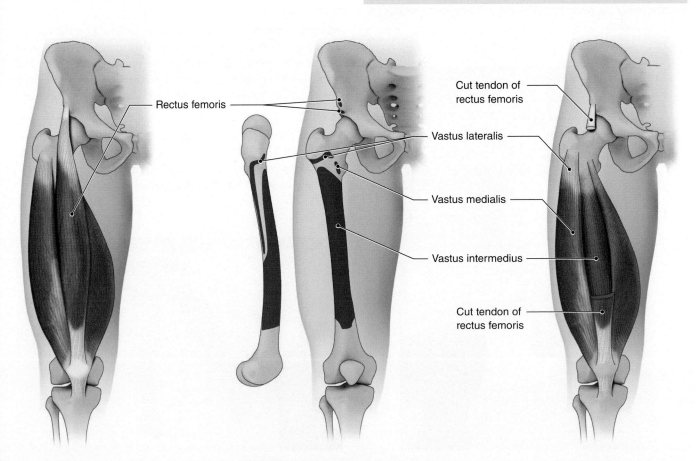

Rectus femoris

Cut tendon of rectus femoris

Vastus lateralis

Vastus medialis

Vastus intermedius

Cut tendon of rectus femoris

FIGURE 9-109 Quadriceps femoris muscle.

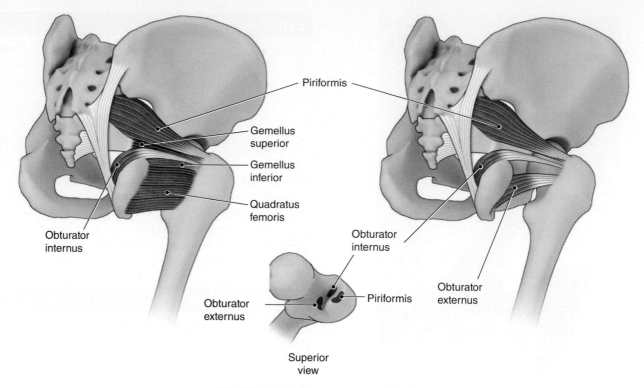

Piriformis

Gemellus superior

Gemellus inferior

Quadratus femoris

Obturator internus

Obturator internus

Obturator externus

Obturator externus

Obturator externus

Piriformis

Superior view

FIGURE 9-110 External rotators of the hip.

Hip Internal Rotators. The hip's internal rotators consist of the TFL, gluteus minimus, and gluteus medius (anterior fibers). These muscles are tested as a group. The patient is positioned in sitting with the thigh supported on the table and the lower leg over the table's edge. The patient rotates the

hip internally such that the foot moves away from the contralateral side. Using one hand, the clinician stabilizes the patient's thigh while, with the other hand, generating a force of external rotation of the hip by applying pressure to the outer aspect of the leg (Figure 9-112).

Hip Adductors. The hip adductors are found on the medial aspect of the joint (Figure 9-113). This muscle group's main action is to adduct the thigh in the open kinetic chain and stabilize the lower extremity to perturbation in the closed kinetic chain. Each muscle can also assist in hip flexion and rotation.[134]

▶ *Adductor magnus.* The adductor magnus (see Figure 9-113) is the most powerful adductor, and it is active to varying degrees in all hip motions except abduction. The posterior portion of the adductor magnus is

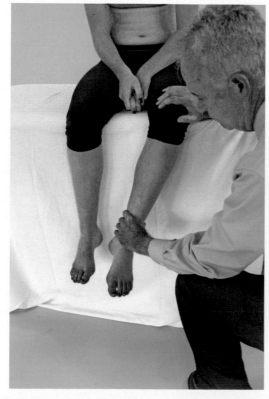

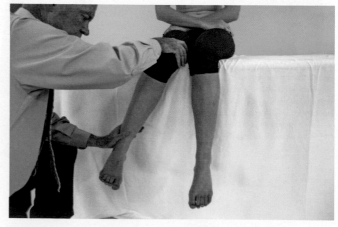

FIGURE 9-111 Test position for external rotators of the hip.

FIGURE 9-112 Test position for internal rotators of the hip.

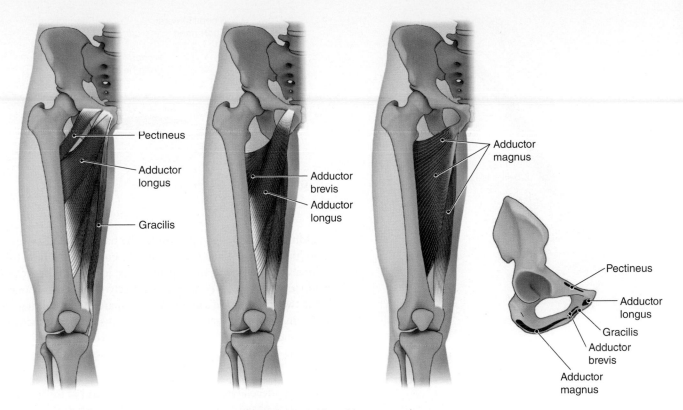

FIGURE 9-113 Hip adductor muscles.

sometimes considered functionally as a hamstring due to its anatomic alignment. Due to its size and anatomic alignment, the adductor magnus is less likely to be injured than the other hip adductors.[135]

▶ *Adductor longus.* During resisted adduction, the adductor longus (see Figure 9-113) is the most prominent adductor muscle and forms the medial border of the femoral triangle. The adductor longus also assists with external rotation, in extension, and internal rotation in other positions. The adductor longus is the most commonly strained adductor muscle.[136]

▶ *Gracilis.* The gracilis (see Figure 9-113) is the most superficial and medial of the hip adductor muscles. It is also the longest. The gracilis functions to adduct and flex the thigh and flex and internally rotate the leg.

▶ *Pectineus.* The pectineus (see Figure 9-113) is an adductor, flexor, and internal rotator of the hip. Like the iliopsoas, the pectineus attaches to and supports the joint capsule of the hip.

The other adductors of the hip include the adductor brevis and obturator externus muscles.

The hip adductors are tested as a group. The patient is positioned in side lying with the tested side closest to the table. The clinician supports the uppermost leg in hip abduction, and the patient is asked to adduct the lower leg off the table (Figure 9-114) while the clinician applies a downward force. The gravity-minimized/eliminated position for this muscle group is with the patient positioned supine.

Sartorius. The sartorius muscle (see Figure 9-115) is the longest muscle in the body. The sartorius is responsible for flexion, abduction, and external rotation of the hip, and some degree of knee flexion.[137] Given its numerous actions, this muscle has numerous synergists and antagonists.[136]

To specifically test this muscle, the patient is positioned supine. The patient is asked to externally rotate, abduct, and flex the hip, while also flexing the knee. The clinician places one hand on the patient's knee's outer aspect and uses the other hand to cup the patient's ankle. The patient is asked to prevent any motion as the clinician applies an extension, internal rotation, and adduction force to the hip while also applying an extension force to the knee (Figure 9-116).

Hamstrings. The hamstrings muscle group consists of the biceps femoris, the semimembranosus, and the semitendinosus.

▶ *Biceps femoris.* The long head of the biceps femoris (Figure 9-117) is the only portion that acts on the hip. It

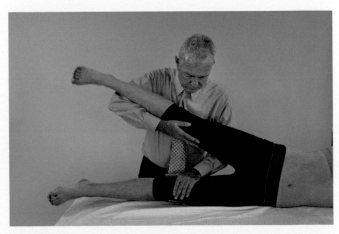

FIGURE 9-114 Test position for hip adductor muscle group.

253

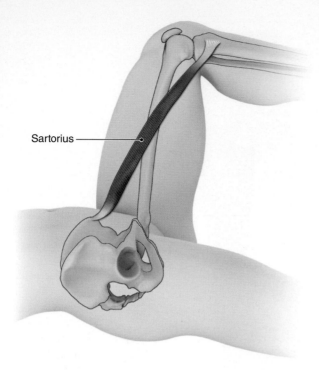

Sartorius

FIGURE 9-115 Sartorius muscle.

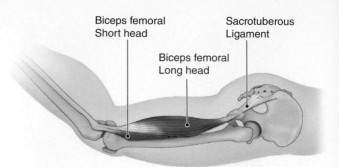

Biceps femoral Short head

Biceps femoral Long head

Sacrotuberous Ligament

FIGURE 9-117 Biceps femoris muscle.

is active during conditions that require lesser amounts of force, such as decelerating the limb at the end of the swing phase and during forceful hip extension.[138] As a whole, the biceps femoris extends the hip, flexes the knee, and externally rotates the tibia. The biceps femoris (53%) is the most commonly strained muscle of the hamstring complex.

▶ *Semimembranosus.* The semimembranosus (Figure 9-118), the most medial of the hamstrings, assists with hip extension, knee flexion, and internal rotation of the tibia.

▶ *Semitendinosus.* The semitendinosus (see Figure 9-118) has the longest tendinous insertion of the hamstrings. It assists with hip extension, knee flexion, and internal rotation of the tibia.

All three muscles of the hamstring complex (except for the short head of the biceps) work with the posterior adductor magnus and the gluteus maximus to extend the hip. In

addition to the actions just listed, the hamstrings also weakly adduct the hip. When the hamstrings contract as a unit, their forces are exerted at the hip and knee joints simultaneously; functionally, however, they can actively mobilize only one of the two joints at the same time. Compared with walking and jogging, running is stressful for the hamstrings and increases the high demands on their tendon attachments, especially during eccentric contractions. During running, the hamstrings have three main functions:

1. They decelerate knee extension at the end of the forward swing phase of the gait cycle. The hamstrings decelerate the forward momentum (ie, leg swing) at approximately 30° short of full knee extension through an eccentric contraction. This action helps provide dynamic stabilization to the weight-bearing knee.

2. At foot strike, the hamstrings elongate to facilitate hip extension through an eccentric contraction, thus further stabilizing the leg for weight-bearing.

3. The hamstrings help the gastrocnemius by paradoxically extending the knee during the running cycle's takeoff phase.

The specific tests for these muscles are described in the section Muscle Testing of the Knee.

MUSCLE TESTING OF THE KNEE

The major muscles that act on the knee joint complex are the quadriceps, the hamstrings (semimembranosus, semitendinosus, and biceps femoris), the gastrocnemius, the popliteus, and the hip adductors.

Quadriceps. The quadriceps muscles can act to extend the knee when the foot is off the ground, although more commonly, they work as decelerators, preventing the knee from buckling when the foot strikes the ground.[124,139] The four muscles that make up the quadriceps are the rectus femoris, the vastus intermedius, the vastus lateralis (VL), and the vastus medialis (Figure 9-109). The quadriceps tendon represents the convergence of all four muscle-tendon units, and it inserts at the anterior aspect of the patella's superior pole. The femoral nerve innervates the quadriceps muscle group.

▶ *Rectus femoris.* The rectus femoris (see Figure 9-109) is the only quadriceps muscle that crosses the hip joint. It originates at the anterior inferior iliac spine. The other

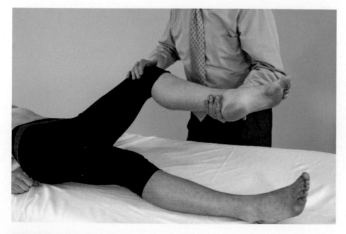

FIGURE 9-116 Test position for sartorius.

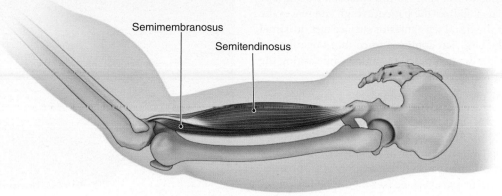

Semimembranosus

Semitendinosus

Right extrenity, posterolateral view

FIGURE 9-118 Semitendinosus and semimembranosus muscles.

quadriceps muscles originate on the femoral shaft. The line of pull of the rectus femoris, concerning the patella, is at an angle of about 5° with the femoral shaft.[124]

▶ *Vastus intermedius.* The vastus intermedius (see Figure 9-109) has its origin on the femur's proximal part, and its line of action is directly in line with the femur.

▶ *Vastus lateralis.* The VL (see Figure 9-109) comprises two functional parts: the VL and the vastus lateralis obliquus (VLO).[139] The VL has a line of pull of about 12–15° to the femur's long axis in the frontal plane, whereas the VLO has a pull of 38–48°.[124]

▶ *Vastus medialis.* The vastus medialis (see Figure 9-109) is composed of two functional parts that are anatomically distinct[139]: the vastus medialis obliquus (VMO) and the vastus medialis proper or longus (VML).[140]

■ *Vastus medialis obliquus.* The VMO (see Figure 9-109) arises from the adductor magnus tendon.[141] The insertion site of the normal VMO is the medial border of the patella, approximately one-third to one-half of the way down from the proximal pole. If the VMO remains proximal to the proximal pole of the patella and does not reach the patella, there is an increased potential for patellar malalignment.[142]

The vector of the VMO is directed medially, and it forms an angle of 50–55° with the mechanical axis of the leg.[139,141,143,144] The VMO is least active in the fully extended position[145-147] and plays little role in extending the knee, acting instead to realign the patella medially during the extension maneuver. It is active in this function throughout the whole range of extension.

According to Fox,[148] the vastus medialis is the weakest of the quadriceps group and appears to be the first muscle of the quadriceps group to atrophy and the last to rehabilitate.[149] The normal VMO/VL ratio of EMG activity in standing knee extension from 30° to 0° is 1:1,[150] but in patients with patellofemoral pain, the activity in the VMO decreases significantly; instead of being tonically active, it becomes phasic in action.[151] The presence of swelling also inhibits the VMO, and it requires almost half of the volume of effusion to inhibit the VMO as it does to inhibit the rectus femoris and VL muscles.[152]

The VMO is frequently innervated independently from the rest of the quadriceps by a separate branch from the femoral nerve.[139]

■ *Vastus medialis longus.* The VML originates from the upper femur's medial aspect and inserts anteriorly into the quadriceps tendon, giving it a line of action of approximately 15–17° off the long axis of the femur in the frontal plane.[124]

Because the quadriceps group is aligned anatomically with the femoral shaft and not with the lower extremity's mechanical axis, any quadriceps muscle contraction (regardless of knee flexion angle) results in compressive forces acting on the patellofemoral joint.[153] The quadriceps group is particularly important when climbing stairs, walking up inclines, or standing from a seated position.

This muscle group's synergists include the gluteus maximus, TFL, iliopsoas, pectineus, gluteus minimus, gluteus medius sartorius, adductor brevis and longus, and adductor magnus (anterior portion). This muscle group's antagonists include the hamstrings, gracilis, sartorius, popliteus, gastrocnemius, TFL, gluteus maximus, adductor magnus (posterior portion), piriformis, and gluteus medius.

To specifically test this muscle group, the patient is positioned sitting at the edge of the table with the thigh supported and the leg hanging over the edge (Figure 9-119). The patient is asked to lean backward to relax the hamstrings and then to

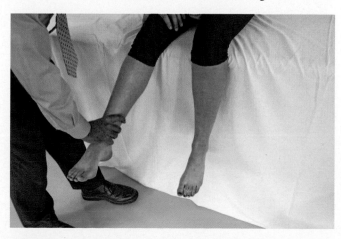

FIGURE 9-119 Test position for the quadriceps femoris group.

255

straighten the knee to just short of full extension. Using one hand, the clinician stabilizes the patient's thigh and places the other hand over the distal leg's anterior surface just proximal to the ankle. The clinician applies a force into knee flexion with the hand slightly proximal to the ankle while asking the patient to resist the movement.

Hamstrings. As previously mentioned, the hamstrings primarily function to extend the hip and flex the knee.

▶ *Semimembranosus.* At the knee, this muscle inserts on the posterior medial aspect of the medial condyle of the tibia and has an important expansion that reinforces the posteromedial corner of the knee capsule (see Figure 9-118). During knee flexion, the semimembranosus pulls the meniscus posteriorly and internally rotates the tibia on the femur.

▶ *Semitendinosus.* Passing over the MCL, the semitendinosus (see Figure 9-118) inserts into the medial surface of the tibia and deep fascia of the lower leg, distal to the attachment of the gracilis, and posterior to the attachment of the sartorius. These three structures are collectively called the *pes anserinus* ("goose's foot") at this point.

▶ *Biceps femoris.* The biceps femoris (see Figure 9-117) inserts on the tibia's lateral condyle and the fibular head. The superficial layer of the common tendon has been identified as the major force creating external tibial rotation and controlling internal rotation of the femur.[154] The pull of the biceps on the tibia retracts the joint capsule and pulls the iliotibial tract posteriorly, keeping it taut throughout flexion.

The hamstrings are specifically tested based on their anatomy—the semimembranosus and semitendinosus are tested together, and the biceps femoris is tested separately. The gravity-minimized/eliminated position for this muscle group is with the patient positioned in side lying with the tested leg on a friction-free surface.

▶ To specifically test the semimembranosus and semitendinosus, the patient is positioned in prone with the knee flexed to approximately 45°. The tibia is internally rotated so that the toes are pointing inward (Figure 9-120). Using one hand to stabilize the patient's thigh, the clinician places the other hand just proximal to the ankle on the posterior aspect of the patient's leg and applies a force

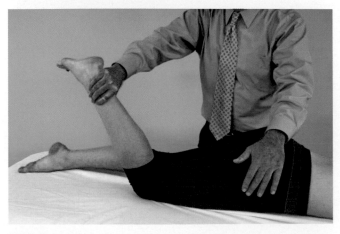

FIGURE 9-120 Test position for the biceps femoris.

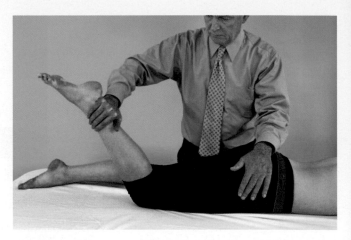

FIGURE 9-121 Test position for the semitendinosus and semimembranosus.

into knee extension while asking the patient to resist the motion (see Figure 9-120).

▶ To specifically test the biceps femoris, the patient is positioned in prone with the knee flexed to approximately 45°, and the tibia in slight external rotation so that the toes are pointing outward (Figure 9-121). Using one hand to stabilize the patient's thigh, the clinician places the other hand just proximal to the ankle on the posterior aspect of the patient's leg and applies a force into knee extension while asking the patient to resist the motion (see Figure 9-121).

Gastrocnemius. The gastrocnemius originates from above the knee by two heads, each head connected to a femoral condyle and the joint capsule (Figure 9-122). Approximately halfway down the leg, the gastrocnemius muscles blend to form an aponeurosis. As the aponeurosis progressively contracts, it accepts the soleus tendon, a flat, broad muscle deep to the gastrocnemius. The aponeurosis and the soleus tendon end in a flat tendon called the Achilles tendon, which attaches to the calcaneus's posterior aspect. The two heads of the gastrocnemius and the soleus are collectively known as the *triceps surae.*

At the knee, the gastrocnemius functions to flex or extend the knee, depending on whether the lower extremity is weight-bearing or not. Kendall and colleagues[155] have proposed that a weakness of the gastrocnemius may cause knee hyperextension.

In addition, it has been proposed that the gastrocnemius acts as an antagonist of the anterior cruciate ligament (ACL), exerting an anteriorly directed pull on the tibia throughout the range of knee flexion–extension motion, particularly when the knee is near extension.[156,157]

The specific test for this muscle is described in the Muscles of the Leg and Foot section later.

Popliteus. The popliteus (Figure 9-123) originates from the lateral femoral condyle near the LCL. The muscle has several attachments, including the lateral aspect of the lateral femoral condyle, the posterior-medial aspect of the fibular head, and the posterior horn of the lateral meniscus.[158] The larger base of this triangular muscle inserts obliquely into the posterosuperior part of the tibia above the soleal line. The muscle has several important functions, including reinforcing the posterior third of the lateral capsular ligament[159] and the unlocking

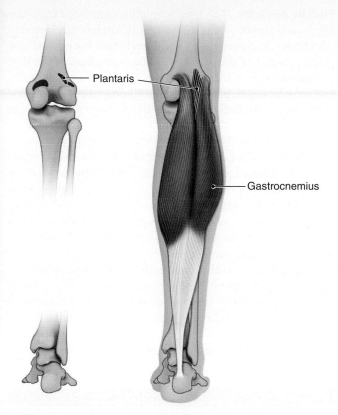

Plantaris

Gastrocnemius

FIGURE 9-122 Gastrocnemius and plantaris muscles.

of the knee during flexion from terminal knee extension during gait. It performs this latter task by internally rotating the tibia on the femur, preventing impingement of the posterior horn of the lateral meniscus by drawing it posteriorly, and, with the posterior cruciate ligament, preventing a posterior glide of the tibia.[159,162] Because knee joint injury frequently involves some component of transverse plane rotation and the popliteus muscle has been described as an important, primary, dynamic, transverse plane, rotatory knee-joint stabilizer, an understanding of its function concerning other posterolateral knee joint structures is important.[163] Attached to the popliteus tendon is the popliteofibular ligament, which forms a strong attachment between the popliteal tendon and the fibula. This ligament adds to posterolateral stability.[164-167]

> ### CLINICAL PEARL
>
> A medial portion of the popliteus penetrates the joint, becoming intracapsular with the lateral meniscus. This part of the popliteus tendon is pain-sensitive, and an injury here can often mimic a meniscal injury on the lateral aspect of the joint line.[168] Differentiation between these two lesions can be elucidated with the reproduction of pain with resisted knee flexion in an extended and externally rotated tibial position if the popliteus is involved.

The tibial nerve innervates the popliteus muscle. This muscle's synergists include the hamstrings, gracilis, sartorius, gastrocnemius, and TFL. The antagonists of this muscle include the biceps femoris and the quadriceps.

To test this muscle specifically, the patient is positioned in sitting with the knee flexed to 90°. The patient is asked to internally rotate the tibia (Figure 9-124). There is no

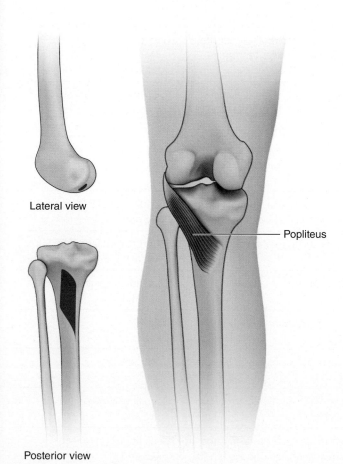

Lateral view

Popliteus

Posterior view

FIGURE 9-123 Popliteus muscle.

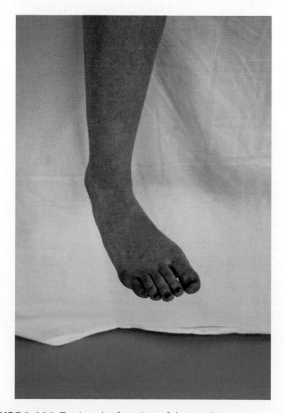

FIGURE 9-124 Testing the function of the popliteus.

resistance applied for this test—the test is used to determine whether the muscle is active and capable of internally rotating the tibia.

Tensor Fasciae Latae (TFL). In addition to its actions at the hip, the TFL is also a weak extensor of the knee, but only when the knee is already extended. The specific test for this muscle is described in the Muscles of the Hip section.

MUSCLE TESTING OF THE LEG AND FOOT

Extrinsic Muscles of the Leg and Foot

The foot's extrinsic muscles (Table 9-8) can be divided into anterior, posterior superficial, posterior deep, and lateral compartments.

Anterior Compartment

This compartment contains the dorsiflexors (extensors) of the foot. These include the tibialis anterior, extensor digitorum longus, extensor hallucis longus, and fibularis (peroneus) tertius.

Tibialis Anterior. The tibialis anterior originates from the upper two-thirds of the tibia's lateral surface, interosseous membrane, and deep fascia and inserts into the medial and plantar surface of the medial cuneiform and base of the first metatarsal bone of the foot (Figure 9-125). The tibialis anterior muscle, which is the first large tendon palpated anterior to the medial malleolus, produces the motion of dorsiflexion and inversion.

The tibialis anterior is innervated by the deep fibular (peroneal) nerve. The synergists of this muscle include the extensor digitorum longus, extensor hallucis longus, fibularis tertius, tibialis posterior, flexor digitorum longus (FDL), flexor hallucis longus (FHL), gastrocnemius, and soleus. The antagonists for this muscle include the tibialis posterior, fibularis longus and brevis, gastrocnemius, soleus, FDL, FHL, fibularis tertius, and extensor digitorum longus.

To specifically test this muscle, the patient is positioned in supine or sitting, and the patient's foot is positioned in dorsiflexion and inversion, with the great toe pointing downward (to minimize activation of the extensor hallucis longus). The knee must remain flexed during the test to allow complete dorsiflexion. Using one hand, the leg is stabilized by the

TABLE 9-8	Extrinsic Muscle Attachments and Innervation		
Muscle	**Proximal**	**Distal**	**Innervation**
Gastrocnemius	Medial and lateral condyle of the femur	The posterior surface of the calcaneus through the Achilles tendon	Tibial (S1-S2)
Plantaris	Lateral supracondylar line of femur	The posterior surface of the calcaneus through the Achilles tendon	Tibial (S1-S2)
Soleus	Head of fibula, the proximal third of the shaft, the soleal line, and the midshaft of the posterior tibia	The posterior surface of the calcaneus through the Achilles tendon	Tibial (S1-S2)
Tibialis anterior	Distal to the lateral tibial condyle, proximal half of lateral tibial shaft, and interosseous membrane	First cuneiform bone, medial and plantar surfaces, and base of first metatarsal	Deep fibular (peroneal) L4, (L5), S1
Tibialis posterior	The posterior surface of the tibia, proximal two-thirds posterior of fibula, and interosseous membrane	Tuberosity of navicular bone and tendinous expansion to other tarsals and metatarsals	Tibial (L4 and L5)
Fibularis (peroneus) longus	Lateral condyle of tibia, head, and proximal two-thirds of fibula	Base of first metatarsal and first cuneiform, lateral side	Superficial fibular (peroneal) (L5 and S1)
Fibularis (peroneus) brevis	Distal two-thirds of lateral fibular shaft	Tuberosity of fifth metatarsal	Superficial fibular (peroneal) (L5 and S1)
Fibularis (peroneus) tertius	Lateral slip from extensor digitorum longus	Tuberosity of fifth metatarsal	Deep fibular (peroneal) (L5 and S1)
Flexor hallucis longus	Posterior distal two-thirds fibula	The base of the distal phalanx of the great toe	Tibial (S2-S3)
Flexor digitorum longus	Middle three-fifths of the posterior tibia	The base of distal phalanx of lateral four toes	Tibial (S2-S3)
Extensor hallucis longus	The middle half of the anterior shaft of the fibula	The base of the distal phalanx of the great toe	Deep fibular (peroneal) (L5 and S1)
Extensor digitorum longus	Lateral condyle of tibia, proximal anterior surface of shaft of fibula	One tendon to each lateral four toes, to the middle phalanx, and extending to distal phalanges	Deep fibular (peroneal) (L5 and S1)

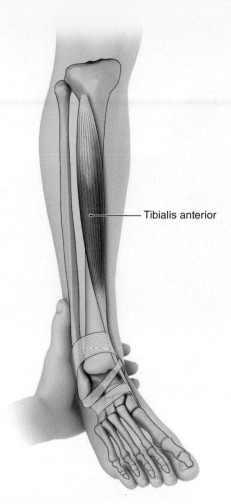

FIGURE 9-125 Tibialis anterior muscle.

Tibialis anterior

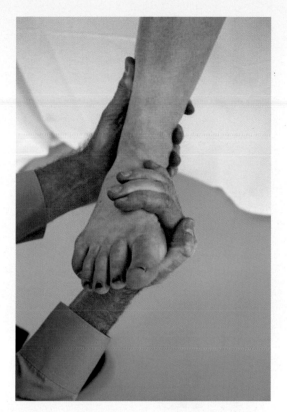

FIGURE 9-126 Testing position for tibialis anterior.

clinician, while resistance is applied to the medial posterior aspect of the forefoot in an inferior/lateral direction into plantarflexion and eversion (Figure 9-126).

Extensor Digitorum Longus (EDL). The EDL arises from the lateral condyle of the tibia, the proximal three-fourths of the anterior surface of the fibula's body, the proximal portion of the interosseous membrane, the deep fascia, and the adjacent intermuscular septa (Figure 9-127). The muscle divides into four slips that insert into the middle and distal phalanges of the lateral four toes. The EDL functions to produce ankle dorsiflexion, foot eversion, and extension of the metatarsophalangeal (MTP), proximal, and DIP joints of the lateral four toes.

The EDL is innervated by the deep fibular (peroneal) nerve. The synergists of this muscle include the extensor digitorum brevis, extensor hallucis longus, tibialis anterior, fibularis tertius, and fibularis longus and brevis. The antagonists of this muscle include the FDL, lumbricals, anterior interossei, posterior interossei, tibialis posterior, flexor digitorum brevis, gastrocnemius, soleus, FHL, fibularis longus and brevis, tibialis anterior, and extensor hallucis longus.

To test this muscle specifically, the patient is positioned sitting or supine, and is asked to extend the toes. Using one hand to stabilize the metatarsals and keeping the foot in slight plantarflexion, the clinician uses the other hand to apply force against the proximal phalanges of toes 2–5 in the direction of toe flexion (Figure 9-128).

Extensor Hallucis Longus (EHL). The EHL arises from the anterior, middle third of the surface of the fibula and interosseous membrane. As the muscle fibers descend, they become a tendon that inserts on the base of the great toe's distal phalanx (Figure 9-129). The EHL functions to extend the great toe and dorsiflex the foot, assisting with foot inversion.

The EHL is innervated by the deep fibular (peroneal) nerve. The synergists of this muscle include the extensor digitorum brevis, tibialis anterior, extensor digitorum longus, and fibularis tertius. The antagonists of this muscle include the FHL, gastrocnemius, soleus, tibialis posterior, FDL, FHL, fibularis longus and brevis, and abductor hallucis.

To test this muscle specifically, the patient is positioned supine or sitting, and the ankle is positioned in a neutral position. The patient is asked to extend the MTP and interphalangeal joints of the great toe and hold a position while the clinician applies pressure on the distal phalanx in a plantarflexion direction (Figure 9-130).

Fibularis (Peroneus) Tertius. The fibularis tertius arises from the lower third of the anterior surface of the fibula, the lower part of the interosseous membrane, and the adjacent intermuscular septum. Working alone, the muscle functions to provide ankle dorsiflexion and foot eversion.

The fibularis tertius is innervated by the deep fibular (peroneal) nerve. The synergists for this muscle include the extensor digitorum longus, extensor hallucis longus, tibialis anterior, and fibularis longus and brevis. The antagonists of this muscle include the FDL, tibialis posterior, gastrocnemius, soleus, FHL, fibularis longus and brevis, tibialis anterior, and extensor hallucis longus.

To test this muscle specifically, the patient is positioned sitting or supine, and the patient is asked to dorsiflex and then

259

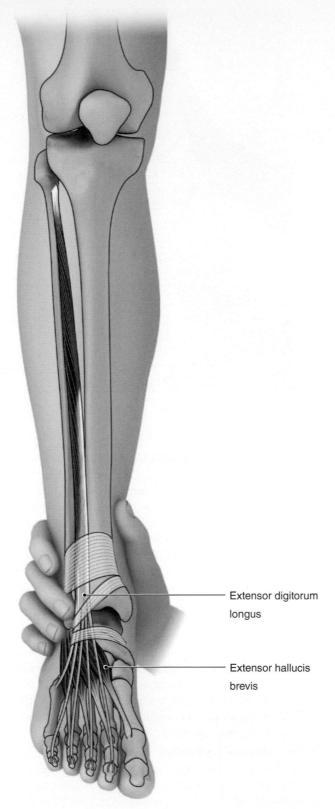

FIGURE 9-127 Extensor digitorum longus and hallucis brevis muscles.

Extensor digitorum longus

Extensor hallucis brevis

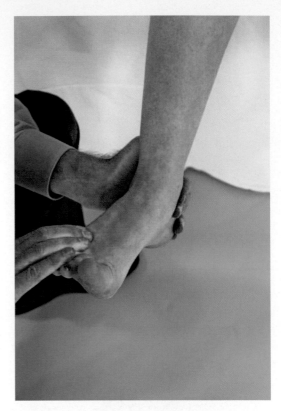

FIGURE 9-128 Test position for extensor digitorum longus.

Posterior Superficial Compartment

This compartment, located posterior to the interosseous membrane, contains the calf muscles that plantarflex the foot. These include the gastrocnemius, soleus (Figure 9-132), and plantaris muscles (see Figure 9-122).

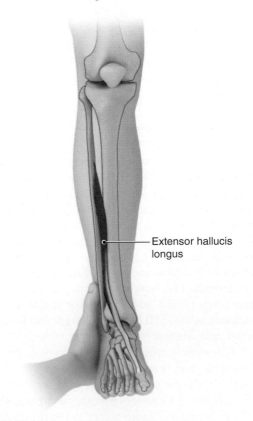

Extensor hallucis longus

FIGURE 9-129 Extensor hallucis longus muscles.

evert the foot (Figure 9-131). While using one hand to stabilize the patient's lower leg, the clinician uses the other hand to apply pressure along the dorsal and lateral aspects of the foot into a plantarflexion and inversion direction while asking the patient to prevent the motion.

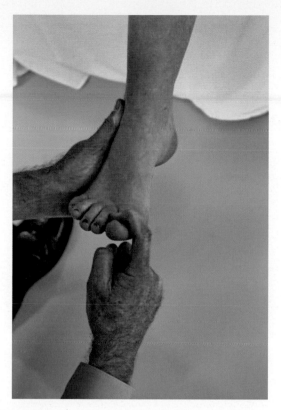

FIGURE 9-130 Test position for the extensor hallucis longus.

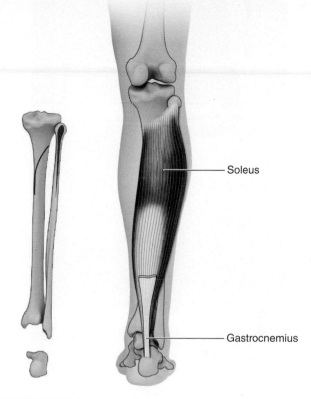

FIGURE 9-132 Soleus muscle.

Gastrocnemius. The two heads of the gastrocnemius arise from the posterior aspects of the distal femur (see Figure 9-122).[169] As the two muscles descend, they form the Achilles tendon along with the soleus muscle. The Achilles tendon courses distally to attach about three-quarters of an inch below the superior portion of the os calcis, on the medial aspect of the calcaneus. The medial head of the gastrocnemius is by far the largest component and, according to electromyographic studies, is the most active of the two during running.[170,171]

> **CLINICAL PEARL**
>
> The Achilles tendon is formed from the conjoint tendons of the gastrocnemius and soleus muscles. The fibers from the gastrocnemius and soleus interweave and twist as they descend, producing an area of high stress 2–6 cm above the distal tendon insertion.[172] A region of relative avascularity exists in the same area,[173] which correlates well with the site of some Achilles tendon injuries, including complete spontaneous rupture.[170,174,175] The Achilles tendon is the thickest, strongest tendon in the body.[169]

The gastrocnemius functions to provide ankle plantarflexion, knee flexion, and mild ankle inversion.

The tibial nerve innervates the gastrocnemius. The synergists of this muscle include the FDL, tibialis posterior, flexes hallucis longus, fibularis longus and brevis, soleus, hamstrings, gracilis, sartorius, TFL, popliteus, tibialis anterior, and extensor hallucis longus. The antagonists of this muscle include the extensor digitorum longus, extensor hallucis longus, tibialis anterior, fibularis tertius, quadriceps, and peroneus longus and brevis.

To specifically test the gastrocnemius, the patient is positioned standing on one leg, holding onto something for

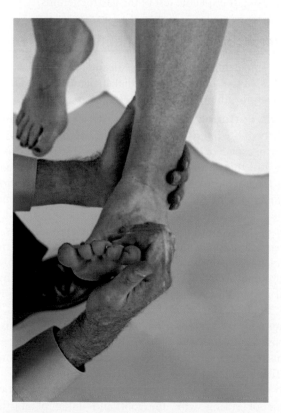

FIGURE 9-131 Test position for the peroneus tertius.

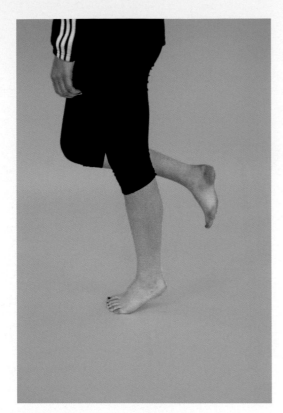

FIGURE 9-133 Test position for the gastrocnemius.

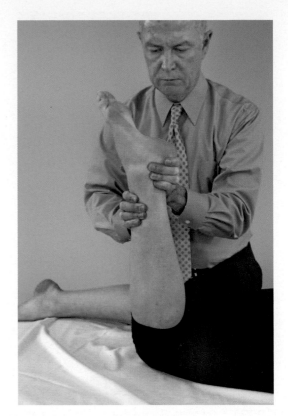

FIGURE 9-134 Test position for the soleus.

balance. Keeping the knee straight, the patient is asked to raise up on the toes (Figure 9-133). For a normal grading, the patient should be able to repeat this 10 times.

Soleus. The soleus muscle arises from the posterior proximal one-third of the fibula and the middle third of the tibia (see Figure 9-132). It conjoins with the gastrocnemius tendon to form the Achilles tendon. The soleus muscle, which is innervated by the tibial nerve, produces ankle plantarflexion. The synergists of this muscle include the FDL, tibialis posterior, FHL, fibularis longus and brevis, gastrocnemius, tibialis anterior, and extensor hallucis longus. The antagonists of this muscle include the extensor digitorum longus, extensor hallucis longus, tibialis anterior, fibularis tertius, and fibularis longus and brevis.

> ### CLINICAL PEARL
>
> The soleus, unlike the gastrocnemius, does not cross the knee joint and is subject to early disuse atrophy with undertraining and/or immobilization.[170]

To test this muscle specifically, the patient is positioned prone with the knee flexed to 90°. Using one hand, the clinician stabilizes the distal leg of the patient by holding the proximal ankle. The patient is asked to plantarflex the ankle without inversion or eversion of the foot, and the clinician applies a dorsiflexion force to the posterior calcaneus (Figure 9-134).

Plantaris. The plantaris muscle originates from the distal portion of the lateral supracondylar line of the femur, the adjacent part of the popliteal surface, and the oblique popliteal ligament (see Figure 9-122). Its tendon inserts on the posterior calcaneus. The plantaris muscle, which has its own tendon and contributes no fibers to the Achilles tendon, works with the gastrocnemius to plantarflex the ankle and assists in flexion of the knee joint.[176] The plantaris muscle is tested using the specific test of the gastrocnemius.

Posterior Deep Compartment

This compartment contains the flexors of the foot. These muscles course behind the medial malleolus. They include the posterior tibialis, FDL, and FHL.

Tibialis Posterior. The tibialis posterior arises from the majority of the interosseous membrane, lateral portion of the posterior aspect of the tibia, proximal two-thirds of the medial surface of the fibula, the adjacent intermuscular septa, and deep fascia (Figure 9-135). Its extensive insertions include the tuberosity of the navicular bone, by fibrous expansions to the sustentaculum tali, three cuneiforms, the cuboid, and bases of the second, third, and fourth metatarsal bones. The primary function of the tibialis posterior muscle is to invert and plantarflex the foot. It also provides support to the medial longitudinal arch.[177] The tibialis posterior is innervated by the tibial nerve. The synergists of this muscle include the FDL, FHL, fibularis longus and brevis, gastrocnemius, soleus, tibialis anterior, and extensor hallucis longus. The antagonists of this muscle include the fibularis longus and brevis, fibularis tertius, extensor digitorum longus, extensor hallucis longus, and tibialis anterior.

To specifically test this muscle, the patient is positioned supine or sitting with the foot and ankle plantarflexed and inverted. The patient is asked to sustain this position

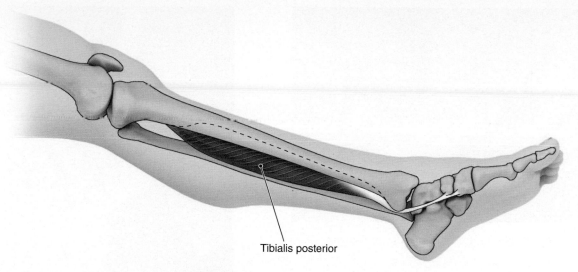

Tibialis posterior

FIGURE 9-135 Tibialis posterior muscle.

throughout the test. Using one hand, the clinician stabilizes the proximal to the patient's ankle while using the other hand to apply an eversion and dorsiflexion force to the patient's foot and ankle (Figure 9-136).

Flexor Digitorum Longus (FDL). The FDL originates from the tibia's posterior aspect and inserts on the distal phalanges of toes 2 to 5 (Figure 9-137). The FDL functions to flex the phalanges of the lateral four toes and assists with plantarflexion of the foot. The tibial nerve innervates the FDL. The synergists of this muscle include the lumbricals, anterior interossei, posterior interossei, tibialis posterior, FHL, fibularis longus and brevis, gastrocnemius, soleus, tibialis anterior, and extensor hallucis longus. The antagonists of this muscle include the extensor digitorum longus, extensor hallucis longus, extensor digitorum brevis, tibialis anterior, fibularis tertius, and fibularis longus and brevis.

To specifically test this muscle, the patient is positioned supine or sitting. The patient is asked to flex the toes and to sustain the position throughout the test. Using one hand to stabilize the midfoot, the clinician applies an extension force to the toes (Figure 9-138).

Flexor Hallucis Longus (FHL). The FHL originates from the distal two-thirds of the fibula and inserts on the distal

phalanx of the great toe (Figure 9-139). The FHL flexes the great toe and also assists with plantarflexion of the foot. The tibial nerve innervates the FHL. The synergists of this muscle include the abductor hallucis, FDL, tibialis posterior, fibularis longus and brevis, gastrocnemius, soleus, tibialis anterior, and extensor hallucis longus. The antagonists of this muscle include the extensor hallucis longus, extensor digitorum brevis, extensor digitorum longus, tibialis anterior, fibularis tertius, and fibularis longus and brevis.

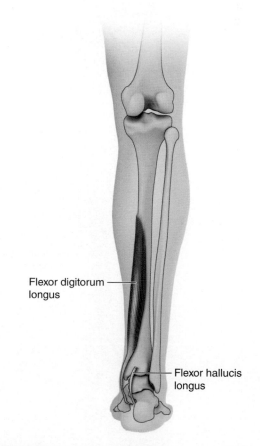

Flexor digitorum longus

Flexor hallucis longus

FIGURE 9-137 Flexor digitorum longus.

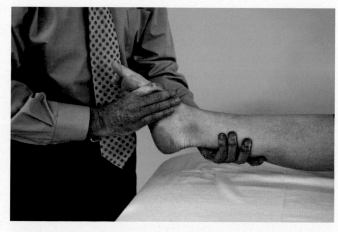

FIGURE 9-136 Test position for the tibialis posterior.

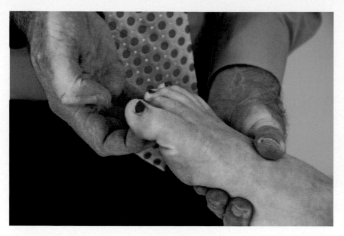

FIGURE 9-138 Test position for the flexor digitorum longus.

To test this muscle specifically, the patient is positioned supine or sitting and is asked to flex the great toe. It is important to note that the patient may have difficulty isolating this toe's motion from the other toes. Using one hand to stabilize the patient's ankle, the clinician uses the other hand to stabilize the metatarsals while applying an extension force to the great toe (Figure 9-140).

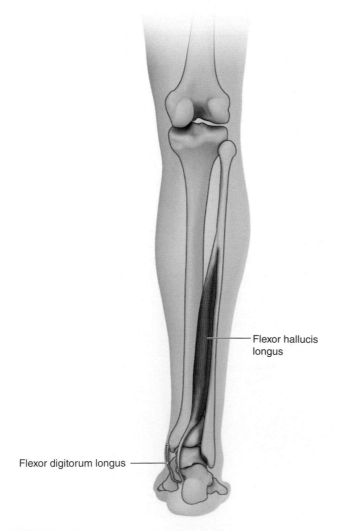

FIGURE 9-139 Flexor hallucis longus muscle.

Flexor hallucis longus

Flexor digitorum longus

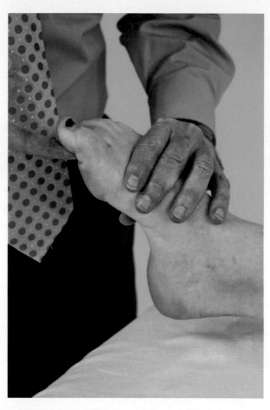

FIGURE 9-140 Test position for the flexor hallucis longus.

Lateral Compartment

This compartment contains the fibularis (peroneus) longus and brevis (Figure 9-141). The fibularis (peroneal) tendons lie behind the lateral malleolus in a fibro-osseous tunnel formed by a groove in the fibula and the superficial fibular (peroneal) retinaculum.

Fibularis (Peroneus) Longus and Brevis. The fibularis longus arises from the lateral condyle of the tibia, the proximal two-thirds of the fibula, and the adjacent intermuscular septum and inserts at the base of the first metatarsal and the medial cuneiform bone. The fibularis brevis arises from the distal two-thirds of the fibula and the adjacent intermuscular septum and inserts on the tuberosity on the base of the fifth metatarsal. The two muscles work in combination to produce ankle plantarflexion, foot eversion, and first metatarsal depression (longus).

Both of the muscles are innervated by the superficial fibular (peroneal) nerve. The synergists to these two muscles include the fibularis tertius, FDL, tibialis posterior, FHL, gastrocnemius, soleus, and extensor digitorum longus. The antagonist of these two muscles includes the tibialis anterior, tibialis posterior, FDL, FHL, extensor hallucis longus, extensor digitorum longus, fibularis tertius, gastrocnemius, and soleus.

CLINICAL PEARL

The fibularis (peroneal) muscles serve as both plantar flexors and evertors of the foot.[178,179] The fibularis (peroneus) longus also abducts the forefoot in the transverse plane, thereby serving as a support for the medial longitudinal arch.[180]

The fibularis longus and fibularis brevis are the only muscles innervated by the superficial fibular (peroneal) nerve.

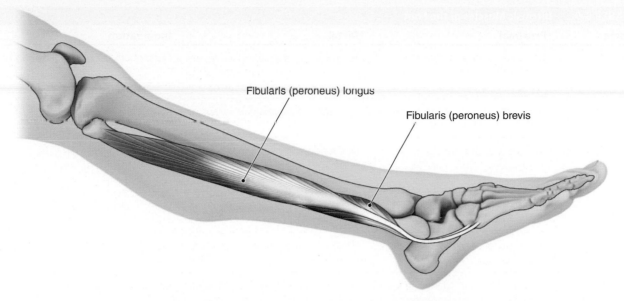

FIGURE 9-141 Fibularis (peroneus) longus and brevis muscles.

Fibularis (peroneus) longus

Fibularis (peroneus) brevis

Both of these muscles are tested together. The patient is positioned in sitting or supine and is asked to plantarflex and evert the foot (Figure 9-142). Using one hand, the clinician stabilizes the distal leg and, using the other hand, applies a force on the lateral aspect of the foot into inversion and dorsiflexion.

Intrinsic Muscles of the Foot

Beneath the plantar aponeurosis–plantar fascia are the four muscular layers of the intrinsic muscles of the plantar foot (Table 9-9), as well as the plantar ligaments of the rear and mid-foot. The intrinsic muscles provide support to the foot during propulsion.[181]

The intrinsic muscles of the foot include the following:

▶ *Abductor hallucis.* This muscle arises from the medial process of the calcaneal tuberosity and inserts into the medial side of the base of the proximal phalanx of the great toe (Figure 9-143). The muscle, which is innervated by the medial plantar nerve, functions to abduct the great toe

and to stabilize the first metatarsal. The synergist of this muscle is the FHL. The antagonists of this muscle are the adductor hallucis, extensor hallucis longus, and extensor digitorum brevis.

To specifically test this muscle, the patient is positioned supine or sitting. Using one hand, the clinician stabilizes the patient's foot while using the other hand to apply adduction force to the great toe and while asking the patient to prevent the motion (Figure 9-144). It is important to remember that this muscle is difficult for many people to isolate.

▶ *Abductor digiti minimi.* This muscle arises from the lateral process of the calcaneal tuberosity and the plantar aponeurosis and inserts into the lateral side of the base of the proximal phalanx of the little toe. The muscle functions to assist in flexion of the interphalangeal joint of the fifth digit and to stabilize the forefoot. The synergists of this muscle include the FDL and the fourth lumbrical. The antagonist to this muscle is the fifth anterior interossei.

▶ *Flexor digitorum brevis* (Figure 9-145). This muscle arises from the medial process of the calcaneal tuberosity, lateral to the abductor hallucis and deep to the central portion of the plantar fascia, and inserts into the middle phalanx of the lateral four toes. The flexor digitorum brevis flexes the PIP joints and assists in flexing the MTP joints of the second through fifth digits.

To specifically test this muscle, the patient is positioned in sitting or supine. Using one hand to stabilize the patient's midfoot, the clinician uses the other hand to apply pressure against the plantar surface of the PIP joints of the second through fifth digits (Figure 9-146).

▶ *Flexor digitorum accessorius (quadratus plantae; Figure 9-147).* This muscle arises from the calcaneal tuberosity via two heads. The medial head arises from the medial surface of the calcaneus and the medial border of the long plantar ligament, whereas the lateral head arises from the lateral border of the plantar surface of the calcaneus and the

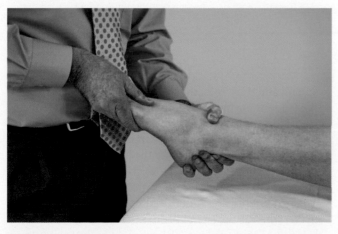

FIGURE 9-142 Test position for the peroneus longus and brevis.

265

TABLE 9-9	Intrinsic Muscles of the Foot		
Muscle	**Proximal**	**Distal**	**Innervation**
Extensor digitorum brevis	The distal superior surface of the calcaneus	The posterior (dorsal) surface of the second through fourth toes and base of the proximal phalanx	Deep fibular (peroneal) (L5 and S1)
Flexor hallucis brevis	The plantar surface of the cuboid and third cuneiform bones	The base of the proximal phalanx of the great toe	Medial plantar (S2-S3)
Flexor digitorum brevis	Tuberosity of calcaneus	One tendon slips into the base of the middle phalanx of each of the lateral four toes	Medial plantar (S1-S3)
Extensor hallucis brevis	Distal superior and lateral surfaces of calcaneus	The posterior (dorsal) surface of the proximal phalanx	Deep fibular (peroneal) (S1 and S2)
Abductor hallucis	Tuberosity of calcaneus and plantar aponeurosis	The base of the proximal phalanx and medial side	Medial plantar (S1-S3)
Adductor hallucis	The base of second, third, and fourth metatarsals and deep plantar ligaments	Proximal phalanx of first digit lateral side	Lateral plantar (S2-S3)
Lumbricales	Lumbricales medial and adjacent sides of flexor digitorum longus tendon to each lateral digit	The medial side of the proximal phalanx and extensor hood	Lumbrical 1: Medial plantar nerve (S2,S3) Lumbricals 2-4: Lateral plantar nerve (S2-S3)
Plantar interossei			
First	Base and medial side of the third metatarsal	The base of the proximal phalanx and extensor hood of the third digit	Lateral plantar nerve (S2-S3)
Second	Base and medial side of the fourth metatarsal	The base of the proximal phalanx and extensor hood of the fourth digit	Lateral plantar nerve (S2-S3)
Third	Base and medial side of the fifth metatarsal	The base of the proximal phalanx and extensor hood of the fifth digit	Lateral plantar nerve (S2-S3)
Dorsal interossei			
First	First and second metatarsal bones	Proximal phalanx and extensor hood of second digit medially	Lateral plantar nerve (S2-S3)
Second	Second and third metatarsal bones	Proximal phalanx and extensor hood of the second digit laterally	Lateral plantar nerve (S2-S3)
Third	Third and fourth metatarsal bones	Proximal phalanx and extensor hood of the third digit laterally	Lateral plantar nerve (S2-S3)
Fourth	Fourth and fifth metatarsal bones	Proximal phalanx and extensor hood of the fourth digit laterally	Lateral plantar nerve (S2-S3)
Abductor digiti minimi	The lateral side of the fifth metatarsal bone	Proximal phalanx of the fifth digit	Lateral plantar nerve (S1-S3)

lateral border of the long plantar ligament. The muscle terminates in tendinous slips, joining the long flexor tendons to the second, third, fourth, and occasionally fifth toes. This muscle modifies the line of pull of the FDL tendons and assists in flexing the second through fifth digits. There is no specific test for this muscle.

▶ *Lumbricales.* There are four lumbricales (see Figure 9-148), all of which arise from the tendon of the FDL. The first arises from the medial side of the tendon of the second toe, the second from adjacent sides of the tendons for the second and third toes, the third from adjacent sides of the tendons for the third and fourth toes, and the fourth from adjacent sides of tendons for the fourth and fifth toes. They insert with the tendons of the extensor digitorum longus and interossei into the bases of the terminal phalanges of the four lateral toes. The function of the lumbricales is to flex the MTP joint and extend the PIP joint. The first lumbrical is innervated by the medial plantar nerve, whereas the lateral plantar nerve innervates lumbricals two through four. The synergist to these muscles

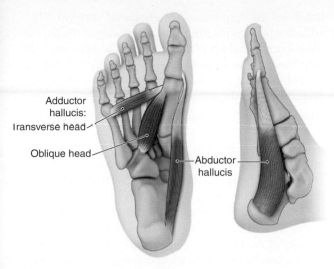

FIGURE 9-143 Abductor hallucis and adductor hallucis muscles.

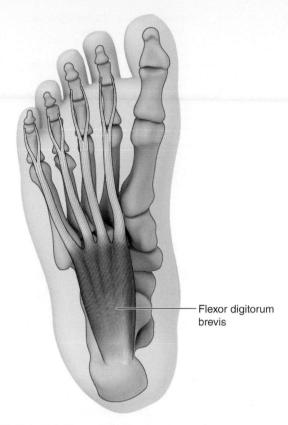

FIGURE 9-145 Flexor digitorum brevis muscle.

is the FDL. The antagonists of this muscle group include the extensor digitorum longus and the extensor digitorum brevis.

To specifically test these muscles, the patient is positioned supine or sitting and is asked to flex the MTP joints of the feet. While using one hand to stabilize the patient's foot, the clinician uses the other hand to apply an extension force under the MTP joints of toes 2 through 4 (Figure 9-149).

▶ *Flexor hallucis brevis (Figure 9-150)*. This muscle arises from the medial part of the cuboid bone's plantar surface, the adjacent portion of the lateral cuneiform, and the

posterior tibialis tendon, and inserts on the medial and lateral side of the proximal phalanx of the great toe. This muscle functions to flex the MTP joint of the great toe and is innervated by the tibial nerve.

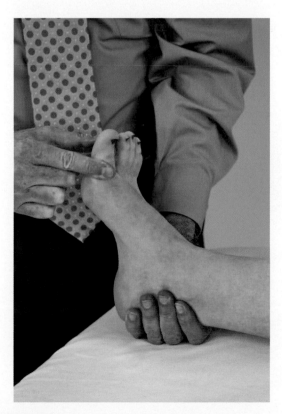

FIGURE 9-144 Test position for the abductor hallucis.

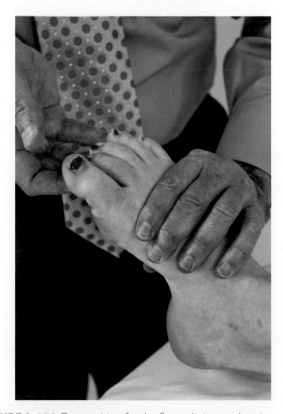

FIGURE 9-146 Test position for the flexor digitorum brevis.

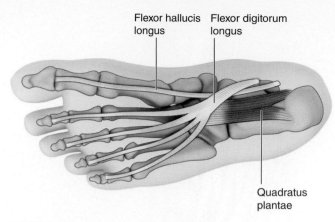

FIGURE 9-147 Quadratus plantae muscle.

To specifically test this muscle, the patient is positioned in supine or sitting. Using one hand to stabilize the foot proximal to the MTP joint and maintaining a neutral position of the foot and ankle, the clinician uses the other hand to apply an extension force at the MTP joints of the great toe (Figure 9-151).

▶ *Adductor hallucis (see Figure 9-143)*. This muscle arises via two heads: an oblique and a transverse head. The oblique head arises from the bases of the second, third, and fourth metatarsal bones and the sheath of the fibularis (peroneus) longus. The transverse head arises from the joint capsules of the second, third, fourth, and fifth MTP

heads and the deep transverse metatarsal ligament. The adductor hallucis inserts on the lateral side of the base of the proximal phalanx of the great toe. The adductor hallucis functions to adduct and assists in flexion of the MTP joint of the great toe, and is innervated by the tibial nerve. There is no specific test for this muscle.

▶ *Posterior (dorsal) interossei (see Figure 9-148)*. The four posterior (dorsal) interossei are bipennate, and they arise from adjacent sides of the metatarsal bones. The first inserts into the medial side of the proximal phalanx of the second toe. The second inserts into the lateral side of the proximal phalanx of the second toe. The third inserts into the lateral side of the proximal phalanx of the third toe, and the fourth inserts into the lateral side of the proximal phalanx of the fourth toe. The posterior (dorsal) interossei function to abduct the second, third, and fourth toes around an axis through the second metatarsal ray. The lateral plantar nerve innervates the posterior interossei. The synergists of these muscles include the FDL, FHL, and lumbricals 2 through 4. The antagonists of these muscles are the anterior interossei.

▶ *Plantar interossei (see Figure 9-148)*. The three plantar interossei are unipennate and arise from the bases and medial sides of the third, fourth, and fifth metatarsal bones. They insert into the medial sides of the bases of the proximal phalanges of the third, fourth, and fifth toes. The plantar interossei function to adduct the lateral three toes from the midline and are innervated by the lateral plantar

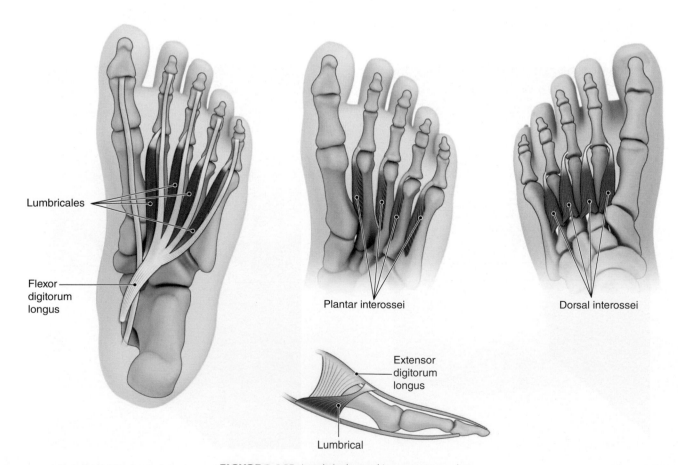

FIGURE 9-148 Lumbricales and interossei muscles.

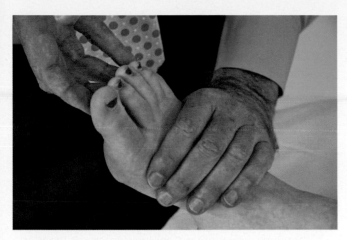

FIGURE 9-149 Test position for the lumbricales.

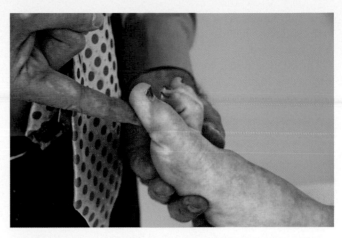

FIGURE 9-151 Test position for the flexor hallucis brevis.

nerve. The synergists of this muscle include the FDL, FHL, and lumbricals 2 through 4. The antagonists of this muscle are the posterior interossei.

To specifically test these muscle groups, the patient is positioned supine or sitting and is asked to extend the interphalangeal joints of the four lateral toes. The clinician stabilizes the MTP joints and places a finger on the posterior surface of the distal phalanges of each toe in the direction of flexion (Figure 9-152).

Posterior (Dorsal) Intrinsic Muscles

The posterior (dorsal) intrinsic muscles of the foot are the extensor hallucis brevis (EHB) and extensor digitorum brevis (EDB).

Extensor Hallucis Brevis. The EHB inserts into the base of the proximal phalanx of the great toe. The muscle is innervated by the lateral terminal branch of the deep fibular (peroneal) nerve. The EHB is tested along with the extensor hallucis longus. Unless innervation to the extensor hallucis longus is absent, a weakness of the extensor digitorum brevis cannot be determined accurately.

Extensor Digitorum Brevis. The EDB originates from the superior lateral aspect of the calcaneus and inserts into the base of the second, third, and fourth proximal phalanges (see Figure 9-127). The EDB functions to extend the MTP joints of toes 1 through 4.

The EDB is innervated by the lateral terminal branch of the deep fibular (peroneal) nerve. The synergists of this muscle include the extensor hallucis longus and the extensor

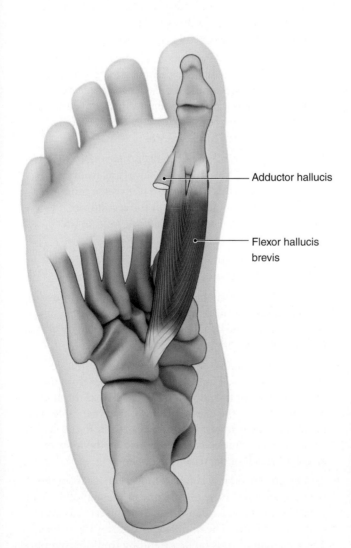

FIGURE 9-150 Flexor hallucis brevis muscle.

Adductor hallucis

Flexor hallucis brevis

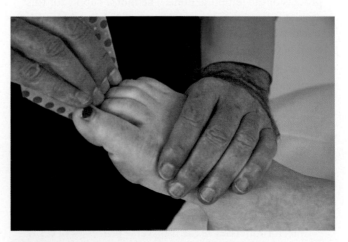

FIGURE 9-152 Test position for the interossei muscles.

digitorum longus. This muscle's antagonists include the FDL, FHL, abductor hallucis, lumbricals, anterior interossei, and dorsal interossei.

The EDB is tested together with the extensor digitorum longus (see Figure 9-128).

MUSCLE TESTING OF THE TRUNK

Various manual muscle testing methods have been used to assess adult abdominal strength clinically:

▶ Kendall and colleagues[39] have proposed two different procedures to measure abdominal muscle strength.

1. An assessment of a person's ability to keep the lumbar spine flat against the table while lowering both legs, with knees extended, from an initial position of 90° of hip flexion. The point in the range of motion at which the lumbar spine begins to demonstrate lordosis determines the muscle grade.

2. An assessment of strength based on the ability to flex the vertebral column and come to a sitting position while the legs remain stabilized in extension.

▶ Daniels and Worthingham[182] assign trunk flexor strength grades by having the person clear the scapulae from the table during trunk flexion. The lower extremities are stabilized in extension during their Normal (Grade 5), Good (Grade 4), and Fair (Grade 3) muscle test positions.

▶ Harvey and Scott[183] used a timed curl-down (reverse sit-up) test to measure abdominal muscle strength in young women.

The Specific Tests

Neck Flexors. The neck flexors include the following muscles:

▶ *Sternocleidomastoid (SCM).* The SCM, the largest muscle in the anterior neck, is attached inferiorly by two heads, arising from the posterior aspect of the medial third of the clavicle and the manubrium of the sternum. From here, it passes superiorly and posteriorly to attach to the mastoid process of the temporal bone. The motor supply for this muscle is from the accessory nerve (CN XI), whereas the sensory innervation is supplied from the anterior (ventral) rami of C2 and C3.[184]

▶ *Prevertebral muscles* (longus colli, longus capitis, rectus capitis anterior, and rectus capitis lateralis).

■ *Longus colli.* The longus colli consists of a vertical portion that originates from the bodies of the first three thoracic and last three cervical vertebrae, an inferior oblique portion that originates from the bodies of the first three thoracic vertebrae, and the superior oblique portion that originates from anterior tubercles of the transverse processes of C3-5. The various portions of the longus colli insert into the bodies of C2-4, the anterior tubercles of the transverse processes of C5-6, and the anterior tubercle of the atlas. The longus colli

is innervated by branches of the anterior primary rami of C2-8.

■ *Longus capitis.* The longus capitis originates from the anterior tubercles of the transverse processes of C3-6 and inserts onto the inferior surface of the basilar part of the occipital bone. The longus capitis is innervated by the muscular branches of C1-4.

■ *Rectus capitis anterior (RCA).* The RCA originates from the lateral mass of the atlas and inserts onto the base of the occipital bone in front of the foramen magnum. The RCA is innervated by the muscular branches of C1-2.

■ *Rectus capitis lateralis (RCL).* The RCL originates from the upper surface of the transverse process of the atlas and inserts onto the inferior surface of the jugular process of the occipital bone. The RCL is innervated by branches of the anterior rami of C1-2.

▶ *Scalenus anterior, medius, and posterior.* The scalenes extend obliquely like ladders (*scala* means ladder in Latin).

■ *Scalenus anterior.* The scalenus anterior runs vertically behind the SCM on the lateral aspect of the neck. Arising from the anterior tubercles of the C3-6 transverse processes, it travels to the scalene tubercle on the inner border of the first rib. It is supplied by the anterior (ventral) rami of C4, C5, and C6.

■ *Scalenus medius.* The scalenus medius is the largest and longest of the scalenus group, attaching to the transverse processes of all cervical vertebrae except the atlas (although it often attaches to this) and running to the upper border of the first rib. It is innervated by the anterior (ventral) rami of C3-8.

■ *Scalenus posterior.* The scalenus posterior, the smallest and deepest of the scalenus group, runs from the posterior tubercles of the C4-6 transverse processes to attach to the outer aspect of the second rib. It is innervated by the anterior (ventral) rami of C5, C6, and C7.

▶ *Suprahyoid.* The suprahyoid muscles include digastric, stylohyoid, geniohyoid, and mylohyoid.

▶ *Geniohyoid.* The geniohyoid muscle is a narrow muscle situated under the mylohyoid muscle. The muscle functions to elevate the hyoid bone. It is innervated by C1 via the hypoglossal nerve (CN XII).

▶ *Digastric.* As its name suggests, the digastric muscle consists of two bellies. The posterior belly arises from the mastoid notch of the temporal bone, whereas the anterior belly arises from the digastric fossa of the mandible. The posterior belly is innervated by a branch from the facial nerve. The anterior belly is innervated by the inferior alveolar branch of the trigeminal nerve.

▶ *Mylohyoid.* This flat, triangular muscle arises from the whole length of the mylohyoid line of the mandible. The posterior fibers pass inferomedially to insert into the body of the hyoid bone. The middle and anterior fibers insert into a median fibrous raphe extending from the symphysis menti to the hyoid bone, where they join at an angle with the fibers of the opposite muscle. The mylohyoid muscle is innervated by the mylohyoid nerve, a branch of the inferior alveolar nerve, which is a branch of the mandibular nerve, a division of the trigeminal nerve.

▶ *Stylohyoid.* The stylohyoid muscle arises from the posterior and lateral surface of the styloid process of the temporal bone, near the base, and, passing inferiorly and anteriorly, inserts into the body of the hyoid bone at its junction with the greater cornu and just superior the omohyoid muscle. It is innervated by the facial nerve (CN VII).

▶ *Infrahyoid.* The infrahyoid muscles comprise the sternohyoid, omohyoid, sternothyroid, and thyrohyoid muscles.

- *Sternohyoid.* The sternohyoid muscle is a straplike muscle that originates from the sternum and inserts on the hyoid bone.

- *Omohyoid.* The omohyoid muscle, situated lateral to the sternohyoid, consists of two bellies. The superior belly arises from the intermediate tendon and inserts on the hyoid bone, whereas the inferior belly arises from the superior border of the scapular and inserts on the intermediate tendon.

- *Sternothyroid.* The sternothyroid muscle arises from the sternum and inserts on the thyroid cartilage.

- *Thyrohyoid.* The thyrohyoid muscle arises from the thyroid cartilage and inserts on the hyoid bone.

Fibers from the upper cervical nerves innervate these infrahyoid muscles. The nerves to the lower part of these muscles are given off from a loop, the ansa cervicalis.

To test this muscle group specifically, the patient is positioned supine with the head in the anatomic position. The patient is asked to lift the head of the treatment table while keeping the chin tucked. Grading can be done as follows[185]:

▶ 10   N   5/5: 5 repetitions
▶ 5   F   3/5: 3–4 repetitions
▶ 2   P   2/5: 1–2 repetitions
▶ 0   Zero   0/5: 0 repetitions

Neck Extensors. The neck extensors include the following muscles:

▶ *Upper trapezius.* See Muscle Testing of the Shoulder.

▶ *Splenius capitis.* The splenius capitis extends upward and laterally, from the posterior (dorsal) edge of the nuchal ligament and the spinous processes of the lower cervical and upper thoracic vertebrae (T4-C7) to the mastoid process of the occipital bone just inferior to the superior nuchal line and deep to the SCM muscle. This muscle is segmentally innervated by the lateral branches of the posterior (dorsal) rami of the spinal nerves.

▶ *Splenius cervicis.* The splenius cervicis is just inferior and appears continuous with the capitis, extending from the spines of the third to the sixth thoracic vertebrae to the posterior tubercles of the transverse processes of the upper cervical vertebrae. This muscle is segmentally

innervated by the lateral branches of the posterior (dorsal) rami of the spinal nerves.

▶ *Erector spinae (cervical).* The erector spinae complex spans multiple segments, forming a large musculotendinous mass consisting of the iliocostalis, longissimus, and spinalis muscles. This muscle group is segmentally innervated by the lateral branches of the posterior (dorsal) rami of the spinal nerves.

▶ *Transversospinalis.* The transversospinalis muscles are a group of muscles that include the semispinalis, the multifidus, and the rotatores. This muscle group is segmentally innervated by the posterior (dorsal) rami of the spinal nerves.

To specifically test this muscle group, the patient is positioned prone with the head in the anatomic position. The patient is asked to lift the head of the treatment table and to hold it against gravity. Grading can be done as follows[185]:

▶ 10   N   5/5: 20 seconds
▶ 5   F   3/5: 10–19 seconds
▶ 2   P   2/5: 1–9 seconds
▶ 0   Zero   0/5: 0 seconds.

Anterior Trunk (Upper Abdominal) Flexors. The anterior trunk flexors include the rectus abdominis, transversus abdominis, and internal and external abdominal obliques.

▶ *Rectus abdominis.* The rectus abdominis originates from the cartilaginous ends of the fifth through seventh ribs and xiphoid and inserts on the superior aspect of the pubic bone.

▶ *Transversus abdominis.* The transverse abdominis muscle originates from the lateral one-third of the inguinal ligament, the anterior two-thirds of the iliac crest's inner lip, the lateral raphe of the thoracolumbar fascia, and the internal aspects of the lower six costal cartilages, where it interdigitates with the diaphragm.[186] Its upper and middle fibers run transversely around the trunk and blend with the fascial envelope of the rectus abdominis muscle, while the lower fibers blend with the insertion of the internal oblique muscle on the pubic crest.

▶ *Internal oblique.* The internal oblique, which forms the middle layer of the lateral abdominal wall, is located between the transversus abdominis and the external oblique muscles.[187] It has multiple attachments to the inguinal ligament, lateral raphe, iliac crest, pubic crest, transverse abdominis, and costal cartilages of the seventh through ninth costal cartilages.

▶ *External oblique.* The external oblique originates from the lateral aspect of the fifth through twelfth ribs and via interdigitations with the serratus anterior and latissimus dorsi. The muscle travels obliquely, medially, and inferiorly to insert into the linea alba, inguinal ligament, anterior–superior iliac spine, iliac crest, and pubic tubercle.

To specifically test this muscle group, the patient is positioned in the supine with the hips and knees flexed, the feet flat on the table, and the shoulder joints flexed to 90°. The patient is asked to assume a sitting position without using the upper extremities. Grading can be done as follows:

10	N	5/5	Able to correctly complete the test movement (flex the vertebral column and keep it flexed while entering the hip-flexion phase and coming to a sitting position) with the hands clasped behind the head
9	G+	4+/5	Able to correctly complete test movement with the hands at the shoulders
8	G	4/5	Able to correctly complete test movement with the arms crossed at the chest
7	G−	4−/5	Able to correctly complete test movement with the arms crossed at the abdomen
6	F+	3+/5	Able to correctly complete test movement with the arms extended forward
5	F	3/5	Able to correctly perform posterior pelvic tilt and flex the vertebral column with arms extended forward, but is unable to maintain the trunk flexion when attempting to enter the hip-flexion phase of the test movement
4	F−	3−/5	Able to tilt the pelvis posteriorly and keep the pelvis and thorax approximated as the head is raised from the table
2	P	2/5	The same position as 3−/5 grade: able to tilt the pelvis posteriorly but unable to maintain it as the head is raised from the table
1	T	1/5	Same position as 3−/5 grade: when the patient attempts to depress the chest or tilt the pelvis posteriorly, a contraction can be felt in the anterior abdominal muscles, but there is no approximation of the pelvis and thorax
0	Zero	0/5	No palpable muscle contraction

Lateral Trunk Flexors. The lateral trunk flexors include the erector spinae and the abdominals on the same side as the direction of side flexion. To specifically test this muscle group, the patient is positioned in side lying with the leg straight and a pillow between the legs. The clinician stabilizes the legs and, while maintaining the upper arm along the side and the other arm across the chest, the patient is asked to lift the body off the floor toward the ceiling. This test can be graded as follows:

▶ *Normal:* able to fully lift and bend the back sideways

▶ *Good:* able to lift and then the back sideways with the shoulder 4 inches from the floor

▶ *Fair:* able to lift and bend the back sideways with the shoulder 2 inches from the floor

▶ *Poor:* unable to lift and bend the back sideways

Anterior Trunk (Lower Abdominals) Flexors. To specifically test this muscle group, the patient is positioned supine with both of the legs straight and the arms folded across the chest. The patient is asked to raise the legs to a vertical position one at a time while keeping the back flat on the floor and then to lower the legs together to the floor slowly. This test can be graded based on the height at which the patient is unable to maintain the low back flat on the floor, as follows:

10	N	5/5	Able to perform posterior pelvic tilt and hold low back flat on the table while lowering the legs to the fully extended position 0–15° (table level)
9	G+	4+/5	Able to perform posterior pelvic tilt and hold low back flat on the table while lowering the legs to an angle of 15–30° with the table
8	G	4/5	Able to perform posterior pelvic tilt and hold low back flat on the table while lowering the legs to an angle of 30–45° with the table
7	G−	4−/5	Able to perform posterior pelvic tilt and hold low back flat on the table while lowering the legs to an angle of 45–60° with the table
6	F+	3+/5	Able to perform posterior pelvic tilt and hold low back flat on the table while lowering the legs to an angle of 60–75° with the table
5	F	3/5	Able to perform posterior pelvic tilt and hold low back flat on the table while lowering the legs to an angle of >75° with the table
4	F−	3−/5	The leg lowering test is not performed

The clinician should note if the patient exhibits any of the following faulty movement patterns:

▶ Excessive participation of the rectus abdominis throughout leg lowering

▶ Excessive participation of head and neck for stabilization

▶ Increased intra-abdominal pressure to stabilize the lumbar spine (holding breath)

Back Extensors. The muscles that provide back extension are numerous and very difficult to isolate. To specifically test this muscle group, the patient is positioned in prone with the hands clasped behind the back. The patient is asked to raise the trunk off the floor. According to Kendall and colleagues,[39] back extensor strength is best graded as slight, moderate, or marked, based on the examiner's judgment. For example:

▶ *Slight:* able to complete test movement with hands behind the head

▶ *Moderate:* able to complete test movement with hands clasped behind the back

▶ *Marked:* able to partially complete the test movement to the point where the xiphoid process is raised slightly, with the hands clasped behind the back

McGill and colleagues[187,188] have published normative data for the lateral, flexor, and extensor tests for young (mean age 21 years), healthy individuals (Table 9-10).

The following tests can be used to assess the strength of the lumbar stabilizers.

Lower Abdominal Hollowing. The abdominal hollowing exercise tests the ability of the multifidus and transverse

TABLE 9-10	Endurance Times and Flexion/Extension Ratios for the Flexor Endurance Test, Lateral Endurance Test, and Extensor Endurance Test		
Test	**Men (mean age 21 years)**	**Women (mean age 21 years)**	**Men (mean age 34 years)**
Extension	162 seconds	185 seconds	103
Flexion	136 seconds	134 seconds	66
Right lateral endurance (SB) test	95 seconds	75 seconds	54
Left lateral endurance (SB) test	99 seconds	78 seconds	54
Flexion/extension ratio	0.84	0.72	0.71
RSB/LSB ratio	0.96	0.96	1.05
RSB/extension ratio	0.58	0.40	0.57
LSB/extension ratio	0.61	0.42	0.58

abdominis to co-contract.[189,190] These muscles are important for the provision of segmental control to the spine, because they provide an important stiffening effect on the lumbar spine, thereby enhancing dynamic stability.[188]

The patient is positioned supine. The patient is instructed to contract the deep abdominal muscles and to draw the navel up toward the chest and in toward the spine, so as to hollow the abdomen. When the muscle contracts properly, an increase in tension can be felt at a point 2 cm medial and inferior to the anterior superior iliac spine. If a bulging is felt at this point, the internal oblique is contracting rather than the transverse abdominis.[189,190] The multifidus is palpated simultaneously and should be felt to swell at a point just lateral to the spinous process.[189,190] The patient's head and upper trunk must remain stable, and he or she is not permitted to flex forward, push through the feet, or tilt the pelvis.

Spine Rotators and Multifidus Test. This test is designed to assess the ability of the spinal rotators and multifidus to stabilize the trunk during dynamic extremity movements.[191] The patient is positioned in the quadruped position, with the pelvis positioned in neutral using muscular control. The patient is then asked to perform the following maneuvers: (1) single straight arm and hold, (2) single straight leg lift and hold, and (3) contralateral straight arm and straight leg lift and hold. The scoring for this test is as follows[191]:

Normal (5) = able to perform contralateral arm and leg lift, both sides, while maintaining neutral pelvis (20–30-second hold)
Good (4) = able to maintain neutral pelvis while performing single leg lift, but not able to hold the pelvis in neutral when doing contralateral arm and leg lift (15–20-second hold)
Fair (3) = Able to do single-arm lift and maintain neutral pelvis (15–20-second hold)
Poor (2) = Unable to maintain neutral pelvis while doing a single-arm lift
Trace (1) = Unable to raise arm or leg off the table to the straight position

Abdominal Endurance Test. This test measures the endurance of the abdominals. The patient is positioned supine, with

the hips flexed to approximately 45°, the feet flat on the bed, and the arms by the side. A line is drawn 8 cm (for patients 40 years and older) or 12 cm (for patients younger than 40 years of age) distal to the fingers.[192] The patient is asked to tuck in the chin and to curl the trunk, and touch the line with the fingers. The patient holds this position for as long as possible. The test is graded as follows[155,193]:

Normal (5) = 20–30-second hold
Good (4) = 15–20-second hold
Fair (3) = 10–15-second hold
Poor (2) = 1–10-second hold
Trace (1) = Unable to raise more than the head off the table

Side Support or Side Bridge Test. The so-called side support or side bridge position has been identified as optimizing the challenge to the quadratus lumborum while minimizing the load on the lumbar spine.[194] The patient is in the side-lying position, with the knees flexed to 90° and resting the upper body on the elbow. The test can be made more difficult by having the knees extended so that the legs are straight. The patient is asked to lift the pelvis off the table and to straighten the curve of the spine without rolling forward or backward. This position is then held.

The test is graded as follows:

Normal (5) = Able to lift the pelvis off the table and hold the spine straight for a 20–30-second hold
Good (4) = Able to lift the pelvis off the table but has difficulty holding the spine straight for a 15–20-second hold
Fair (3) = Able to lift the pelvis off the table but has difficulty holding the spine straight for a 10–15-second hold
Poor (2) = Able to lift the pelvis off the table but cannot hold the spine straight for a 1–10-second hold
Trace (1) = Unable to lift the pelvis off the table

Double Straight Leg Lowering Test. The straight leg lowering test can be used to assess core strength.[189,195-201] The patient is in the supine hooklying position, with the hips flexed to 90°, and with a pressure cuff placed under the lumbar spine at the level of L4–L5. The cuff is inflated to 40 mm Hg. The clinician raises the patient's legs until the pelvis is seen to rotate posteriorly, and the needle on the pressure monitor begins to move. The patient is asked to perform the lower abdominal hollowing maneuver to prevent further pelvic motion and is then asked to lower the legs toward the bed while maintaining the lower abdominal hollowing. At the point when the cuff pressure is seen to increase or decrease, or when the pelvis anteriorly rotates, the test is over, and the hip angle at which this occurs is measured. This test may also be graded using the following scoring[193]:

Normal (5) = Able to reach 0–15° from the table before pelvis tilts

Good (4) = Able to reach 16–45° from the table before pelvis tilts

Fair (3) = Able to reach 46–75° from the table before pelvis tilts

Poor (2) = Able to reach 75–90° from the table before pelvis tilts

Trace (1) = Unable to hold the pelvis in neutral

A study by Youdas and colleagues[201] found that the odds of a patient having chronic low back pain is increased if the score on the leg lowering test for the abdominal muscles exceeds 50° for men and 60° for women. Another study[202] found that there is a natural tendency for the pelvis to rotate anteriorly from very early on during this test, and that, as healthy, young subjects were unable to prevent the tilting, the preceding scoring system may be questionable.

The Bent Knee Lowering Test. The lower abdominal musculature can be assessed similarly.[195,196,199] The patient is positioned supine with the knees and hips flexed to approximately 90°. A pressure cuff, inflated to 40 mm Hg, is placed under the L4–L5 segment. The patient is asked to perform the abdominal hollowing maneuver and slowly lower the legs to the bed until the monitor's pressure is seen to decrease. The hip angle is again measured at the point where there is a change in the pressure cuff reading or where the anterior tilt of the pelvis occurred.

Normal (5) = Able to reach 0–15° from the table before pelvis tilts

Good (4) = Able to reach 16–45° from the table before pelvis tilts

Fair (3) = Able to reach 46–75° from the table before pelvis tilts

Poor (2) = Able to reach 75–90° from the table before pelvis tilts

Trace (1) = Unable to hold the pelvis in neutral

Trunk Raise. The trunk raise test can be used to assess the endurance of the iliocostalis lumborum (erector spinae) and the multifidus.[195,199,203,204] The patient is positioned prone, with the hands behind the back or by the sides. The patient is instructed to extend at the lumbar spine by raising the chest off the bed to approximately 30° (the axilla can be used as the reference for the axis if a goniometer is used) and hold the position as long as possible. The clinician times the test[195]:

Normal (5) = 20–30-second hold
Good (4) = 15–20-second hold
Fair (3) = 10–15-second hold

Poor (2) = 1–10-second hold
Trace (1) = Unable to raise more than the head off the table

Lunge. The patient is asked to perform a lunge. The clinician notes the quality and quantity of the motion and the patient's ability to sustain the position for 30 seconds.[205] Excessive shaking of the legs with this maneuver may indicate weakness of the lumbopelvic stabilizers or poor balance and proprioception.

MUSCLE TESTING THE TRUNK IN THE ATHLETIC POPULATION

According to McGill and colleagues,[189,190] the torso flexors, extensors, and lateral musculature are involved in spine stability during virtually any task, and therefore the endurance of each of these muscle groups should be measured. The following tests are recommended:

▶ *Flexor endurance test.* The patient is positioned in sitting with the back supported at an angle of approximately 60° from the floor (Figure 9-153), with both knees and hips flexed to 90° and the arms folded across the chest. The patient's foot can be stabilized manually or by using a belt (see Figure 9-153). Once the patient is ready, the support is removed from the back (Figure 9-154), and the patient attempts to maintain the isometric posture for as long as possible. Failure occurs when the patient is no longer able to maintain the position.

▶ *Lateral endurance test.* The patient is positioned in the full side bridge position (Figure 9-155). The patient attempts to maintain this position for as long as possible. Failure occurs when the patient loses the straight-backed posture and the hip returns to the table. The test is then repeated on the other side.

▶ *Extensor endurance test.* The patient is positioned in prone with the lower extremity supported so that the trunk and upper extremities are over the edge of the table (Figure 9-156). The upper extremities are held across the chest. Failure occurs when the upper body drops from the horizontal position.

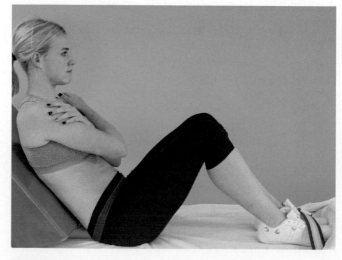

FIGURE 9-153 Flexor endurance test—start position.

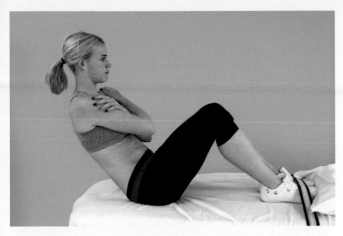

FIGURE 9-154 Flexor endurance test—support removed.

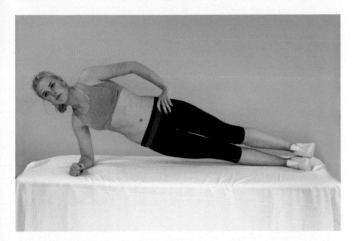

FIGURE 9-155 Lateral endurance test.

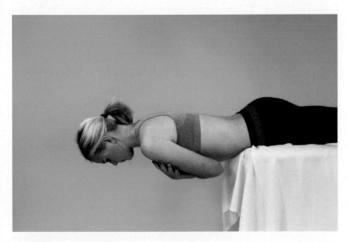

FIGURE 9-156 Extensor endurance test.

TABLE 9-11	Asymmetrical Unbalances	
Right side bridge/left side bridge endurance		>0.05
Flexion/extension endurance		>1.0
Side bridge (either side)/extension endurance		>0.75
Extensor strength (N. m)/extensor endurance (seconds)—strength to endurance ratio		>4.0

McGill used these tests on young, healthy individuals (92 men and 137 women with a mean age of 21 years) and with a group of men with a mean age of 34 years with no history of back trouble. The results are depicted in Table 9-10. According to McGill, the interpretation of absolute endurance should be secondary to interpreting the imbalance among the three muscle groups, and the discrepancies outlined in Table 9-11 suggest unbalanced endurance, which increases the potential for injury and should thus be the focus of the intervention.

REFERENCES

1. Dutton M. Improving muscle performance. In: Dutton M, ed. *Dutton's Orthopaedic: Examination, Evaluation and Intervention*, 4th ed. New York: McGraw-Hill; 2016:463-520.
2. Dutton M. The musculoskeletal system. In: Dutton M, ed. *Dutton's Orthopaedic: Examination, Evaluation and Intervention*, 4th ed. New York: McGraw-Hill; 2016:3-28.
3. American Medical Association. The spine. In: Cocchiarella L, Andersson GBJ, eds. *Guides to the Evaluation of Permanent Impairment*, 5th ed. Chicago: American Medical Association; 2001:373-432.
4. Beasley WC. Quantitative muscle testing: Principles and applications to research and clinical services. *Arch Phys Med Rehab*. 1961;42:398-425.
5. MacConnail MA, Basmajian JV. Muscles and Movements: *A Basis for Human Kinesiology*. New York: Robert Krieger Pub Co; 1977.
6. White DJ. Musculoskeletal examination. In: O'Sullivan SB, Schmitz TJ, eds. *Physical Rehabilitation*, 5th ed. Philadelphia: FA Davis; 2007:159-192.
7. Florence JM, Pandya S, King WM, Robison JD, Baty J, Miller JP, et al. Intrarater reliability of manual muscle test (Medical Research Council scale) grades in Duchenne's muscular dystrophy. *Phys Ther*. 1992;72:115-122; discussion 22-26.
8. Barr AE, Diamond BE, Wade CK, Harashima T, Pecorella WA, Potts CC, et al. Reliability of testing measures in Duchenne or Becker muscular dystrophy. *Arch Phys Med Rehabil*. 1991;72:315-319.
9. Nadler SF, Rigolosi L, Kim D, Solomon J. Sensory, motor, and reflex examination. In: Malanga GA, Nadler SF, eds. *Musculoskeletal Physical Examination—an Evidence-based Approach*. Philadelphia: Elsevier-Mosby; 2006:15-32.
10. Bohannon RW. Make tests and break tests of elbow flexor muscle strength. *Phys Ther*. 1988;68:193-194.
11. Stratford PW, Balsor BE. A comparison of make and break tests using a hand-held dynamometer and the Kin-Com. *J Orthop Sports Phys Ther*. 1994;19:28-32.
12. Andrews AW, Thomas MW, Bohannon RW. Normative values for isometric muscle force measurements obtained with hand-held dynamometers. *Phys Ther*. 1996;76:248-259.
13. Sapega AA. Muscle performance evaluation in orthopedic practice. *J Bone Joint Surg*. 1990;72A:1562-1574.
14. Iddings DM, Smith LK, Spencer WA. Muscle testing: part 2. Reliability in clinical use. *Phys Ther Rev*. 1961;41:249-256.
15. Silver M, McElroy A, Morrow L, Heafner BK. Further standardization of manual muscle test for clinical study: Applied in chronic renal disease. *Phys Ther*. 1970;50:1456-1465.
16. Marx RG, Bombardier C, Wright JG. What we know about the reliability and validity of physical examination tests used to examine the upper extremity. *J Hand Surg Am*. 1999;24A:185-193.
17. Astrand PO, Rodahl K. *Textbook of Work Physiology*. New York: McGraw-Hill; 1973.
18. Astrand PO, Rodahl K. *The Muscle and Its Contraction: Textbook of Work Physiology*. New York: McGraw-Hill; 1986.
19. Muller EA. Influences of training and inactivity of muscle strength. *Arch Phys Med Rehab*. 1970;51:449-462.
20. Phillips BA, Lo SK, Mastaglia FL. Muscle force measured using "break" testing with a hand-held myometer in normal subjects aged 20 to 69 years. *Arch Phys Med Rehabil*. 2000;81:653-661.
21. Beck M, Giess R, Wurffel W, Magnus T, Ochs G, Toyka KV. Comparison of maximal voluntary isometric contraction and Drachman's hand-held dynamometry in evaluating patients with amyotrophic lateral sclerosis. *Muscle & Nerve*. 1999;22:1265-1270.
22. Roy MA, Doherty TJ. Reliability of hand-held dynamometry in assessment of knee extensor strength after hip fracture. *Am J Phys Med Rehabil*. 2004;83:813-818.

23. Hutten MM, Hermens HJ. Reliability of lumbar dynamometry measurements in patients with chronic low back pain with test-retest measurements on different days. *Eur Spine J.* 1997;6:54-62.
24. Stokes HM, Landrieu KW, Domangue B, et al. Identification of low effort patients through dynamometry. *J Hand Surg Am.* 1995;20A:1047-1056.
25. Bohannon RW. Hand-held compared with isokinetic dynamometry for measurement of static knee extension torque (parallel reliability of dynamometers). *Clin Phys Physiol Meas.* 1990;11:217-222.
26. Hartsell HD, Forwell L. Postoperative eccentric and concentric isokinetic strength for the shoulder rotators in the scapular and neutral planes. *J Orthop Sports Phys Ther.* 1997;25:19-25.
27. Hartsell HD, Spaulding SJ. Eccentric/concentric ratios at selected velocities for the invertor and evertor muscles of the chronically unstable ankle. *Br J Sports Med.* 1999;33:255-258.
28. Griffin JW. Differences in elbow flexion torque measured concentrically, eccentrically and isometrically. *Phys Ther.* 1987;67:1205-1208.
29. Hortobagyi T, Katch FI. Eccentric and concentric torque-velocity relationships during arm flexion and extension. *J Appl Physiol.* 1995;60:395-401.
30. Trudelle-Jackson E, Meske N, Highenboten C, et al. Eccentric/concentric torque deficits in the quadriceps muscle. *J Orthop Sports Phys Ther.* 1989;11:142-145.
31. Rothstein JM, Lamb RL, Mayhew TP. Clinical uses of isokinetic measurements. Critical issues. *Phys Ther.* 1987;67:1840-1844.
32. Bohannon RW. Manual muscle test scores and dynamometer test scores of knee extension strength. *Arch Phys Med Rehabil.* 1987;67:390-392.
33. Mulroy SJ, Lassen KD, Chambers SH, Perry J. The ability of male and female clinicians to effectively test knee extension strength using manual muscle testing. *J Orthop Sports Phys Ther.* 1997;26:192-199.
34. Jobe FW, Pink M. Classification and treatment of shoulder dysfunction in the overhead athlete. *J Orthop Sports Phys Ther.* 1993;18:427-431.
35. Haymaker W, Woodhall B. *Peripheral Nerve Injuries. Principles of Diagnosis.* London: WB Saunders; 1953.
36. Brodal A. *Neurological Anatomy.* London: Oxford University Press; 1981.
37. Mercer S, Campbell AH. Motor innervation of the trapezius. *J Man & Manip Ther.* 2000;8:18-20.
38. Ayub E. Posture and the upper quarter. In: Donatelli RA, ed. *Physical Therapy of the Shoulder,* 2nd ed. New York: Churchill Livingstone; 1991:81-90.
39. Kendall FP, McCreary EK, Provance PG, McIntyre-Rodgers M, Romani WA. *Muscles: Testing and Function, with Posture and Pain.* Baltimore: Williams & Wilkins; 2005.
40. Neumann DA. Shoulder complex. In: Neumann DA, ed. *Kinesiology of the Musculoskeletal System: Foundations for Physical Rehabilitation.* St. Louis: Mosby; 2002:91-132.
41. White SM, Witten CM. Long thoracic nerve palsy in a professional ballet dancer. *Am J Sports Med.* 1993;21:626-629.
42. Jobe CM. Gross anatomy of the shoulder. In: Rockwood CA, Matsen FA, eds. *The Shoulder,* 2nd ed. Philadelphia: WB Saunders; 1998:35-97.
43. Connor PM, Yamaguchi K, Manifold SG, et al. Split pectoralis major transfer for serratus anterior palsy. *Clin Orthop.* 1997;341:134-142.
44. Schultz JS, Leonard JA. Long thoracic neuropathy from athletic activity. *Arch Phys Med Rehab.* 1992;73:87-90.
45. Gregg JR, Labosky D, Hearty M, Lotke P, Ecker M, DiStefano V, et al. Serratus anterior paralysis in the young athlete. *J Bone and Joint Surg.* 1979;61A:825-832.
46. Marks PH, Warner JJP, Irrgang JJ. Rotator cuff disorders of the shoulder. *J Hand Ther.* 1994;7:90-98.
47. Warner JJ, Navarro RA. Serratus anterior dysfunction. Recognition and treatment. *Clin Orthop Relat Res.* 1998;349:139-148.
48. Leffert RD. Neurological problems. In: Rockwood CA, Jr., Matsen FR, III., eds. *The Shoulder.* Philadelphia: WB Saunders; 1990:750-773.
49. Perry J. Biomechanics of the shoulder. In: Rowe CR, ed. *The Shoulder.* New York: Churchill Livingstone; 1988:1-15.
50. Warner JJP, Micheli LJ, Arslanian LE, Kennedy J, Kennedy R. Scapulothoracic motion in normal shoulders and shoulders with glenohumeral instability and impingement syndrome. A study using Moire topographic analysis. *Clin Orthop.* 1992;285:191-199.
51. Post M. Pectoralis major transfer for winging of the scapula. *J Shoulder Elbow Surg.* 1995;4:1-9.
52. Kapandji IA. *The Physiology of Joints.* New York, NY: Churchill Livingstone; 1974.
53. Dunleavy K. *Relationship Between the Shoulder and the Cervicothoracic Spine.* La Crosse, WI: Orthopedic Section, APTA; 2001.
54. Porterfield, J, De Rosa C. *Mechanical Neck Pain: Perspectives in Functional Anatomy.* Philadelphia: WB Saunders; 1995.
55. Murray MP, Gore DR, Gardner GM, Mollinger LA. Shoulder motion and muscle strength of normal men and women in two age groups. *Clin Orthop Relat Res.* 1985:268-273.
56. Mikesky AE, Edwards JE, Wigglesworth JK, Kunkel S. Eccentric and concentric strength of the shoulder and arm musculature in collegiate baseball pitchers. *Am J Sports Med.* 1995;23:638-642.
57. Perry J. Muscle Control of the Shoulder. In: Rowe CR, ed. *The Shoulder.* New York: Churchill Livingstone; 1988:17-34.
58. Culham E, Peat M. Functional anatomy of the shoulder complex. *J Orthop Sports Phys Ther.* 1993;18:342-350.
59. Blackburn TA, McLeod WD, White B, Wofford L. EMG analysis of posterior rotator cuff exercises. *Athl Training.* 1990;25:40-45.
60. Bradley JP, Tibone JE. Electromyographic analysis of muscle action about the shoulder. *Clin Sports Med.* 1991;4:789-805.
61. Perry J, Glousman RE. Biomechanics of throwing. In: Nicholas JA, Hershman EB, eds. *The Upper Extremity in Sports Medicine.* St Louis: CV Mosby; 1990:727-751.
62. Sharkey NA, Marder RA. The rotator cuff opposes superior translation of the humeral head. *Am J Sports Med.* 1995;23:270-275.
63. Sharkey NA, Marder RA, Hanson PB. The role of the rotator cuff in elevation of the arm. *Trans Orthop Res Soc.* 1993;18:137.
64. Turkel SJ, Panio MW, Marshall JL, et al. Stabilizing mechanisms preventing anterior dislocation of the glenohumeral joint. *J Bone Joint Surg [Am].* 1981;63:1208-1217.
65. Chepeha JC. Shoulder trauma and hypomobility. In: Magee DJ, Zachazewski JE, Quillen WS, eds. *Pathology and Intervention in Musculoskeletal Sehabilitation.* St. Louis, MI: Saunders; 2009:92-124.
66. Vangsness CT, Jr., Jorgenson SS, Watson T, Johnson DL. The origin of the long head of the biceps from the scapula and glenoid labrum. An anatomical study of 100 shoulders. *J Bone Joint Surg Br.* 1994;76:951-954.
67. Altchek D, Wolf B. Disorders of the biceps tendon. In: Krishnan S, Hawkins R, Warren R, eds. *The Shoulder and the Overhead Athlete.* Philadelphia, PA: Lippincott, Williams & Wilkins; 2004:196-208.
68. Habermeyer P, Magosch P, Pritsch M, Scheibel MT, Lichtenberg S. Anterosuperior impingement of the shoulder as a result of pulley lesions: a prospective arthroscopic study. *J Shoulder Elbow Surg.* 2004;13:5-12.
69. Krupp RJ, Kevern MA, Gaines MD, Kotara S, Singleton SB. Long head of the biceps tendon pain: differential diagnosis and treatment. *J Orthop Sports Phys Ther.* 2009;39:55-70.
70. Mathes SJ, Nahai F. Biceps brachii. In: Mathes SJ, Nahai F, eds. *Clinical Atlas of Muscle and Musculocutaneous Flaps.* St. Louis: Mosby; 1979:426–432.
71. Matsen FA, III., Arntz CT. Subacromial impingement. In: Rockwood CA, Jr., Matsen FA, III., eds. *The Shoulder.* Philadelphia, Pa: WB Saunders; 1990:623-648.
72. Neer CS, II. Anterior acromioplasty for the chronic impingement syndrome in the shoulder: a preliminary report. *The J Bone Joint Surg Am.* 1972;54:41-50.
73. Neer C. Impingement lesions. *Clin Orthop.* 1983;173:71-77.
74. Lucas DB. Biomechanics of the shoulder joint. Arch Surg. 1973;107:425-432.
75. Levy AS, Kelly BT, Lintner SA, et al. Function of the long head of the biceps at the shoulder: electromyographic analysis. *J Shoulder Elbow Surg.* 2001;10:250-255.
76. Andrews JR, Carson WG, McLeod WD. Glenoid labrum tears related to the long head of the biceps. *Am J Sports Med.* 1985;13:337-341.
77. Basmajian JV, Deluca CJ. Muscles Alive: Their Functions Revealed by Electromyography. Baltimore: Williams & Wilkins; 1985.
78. Basmajian JV, Bazant FJ. Factors preventing downward dislocation of the adducted shoulder joint: An electromyographic and morphological study. *J Bone and Joint Surg.* 1959;41A:1182-1186.
79. Itoi E, Kuechle DK, Newman SR, et al. Stabilising function of the biceps in stable and unstable shoulders. *J Bone and Joint Surg Am.* 1993;75B:546-550.
80. Rodosky MW, Harner CD, Fu FH. The role of the long head of the biceps muscle and superior glenoid labrum in anterior stability of the shoulder. *Am J Sports Med.* 1994;22:121-130.
81. Norkin C, Levangie P. *Joint Structure and Function: A Comprehensive Analysis.* Philadelphia: F.A. Davis Company; 1992.
82. Pagnani M, Deng X-H, Warren RF, Torzilli PA, Altchek D. Effect of lesions of the superior portion of the glenoid labrum on glenohumeral translation. *J Bone and Joint Surg.* 1995;77A:1002-1010.
83. Payne LZ, Deng X, Craig EV, Torzilli PA, Warren RF. The combined dynamic and static contributions to subacromial impingement. *Am J Sports Med.* 1997;25:801-808.

84. Warner JJP, McMahon PJ. The role of the long head of the biceps brachii in superior stability of the glenohumeral joint. *J Bone and Joint Surg.* 1995;77A:366-372.

85. Kido T, Itoi E, Konno N, Sano A, et al. The depressor function of biceps on the head of the humerus in shoulders with tears of the rotator cuff. *J Bone and Joint Surg.* 2000;82B:416-419.

86. Itoi E, Hsu HC, Carmichael SW, Morrey BF, An K-N. Morphology of the torn rotator cuff. *J Anat.* 1995;186:429-434.

87. Jobe FW, Nuber G. Throwing injuries of the elbow. *Clin Sports Med.* 1986;5;621.

88. Ryan J. Elbow. In: Wadsworth C, ed. *Current Concepts of Orthopedic Physical Therapy—Home Study Course.* La Crosse, WI: Orthopaedic Section, APTA; 2001.

89. Neumann DA. Elbow and forearm complex. In: Neumann DA, ed. *Kinesiology of the Musculoskeletal System: Foundations for Physical Rehabilitation.* St. Louis: Mosby; 2002:133-171.

90. Schuind F, Garcia-Elias M, Cooney WP, et al. Flexor tendon forces: In vivo measurements. *J Hand Surg Am.* 1992;17A:291-298.

91. Schuind FA, Goldschmidt D, Bastin C, Burny F. A biomechanical study of the ulnar nerve at the elbow. *J Hand Surg Br.* 1995;20:623-627.

92. Pauly JE, Rushing JL, Schering LE. An electromyographic study of some muscles crossing the elbow joint. *Anat Rec.* 1967;159:47-53.

93. Basmajian JV, Latif A. Integrated actions and functions of the chief flexors of the elbow: A detailed electromyographic analysis. *J Bone Joint Surg Am.* 1957;39A:1106-1118.

94. Funk DA, An KA, Morrey BF, Daube JR. Electromyographic analysis of muscles across the elbow joint. J Orthop Res. 1987;5:529-538.

95. Basmajian JV, Deluca CJ. *Muscles Alive*, 5th ed. Baltimore: Williams & Wilkins; 1985:268-269.

96. Thepaut-Mathieu C, Maton B. The flexor function of the muscle pronator teres in man: a quantitative electromyographic study. *Occup Physiol.* 1985;54:116-121.

97. An KN, Morrey BF. Biomechanics of the Elbow. In: Morrey BF, ed. *The Elbow and Its Disorder*, 2nd ed. Philadelphia: WB Saunders Co; 1993:53-73.

98. Jackson-Manfield P, Neumann DA. Structure and function of the elbow and forearm complex. In: Jackson-Manfield P, Neumann DA, eds. *Essentials of Kinesiology for the Physical Therapist Assistant.* St. Louis, MO: Mosby Elsevier; 2009:91-122.

99. An KN, Hui FC, Morrey BF, Linscheid RL, Chao EY. Muscles across the elbow joint: A biomechanical analysis. J Biomech. 1981;14:659-669.

100. Davidson PA, Pink M, Perry J, et al. Functional anatomy of the flexor pronator muscle group in relation to the medial collateral ligament of the elbow. *Am J Sports Med.* 1995;23:245-250.

101. Reid DC. *Functional Anatomy and Joint Mobilization,* 2nd ed. Edmonton: University of Alberta Press; 1975.

102. Hirasawa Y, Sawamura H, Sakakida K. Entrapment neuropathy due to bilateral epitrochlearis muscles: A case report. *J Hand Surg Am.* 1979;4:181-184.

103. Onieal M-E. Common wrist and elbow injuries in primary care. Lippincott's Primary Care Practice Musculoskeletal Conditions. 1999;3:441-450.

104. Brand PW, Hollister AM, Agee JM. Transmission. In: Brand PW, Hollister AM, eds. *Clinical Mechanics of the Hand.* St Louis: Mosby; 1999:61-99.

105. Wadsworth C. Wrist and hand. In: Wadsworth C, ed. *Current Concepts of Orthopedic Physical Therapy—Home Study Course.* La Crosse, WI: Orthopaedic Section, APTA; 2001.

106. Kaplan EB. Anatomy and kinesiology of the hand. In: Flynn JE, ed. *Hand Surgery,* 2nd ed. Baltimore: Williams and Wilkins; 1975.

107. Linburg RM, Comstock BE. Anomalous tendon slips from the pollicis longus to the flexor digitorum profundus. *J Hand Surg Am.* 1979;4:79-83.

108. Rennie WRJ, Muller H. Linburg syndrome. *Can J Surg.* 1998;41:306-308.

109. Brand PW. *Clinical Mechanics of the Hand.* St. Louis: CV Mosby; 1985.

110. Tubiana R, Thomine J-M, Mackin E. *Examination of the Hand and Wrist.* London: Mosby; 1996.

111. Ketchum LD, Thompson DE. An experimental investigation into the forces internal to the human hand. In: Brand PW, Hollister A, eds. *Clinical Mechanics of the Hand.* St. Louis: CV Mosby; 1993:66-96.

112. Hollinshead WH. *Anatomy for Surgeons,* 2nd ed. New York: Harper & Row; 1969.

113. Wadsworth CT. Anatomy of the hand and wrist. *Manual Examination and Treatment of the Spine and Extremities.* Baltimore, MD: Williams & Wilkins Co; 1988:128-138.

114. Neumann DA. Kinesiology of the hip: A focus on muscular actions. *J Orthop Sports Phys Ther.* 2010;40:82-94.

115. Delp SL, Hess WE, Hungerford DS, Jones LC. Variation of rotation moment arms with hip flexion. *J Biomech.* 1999;32:493-501.

116. Yoshio M, Murakami G, Sato T, Sato S, Noriyasu S. The function of the psoas major muscle: Passive kinetics and morphological studies using donated cadavers. *J Orthop Sci.* 2002;7:199-207.

117. Hall SJ. The biomechanics of the human lower extremity. *Basic Biomechanics,* 3rd ed. New York: McGraw-Hill; 1999:234-81.

118. Janda V. On the concept of postural muscles and posture in man. *Aust J Physiother.* 1983;29:83-84.

119. Fagerson TL. Hip pathologies: diagnosis and intervention. In: Magee DJ, Zachazewski JE, Quillen WS, eds. *Pathology and Intervention in Musculoskeletal Rehabilitation.* St. Louis, MO: Saunders; 2009:497-527.

120. Gordon EJ. Trochanteric bursitis and tendinitis. *Clin Orthop.* 1961;20:193-202.

121. Renne JW. The iliotibial band friction syndrome. *J Bone and Joint Surg.* 1975;57:1110-1111.

122. Evans P. The postural function of the iliotibial tract. *Ann Royal Coll Surg Eng.* 1979;61:271-280.

123. Pease BJ, Cortese M. Anterior Knee Pain: *Differential Diagnosis and Physical Therapy Management.* La Crosse, WI: Orthopaedic Section, APTA, Inc; 1992.

124. Grelsamer RP, McConnell J. *Normal and Abnormal Anatomy of the Extensor Mechanism. The Patella: A Team Approach.* Maryland: Aspen; 1998:11-24.

125. Kapandji IA. *The Physiology of the Joints, Lower Limb.* New York: Churchill Livingstone; 1991.

126. Durrani Z, Winnie AP. Piriformis muscle syndrome: An underdiagnosed cause of sciatica. *J Pain and Symptom Manage.* 1991;6:374-379.

127. Julsrud ME. Piriformis syndrome. *J Am Podiat Med Assn.* 1989; 79:128-131.

128. Pace JB, Nagle D. Piriformis syndrome. *Western J Med.* 1976;124:435-439.

129. Steiner C, Staubs C, Ganon M, Buhlinger C. Piriformis syndrome: Pathogenesis, diagnosis, and treatment. *J Am Osteopath Assn.* 1987; 87:318-323.

130. Harvey G, Bell S. Obturator neuropathy. An anatomic perspective. *Clin Orthop Relat Res.* 1999;363:203-211.

131. Williams PL, Warwick R, Dyson M, Bannister LH. *Gray's Anatomy,* 37th ed. London: Churchill Livingstone; 1989.

132. Dixon MC, Scott RD, Schai PA, Stamos V. A simple capsulorrhaphy in a posterior approach for total hip arthroplasty. *J Arthroplasty.* 2004;19:373-376.

133. Mihalko WM, Whiteside LA. Hip mechanics after posterior structure repair in total hip arthroplasty. *Clin Orthop Relat Res.* 2004;420:194-198.

134. Lynch SA, Renstrom PA. Groin injuries in sport: Treatment strategies. *Sports Med.* 1999;28:137-144.

135. Holmich P. Adductor related groin pain in athletes. *Sports Med Arth Rev.* 1998;5:285-291.

136. Hasselman CT, Best TM, Garrett WE. When groin pain signals an adductor strain. *Physician Sports Med.* 1995;23:53-60.

137. Johnson CE, Basmajian JV, Dasher W. Electromyography of the sartorius muscle. *Anat Rec.* 1972;173:127-130.

138. Anderson MA, Gieck JH, Perrin D, Weltman A, Rutt R, Denegar C. The relationship among isokinetic, isotonic, and isokinetic concentric and eccentric quadriceps and hamstrings force and three components of athletic performance. *J Orthop Sports Phys Ther.* 1991;14:114-120.

139. Lieb F, Perry J. Quadriceps function. *J Bone and Joint Surg Am.* 1968; 50:1535.

140. Hallisey MJ, Doherty N, Bennett WF, Fulkerson JP. Anatomy of the junction of the vastus lateralis tendon and the patella. *J Bone Joint Surg Am.* 1987;69:545-549.

141. Bose K, Kanagasuntheram R, Osman MBH. Vastus medialis oblique: an anatomic and physiologic study. *Orthopedics.* 1980;3:880-883.

142. Grelsamer RP. Patellar Malalignment. *J Bone Joint Surg Am.* 2000; 82-A:1639-1650.

143. Koskinen SK, Kujala UM. Patellofemoral relationships and distal insertion of the vastus medialis muscle: A magnetic resonance imaging study in nonsymptomatic subjects and in patients with patellar dislocation. *Arthroscopy.* 1992;8:465-458.

144. Raimondo RA, Ahmad CS, Blankevoort L, April EW, Grelsamer RP, Henry JH. Patellar stabilization: A quantitative evaluation of the vastus medialis obliquus muscle. *Orthopedics.* 1998;21:791-795.

145. Nakamura Y, Ohmichi H, Miyashita M, eds. EMG relationship during maximum voluntary contraction of the quadriceps. IX Congress of the International Society of Biomechanics; 1983; Waterloo, Ontario.

146. Knight KL, Martin JA, Londerdee BR. EMG comparison of quadriceps femoris activity during knee extensions and straight leg raises. *Am J Phys Med.* 1979;58:57-69.

147. Brownstein BA, Lamb RL, Mangine RE. Quadriceps torque and integrated electromyography. *J Orthop Sports Phys Ther.* 1985;6:309-314.

148. Fox TA. Dysplasia of the quadriceps mechanism: hypoplasia of the vastus medialis muscle as related to the hypermobile patella syndrome. *Surg Clin North Am.* 1975;55:199-226.

149. Tria AJ, Palumbo RC, Alicia JA. Conservative care for patellofemoral pain. *Orthop Clin N Am.* 1992;23:545-554.

150. Reynolds L, Levin TA, Medeiros JM, Adler NS, Allum A. EMG activity of the vastus medialis oblique and the vastus lateralis in the their role in patellar alignment. *Phys Med.* 1983;62:62-70.

151. Moller BN, Krebs B, Tideman-Dal C, Aaris K. Isometric contractions in the patellofemoral pain syndrome. *Arch Orthop Trauma Surg.* 1986;105:124.

152. Reid DC. Anterior knee pain and the patellofemoral pain syndrome. *Sports Injury Assessment and Rehabilitation.* New York: Churchill Livingstone; 1992:345-398.

153. Larson RL, Jones DC. Dislocations and ligamentous injuries of the knee. In: Rockwood CA, Green DP, eds. *Fractures in Adults,* 2nd ed. Philadelphia: JB Lippincott; 1984:1480-1591.

154. Gill DM, Corbacio EJ, Lauchle LE. Anatomy of the knee. In: Engle RP, ed. *Knee Ligament Rehabilitation.* New York: Churchill Livingstone; 1991:1-15.

155. Kendall FP, McCreary EK, Provance PG. *Muscles: Testing and Function.* Baltimore: Williams & Wilkins; 1993.

156. O'Connor JJ. Can muscle co-contraction protect knee ligaments after injury or repair? *J Bone and Joint Surg.* 1993;75-B:41-48.

157. Fleming BC, Renstrom PA, Goran O, Johnson RJ, Peura GD, Beynnon BD, et al. The gastrocnemius muscle is an antagonist of the anterior cruciate ligament. *J Orthop Res.* 2001;19:1178-1184.

158. Timm KE. Knee. In: Richardson JK, Iglarsh ZA, eds. *Clinical Orthopaedic Physical Therapy.* Philadelphia: WB Saunders; 1994:399-482.

159. Sudasna S, Harnsiriwattanagit K. The ligamentous structures of the posterolateral aspect of the knee. *Bull Hosp Joint Dis Orthop Institute.* 1990;50:35-40.

160. Brownstein B, Noyes FR, Mangine RE, Kryger S. Anatomy and biomechanics. In: Mangine RE, ed. *Physical Therapy of the Knee.* New York: Churchill Livingstone; 1988:1-30.

161. Magee DJ. *Orthopedic Physical Assessment,* 2nd ed. Philadelphia: WB Saunders Company; 1992.

162. Reid DC. Knee ligament injuries, anatomy, classification, and examination. In: Reid DC, ed. *Sports Injury Assessment and Rehabilitation.* New York: Churchill Livingstone; 1992:437-493.

163. Nyland J, Lachman N, Kocabey Y, Brosky J, Altun R, Caborn D. Anatomy, function, and rehabilitation of the popliteus musculotendinous complex. *J Orthop Sports Phys Ther.* 2005;35:165-179.

164. Veltri DM, Deng XH, Torzilli PA, Warren RF, Maynard MJ. The role of the cruciate and posterolateral ligaments in stability of the knee. A biomechanical study. *Am J Sports Med.* 1995;23:436-443.

165. Veltri DM, Deng XH, Torzilli PA, Maynard MJ, Warren RF. The role of the popliteofibular ligament in stability of the human knee. A biomechanical study. *Am J Sports Med.* 1996;24:19-27.

166. Maynard MJ, Deng XH, Wickiewicz TL, Warren RF. The popliteofibular ligament. Rediscovery of a key element in posterolateral stability. *Am J Sports Med.* 1996;24:311-316.

167. Veltri DM, Warren RF, Wickiewicz TL, O'Brien SJ. Current status of allograft meniscal transplantation. *Clin Orthop Relat Res.* 1994;303:44-55.

168. Last RJ. The popliteus muscle and the lateral meniscus. *J Bone Joint Surg.* 1950;32B:93-99.

169. Scioli MW. Achilles tendinitis. *Orthop Clin North Am.* 1994;25:177-182.

170. Soma CA, Mandelbaum BR. Achilles tendon disorders. *Clin Sports Med.* 1994;13:811-823.

171. Gerdes MH, Brown TW, Bell A, et al. A flap augmentation technique for Achilles tendon repair. Postoperative strength and functional outcome. *Clin Orthop.* 1992;280:241-246.

172. Reynolds NL, Worrell TW. Chronic Achilles peritendinitis: etiology, pathophysiology, and treatment. *J Orthop Sports Phys Ther.* 1991;13:171-176.

173. Carr AJ, Norris SH. The blood supply of the calcaneal tendon. *J Bone and Joint Surg.* 1989;71B:100-111.

174. Lagergren C, Lindholm A. Vascular distribution in the Achilles tendon: An angiographic and microangiographic study. *Acta Chir Scand.* 1958;116:491-495.

175. Nelen G, Martens M, Bursens A. Surgical treatment of chronic Achilles tendinitis. *Am J Sports Med.* 1989;17:754-759.

176. Nichols AW. Achilles tendinitis in running athletes. *J Am Bd Fam Pract.* 1989;2:196-203.

177. Conti SF. Posterior tibial tendon problems in athletes. *Orthop Clin North America.* 1994;25:109-121.

178. Clarke HD, Kitaoka HB, Ehman RL. Peroneal tendon injuries. *Foot Ankle Int.* 1998;19:280-288.

179. Brage ME, Hansen ST. Traumatic subluxation/dislocation of the peroneal tendons. *Foot Ankle Int.* 1992;13:423-431.

180. Thordarson DB, Schotzer H, Chon J, et al. Dynamic support of the human longitudinal arch. *Clin Orthop.* 1995;316:165-172.

181. Mann R, Inman V. Phasic activity of intrinsic muscles of the foot. *J Bone Joint Surg Am.* 1964;46:469-481.

182. Daniels K, Worthingham C. *Muscle Testing Techniques of Manual Examination,* 5th ed. Philadelphia: WB Saunders; 1986.

183. Harvey VP, Scott GD. An investigation of the curl-down test as a measure of abdominal strength. *Res Q.* 1967;38:22-27.

184. Fitzgerald MJT, Comerford PT, Tuffery AR. Sources of innervation of the neuromuscular spindles in sternomastoid and trapezius. *J Anat.* 1982;134:471-490.

185. Palmer ML, Epler M. *Clinical Assessment Procedures in Physical Therapy.* Philadelphia: JB Lippincott; 1990.

186. Huijbregts PA. Lumbopelvic region: Anatomy and biomechanics. In: Wadsworth C, ed. *Current Concepts of Orthopaedic Physical Therapy—Home Study Course.* La Crosse, WI: Orthopaedic Section, APTA; 2001.

187. Lee DG. *The Pelvic Girdle: An Approach to the Examination and Treatment of the Lumbo-Pelvic-Hip Region,* 2nd ed. Edinburgh: Churchill Livingstone; 1999.

188. Aspden RM. Review of the functional anatomy of the spinal ligaments and the lumbar erector spinae muscles. *Clin Anat.* 1992;5:372-387.

189. Jull G, Richardson CA, Hamilton C, et al. Towards the validation of a clinical test for the deep abdominal muscles in back pain patients: Manipulative Physiotherapists Association of Australia Ninth Biennial Conference. Gold Coast, Queensland. 1995;65-67.

190. Richardson CA, Jull GA, Hodges P, Hides J. *Therapeutic Exercise for Spinal Segmental Stabilization in Low Back Pain.* London: Churchill Livingstone; 1999.

191. Magee DJ. Lumbar spine. In: Magee DJ, ed. *Orthopedic Physical Assessment,* 4th ed. Philadelphia: W.B. Saunders; 2002:467-566.

192. Moreland J, Finch E, Stratford P, et al. Interrater reliability of six tests of trunk muscle function and endurance. *J Orthop Sports Phys Ther.* 1997;26:200-208.

193. Reese NB. *Muscle and Sensory Testing.* Philadelphia: WB Saunders; 1999.

194. McGill SM, Childs A, Liebenson C. Endurance times for low back stabilization exercises: Clinical targets for testing and training from a normal database. *Arch Phys Med Rehab.* 1999;80:941-944.

195. Ashmen KJ, Swanik CB, Lephart SM. Strength and flexibility characteristics of athletes with chronic low back pain. *J Sport Rehab.* 1996;5:372-387.

196. Hodges P, Richardson C, Jull G. Evaluation of the relationship between laboratory and clinical tests of transversus abdominis function. *Physiother Res Int.* 1996;1:30-40.

197. O'Sullivan P, Twomey L, Allison G. Evaluation of specific stabilizing exercise in the treatment of chronic low back pain with radiologic diagnosis of spondylolysis or spondylolisthesis. *Spine.* 1997;22:2959-2967.

198. O'Sullivan P, Twomey L, Allison G. Altered patterns of abdominal muscle activation in chronic back pain patients. *Aust J Physiother.* 1997;43:91-98.

199. Clark MA. *Integrated Training for the New Millenium.* Thousand Oaks, CA: National Academy of Sports Medicine; 2001.

200. Clarkson HM. *Musculoskeletal Assessment,* 2nd ed. Philadelphia: Lippincott Williams & Wilkins; 2000.

201. Youdas JW, Garrett TR, Egan KS, Therneau TM. Lumbar lordosis and pelvic inclination in adults with chronic low back pain. *Phys Ther.* 2000;80:261-275.

202. Zannotti CM, Bohannon RW, Tiberio D, et al. Kinematics of the double-leg-lowering test for abdominal muscle strength. *J Orthop Sports Phys Ther.* 2002;32:432-436.

203. Gracovetsky S, Farfan HF. The optimum spine. *Spine.* 1986;11:543.

204. Gracovetsky S, Farfan HF, Helleur C. The abdominal mechanism. *Spine.* 1985;10:317-324.

205. Hyman J, Liebenson C. Spinal stabilization exercise program. In: Liebenson C, ed. *Rehabilitation of the Spine: A Practitioner's Manual.* Baltimore: Lippincott Williams & Wilkins; 1996:293-317.

CHAPTER 10

Patient Transfers and Mobility

CHAPTER OBJECTIVES

At the completion of this chapter, the reader will be able to:

1. Understand the importance of choosing the most efficient and safest method of transfer and mobility task

2. Determine the best transfer or mobility procedure based on the level of patient dependence or independence

3. Discuss the importance of patient safety during transfers and mobility tasks

4. Discuss the importance of clinician safety during transfers and mobility tasks

5. Transfer a patient to and from many different types of surfaces

6. Perform a variety of mobility tasks

7. Describe the various wheelchair components and their functions

8. Measure a patient for a wheelchair

9. Train a patient in how to use a wheelchair

OVERVIEW

A transfer can be viewed as the safe movement of a person from one place or surface to another and an opportunity to train an individual to enhance independent function. In both cases, the clinician must choose the most efficient and safest method.

Controlling a patient's movement while moving them from one position or surface to another or preventing a patient from falling requires that the clinician be close to the patient's center of motion (COM), which is typically located between the shoulders and the pelvis. When these control points are used, patient transfers are more efficient, and patient safety is enhanced. The most efficient way to enhance the patient's movement (unless they are completely dependent) is to encourage movement of the body's distal component—the part of the body farthest from the trunk. For example, when assisting a patient to stand from a seated position, a common verbal cue is to ask the patient to lean their trunk forward. It is also important to have the patient look in the direction of the transfer's destination to encourage correct head-turning.

PATIENT TRANSFERS

One of the main purposes of transfers is to permit a patient to function in different environments and increase their independence level. Several moving and lifting devices (total body lifts and sit-to-stand lifts) have been designed and incorporated into the healthcare system because of advancements in recent years. However, because of the expense and sometimes the inconvenience of these devices, manual transfers continue to be commonly used. In these cases, the best body mechanics possible should be used to maximize the ability to encompass a task with minimal effort and maximum safety (see Chapter 7). It is important to note that certain transfers increase the risk for injury (Table 10-1), necessitating additional care and attention. Depending on the patient's functional ability, a transfer may be performed independently by the patient, with assistance from the clinician (minimal, moderate, maximal, or standby supervision) or dependently (Table 10-2).

CLINICAL PEARL

During a sit-to-stand transfer, several forces are at play. These include:

▶ Gravity.

▶ The combined weight of the clinician's trunk, arms, and head (TAH), which is approximately 65% of the total weight of the body. The moment arm (MA) for TAH (TAH_{MA}) is the perpendicular distance between gravity's line of action acting on the TAH to the axis.

▶ The force required to extend the clinician's trunk, which is borne by the erector spinae muscles (Mu). The moment arm for Mu is the perpendicular distance between the line of action of Mu and the axis (MA_{Mu}).

▶ The weight of the patient (depends on the level of assistance required).

There are two options for the lower extremities:

▶ Keeping the knees extended.

▶ Flexing the knees.

To calculate the difference in forces that the erector spinae muscles of the trunk of an individual weighing 160 lbs (712 N) must generate between the two lower extremity positions (excluding the weight of the patient), a few simple mathematical equations can be used:

Knees extended:

$$TAH = 712 * 0.65 = 463$$

$$NMA_{TAH} = 0.5\ m;\ MA_{Mu} = 0.04\ m$$

$$Mu = (TAH * MA_{TAH})/MA_{Mu} = (463\ N * 0.5\ m)/0.04\ m = 5782\ N\ (approximately\ 1300\ lbs)$$

Knees flexed:

$$TAH = 712 * 0.65 = 463\ N$$

$$MA_{TAH} = 0.25\ m;\ MA_{Mu} = 0.04\ m$$

$$Mu = (TAH * MA_{TAH})/MA_{Mu} = (463\ N * 0.25\ m)/0.04\ m = 2894\ N\ (approximately\ 650\ lbs)$$

Several factors influence the decision on how a transfer is to be performed and how many helpers are needed (Table 10-3). In addition to the factors listed in Table 10-3, the clinician should consider the following before performing a transfer:

TABLE 10-1	Transfer Techniques and Their Risk for Injury from the Least to Most Stressful

Transferring a patient from bathtub to chair
Transferring a patient from bed to chair
Transferring a patient from chair to bed
Transferring a patient from chair to toilet
Transferring a patient from toilet to chair

Reproduced with permission from Garg A, Owen BD, Carlson B: An ergonomic evaluation of nursing assistants' job in a nursing home, *Ergonomics*. 1992 Sep;35(9):979-995.

▶ The patient's level of cognition, emotional capability, and physical ability.

▶ How much assistance the clinician requires. When in doubt, a second person should be used.

▶ The appropriate equipment should be arranged before the transfer.

▶ Correct positioning of both the patient and the clinician. The clinician should maintain a large base of support (BOS) and use proper body mechanics throughout the transfer.

A patient's medical or physical condition may require modification to a transfer technique. For example, range of motion (ROM) restrictions, decreased muscle control, and poor balance may require an adaptation to the transfer technique. In the case of decreased muscle control, it is generally easier for the patient to transfer toward the stronger side.

TABLE 10-2	Levels of Physical Dependence and Recommended Assists	
Level of Dependence	**Definition**	**Recommended Assist**
Independent	The patient does not require any form of assistance (physical or verbal) to complete the task safely and in an acceptable time frame.	None
Modified independent assisted	The patient uses adaptive or assistive equipment (furniture, bed rail, grab bars, transfer board) but can perform the task without assistance, including verbal or tactile cues.	Gait or transfer belt Assistive device
Assisted	The patient requires assistance (oral or tactile cues) from another person to perform the activity safely and in an acceptable time frame.	Gait or transfer belt Assistive device
Standby assist (supervision)	The patient requires oral or tactile cues from another person positioned close to but not touching to perform the activity safely and in an acceptable time frame.	Gait or transfer belt Assistive device
Contact guard	The patient requires the clinician to maintain contact with the patient or safety belt to complete the task. A contact guard is usually needed to assist if there is a loss of balance.	Gait or transfer belt Assistive device
Minimal assist	The patient can perform approximately 75% of the task but requires approximately 25% of assistance from the clinician to complete the task.	Stand-assist lift Transfer board Gait or transfer belt
Moderate assist	The patient can perform approximately 50% of the task but requires approximately 50% of assistance from the clinician to complete the task.	Stand-assist lift
Maximal assist	The patient can perform approximately 25% of the task but requires approximately 75% of assistance from the clinician to complete the task.	Mechanical lift with a full sling Stand-assist lift
Dependent	The patient cannot participate, and the clinician must provide all of the effort to perform the task.	Mechanical lift with a full sling Transfer chair that can be converted into a stretcher

TABLE 10-3	Factors That Influence Decision Making for Transfers	
Factor	**Example**	**Influences on Decision**
Patient	Weight, strength, endurance, cooperation, level of fear, cognition level, weight-bearing status, physical capabilities/limitations, sitting or standing balance, movement precautions, current transfer ability, head control, pain level, footwear, and any required external device	Small movements generally allow for greater control over both the movement and any equipment. More assistance generally allows for greater control and support.
Environment	The proximity of the transfer surfaces, equipment needed, floor surface (carpet, tile, etc) the height differences between the two surfaces, and the width of the two transfer surfaces	The two transfer surfaces should be arranged so that the clinician can maintain an upright position that minimizes trunk flexion, can achieve good trunk stability and can perform the transfer with an unobstructed path.
Task	The type of transfer and the objective of the transfer	This type of transfer is largely determined by the patient's capabilities to assist as much as possible.

Before meeting the patient, the clinician should review the medical record to determine their limitations and abilities. When appropriate, the clinician should interview the patient's family for information as to their abilities. Physical abilities to consider include gross motor strength and control, joint and soft tissue flexibility, sitting and standing endurance, and sitting and standing balance. The major muscle groups involved with transfers include the patient's elbow extensors and flexors, the shoulder extensors and flexors, and the hip and knee extensors. Having reviewed the medical record and talked to the patient's family, and considered the goals of the treatment, the clinician must determine whether mechanical or human assistance will be needed. The types of equipment used in transfers include but are not limited to a trapeze bar, a transfer board, a transfer/gait belt, and a hydraulic or pneumatic lift/hoist.

▶ *Trapeze bar.* Consists of a metal triangle, a chain, and clamps and is used to assist patients to maneuver in bed by pulling with one or both upper extremities.

▶ *Transfer boards.* These items, which come in various shapes and sizes, are most commonly used for horizontal transfers, such as transferring from the bed to a wheelchair or a wheelchair to a mat table.

▶ *Transfer/gait belt.* As a patient's activities advance to those requiring a higher COM, a smaller BOS, and a higher demand for dynamic stability, the risk of falling increases. These belts provide an alternative method of providing a control point near the center of the patient's body during transfers when direct manual contacts cannot be safely maintained. In some settings, transfer belts may be required equipment.

▶ *Hydraulic or pneumatic lift/hoist.* These pieces of equipment (Figure 10-1), commonly referred to as Hoyer lifts, are designed for many uses to help transport patients from a bed to a chair, wheelchair, or toilet, or assist a patient in standing from a seated position. Their operation can be manual, through the use of a pump handle, or electric. Each lift is fitted with caster wheels to aid in positioning and maneuvering, and the base of the lift can be widened to fit around a wheelchair or other equipment. Also, each

lift has a sling made of various fabrics and designs on which the patient rests. The sling is attached to a spreader bar on the lift by two chains with hooks, and the length of the chain can be adjusted to accommodate the patient's height.

CLINICAL PEARL

Documentation concerning transfers must include the equipment or devices used, the amount or type of assistance a patient requires to perform the transfer, the amount of time to complete it, the level of safety demonstrated, and the level of consistency of the performance.

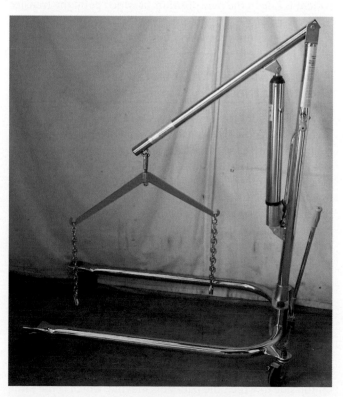

FIGURE 10-1 Hydraulic or pneumatic lift/hoist.

Transfers require movements that move the center of gravity (COG) away from the BOS for both the patient and the clinician. These movements have the potential of causing a loss of balance. After the introductions between the clinician and the patient, it is important to inform the patient what transfer is to occur and why.

CLINICAL PEARL

During a transfer, the clinician's primary responsibility is to avoid patient injury or injury to himself or herself.

Setting the feet in stride and slightly apart provides a larger BOS. The clinician's feet should also be unencumbered to move as the situation requires, always allowing the BOS to be re-established under the moving COG as necessary. Any crossing of the clinician's legs during movement should be avoided, because it decreases the BOS size and constrains foot movement.

Patients must know what they are to do and when they are to do it during transfers to participate effectively. Any instructions must be kept simple and informative, using terminology that the patient can understand. Verbal explanations and physical demonstrations should be used to highlight the expectations and transfer sequence. Having the patient repeat the instructions ensures that the patient understands them. If necessary, the patient is taught smaller segments of the transfer before performing the entire transfer. Manual contacts can be used with the patient to direct his or her participation during the transfer.

Commands and counts can be used to help synchronize the various components of the transfer. The typical command and count used is "one, two, three, lift." It is important to remember that a transfer is not considered complete until the patient is safe in the new position, at which point the transfer team can release control of the patient.

The most common transfers are described in this chapter.

Transfer from Bed to Wheeled Stretcher—Sliding Method

The clinician informs the patient about what is to occur and then positions the wheeled stretcher parallel to, against, and at approximately the same height as the bed. Whenever possible, the target transfer surface should be lower than the surface the patient is being transferred from. It is also important to ensure that the transfer surface's height is appropriate for the clinician. As a general rule, this is at waist level. The cart is positioned on the patient's uninvolved side. The bed rails and stretcher rails are lowered, and both the bed and the stretcher are secured using wheel locks or other appropriate devices. If the patient can move without assistance, the stretcher is stabilized, and the clinician merely provides verbal assistance. If the patient cannot assist in the transfer, three or more able-bodied individuals are needed to perform the transfer using a draw sheet. The draw sheet is placed under the patient and then rolled and grasped close to the patient by each clinician (Figure 10-2). If three clinicians are used, two of them are on the side to which the patient is moving, which is the same side as the wheeled stretcher (see Figure 10-2), and the other

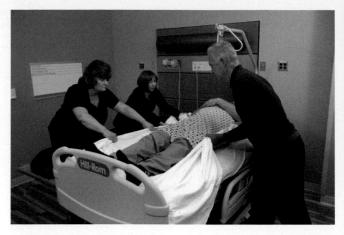

FIGURE 10-2 Clinician positioning in preparation for sliding transfer.

clinician, whose main function is to help guide the direction of the transfer, is on the other side of the bed (VIDEO 10-1). When all three clinicians are positioned correctly, the clinician at the head of the bed takes responsibility for coordinating the transfer and issuing the various commands. During the first lift, the patient is pulled toward the edge of the side of the bed in the direction of the transfer (Figure 10-3), then to the edge of the bed (Figure 10-4), and finally onto the cart (Figure 10-5).

Video Description

Note how the clinicians roll the edges of the sheet to form a handle. One clinician is designated to coordinate the transfer. Whenever there is an odd number of helpers, the majority are positioned on the side toward which the patient is being moved. Depending on the bed and stretcher's width and the patient's size, it may be necessary for one or more of the clinicians to assume a kneeling position on one of the transfer surfaces. Note how the clinician on the side opposite the direction of the transfer leans forward over the transfer surface while securing the thighs against the side of the bed to maintain good trunk stability and enhance leverage.

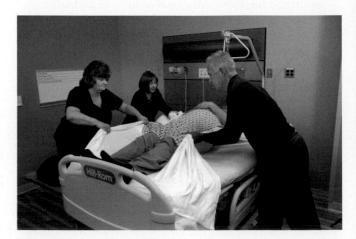

FIGURE 10-3 Patient is moved toward the wheeled stretcher.

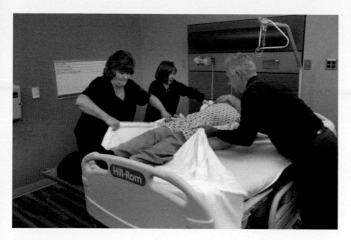

FIGURE 10-4 Patient is moved to the edge of the bed.

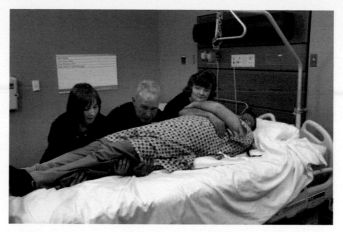

FIGURE 10-6 Clinician positioning for three-person carry.

Several devices have recently been introduced that minimize the level of physical assistance by the clinician. These include:

▶ *Rigid or semirigid transfer boards.* These friction-reducing devices are made of various materials and have handles along the board's edge in the form of openings.

▶ *Patient roller.* This mechanical device consists of multiple rollers placed within a rigid frame and enclosed in a cover. This device is commonly used to transfer patients from wheel stretchers to surgical tables.

▶ *Slippery sheet.* This is essentially a flat nylon sheet, coated with a low-friction solution, with handles on the sides.

▶ *Air assistive device.* This device consists of an upper and a lower air chamber, both of which are mechanically inflated to create a cushioned film of air underneath the patient, thereby reducing friction.

Transfer from Bed to Wheeled Stretcher—Three-Person Carry

This technique is used when the bed and wheeled stretcher cannot be situated parallel to each other or at a safe height distance. The clinicians involved in the transfer must remove

all jewelry to prevent scratching the patient. One of the three clinicians positions the cart perpendicular to the bed with the head of the cart at the foot end of the bed. Alternatively, the cart can be positioned perpendicular to the bed with the foot of the cart at the head of the bed. The three clinicians stand on the same side of the bed and are positioned in such a way that one can support the head and upper trunk of the patient, one can support the midsection of the patient, and one can support the lower extremities (Figure 10-6). Ideally, the strongest clinician is in the middle position or at the head. The clinician at the head of the bed takes responsibility for coordinating the transfer and issuing the various commands. When the three clinicians are positioned correctly, each of them slides both arms under the patient so that the elbows rest on the treatment table and the patient is cradled from head to foot (Figure 10-7). Each clinician places one foot in front of the other, and, on the first lift command, the patient is moved to the edge of the bed. Then, by flexing the elbows, the clinicians roll the patient onto his or her side as in a log roll, so that the patient is now cradled in the bend of the clinicians' elbows, which brings the weight of the patient closer to the center of the clinicians' BOS (Figure 10-8). On the second lift command, the clinicians simultaneously stand and lift the patient. On the command to pivot, the clinicians pivot and line up parallel to the cart, moving forward in a straight line until all

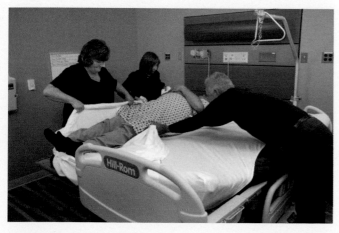

FIGURE 10-5 Patient is moved onto the wheeled stretcher.

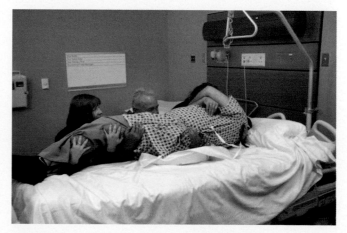

FIGURE 10-7 Patient is cradled in clinicians' arms.

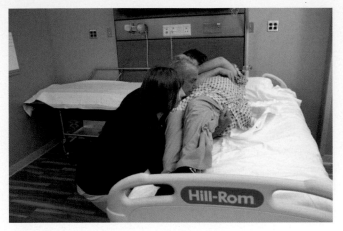

FIGURE 10-8 Patient is rolled toward the clinicians.

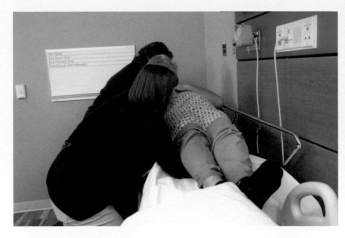

FIGURE 10-10 Patient is rolled onto the wheeled stretcher.

three clinicians feel the edge of the wheeled stretcher against their thighs. Again, each clinician places one foot in front of the other and, on the command to lower the patient, the clinicians bend their legs until the elbows rest on the edge of the stretcher (Figure 10-9) and then slowly lower the patient onto the center of the wheeled stretcher (Figure 10-10). Once the patient is positioned correctly, the clinicians remove their arms from under the patient, and the rails of the stretcher are raised (Figure 10-11).

Transfer from Bed to Chair Using Hydraulic/ Pneumatic Lift

The clinician moves the lift close to the patient and detaches the sling. The clinician first places a rolled sling under the patient by rolling the patient onto one side. The sling is positioned so that the seams are outside, away from the patient, to avoid pressure areas. Once the rolled sling is positioned correctly, the patient is then rolled to the other side, and the sling is unrolled. The clinician positions the lift so that the spreader bar is across the patient, and both ends of the chain are then attached to their respective sides of the sling. The shorter segment of each chain is attached to the upper part of the sling, which is the part that supports the patient's back.

The longer segment of each chain is attached to the lower part of the sling, which is the part that supports the patient's lower extremities. The chain hooks are attached from inside the sling to the outside to reduce patient injury by the hook. Once the chains have been attached, the clinician begins lifting the patient, using the lift to move the patient into a sitting position. Once the patient is secured in the sitting position, the clinician uses one arm under the patient's lower extremities to assist the patient's lower extremities off the bed so that the lift fully suspends the patient. While the clinician prevents the patient from swaying excessively, the patient is moved to a locked wheelchair, the base of the lift is placed in the wide position, and the lift is maneuvered so that the patient is over the seat of the locked wheelchair. The clinician then operates the lift to slowly lower the patient into the wheelchair while applying a slight pressure at the patient's knees or thighs to steer the patient into the wheelchair so that the patient's back is resting firmly against the back of the wheelchair. Once the patient is correctly and safely seated in the wheelchair, the chains are removed from the sling and, after checking that the patient is capable of sitting without assistance, the clinician moves the hydraulic lift safely away from the patient. Depending on when the next transfer is to occur, the sling may be left in situ depending on the sling design. For example, one-piece slings

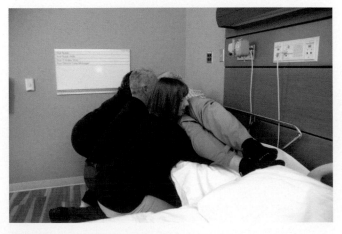

FIGURE 10-9 Patient is lowered onto the wheeled stretcher.

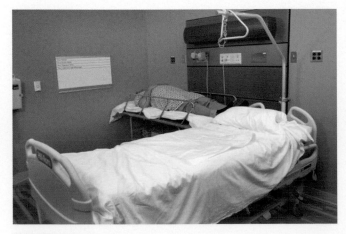

FIGURE 10-11 Patient position after transfer.

are left in place under the patient, whereas the portion behind the patient's back in a two-piece sling can be removed.

WHEELCHAIR MOBILITY

A wheelchair is a postural support system on wheels used by people for whom walking is difficult or impossible because of illness or disability. Whenever possible, every attempt should be made to design the wheelchair to provide the patient with maximum function, comfort, stability, safety, and protection, while also reducing the amount of force required to propel the wheelchair. Fortunately, wheelchairs are now available in various sizes and styles, and wheelchair design continues to improve in both safety and construction.

Wheelchairs can be grouped into several classes: indoor (small wheelbase to allow maneuvering in confined spaces, but lacks the ability or power to negotiate obstacles), indoor/outdoor (provides mobility for those who stay on finished surfaces, such as sidewalks, driveways, and flooring), and active indoor/outdoor (provides the ability to travel long distances, move fast, and drive over unstructured environments such as grass, gravel, and uneven terrain) (Table 10-4).

Wheelchair fitting is highly individualized and requires a team effort among the physiatrist, neurologist, orthopedist, occupational or physical therapist, a specialist in assistive

TABLE 10-4	Types of Wheelchairs	
Type	**Description**	**Comments**
Standard	Designed for temporary use for individuals under 200 lbs	Requires manual propulsion Ideal for smooth surfaces only May or may not have removable armrests/leg rests Although foldable and therefore transportable, they are generally heavy (average weight = 50 lbs)
Pediatric	Essentially a smaller version of the standard wheelchair	Lighter and therefore easier to transport
Bariatric	Similar to standard wheelchair design except sturdier Appropriate for individuals over 200 lbs	Very heavy
Hemiplegic	Designed for patients who have a one-sided weakness, eg, following a cerebrovascular accident (stroke). Wheelchair height is usually 2 inches lower than standard wheelchair to allow the patient to propel the wheelchair with their feet Some allow for a single-hand drive to propel and turn the chair Usually fitted with a double handrim—the outer rim controls the wheel on the same side, and the smaller rim controls the wheel on the other side	Tend to be more difficult to transport than a standard wheelchair. May require a chairlift and therefore a transport-type van
Amputee	Drive wheels positioned two inches posterior to the normal position, which produces a wider base of support	Built-in counterbalance compensates for the loss of lower extremities, increasing stability
Sport	Designed with lightweight materials (aircraft aluminum alloys, titanium, or graphite), low seatbacks, and angled wheels. Some racing wheelchairs weigh only 15 lbs Folding frames, with or without crossbars, usually fitted with locks to prevent even minor folding during activity	Very maneuverable Many color choices
Ultralight	Lighter than a standard wheelchair (~25 lbs) Rigid or collapsible Fixed or removable leg rests	Easier to transport Increased mobility Very light (~25 lbs)
Motorized	Powered by electric/battery motors Controlled by mouth/chin pieces or joysticks Fixed or adjustable speeds	Frequently prescribed for people with severe neuromusculoskeletal disabilities or poor endurance due to cardiopulmonary disease Extremely heavy Batteries need replacing
Tilting space/reclining	Reclining chairs offer fully or semi-reclining chair back Tilting space chairs allow the entire chair to be tilted at different angles Both types of chairs require headrests and elevating leg rests but can be customized with various accessories (lateral trunk support, seat cushions, etc)	Very large and difficult to transport

technology and driver training, and rehabilitation technology providers. When helping choose a wheelchair, a few patient and design-based considerations must be taken into account. The patient considerations include:

▶ *Patient needs.* These needs can include recreational, social, or vocational needs. Depending on the patient's age, peer acceptance may be a patient need. An individual's needs can change with time, so it is well worth anticipating future needs, prognosis, or change.

▶ *Mobility needs.* The team needs to observe the patient and the current wheelchair to determine how well the wheelchair serves the patient's mobility needs, including locomotion requirements for the home and community.

▶ *Physical abilities.* Manual wheelchairs require a significant amount of strength and endurance to operate, so the team needs to help choose a wheelchair that will not hinder mobility because of a patient's physical limitations. It is also important to determine the patient's ability to alter their position, especially over bony prominences.

▶ *Sensory awareness.* The team must determine whether the patient has any impaired peripheral circulation, abnormal skin integrity, or neurologic dysfunction.

▶ *Dexterity and coordination.* Many of the components of the wheelchair, such as the brakes and seatbelt on a standard wheelchair, require a fair degree of dexterity and coordination on the part of the patient.

▶ *Anthropometric characteristics.* Of particular importance are the patient's height and weight (see Wheelchair Measurements, later).

The design considerations (see Wheelchair Components, later) include:

▶ Wheelchair weight
▶ Seating system
▶ Armrest style
▶ Front rigging (leg rests and footplates)
▶ Frame
▶ Drive wheels
▶ Tires
▶ Casters
▶ Manual versus power source
▶ Expected use of the chair
▶ Length of time the chair will be used—temporary or permanent

When combined, all of the listed design components add to the overall weight of a wheelchair. The more popular wheelchairs range in weight from 25 lbs (ultralight) to 45 lbs (standard).

All wheelchairs should be kept in good working order to ensure patient safety, ease of use, control of repair costs, and extended life of the chair. This may include regular lubrication, tire care, spoke maintenance, and lock maintenance. The owner's manual is an important resource and provides information about which parts of the wheelchair have a warranty, how to take care of the wheelchair, and where to buy replacements or accessories.

WHEELCHAIR COMPONENTS

The choice of which of the various wheelchair components should be used is based on the patient's needs and abilities. With each choice, there are positives and negatives. For example, the team often has to choose between stability and mobility or between size and maneuverability. Therefore, the team needs to make the patient aware of the available options and the advantages and disadvantages of each.

Frame

Stainless steel tubing used to be the only frame material available, and it made the wheelchair very heavy. However, wheelchair users today have their choice of aluminum, airplane steel, graphite, and titanium. A standard wheelchair (Figure 10-12) with a fixed box frame can be designed to support up to 250 lbs. However, because the frame is fixed, it results in less shock absorption and is difficult to transport. Next in terms of durability are wheelchairs with folding frames, which are constructed with a cross-brace design. This design allows the right and left sides of the chair to be brought together by pulling at the center of the sling seat or on the seat rail for ease in transportation and compact storage. Although the folding-frame wheelchair provides better suspension than a fixed box-frame wheelchair, it requires more energy to propel than the rigid frame design ones.

CLINICAL PEARL

Integrated standing wheelchairs are designed to allow a patient to move between sitting and standing while being supported by the chair.

In general, the lighter the frame's weight, the greater the ease of use, but the less structural strength provided.

CLINICAL PEARL

An antitipping/tipping device can be attached to the frame of the wheelchair. These devices are posterior extensions attached to the low horizontal supports to prevent the patient from tipping the wheelchair too far backward and falling but allowing a caregiver to tip the wheelchair back to negotiate stairs or curbs. These devices, which may need to be removed for a patient working on curb negotiation tasks, can often be tilted up out of the way in some models.

Items such as a headrest, lateral trunk support, back panel, armrest trough, and lower extremity supports can be added to a chair to accomplish specific goals. The team should observe the position of the head, trunk, pelvis, knees, and feet of the patient in the wheelchair, in addition to determining the patient's sitting balance, stability, reaching ability, ability to change positions, transferability, and preferred method of propulsion.

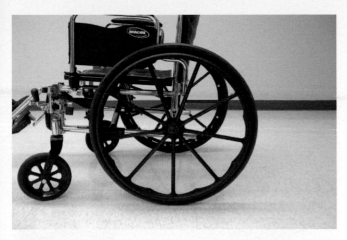

FIGURE 10-12 Standard wheelchair frame.

Upholstery

Upholstery for wheelchairs must withstand daily use in all kinds of weather. Consequently, manufacturers provide various options to users, ranging from cloth to new synthetic fabrics to leather. Many manufacturers also offer a selection of upholstery colors, ranging from black to neon, to allow for individual selection and differing tastes among consumers.

Seating System

The wheelchair seat provides postural support to the patient, so the seating system is considered one of the most important wheelchair components. Most standard wheelchairs come with a rigid or sling seat, which is adequate for an individual who uses the chair for short periods, but not for long-term use. For example, a sling seat encourages a forward head posture, the hips to slide forward, the thighs to adduct and internally rotate, and the patient to sit asymmetrically, reinforcing a poor pelvic position and increasing the potential for skin breakdown over the bony prominences. Proper seating and positioning aim to promote function, prevent secondary complications, prevent deformity, improve body alignment, and prevent tissue damage.

CLINICAL PEARL

It is very important to remember that no cushion design will prevent skin breakdown without frequent repositioning by the patient or caregiver.

Whenever possible, seating must be customized on an individual basis, and in most cases, seating surfaces are purchased separately from the wheelchairs themselves. Generally speaking, there are two types of cushions:

► *Uniform cushions.* These cushions are fabricated from wood or plastic and padded with foam. They create a stable, firm sitting surface, improve pelvic position, and reduce the tendency to slide forward or sit with a posterior pelvic tilt. Foam cushions are lighter but can also be bulky.

► *Contoured cushions.* These cushions can be inflatable or made from a gel-like substance and function to distribute weight-bearing pressures, which helps prevent decubitus ulcers in patients with decreased sensation, prolong wheelchair sitting times, and accommodate moderate to severe postural deformities. The inflatable cushions are light and can be filled or emptied for better customization. Gel cushions, which offer more support than foam cushions, tend to be heavy, more expensive (if customized), and require continuous maintenance. However, gel cushions can be custom-molded, are designed to accommodate moderate to severe postural deformity, and make it easy for caregivers to reposition the patient.

CLINICAL PEARL

The depth of the cushion is an important consideration. One that is too deep may interfere with slide board transfers.

Backrest

As with seat cushion systems, backrests come in rigid and sling varieties and are customizable. The standard-height backrest provides support to the mid-scapula region. Several modifications can be made to suit the user:

► A lower back height may increase functional mobility—typically seen in sports chairs—but may also increase back strain.

► *Lateral trunk supports:* improve trunk alignment for patients with scoliosis or poor stability.

► *Insert or contour backs:* improve trunk extension and overall upright alignment.

► *A high back height:* may be necessary for patients with poor trunk stability or with extensor spasms.

► *Reclining wheelchairs.* These are designed with an extended back and typically with elevating leg rests. The angle of the back is adjusted by releasing knobs on the side of the wheelchair. A head support is required on a reclining wheelchair. A bar across the back of the reclining wheelchair provides support and stability. The purpose of the reclining wheelchair is to allow intermittent or constant reclined positioning. Reclining wheelchairs are indicated for patients who are unable to maintain an upright sitting position independently. The chairs can be controlled either manually or electrically (if the patient cannot do active push-ups or pressure relief maneuvers).

► *Tilt in space.* A chair designed to allow for a reclining position without losing the required 90° of hip flexion and 90° of knee flexion. This chair is indicated for patients with extensor spasms that may throw the patient out of the chair or for pressure relief.

Armrests

Wheelchair armrests can be fixed or removable. Fixed armrests usually result in a lighter and narrower wheelchair, whereas removable armrests are important for patients who

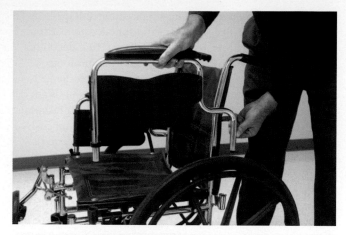

FIGURE 10-13 Removable armrest.

will be performing lateral transfers in and out of a wheelchair or for those who wish to sit closer to a table or desk. The removable armrests (Figure 10-13) are typically released using a lever, latch, or pushbutton. In addition to providing a place to rest the arms and support the upper body, correctly positioned armrests also decrease pressure through the buttocks. Armrests are available in several styles depending on the patient's needs:

▶ *Desk length.* This design, in which one portion of the armrest's length is lower than the remaining portion to allow the user closer access to desks and tables, also allows the patient to remove and reverse the armrest so that the higher part is closer to the front edge to aid in pushing to standing. The disadvantage of this type of armrest is that they provide less forearm support and are generally more expensive.

▶ *Full length.* These are designed to support the entire forearm's entire length and are usually preferable if the patient weighs over 250 lbs.

▶ *Wraparound (space saver).* This design reduces the overall width of the chair by 1½". The height of the armrests can also be adjustable.

▶ *Customizable.* These armrests function as arm troughs (prevent the arm from falling off the armrests and maintain the arm on the armrest) or arm trays (allow the patient to rest both of their arms and place objects on them).

Armrests can be fitted with skirt/clothing guards to prevent the patient's clothes from getting caught in the drive wheels.

CLINICAL PEARL

The need for attachments may determine the choice of armrest height. For example, armrests can be fitted with upper extremity support surface trays or troughs, which help the user who has difficulty with upper body balance or has decreased use of the upper extremities.

Many lightweight manual chairs are designed without armrests, making it easier for the user to roll up to a desk or table and perform transfers and provide a streamlined look.

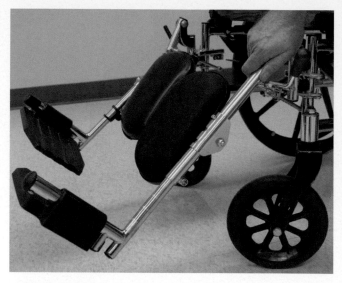

FIGURE 10-14 Front rigging of a wheelchair.

In general, armrests increase the overall width of a wheelchair and decrease the mechanical advantage of the patient's arm position for propelling.

Front Rigging

The front rigging of a wheelchair (Figure 10-14), which consists of a footplate attached to either a footrest or elevating leg rest, supports the lower extremities.

▶ *Footplate.* A footplate (Figure 10-15) is standard equipment on a wheelchair. The footplates are usually incorporated into rigid-frame chairs as part of the design.

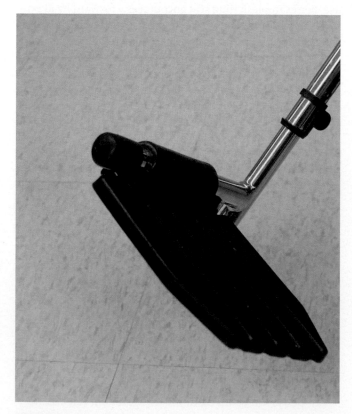

FIGURE 10-15 Wheelchair footplate.

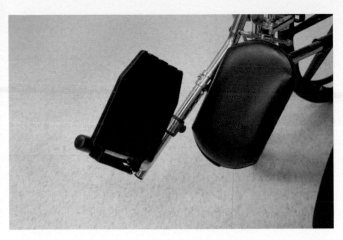

FIGURE 10-16 Wheelchair footplate flipped up.

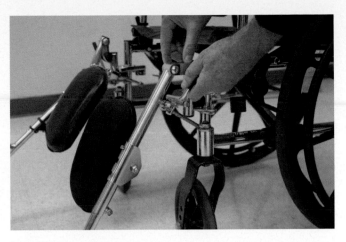

FIGURE 10-18 Elevating leg rest.

Cross-brace folding chairs often have footplates that swivel, flip up (Figure 10-16), and/or can be removed. Footplates can be adjusted to accommodate the patient's foot and provide a resting base for the feet so that the ankles are in neutral with a knee flexed to 90°. The angle of the footplate can be customized depending on a patient's needs. For example, wheelchair athletes prefer to have a slight inward angle for increased maneuverability. Heel loops can be fitted to help maintain the foot position and prevent posterior sliding of the foot. Ankle and calf straps can be added to stabilize the feet onto the footplates. Toe loops may also be used when the patient has difficulty maintaining the foot on the footplate in a forward direction.

▶ *Leg rests.* The standard leg rest positions the lower extremities at an angle of 70° from the horizontal plane. As with other wheelchair components, leg rests also come in various designs, including swing away, removable, and elevating.

■ *Swing away* (Figure 10-17). This design facilitates transfers and a clear front approach to the wheelchair when ambulating. The leg rests are snapped into place during wheelchair mobility. The disadvantage of this

type of leg rest is that the leg rests are not lockable in the away position, allowing the leg rest to swing back against the leg.

■ *Removable.* These can be fully detached from the wheelchair, enabling the patient to maneuver in smaller spaces and make the wheelchair easier to transport. The disadvantage of this type of leg rest is that they may be lost.

■ *Elevating* (Figure 10-18). This design can be used when the patient cannot flex the knee for postural support or when a dependent leg contributes to lower extremity edema. The leg rest position, which can be raised and fixed at any angle from 90° to 0°, is adjusted by pushing down on a lever on the side of the chair. Articulating leg rests allow the leg rest to be adjusted to accommodate the full length of the patient's leg and provide padded calf support. This type of leg rest is suitable for patients with an arthrodesis of the knee, orthostatic hypotension, or a leg cast. Elevating leg rests can typically be released from the wheelchair or pivoted to one side during transfers. Elevated leg rests are contraindicated for patients with hypertonicity or adaptive shortening of the hamstrings. One of the disadvantages of this type of leg rest is that it increases the wheelchair's overall length and weight, negatively impacting maneuverability and transportability.

Wheels

Most wheelchairs use four wheels: two large drive wheels (standard spokes or spokeless) at the back (fitted with an outer rim that allows for hand grip and propulsion) and two smaller ones (casters) at the front (Figure 10-19).

CLINICAL PEARL

Although they require maintenance, spoked wheels are lightweight, and the spokes can be individually adjusted to keep the wheel perfectly round. The mag wheel is a type of spoked wheel with six to eight broad struts connecting the hub to the wheel's outer rim.

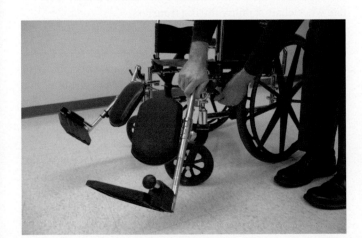

FIGURE 10-17 Swing away leg rest.

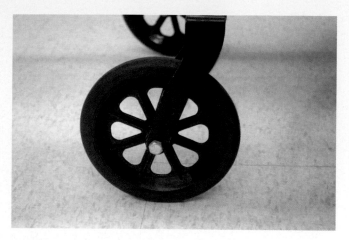

FIGURE 10-19 Wheelchair caster.

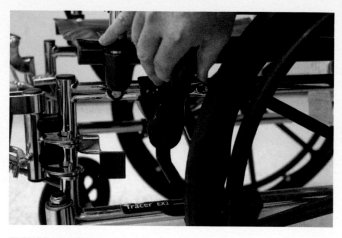

FIGURE 10-20 Wheelchair lock.

The standard sizes for the drive wheel of a manual wheelchair are 22, 24, and 26 inches. However, smaller and larger wheel sizes are also available. For example, powered wheelchairs often incorporate a 10-inch wheel drive design.

Wheels fitted with an outer rim, referred to as a pushrim or handrim, enable patients to propel themselves without placing their hands directly on the tires. The handrims can be coated to increase friction and increase propulsion. For patients with only one functional arm, two outer rims can be fitted on one wheel so that the arm drive achieves both forward and backward propulsion.

Projections (vertical, oblique, or horizontal) can be attached to the rims to facilitate propulsion for patients with poor handgrip. However, horizontal and oblique extensions add to the overall width of the chair and may reduce maneuverability.

The drive wheels are positioned nearly perpendicular to the floor in a standard wheelchair, but in chairs requiring more stability and agility, the wheels are often angled inwards (cambered). Composite mag wheels, manufactured from a nylon/fiberglass-like material that is strong, resilient, and lightweight, are the most common wheelchair wheels and come standard on most wheelchairs.

CLINICAL PEARL

The inward angle of the wheel relative to the vertical position is referred to as the camber. Although a greater camber provides increased stability, the wider position of the wheels near the floor can limit the wheelchair's ability to pass through narrow spaces.

Wheel Locks

Wheel locks (Figure 10-20), sometimes erroneously referred to as brakes as they do not function to slow down a wheelchair, are an important safety feature and must be engaged for all patient transfers in and out of the chair or during wheelchair exercises. The majority of wheel locks consist of a lever system with a toggle, cam, or ratchet. Extensions may be added to increase the ease of both locking and unlocking. When a wheelchair has a reclining back, an additional lock is necessary. A hill holder is a mechanical lock that allows

the chair to go forward but automatically applies it when the chair goes into reverse. A scissor lock, which retracts to a position completely away from the tire and wheel and allows more freedom for the patient's hands, is designed for the more active patients.

Tires

The tires used for the rear wheels may be solid hard rubber, pneumatic inflatable, semi-pneumatic, or radial. In general, solid tires are well suited for indoor use and require less energy to propel, while pneumatic inflatable tires (if fitted with treads) can allow a patient to traverse uneven terrain because of their increased shock absorption. However, pneumatic tires require correct inflation for efficient propulsion and effective application of wheelchair locks. Also, pneumatic tires are subject to blowouts, although newer designs have solid inserts that make them puncture-proof and help maintain inflation at the expense of being heavier.

Casters

Casters, the smaller wheels at the front of the wheelchair, vary in size (ranging 2–8 inches in diameter) and composition (pneumatic, solid rubber, plastic, or a combination of these). The function of the casters is to allow changes in direction. Large casters create more stability, whereas small casters increase maneuverability. Caster locks can be added to facilitate wheelchair stability during transfers.

Axle

The axle position affects the stability and maneuverability of the wheelchair as it determines the drive wheel position. For example, if the front and back wheels are closer together, the wheelchair is more nimble but also more challenging to control. The more recent wheelchair models have adjustable axles.

CLINICAL PEARL

Most modern standard wheelchairs have "dual axle" adjustments for the rear wheel and three placements to adjust the front caster. This allows the chair seat to be lowered or raised 2 inches.

Seat Belts

Seat Belts can be used for safety or positioning:

▶ Restraining belts are used to prevent patients from falling out of the wheelchair.

▶ Seat belts can be fitted to grasp around the pelvis at a 45° angle to the seat to help position the pelvis. An additional belt can also be added to provide lateral or medial support at the hip and knee to maintain lower extremity alignment and/or control spasticity.

Powered Chairs

This type of chair, which uses a power source (battery) that propels the wheelchair is usually prescribed for patients who are not capable of self-propulsion or have very low endurance. The battery is stored on the chair. Microprocessors allow the control of the wheelchair to be adapted to various controls (joystick, head, breath). Recent changes in the power bases have allowed for such innovations as power seat functions (power tilt, recline, elevating leg rest, seat elevator) and control interfaces (mini-joysticks, head controls). Power wheelchair bases can be classified in one of three categories, based on the drive wheel location relative to the system's center of gravity:

▶ *Rear-wheel drive.* In this base design, the drive wheels are located behind the user's COG, and the casters are located in the front, providing predictable drive characteristics and stability. In general, a rear-wheel drive allows a chair to move more rapidly than a front-wheel drive wheelchair.

▶ *Mid-wheel drive.* In this design, the drive wheels are directly below the user's COG, and the chair generally has a set of casters or anti-tippers in the front and rear of the drive wheels. The advantage of this system is a smaller turning radius. The disadvantage is a tendency to rock or pitch forward, especially with sudden stops or fast turns. Also, this type of design can get stuck going over obstacles.

▶ *Front-wheel drive.* In this design, the drive wheels are located in front of the user's COG, which provides stability, a tight turning radius, and the ability to climb obstacles or curbs more easily than a chair with a rear-wheel drive. One of the disadvantages of this design is its rearward COG, making it difficult to drive in a straight line, especially on uneven surfaces.

The disadvantages of power wheelchairs are that they:

▶ Are more expensive

▶ Are difficult to transport

▶ Have a battery that requires charging

▶ Require protection from wet weather

CLINICAL PEARL

▶ Power chairs are more expensive than manual chairs. Power chairs have inherent safety concerns and create issues surrounding transportation and home accessibility.

▶ Manual wheelchairs are easier to transport and lift into a non-accessible home.

Pediatric Wheelchairs

Children with cerebral palsy, spina bifida, or osteogenesis imperfecta may be candidates for either manual or power wheelchairs, depending on upper extremity strength, rate of fatigue, cognitive abilities, and family circumstances. Those with spinal muscular dystrophy, arthrogryposis, or high-level spinal cord injuries and those with progressively worsening Duchenne muscular dystrophy are typically immediate candidates for powered mobility. Key decisions concerning wheelchair design must be a team effort.

A pediatric wheelchair must have approximately 4 inches of available space in the frame to accommodate growth. Also, the seating system should be flexible enough to accommodate tonal or postural changes. Examples of flexibility in the system involve the placement of laterals, which are often attached to tracks, or the backrest can include T-nuts placed throughout the back to allow easy hardware mounting. Pediatric chairs often employ linear seating systems (to accommodate the delicate balance between providing contours in the system and accommodating growth) versus molded seats, which are more difficult to increase in size. Similarly, a contoured backrest is more accommodating and provides more contact surface and thus more comfort. Caregivers should be made aware of the proper use of all accessories, including head supports and upper chest supports.

One must also always consider the aesthetic appeal of the wheelchair. Where possible, the wheelchair should reflect the patient's individuality and personality.

WHEELCHAIR MEASUREMENTS

A correctly sized wheelchair contributes to the patient's overall function and well-being by preventing complications, enhancing posture, and optimizing mobility. Five measurements are required: seat height, seat depth, seat width, seatback height, and armrest height (Table 10-5).

The range of available pelvic and hip movements related to spinal and pelvic alignment should be determined. To measure a patient for a wheelchair, the patient should be well supported in supine on a firm surface in the 90-90-90 position (90° of hip flexion, 90° to 100° knee flexion, and neutral 90° of ankle position). The degree of knee flexion must be determined so that the hamstring muscle group's influence is eliminated.[1] The clinician must support the lower extremities well in this position. It is important that the clinician maintain the tape measure in a straight line from one endpoint to the other, rather than allowing the tape to follow the contours of the patient's body, as the latter method will distort the results. ROM measurements should include hip flexion, abduction, adduction, and internal and external rotation; their effect on pelvic position and general body alignment should be noted as well.

CLINICAL PEARL

Along with seat depth, seat width is the most important wheelchair measurement because of the effect the wheelchair's width has on the position of the arms for propelling the wheelchair.

TABLE 10-5	Wheelchair Measurements	
Dimension	**Guidelines**	**Average Size**
Seat height	The seat-to-floor height affects many functional activities, including the ability to eat and work at standard-height tables and desks and the ability to use the lower extremities to propel the wheelchair. The measurement is taken from the sole of the patient's usual footwear to the popliteal fold. If the wheelchair is to be propelled, this distance will be used as a seat height. However, if the patient will not be using the feet to propel the wheelchair, 2 inches is added to this measurement to allow clearance between the footplate and the floor. If the patient will be sitting on a cushion, the cushion's thickness needs to be considered in the measurement, bearing in mind that a 3-inch-thick cushion may compress to 1 inch under the patient's body weight.	Bariatric: 19.5–20.5 inches Adult: 18–20.5 inches. Sports: Front, 16–22 inches; rear, 13–23 inches Pediatric: 15–21 inches Hemi/low seat: 15.5–17.5 inches. Reclining: 19.5–19.75 inches
Seat depth	This is the most critical measurement for the pelvic position and is also the most common measurement for error because the upper leg length varies according to how the patient is sitting. If the patient is allowed to sacral sit during the measurement, the upper leg measurement will be falsely high; this measurement should be made with the patient positioned supine. The measurement is taken from the patient's posterior buttock/mat surface along the lateral thigh to the popliteal fold. Approximately 2 inches are subtracted from this measurement to avoid pressure from the seat's edge against the popliteal space.	Bariatric: 15.75–17.5 inches Adult: 16–18 inches Sports: 10–20 inches Pediatric: 8–18 inches Hemi/low seat: 15.5–17.5 inches Reclining: 16–18 inches
Seat width	Measurement is taken of the widest aspect of the patient's buttocks, hips, or thighs while taking into account the patient's customary clothing. 1–2 inches are added to this measurement to provide space for bulky clothing, orthoses, or clearance of the trochanters from the armrest side panel. It is important to remember that the greater the seat width, the more difficult it is to propel the chair and to navigate it through small spaces. To improve this measurement's accuracy, a book can be placed against each of the patient's hips and a measurement taken between the inner edges of the books.	Bariatric: 16–30 inches Adult: 14–18 inches Sports: 12–20 inches Pediatric: 10–16 inches Hemi/low seat: 16–30 inches Reclining: 14–22 inches
Seatback height	The height of the seat back determines the level of postural support provided to the patient. For a medium-height back, the measurement is taken from the chair seat to the base of the axilla. The patient's shoulder is flexed to 90°. 4 inches are subtracted from this measurement, so the final back height is below both inferior angles of the scapulae. NB: this measurement will be affected if a seat cushion is to be used—the patient should be measured while seated on the seat cushion, or the thickness of the cushion must be considered by adding that value to the actual measurement.	Bariatric: 16 inches Adult: As required Sports: 9–20 inches Pediatric: 8–16 inches Hemi/low seat: 16 inches Reclining: 22–24 inches
Armrest height	The measurement is taken from the chair seat to the olecranon process with the patient's elbow flexed to 90°. 1 inch is added to this measurement. NB: this measurement will be affected if a seat cushion is to be used—the patient should be measured while seated on the seat cushion, or the thickness of the cushion must be considered by adding that value to the actual measurement.	Bariatric: As required Adult: 5–12 inches Sports: None Pediatric: 4.5–6.75 inches Hemi/low seat: 5–12 inches Reclining: 5–12 inches

Data from Dreeben, O: *Physical Therapy Clinical Handbook for PTAs*. London, Jones & Bartlett; 2008.

Once the ROM is documented, a linear measurement of seat depth should be determined.

Once measurement in the supine position is completed, the patient should be placed in a supported sitting position with the knees flexed to 100° (or more) to eliminate the hamstring muscle group's influence. Ideally, the seated measurement should be done on a simulator—a chair specifically designed for planar seated examinations. If a simulator is not available, the measurement can be done on the mat table with a thin front edge to allow 100° of knee flexion. The physical therapist confirms the fit of a new or existing wheelchair by observation, questioning the patient, and physical assessment of the patient's posture and mobility.

CLINICAL PEARL

Many patients sacral sit—sit with the pelvis posteriorly rotated and the trunk resting on the sacrum rather than on the ischial tuberosities. Taking measurements when the patient is in this position will result in errors (see Table 10-5). As a quick check, measurements of the upper leg (from the popliteal fold to the most posterior point of the body) and lower leg (from the sole of the foot to the popliteal fold) should be within 1 inch of each other if the patient is sitting correctly.

The two-finger rule can be used to check for the approximate fit of a standard wheelchair:

▶ *Seat depth:* leave no more or less than two finger-widths of space behind the back of the calf and the front edge of the wheelchair.

▶ *Seat width:* leave no more or less than two finger-widths of space between the hip and the inside of the wheelchair arm.

▶ *Seat height:* leave no more or less than two finger-widths of space between the floor and floor plates.

CLINICAL PEARL

A lower seat height allows for greater upper extremity motions.

▶ *Seat back height:* leave no more or less than two finger-widths of space between the top of the wheelchair back and the patient's axilla.

▶ *Armrest height:* leave no more or less than two finger-widths of space between the top of the drive wheel and the underside of the patient's forearm.

The patient needs to maintain good posture in the wheelchair, and an ill-fitting wheelchair can produce several undesirable effects (Table 10-6). He or she should be seated well back in the chair, with the lower extremities on the foot or leg rests. Wheelchair users are susceptible to muscle imbalances. Nearly every motion and/or repetitive motion is forward, working such areas as the shoulder flexors (pectoralis major and anterior deltoid) and shoulder internal rotators. These anterior muscles can become adaptively shortened, while the

TABLE 10-6	Negative Impacts and Solutions for an Ill-fitting Wheelchair	
Measurement	**Negative impact**	**Solution**
Seat height		
Too low	Sacral sitting/posterior pelvic rotation	Add rigid insert or consult with physical therapist about the need for a different wheelchair
Too high	Insufficient trunk support Difficulty positioning knees under table/desk	Suggest lower profile cushion or consult with physical therapist about the need for a different wheelchair
Seat depth		
Too deep	Sacral sitting/posterior pelvic rotation Increased pressure on the popliteal space	Re-measure upper leg length minus 2"
Too shallow	Windswept posture (decreased femoral contact and trunk stability) Abduction, or adduction of lower extremities Poor trunk balance Increased weight bearing on ischial tuberosities	Use a cushion with medial abduction and lateral adduction contours
Seat width		
Too wide	Hips internally rotated Lower extremities excessively adducted Pelvic obliquity/leaning to one side Hands unable to reach the drive wheels	Use a cushion with medial abduction and lateral adduction contours
Too narrow	Excess pressure on greater trochanters Difficulty changing positions Windswept position of the lower extremities (positioned to one side)	Consult with physical therapist about the need for a wider wheelchair
Seatback height		
Too high	Difficulty propelling the wheelchair Increase pressure on scapulae	Consult with physical therapist about the need for a wheelchair with a lower seatback
Too low	Decreased trunk stability Postural deviations	Consult with physical therapist about the need for a wheelchair with a higher seatback
Armrest height		
Too high	Difficulty propelling the wheelchair Elevated shoulders	Consult with physical therapist about the need for a different wheelchair
Too low	Decreased trunk stability Depressed shoulders	Consult with physical therapist about the need for a different wheelchair

upper back muscles become weak and elongated. The typical posture of the wheelchair user has rounded shoulders with mild thoracic kyphosis and a forward head. This posture can result in impingement of the soft tissue structures of the acromiohumeral space. The patient should be able to maintain a seated position when his or her balance is challenged.

WHEELCHAIR TASKS

Several wheelchair transfers can be made easier with the following tasks:

▶ *Forward hip slide.* Most of the transfers from a wheelchair require that the patient maneuver to the seat's front edge, thereby placing their center of mass (COM) over their BOS (**VIDEO 10-2**). To do this, the patient can use one of the following methods:

■ *Upward and forward lift.* The patient pushes down through the arms and/or legs, lifts the hips above the seating surface, and then moves the buttocks forward.

■ *Weight shift.* The patient leans the upper body to one side and then to the other, each time lifting the contralateral hip up and forward until the correct position is attained.

■ *Forward hip slide.* The patient leans back in the chair and, by extending the trunk, slides the hips to the front edge of the seat before grasping the arms of the chair and pulling the trunk forward into an upright position.

Suppose the patient is unable to perform this movement independently. In that case, the clinician can assist by squatting or half-kneeling in front of the patient and placing their hands behind the patient's hip with the fingers or fingertips over the sacroiliac joints. From this position, the clinician pulls the patient's hips forward simultaneously or alternating side to side, with the patient participating as much as possible. At the end of this technique, depending on the level of trunk control that the patient possesses, the clinician may need to place their hands behind the patient's shoulders and assist them in moving the shoulders forward over the pelvis to achieve an erect sitting position.

▶ *Sitting push-up.* This technique, which requires the patient to form a series of sitting push-ups, can assist the patient to the front edge of the seat. After each sitting push-up, the patient lowers themselves closer to the front edge of the wheelchair seat. The clinician may assist by lifting under the patient's buttocks or by guarding at the shoulders. The sitting push-up can also relieve pressure on the buttocks and posterior thighs (**VIDEO 10-3**).

▶ *Weight shifting side to side.* This technique can be used to assist the patient to the front edge of the seat. The clinician places one arm around the patient's shoulders from one side and the other arm under the thigh at the opposite lower extremity. The patient's weight can then be shifted to one side. For example, suppose the clinician places his or her left arm around the patient's right shoulder, and the right hand is placed under the patient's left side. In that case, the patient's weight can be shifted to the right, which

unweights the patient's left buttock, and then the clinician assists the patient in moving the left thigh forward. Once the left lower extremity is lowered to the supporting surface, the patient is returned to an erect sitting position, and the technique is performed to the other side. This sequence is repeated until the patient reaches the front edge of the seat.

▶ *Foot position.* Once the patient's hips are moved to the front edge of the wheelchair seat, the patient's feet must be positioned posteriorly and approximately shoulder-width apart (closer if both knees will be blocked during the transfer) so that the BOS is directly under the patient's new COM. If the patient cannot position his or her feet independently, assistance is provided by the clinician. In certain circumstances, such as a weight-bearing restriction on one of the lower extremities, only one foot is positioned posteriorly, leaving the other extended out in front of the patient.

▶ *Trunk flexion.* As the mass of the trunk is moved forward over the BOS, so that the nose is over the toes, the patient can use the large muscles of the lower extremities more effectively. However, it is important to remember that a patient who has undergone a total hip arthroplasty (posterolateral approach) must limit trunk flexion by maintaining an upright position or lean somewhat posteriorly.

▶ *Hand positioning.* The position of the hands varies greatly depending on the patient's level of independence. If hand positioning can be performed independently, the patient positions the hands posterior to the flexed trunk before initiating a push-off from the armrests. Occasionally, the clinician may ask the patient to hold onto the clinician's forearm or hips. If the patient cannot perform hand positioning independently, the clinician must position the hands and arms inside the armrests in the patient's lap.

▶ *Moving backward.* The patient is asked to lean forward by flexing the trunk and then to place the hands on the armrests posterior to the shoulder. The feet are then placed as far posteriorly as possible while maintaining contact with the floor. The patient is asked to push down through the arms and legs and lift the hips up and back. This sequence is repeated as often as needed to achieve the correct position.

WHEELCHAIR TRANSFERS

Several areas need to be addressed when training a patient on how to be as functionally independent as possible with a wheelchair. The various components of the wheelchair should be reviewed with the patient, and the patient should perform all of the necessary tasks while being supervised by the clinician.

Transfer from Wheelchair to Floor—Two-Person Lift

The two-person lift is used when the patient has some trunk control and upper extremity strength. It is important to ensure that the wheelchair is locked and that the footrests are removed or swung out of the way. The armrest on the side of the wheelchair to which the patient will be transferred is also removed. One of the clinicians is positioned behind the patient, while the other clinician is in front of the patient. The patient is asked to hug himself or herself. The clinician behind the patient reaches under the patient's upper extremities and grasps the patient's opposite wrist (right arm on the left and left on the right) to prevent the patient from abducting their arms during the lift. The clinician in front of the patient cradles the patient's thighs with one hand and the lower legs with the other hand. On the command from the clinician behind the patient, the patient is lifted by both clinicians to a height that clears all parts of the wheelchair, and then, as a unit, the two clinicians step in the required direction before lowering the patient onto the floor. Once the patient is correctly and safely positioned, he or she is released.

Transfer from Floor to Wheelchair— Two-Person Lift

The patient's transfer back from the floor to the wheelchair is essentially the reverse of the previous procedure. The wheelchair is prepared—the brakes are secured, and the armrests and footrests are removed. The patient is positioned in long-sitting. Both clinicians squat down, and then both use the same holding techniques as in the previous transfer. On the command from the clinician at the head of the patient, the patient is lifted to a height that will clear all parts of the wheelchair. Then, as a unit, the two clinicians transfer the patient onto the seat of the wheelchair. Both clinicians ensure that the patient assumes proper sitting posture before replacing the armrests and footrests and placing the patient's feet on the footrests.

Transfer from Wheelchair to Treatment Table—Squat-Pivot Transfer

The squat-pivot transfer is used when a patient can bear weight but has insufficient strength or control of the lower extremities to stand upright. This is a physically demanding transfer for the clinician, who must decide whether extra assistance is required. Before the transfer can begin, the clinician must position the wheelchair near parallel to the treatment table, lock the wheels, and remove the wheelchair armrest on the side toward which the patient is moving. The clinician then removes or swings the footrests away so that the patient's feet can be placed on the floor. The patient is fitted with a transfer belt. If the patient cannot slide his or her hips forward in the wheelchair, the clinician uses one of the methods described under wheelchair tasks or reaches around the back of the patient's pelvis and slides the patient forward in the seat of the wheelchair (VIDEO 10-4). When possible, the patient's feet should be positioned under the COG and slightly apart to maximize the BOS. If feasible, the patient should place each hand on an armrest with the forearms in a near-vertical position so that the pushing force will be vertical. Once the patient is positioned correctly, the clinician places each foot and knee outside of the patient's feet and knees in preparation for blocking both of the patient's

lower extremities by directing the force at the patient's proximal tibia (squeezing the patient's knees together is not recommended).

CLINICAL PEARL

The decision whether to block a patient's knee during a transfer requires a basic understanding of the biomechanics of the process:

- ▶ A combination of the clinician's and patient's feet forms the BOS.
- ▶ The line of gravity (LOG) is posterior to the patient's knees and feet, so during the transfer, the LOG will need to be redirected to fall within the BOS.
- ▶ To stand up, the patient (or clinician) must counteract the forces that are acting to flex the patient's knees and dorsiflex the ankles. Blocking the patient's knee applies a force that counteracts these forces.

Throughout the transfer, the patient's lower extremities are not fully extended at any time. If applicable, the patient is asked to push down on the remaining armrest as the transfer is initiated. The clinician simultaneously pivots on the balls of the feet as the patient is lifted and shifts the COG laterally until the patient's hips are above the treatment table. The clinician then lowers the patient's hips to the table in a controlled manner and then adjusts the patient's position as needed. The transfer from the treatment table back to the wheelchair is essentially the reverse.

CLINICAL PEARL

Specialized equipment, stationary poles, or assistive devices can assist the clinician and patient during a pivot transfer.

- ▶ *Specialized equipment.* Pivot discs, designed for use by patients who can stand but cannot readily move their legs, serve to minimize the force required for a transfer.
- ▶ *Stationary poles.* These are poles attached to the floor and the ceiling, which the patient can hold onto with one or both hands while transferring.
- ▶ *Assistive devices.* A walk or a crutch can help provide stability during a pivot transfer (see Chapter 11). The patient places one hand on the armrest and one hand on the crutch handle or walker. It is important to stress to the patient that the assistive device is to be used for balance only and not to push or pull the patient.

Transfer from Wheelchair to Treatment Table— Standing Pivot

This technique is used for patients who cannot stand independently but can bear some weight through one or both lower extremities. Before the transfer can begin, the clinician must position the wheelchair parallel to the treatment table and then lock the wheels. The clinician then removes or swings the footrests away so that the patient's feet can be placed on the floor. If the patient cannot slide his or her hips forward in the wheelchair, the clinician uses one of the methods described under wheelchair tasks or reaches around the back of the patient's pelvis and slides the patient forward in the seat of the wheelchair. Once the patient is positioned correctly, the clinician places each foot and knee outside of the patient's feet and knees to block one or both of the patient's lower extremities (VIDEO 10-5). Determining how much blocking will be required is a matter of clinical judgment. Patients who are progressing from dependent pivot transfers to assisted pivot transfers may require blocking of both knees, whereas patients transitioning from assisted pivot transfers may require only one or neither knee to be blocked.

▶ *Blocking one knee:* the clinician flexes his or her hips and knees to position his or her proximal tibia against the patient's tibia, just inferior and central to the patient's tibial tuberosity. The clinician can also use both of his or her knees to block one of the patient's knees by placing the medial aspect of both knees on either side of the patient's tibial tuberosity.

▶ *Blocking both knees:* the clinician positions the patient's feet together but slightly staggered and then places the medial aspect of both his or her knees against the antero-lateral aspects of the patient's knees.

The blocking technique produces a counterforce that is necessary once the patient is upright to counteract gravity, which creates a flexion moment at the patient's hips and knees. By placing the feet outside of the patient's feet, the clinician creates a wide BOS, which is designed to help support the dynamic weight of two people once the patient is upright. To assist with the pivot, the patient's foot nearer the target surface should be moved slightly forward relative to the other foot. The clinician's foot placement mimics the patient's—on the side toward which the patient is turning, the clinician places that foot slightly posteriorly and the other slightly anteriorly. Having the patient come to a standing position can occur in several ways:

▶ The clinician places both hands under the patient's buttocks, and the patient is asked to place both of his or her arms around the clinician's upper back (not the neck!) (VIDEO 10-6). On the clinician's count and command, the clinician initiates a rocking motion in time to the counts. On the command "up," the clinician straightens his or her legs and lifts the patient from the wheelchair to a height that is sufficient to clear the wheelchair and any height difference between the wheelchair and the treatment table.

▶ The patient places both hands on the wheelchair armrests and, on the clinician's count and command, pushes down on the armrests to bring himself or herself to the standing position while the clinician guards the patient. If a patient has undergone a total hip arthroplasty (posterolateral approach), pushing to a standing position can prove difficult: the patient must maintain his or her trunk position in an upright or slightly backward position during the transfer, which places the COG posterior to the feet, increasing the potential for falling backward. The clinician must also monitor the amount of internal rotation of the patient's involved hip during the transfer. Having the

patient transfer toward the uninvolved side creates less risk of hip internal rotation, although the patient must be able to transfer toward both sides.

As the patient rises, the clinician leans posteriorly to accommodate the patient's anteriorly moving COG while simultaneously guarding the patient against a fall. Once the patient's trunk is high enough to clear the chair, the clinician and patient begin to pivot toward the treatment table. The actual pivot may need to be performed in a series of small movements for the first few attempts. At the end of the pivot, the patient should be in the correct position for sitting on the table, and as the patient is lowered, he or she should reach back for the target surface. During the lowering process, the patient should be encouraged to maintain trunk flexion so that the patient's COG does not move too quickly in a posterior direction and so that the descent can be performed in a controlled manner. Once the patient is correctly and safely positioned, he or she can be released. The transfer from the treatment table back to the wheelchair is essentially the reverse.

Transfer from Bed to Wheelchair—Assisted Standing Pivot

The assisted standing pivot transfer is similar to the standing pivot transfer, except that the clinician provides less assistance to the patient (VIDEO 10-7). The decision to use this transfer instead of the standing pivot transfer is based on the patient's independence level. The assisted standing pivot can be used when a patient can bear some weight on the lower extremities but has a weakness that necessitates some assistance. The planned transfer is typically set up so that the patient can move toward the uninvolved side during the transfer. The clinician assists the patient by controlling the patient's pelvis. This is accomplished by placing a hand posterior to the pelvis, on the side of the pelvis, or the anterior aspect of the pelvis, depending on where the assistance is needed. The other hand is placed on the posterior aspect of the patient's opposite shoulder. Stability is provided by guarding or blocking the patient's uninvolved lower extremity using the same lower extremity (the patient's right knee is guarded with the clinician's right knee). On the clinician's command, the patient pushes to the standing position. Once in the full upright position and under control, the patient pivots or reaches for the wheelchair before lowering himself or herself with appropriate assistance. Once the patient is correctly and safely positioned, he or she can be released. The transfer from the wheelchair back to the bed is essentially the reverse.

Transfer from Wheelchair to Treatment Table—Sliding Board

A sliding board transfer allows a patient to transfer between numerous sitting surfaces using a series of small shifts of the trunk without bearing weight through the lower extremities. However, such transfers require high levels of trunk and upper body strength and sitting balance. Ideally, the transfer should occur between two surfaces with the same height as each other or from a slightly higher surface to a slightly lower one. Before the transfer is attempted, the clinician or the patient positions the wheelchair parallel to or at a slight angle to the treatment table and locks the wheels. The footrests are then removed or swung away, and the patient's feet are placed on the floor. The patient is asked to move forward on the seat of the wheelchair, and the armrest of the wheelchair on the side nearest the treatment table is removed. The patient is asked to lean away from the treatment table, and the sliding board is positioned well under the patient's buttocks before the patient returns to an upright position. The patient is instructed not to grasp the sliding board's edge to prevent the fingers from being pinched during the technique.

This transfer technique involves a series of seated push-ups—straightening the upper extremities, depressing the shoulders, and lifting the body up and across the sliding board toward the treatment table. If the patient's wrists are unable to weight bear sufficiently, they can use the outside of the fists. After each push-up and slide, the patient repositions his or her hands, and the sequence is repeated until the patient is on the treatment table with only one buttock remaining on the sliding board. At this point, the patient leans away from the wheelchair to remove the sliding board, and the clinician ensures that the patient is in a position that can be maintained independently. During the initial attempts to use this technique, the clinician provides as much assistance as necessary. This assistance can vary from standing in front of the patient, observing, to blocking the patient's knees to prevent them from sliding off the sliding board. The patient may also require assistance from the clinician to lift the buttocks to assist with the sliding technique. The transfer from the treatment table back to the wheelchair is essentially the reverse.

Video Description

VIDEO 10-8 shows a transfer from a hospital bed to a wheelchair using a sliding board. The principles remain the same. Notice how the clinician teaches the patient to position the board and reminds the patient to avoid pinching the fingers under the board during the transfer. Independent sliding board transfers require a high level of trunk and upper body strength and motor control.

Transfer from Wheelchair to Treatment Table—Push-Up

A push-up transfer is similar to the sliding board transfers except that the patient can bear weight through the lower extremities. Before the transfer is attempted, the clinician or the patient positions the wheelchair parallel to or at a slight angle to the treatment table and locks the wheels. The footrests are then removed or swung away, and the patient's feet are placed on the floor. The patient is asked to move forward on the seat of the wheelchair, and the armrest of the wheelchair on the side nearest the treatment table is removed. The

patient is asked to place one hand on the treatment table and the other hand on the remaining armrest of the wheelchair. The patient pushes down on both arms and, while maintaining the hand on the treatment table, moves the hand on the armrest to the seat of the wheelchair while pivoting toward the treatment table so that the backs of the thighs touch the treatment table. The patient then lowers himself or herself onto the table. The transfer from the treatment table back to the wheelchair is essentially the reverse.

Transfer from Floor to Wheelchair— One-Person Dependent

On occasion, a patient can inadvertently fall out of or tip over a wheelchair and be unable to get back into the wheelchair. Depending on the patient's size and the clinician's physical capability, another clinician may be needed for assistance. The following description is for a one-person transfer. The clinician positions the wheelchair on its back and at the patient's feet. Using one arm, the clinician places it under the patient's lower extremities and uses the other arm to wrap around the patient's upper back so that the patient's lower extremities are flexed at the hips and knees. Maintaining good body mechanics, the clinician moves the patient so that the patient's ankles are over the front edge of the wheelchair seat and then uses a series of short lifting and sliding movements to negotiate the patient into the wheelchair. Once the patient is positioned in the wheelchair, the clinician grasps both handles of the wheelchair while maintaining contact with the patient's upper trunk (or one handle of the wheelchair with one hand while supporting the patient's trunk with the other hand), and then lifts the patient and wheelchair as a unit toward the upright position. As the wheelchair and patient approach the upright position, the clinician uses one arm on the anterior aspect of the patient's upper trunk to prevent the patient from falling forward.

Transfer from Wheelchair to Floor—Independent

Patients can use a variety of methods to transfer from the floor to a wheelchair. The transfer selected depends on the patient's strength, agility, confidence, and ROM. The most important strength components for the patient are the strength of the elbow extensors and shoulder extensors. During the initial training sessions, the patient must be guarded and occasionally assisted. In preparation for the transfer, the wheelchair casters are turned forward to prevent the wheelchair from tipping forward, and then the wheelchair is locked.

Anterior Approach

The patient's feet are placed on the floor, the footplates are raised, and the footrests are removed or swung out of the way. The patient moves to the front of the wheelchair seat, and the lower extremities are positioned in extension. Using one hand, the patient positions it on the side, and toward the front edge of the wheelchair seat, while the other hand is placed on the caster or floor. The patient then lowers himself or herself to the floor. To independently return from the floor to the wheelchair, the procedure is reversed.

Posterior Approach

The patient assumes the quadruped position in front of the wheelchair, with the head closest to the seat (VIDEO 10-9). The patient places one hand on the seat toward the front edge and places the other hand in the same position on the opposite side of the wheelchair seat. The patient then moves into a kneeling position by extending the elbows. One hand of the patient is then moved to the top of the armrest while the other remains on the wheelchair seat. Using a combination of upper extremity extension and shoulder girdle depression, the patient lifts himself or herself and starts to turn. The turn is continued until the patient can lower himself or herself onto the seat of the wheelchair. Using a hand on each armrest, the patient pushes down on the armrests and positions himself or herself properly in the wheelchair. The procedure is reversed to independently return to the floor from the wheelchair (VIDEO 10-10).

Dependent Propulsion

To transport a patient in a wheelchair, the clinician must ensure that the patient is seated safely, including sitting well back in the seat, the arms resting on the armrests or in the patient's lap, and the lower extremities supported by the footplates or leg rests. After unlocking the brakes, the clinician should move the wheelchair as smoothly as possible while maintaining good body mechanics and at a speed that is comfortable and safe for the patient. Maneuvering a wheelchair over a smooth surface is much easier than maneuvering a wheelchair on uneven or yielding surfaces such as gravel, sand, grass, and carpet. In such instances, it is recommended that the wheelchair be tipped back to lift the casters off the ground or to pull the wheelchair rather than push it.

Once a clinician has mastered how to maneuver a patient in a wheelchair in various indoor environments and surfaces, further complexities can be added. Although a wide variety of methods can be used for the following tasks, only the safest ones are presented.

- ▶ *Assisted navigation through doorways.* The clinician determines that the patient is sitting safely and then determines the type of door (automatic or manual) and in which direction the door opens (away or toward). If the door is automatic, the clinician must ensure that the wheelchair is clear of the door's path before engaging the door opener and must also be prepared to block the closing door if necessary to prevent the wheelchair or patient from being struck by the door. If the door is manual, the method used will depend on which direction the door opens:

  - ▪ *The door opens away from the patient.* In this scenario, the clinician releases the door latch with his or her back to the doorway, backs the wheelchair through the doorway while keeping the door open with his or her foot or shoulder, and then turns the wheelchair to face the desired direction once the wheelchair has cleared the doorway.

  - ▪ *The door opens toward the patient.* In this scenario, the clinician positions the wheelchair on the handle or left side of the door and then uses one hand to open the

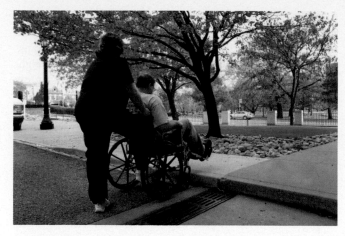

FIGURE 10-21 Wheelchair position to ascend curb.

door while holding one push handle of the wheelchair with the other hand. As soon as the door is open, the clinician locks the door with their foot and pushes the wheelchair forward through the doorway. Once the wheelchair has passed completely to the doorway, the clinician releases the door and moves the wheelchair forward.

- ▶ *Assisted navigation on ascending an incline.* The most efficient way to propel the wheelchair up an incline is to push it forward up the incline with all four wheels in contact with the ground. For very steep slopes, zigzagging may be necessary. If appropriate, the patient can be asked to move the hips forward in the wheelchair, lean the trunk forward, and push equally on both handrims.

- ▶ *Assisted navigation on descending an incline.* The safest way to descend an incline is to roll the wheelchair backward down the slope with all four wheels in contact with the ground while glancing back periodically to be sure the pathway is clear. If appropriate, the patient can be asked to position the hips to the rear of the seat and maintain the trunk erect.

- ▶ *Assisted navigation up a curb moving forward.* The wheelchair is positioned facing the curb (Figure 10-21). The clinician tips the chair back, raising the casters above the curb level, and then rolls the wheelchair forward until the casters are well over the sidewalk before lowering the casters gently onto the sidewalk (Figure 10-22). If

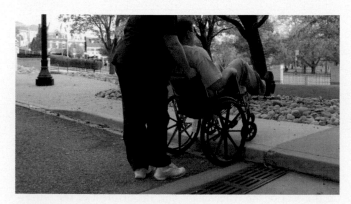

FIGURE 10-22 Casters resting on curb.

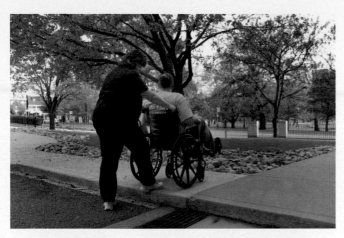

FIGURE 10-23 Wheelchair on top of curb.

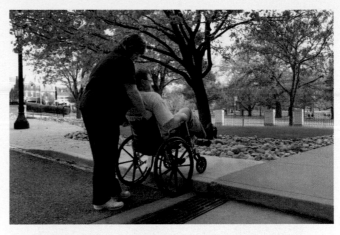

FIGURE 10-25 Drive wheels at bottom of curb.

appropriate, the patient can be asked to lean the trunk forward and push forward on the pushrims on the clinician's command. The wheelchair is then rolled forward until the drive wheels are resting against the curb, at which point the clinician gives the patient the command to push forward on the pushrims (if appropriate), and then rolls the drive wheels up onto the sidewalk by lifting on the push handles of the wheelchair using the power from the legs, and keeping the drive wheels in contact with the curb (Figure 10-23).

▶ *Assisted navigation down a curb moving backward.* This is simply a reverse of the previous procedure. The back of the wheelchair is positioned close to the edge of the curb (Figure 10-24). The clinician then steps off the edge of the curb while holding the push handles of the wheelchair. Maintaining the thigh against the back of the wheelchair, and while gripping the push handles, the clinician slowly rolls the drive wheels down over the curb, making sure that the tires maintain contact with the curb (Figure 10-25). If appropriate, the patient can assist by leaning the trunk forward as the chair rolls over and down the curb. Once the drive wheels are resting on the lower surface, the clinician tips the wheelchair back and rolls it backward until the casters and footplates fully clear the curb before gently

lowering the front casters to the ground in a controlled fashion (Figure 10-26).

▶ *Assisted navigation up a curb moving backward.* The back of the drive wheels of the wheelchair are positioned up against the curb. The clinician stands up on the curb behind the wheelchair, grasps the push handles, and tips the wheelchair backward into a wheelie position. The clinician then pulls the wheelchair back, rolling it up onto the curb while maintaining the wheelie position. The clinician continues to roll the wheelchair back on the sidewalk until the casters are clearly over the sidewalk before slowly lowering the casters to the ground in a controlled manner.

▶ *Assisted navigation ascending steps moving backward.* This task requires two to three transporters and should only be attempted when absolutely necessary. Normally, the strongest clinician is positioned behind the wheelchair and leads the activity while the other assistants help from the sides by grasping the chair frame. However, if both assistants are strong, having the strongest clinician behind the wheelchair is not as critical. Once the clinician and assistants are in position, the wheelchair locks are disengaged, and the wheelchair is backed to the bottom of the stairs until the drive wheels make contact with the bottom step

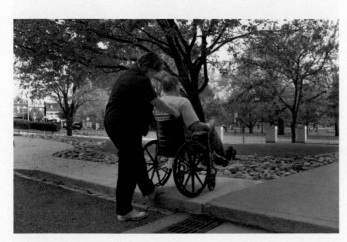

FIGURE 10-24 Wheelchair backed up to edge of curb.

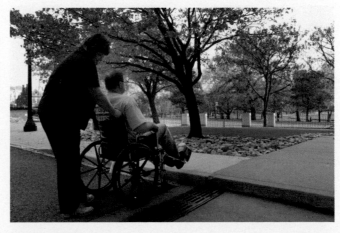

FIGURE 10-26 Wheelchair at bottom of curb.

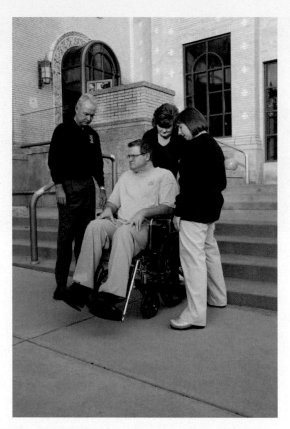

FIGURE 10-27 Wheelchair positioned at bottom of steps.

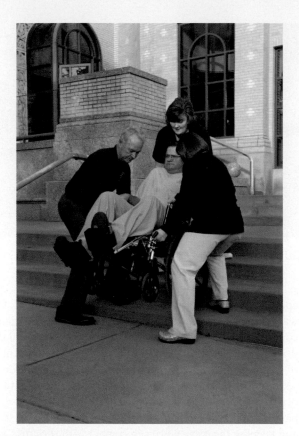

FIGURE 10-29 Wheelchair is moved up to the first step.

(Figure 10-27). The clinician grasps the push handles and tips the wheelchair backward into a wheelie position to elevate the caster wheels (Figure 10-28). This tipped position is maintained throughout the task. On the count of "three," the clinician and the two assistants pull the chair upward by rolling the drive wheels up and over the step (Figure 10-29). This procedure is repeated one step at a time until the top step is reached (Figures 10-30 through 10-35), at which point the wheelchair is rolled backward until the casters are clearly beyond the steps before being slowly lowered in a controlled manner (Figure 10-36).

▶ *Assisted navigation descending steps moving forward.* This task requires two to three transporters and should only be attempted when absolutely necessary. Normally, the strongest clinician is positioned behind the wheelchair and

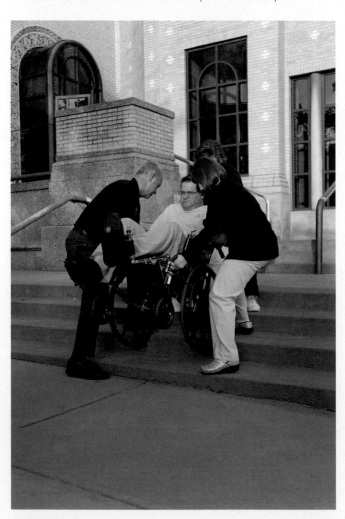

FIGURE 10-30 Wheelchair is gradually moved to the top step.

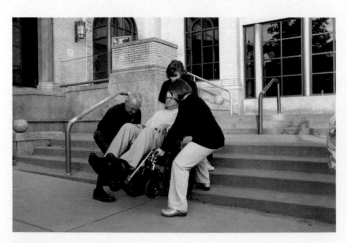

FIGURE 10-28 Wheelchair is tilted back in preparation.

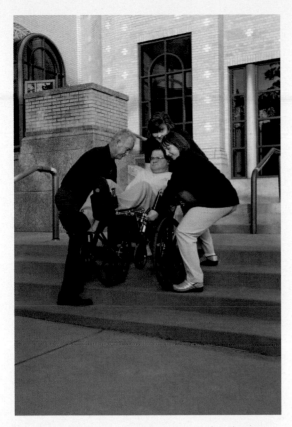

FIGURE 10-31 Wheelchair is gradually moved to the top step.

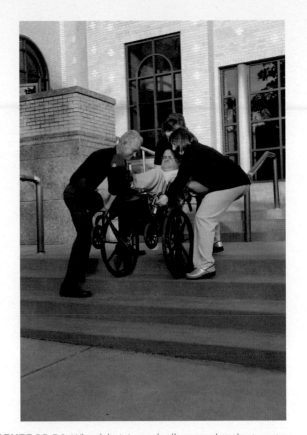

FIGURE 10-34 Wheelchair is gradually moved to the top step.

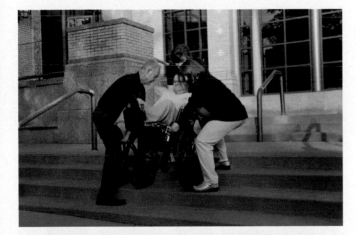

FIGURE 10-32 Wheelchair is gradually moved to the top step.

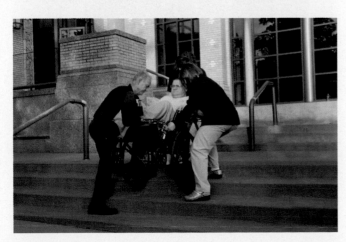

FIGURE 10-33 Wheelchair is gradually moved to the top step.

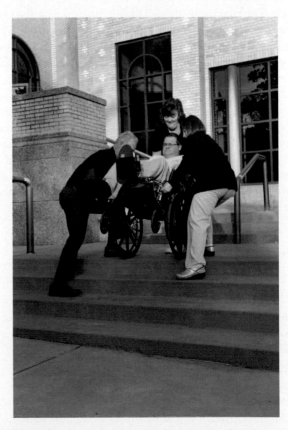

FIGURE 10-35 Wheelchair is gradually moved to the top step.

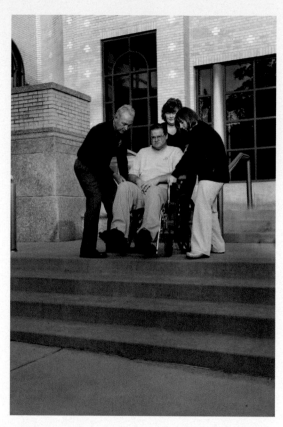

FIGURE 10-36 Wheelchair lowered at the top of the steps.

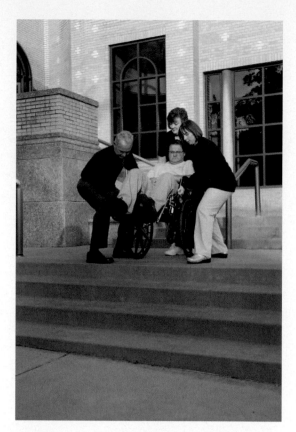

FIGURE 10-37 Wheelchair is tilted back in preparation.

leads the activity while the other assistants help from the sides. However, if both assistants are strong, having the strongest clinician behind the wheelchair is not as important. The chair is positioned facing forward near the top step's edge, and the wheelchair locks are disengaged. The clinician tips the wheelchair back into a wheelie position, elevating the casters, and then slowly and carefully rolls the wheelchair forward until the drive wheels are at the edge of the top step (Figure 10-37). This tipped position is maintained throughout the task. On the count of "three," the clinician and the two assistants control the motion of the rear wheels down to the next step (Figures 10-38 and 10-39). The process is repeated one step at a time until the last step is descended (Figures 10-40 through 10-43), at which point the clinician slowly lowers the casters to the ground in a controlled manner (Figure 10-44).

Independent Propulsion

Depending on the patient's functional level, the patient is instructed on how to:

▶ Operate the wheel locks, foot supports, and armrests, and use the mechanisms safely without tipping forward or sideways out of the chair seat.

▶ Transfer in and out of the chair with the least possible assistance (see the Patient Transfer section). This may involve transfer training from the wheelchair to a car seat. To transfer from a wheelchair to a car seat, the patient applies the same principles as in a bed-to-chair transfer.

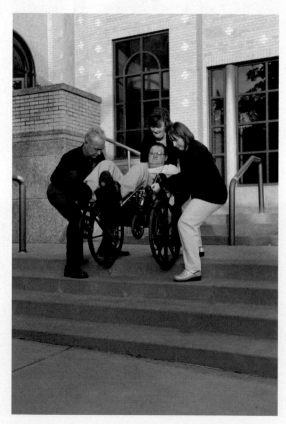

FIGURE 10-38 Wheelchair is lowered down the first step.

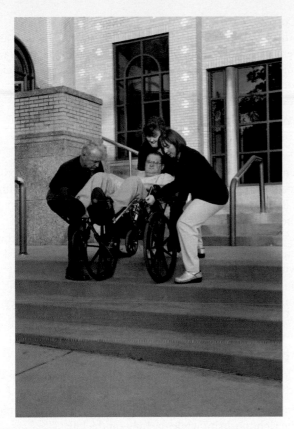

FIGURE 10-39 Wheelchair is lowered down the first step.

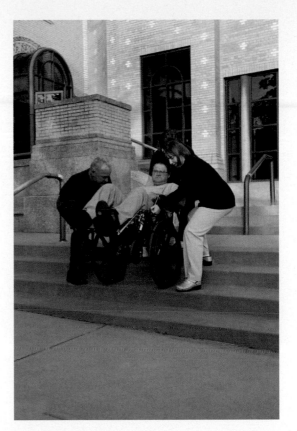

FIGURE 10-41 Wheelchair is gradually moved to the bottom of the steps.

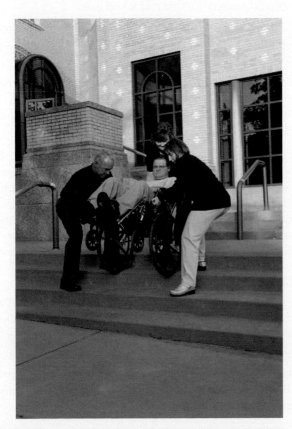

FIGURE 10-40 Wheelchair is gradually moved to the bottom of the steps.

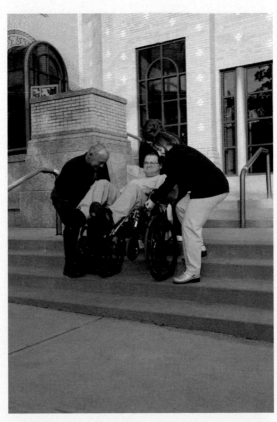

FIGURE 10-42 Wheelchair is gradually moved to the bottom of the steps.

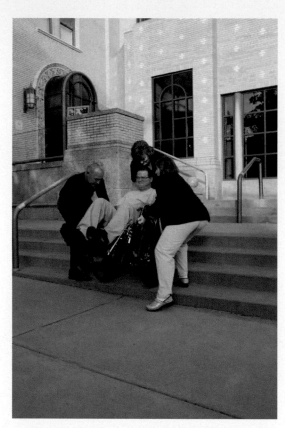

FIGURE 10-43 Wheelchair is gradually moved to the bottom of the steps.

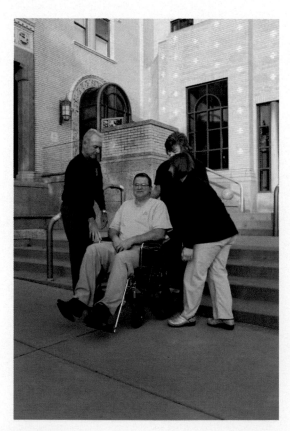

FIGURE 10-44 Casters of the wheelchair are returned to the ground.

Correct positioning of the wheelchair is critical. The wheelchair armrest and leg rest nearest to the car seat are removed, and the wheelchair is positioned so that it is facing forward between the open door and the car seat before locking the wheels. Any hand placement during a car transfer must be on a secure surface.

► Propel the wheelchair in all directions and around corners.

► *Propelling forward.* The patient grasps both pushrims simultaneously behind the apex of the wheel at approximately 10 o'clock position and then pushes forward with a long, smooth stroke, releasing the pushrim at about the 2 or 3 o'clock position on the wheels. As the hands are returned to the start position, they remain below the pushrim. This semicircular pattern has been associated with lower stroke frequency, greater time spent in the push phase relative to the recovery phase, less angular joint velocity and acceleration, and increased efficiency.[2-4]

► *Propelling backward.* The patient grasps both pushrims simultaneously at about the 2 or 3 o'clock position on the wheels and then pulls the wheels posteriorly.

► *Turning to the left.* To turn to the left, the patient holds the left pushrim while pushing on the right.

► *Turning to the right.* To turn to the right, the patient holds the right pushrim while pushing on the left.

More advanced users can benefit from the results of several biomechanical studies[2-8] about the patient's position within the wheelchair during propulsion:

► To increase efficiency, the patient's shoulder axis should be slightly anterior to the rear wheel axle.

► The most efficient push angle can be achieved with a seat alignment that allows 100° to 120° of elbow flexion relative to the apex of the wheel.

Although the most common way to maneuver a wheelchair is to use both upper extremities, the wheelchair can also be propelled using the feet or a combination of the feet and hands.

► If using the feet to propel a wheelchair, the wheelchair footplates are raised and, if possible, the leg rest is moved out of the way. Using shoes with a good grip, the patient places one foot out in front of the chair, pushes down with the foot, and flexes the knee to move the wheelchair forward. To move the wheelchair backward, the patient places one foot slightly underneath the chair, pushes down on the floor, and extends the knee. If the patient is only able to use one leg, the same technique is used.

► A patient may need to use the hands and feet to propel a wheelchair. For example, a patient with one-sided weakness may propel a wheelchair using the arm and leg on the same side.

Once the patient has demonstrated that they can maneuver in all directions independently, the clinician must advance the complexity of the navigational tasks as appropriate.

► *Perform more advanced techniques as necessary or appropriate.* Advanced techniques are necessary when a patient

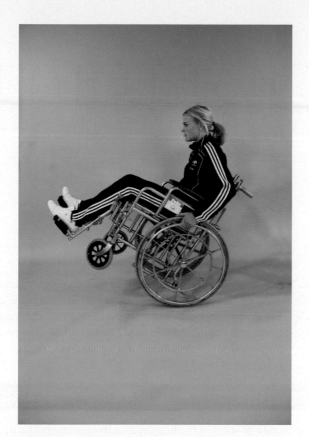

FIGURE 10-45 Wheelchair wheelie.

has to negotiate obstacles independently using a wheelie (Figure 10-45). Wheelies are important for patients who need to go up and down curbs independently when there are no curb ramps. A wheelie is performed by balancing on the rear wheels of a wheelchair while the caster wheels are in the air. Initially, the clinician must be positioned behind the chair and move with the chair, with the hands held beneath the wheelchair handles, ready to catch the wheelchair if it tilts too far backward. To perform a wheelie, the patient is asked to place the hands at 11 o'clock on the wheels, then lean forward and arch the back. Initially, the patient practices bouncing the body off the back of the chair and leaning back while holding the hands still—the front of the chair is raised by pushing backward on the chair back. The patient practices until he or she can bounce the front end off the ground. By changing the COG (by pushing the chair forward while the body is going backward), the patient will achieve a point of equilibrium. Once the patient can bounce the front end off the ground and find a point of equilibrium, they can progress to reaching back and placing the hands at about 10 o'clock on the wheels. From this point, the patient leans forward, arches the back, and then begins to push forward quickly while letting the body come back against the chair (when the back hits the chair, the hands should be in the 12 o'clock position). By continuing to lean back while pushing the chair forward, the front end should

start to leave the ground, and by the time the hands get to the 2 o'clock position, the front end should feel weightless, as the chair balances on the rear axle. To maintain equilibrium, the patient will need to move the chair forward if the front end begins to fall down or backward if the chair begins to fall backward. This may be accomplished by sliding the hands back to about the 1 o'clock position without taking the hands off the wheels. Once the chair is up and balanced, the patient will need to keep just a fraction of weight on the front end so that if balance is lost, the chair will fall forward, not backward.

Once the patient is ready to try a wheelie independently, a good place to begin practicing is on carpeting, grass, or sand. As part of the wheelie training, the patient should be taught how to fall in a controlled manner.

▶ *Falling backward.* This is probably the most common direction of falling. The patient should be taught how to tuck the head into the chest if falling backward so that the back of the head is not hit. Applying a slight braking force to the drive wheels can prevent the wheelchair from sliding too far forward and catching the lower extremities.

▶ *Falling forward.* The patient should be taught how to land as far forward of the chair as possible by extending the arms and trunk to prevent the upper body from landing on the patient's legs.

▶ *Falling sideways.* The patient should be told to tuck the arms close to the chest and to round the shoulder on the side of the fall while side flexing the head away from the ground.

Finally, the patient should be taught how to use his or her wheelie skills to:

▶ Ascend a curb forward.

▶ Descend a curb forward.

REFERENCES

1. Edelstein JE. Prosthetics. In: O'Sullivan SB, Schmitz TJ, eds. *Physical Rehabilitation,* 5th ed. Philadelphia: FA Davis; 2007:1251-1286.
2. Rankin JW, Kwarciak AM, Richter WM, Neptune RR. The influence of wheelchair propulsion technique on upper extremity muscle demand: A simulation study. *Clin Biomech.* 2012;27(9):879-886.
3. Kwarciak AM, Turner JT, Guo L, Richter WM. The effects of four different stroke patterns on manual wheelchair propulsion and upper limb muscle strain. *Disabil Rehabil Assist Technol.* 2012: 7(6):459-463.
4. Boninger ML, Souza AL, Cooper RA, Fitzgerald SG, Koontz AM, Fay BT. Propulsion patterns and pushrim biomechanics in manual wheelchair propulsion. *Arch Phys Med Rehabil.* 2002;83:718-723.
5. Coutts KD. Kinematics of sport wheelchair propulsion. *J Rehabil Res Dev.* 1990;27:21-26.
6. Cowan RE, Nash MS, Collinger JL, Koontz AM, Boninger ML. Impact of surface type, wheelchair weight, and axle position on wheelchair propulsion by novice older adults. *Arch Phys Med Rehabil.* 2009;90:1076-1083.
7. Desroches G, Dumas R, Pradon D, Vaslin P, Lepoutre FX, Cheze L. Upper limb joint dynamics during manual wheelchair propulsion. *Clin Biomech.* 2010;25:299-306.
8. Gorce P, Louis N. Wheelchair propulsion kinematics in beginners and expert users: Influence of wheelchair settings. *Clin Biomech.* 2012;27:7-15.

Gait Training

CHAPTER 11

CHAPTER OBJECTIVES

At the completion of this chapter, the reader will be able to:

1. Describe the various gait parameters

2. Describe the characteristics of normal gait

3. Discuss how to use the various pieces of pre-ambulation equipment, including the tilt table and parallel bars

4. Describe the various types of weight-bearing status and the functions of each

5. Describe the various methods to monitor the weight-bearing status

6. Make a clinical decision as to how well an assistive device is assisting a patient

7. Be able to fit a patient for an assistive device

8. Discuss the importance of patient safety during gait or ambulation activities

9. Provide training to the patient on how to use an assistive device during various transfers

10. Teach a patient how to use an assistive device with varying gait patterns, during stair negotiation, and ambulation in the community

OVERVIEW

It is not clear whether gait is learned or is preprogrammed at the spinal cord level. However, once mastered, gait allows us to efficiently move around our environment, requiring little conscious thought, at least in familiar surroundings. On the surface, gait appears to be a very simple task where the lower kinetic chain has two main functions: to provide a stable base of support (BOS) in standing and to propel the body through space with gait allowing the arms and hands to be free for exploration of the environment. Whereas the objective in standing is to maintain a static equilibrium of forces,

the objective with mobility is to create and control dynamic, unbalanced forces to produce movement.[1] So gait is a complex process that requires control of various neuromuscular, musculoskeletal, cardiopulmonary, and psychological factors to produce controlled instability, making it prone to breakdown.

POSTURE

The transformation of the human race from arboreal quadrupeds to upright bipeds is likely related to the need to have the upper extremities available for carrying a wider variety of foods across fairly long distances.[2] This transformation from quadruped to biped was responsible for changes in the weight-bearing (WB) parts of the musculoskeletal structures and adaptations in the upper extremities, which were now free for the development of a greater variety of manipulative skills.

As the human body develops from infancy to old age, several physical and neurologic factors may affect posture. At birth, a series of primary curves cause the entire vertebral column to be concave forward or flexed, giving a kyphotic posture to the whole spine, although the overall contour in the coronal plane is straight. In contrast, the contour of the sagittal plane changes with growth. With the erect posture development, secondary curves appeared in the cervical and lumbar spines, producing a lordosis in these regions. The curves in the spinal column provide it with increased flexibility and shock-absorbing capabilities. At the other end of the life span, the aging adult tends to alter posture in several ways. A common function of aging, at least in women, is developing a stooped posture associated with osteoporosis, with a resultant kyphosis of the thoracic spine. Also, degeneration of the lumbar spine tends to flatten the lumbar lordosis. The normal coronal and sagittal alignment of the spine can be altered by many conditions, including leg-length inequality, congenital anomalies, developmental problems, or trauma.[3-5] For example, scoliosis represents a progressive disturbance of the intercalated series of spinal segments that produces a three-dimensional deformity (lateral curvature and vertebral rotation) of the spine.

Changes in the body shape's contours or orientation can produce joint dysfunction and require greater energy expenditure during normal activities. Also, pathologic changes to the musculoskeletal system (eg, excessive wearing of the articular surfaces of joints, the development of osteophytes

Figure 11-13 to Figure 11-58 are reproduced with permission from Dutton M: Introduction to Physical Therapy and Patient Skills, 2nd ed. New York, NY: McGraw Hill; 2014.

and traction spurs, and maladaptive changes in the length-tension development and angle of pull of muscles and tendons) may be the result of the cumulative effect of repeated small stresses (microtrauma) over a long phase of time or of constant abnormal stresses (macrotrauma) over a short phase of time. Strong, flexible muscles can resist the detrimental effects of faulty postures for longer periods and unload the structures through a change of position. However, these changes in position are not possible if the joints are stiff (hypomobile) or too mobile (hypermobile), or if the muscles are weak, shortened, or lengthened.

It is difficult to determine why a particular posture becomes dysfunctional in one individual, yet not in another. Differing adaptive potentials of the tissues between individuals may be among the causes, in addition to neurologic, neurodevelopmental, and neurophysiologic factors.

REQUIREMENTS OF GAIT

Although individual gait patterns are characterized by significant variation, three essential requirements have been identified for locomotion: progression, postural control, and adaptation[6]:

▶ *Progression.* The fall that occurs at the initiation of gait to take the first step is controlled by the central nervous system (CNS).[7] The CNS computes in advance the required size and direction of this fall toward the supporting foot. Also, gait relies on the control of limb movements by reflexes. Two such reflexes include the stretch reflex and the extensor thrust. The stretch reflex is involved in the extremes of joint motion, whereas the extensor thrust may facilitate the extensor muscles of the lower extremity during WB.[8] Both the CPG and the reflexes that mediate afferent input to the spinal cord are under the brainstem's

control and are therefore subconscious.[9] This would tend to indicate that verbal coaching (ie, feedback that is processed in the cortex) regarding an aberrant gait pattern might be less effective than a sensory input that will elicit a brainstem-mediated postural response.[1]

▶ *Postural control.* Postural control is dynamically maintained to position the body for efficient gait appropriately.

▶ *Adaptation.* Although central pattern generation occurs independent of sensory input, afferent information from the periphery can influence the central pattern. Adaptation is achieved by adjusting the central pattern generated to meet task demands and environmental demands.

Gait, therefore, is generated grossly in the spinal cord and fine-tuned from higher brain centers.[1] In patients who have developed dysfunctional gait patterns, physical therapy can help restore this exquisite evolutionary gift.[10] Pain, weakness, and disease can all cause a disturbance in the normal gait rhythm. However, except in obvious cases, abnormal gait does not always equate impairment.

Walking involves the alternating action of the two lower extremities. The walking pattern is studied as a gait cycle. The *gait cycle* is defined as the interval of time between any of the repetitive events of walking, such as from the point when the foot first contacts the ground, to the point when the same foot contacts the ground again.[11] The gait cycle consists of two phases (Figure 11-1):

1. **Stance.** This phase constitutes approximately 60–65% of the gait cycle[12,13] and describes the entire time the foot is in contact with the ground and the limb is bearing weight. The stance phase begins when the foot makes contact with the ground and concludes when the ipsilateral foot leaves the ground. The stance phase takes about 0.6 seconds at an average walking speed.

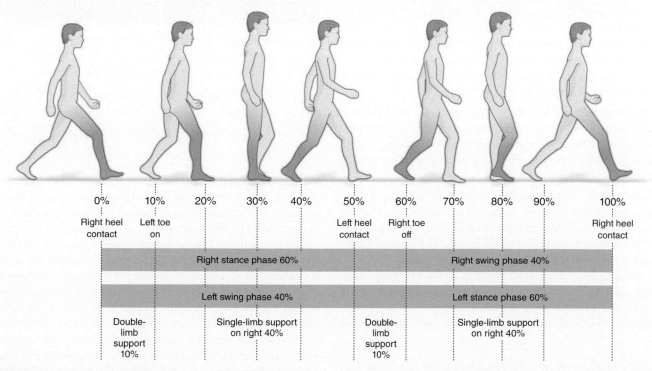

FIGURE 11-1 The gait cycle. (Reproduced with permission from Dutton, M: Dutton's Orthopaedic Examination, Evaluation and Intervention, 5th ed. New York, NY: McGraw Hill; 2017.)

2. *Swing.* The swing phase constitutes approximately 35–40% of the gait cycle[12,13] and describes the phase when the foot is not in contact with the ground. The swing phase begins as the foot is lifted from the ground and ends when the ipsilateral foot makes contact with the ground again.[7]

GAIT PARAMETERS

A normal gait pattern is a factor of several parameters.

Base (Step) Width. The base width is the lateral distance between both feet. The normal BOS is considered to be between 5 and 10 cm (2–4 inches). The size of the BOS and its relation to the center of gravity (COG*) are important factors in maintaining balance and, thus, the object's stability. The COG must be maintained over the BOS if an equilibrium is to be maintained. The BOS includes the part of the body in contact with the supporting surface and the intervening area.[14] As the COG moves forward with each step, it briefly passes beyond the anterior margin of the BOS, resulting in a temporary loss of balance.[14] This temporary loss of equilibrium is counteracted by the advancing foot at initial contact, establishing a new BOS. A larger-than-normal BOS is observed in individuals with muscle imbalances of the lower limbs and trunk and those with overall static-dynamic balance problems.[15] The base width should decrease to around zero with increased speed. If the base width decreases to a point below zero, crossover occurs, whereby one foot lands where the other should, and vice versa.[16] Assistive devices, such as crutches or walkers, can be prescribed to increase the BOS and enhance stability.

Step Length. Step length is measured as the distance between the same part of one foot on successive footprints (ipsilateral to the contralateral footfall). The average step length is about 72 cm (28 inches). The measurement should be equal for both legs.

Stride Length. Stride length is the distance between successive points of foot-to-floor contact of the same foot. A stride equates to one full lower extremity cycle. Two step lengths are added together to make the stride length. The average stride length for normal individuals is 144 cm (56 inches).[17]

Typically, the step and stride lengths do not vary more than a few centimeters between tall and short individuals. Men typically have longer step and stride lengths than women. Step and stride lengths decrease with age, pain, disease, and fatigue.[18] They also decrease as the speed of gait increases.[19] A decrease in step (or stride) length may also result from a forward head posture, a stiff hip, or a decrease in motion availability at the lumbar spine. The decrease in step and stride length that occurs with aging is thought to result from the increased likelihood of falling during the swing phase of ambulation, caused by diminished hip musculature control.[20] This lack of control prevents the aged person from intermittently losing and recovering the same balance that the younger adult can lose and recover.[20]

Cadence. Cadence is defined as the number of separate steps taken within a certain time. Normal cadence is between 90 and 120 steps per minute.[21,22] The cadence of women is usually 6–9 steps per minute slower than that of men.[14] Cadence is also affected by age, decreasing from the age of 4 to the age of 7 years, and then again in advancing years.[23]

Velocity. The primary determinants of gait velocity are the repetition rate (cadence), physical conditioning, and the person's stride length.[17]

Vertical Ground Reaction Forces. Newton's third law states that for every action, there is an equal and opposite reaction. During gait, vertical ground reaction forces (GRFs) are created by gravity, body weight, and the ground's firmness. Under normal conditions, we are mostly unaware of these forces. However, in the presence of joint inflammation or tissue injury, the significance of these forces becomes apparent. Vertical GRFs begin with an impact peak of less than body weight and then exceed body weight at the end of the initial contact interval, dropping during midstance and rising again to exceed body weight, reaching a peak during the terminal stance interval. Thus, two peaks of GRF occur during the gait cycle: the first at maximum limb loading during the loading response and the second during terminal stance.

---

*The COG of the body is located approximately at midline in the frontal plane and slightly anterior (5 cm or 2 inches) to the second sacral vertebra in the sagittal plane.

The GRF vector is anterior to the hip joint at initial contact, then migrates progressively posteriorly until late stance, when the ground reaction force is posterior to the hip.[33,34] Peak flexion torque occurs at initial contact but gradually declines, changing to an extension torque in midstance. The extension torque remains until terminal stance.[33,34]

During the gait cycle, the tibiofemoral joint reaction force has two peaks. The first immediately follows initial contact (2–3 times body weight) and the second during pre-swing (three to four times body weight).[35] Tibiofemoral joint reaction forces increase to 5–6 times body weight during running and stair climbing, and 8 times body weight with downhill walking.[35-37]

It is well established that joint angles and GRF components increase with walking speed.[38] This is not surprising because the dynamic force components must increase as the body is subject to increasing deceleration and acceleration forces when walking speed increases.

CLINICAL PEARL

Because leg length in women is 51.2% of total body height compared with 56% in men, women must strike the ground more often to cover the same distance.[39] Furthermore, because their feet are shorter, women complete the heel-to-toe gait in a shorter time than men do. Therefore, the cumulative GRFs may be greater in women.[24]

Mediolateral Shear Forces. Mediolateral shear in walking gait begins with an initial medial shear (occasionally lateral) after initial contact, followed by lateral shear for the remainder of the stance phase.[33,34] At the end of the stance phase, the shear shifts to a medial direction because of propulsion forces.

Anteroposterior Shear Forces. Anteroposterior shear forces in gait begin with an anterior shear force at initial contact, and the loading response intervals and a posterior shear at the end of the terminal stance interval.

CHARACTERISTICS OF NORMAL GAIT

Much has been written about the criteria for normal and abnormal gait.[11,13,25,33,40-45] Although the presence of symmetry in gait appears to be important, asymmetry in itself does not guarantee impairment. It must be remembered that the definition of what constitutes the so-called normal gait is elusive. Unlike posture, which is a static event, gait is dynamic.

CLINICAL PEARL

Good alignment of the WB segments of the body:

▶ Reduces the likelihood of strain and injury by reducing joint friction and tension in the soft tissues.

▶ Improves the stability of the WB limb and the balance of the trunk. The stability of the body is directly related to the size of the BOS. To be stable, the intersection of the line of gravity with the BOS should be close to the geometric center of the base.[46]

▶ Reduces excess energy expenditure.

Gait involves the displacement of body weight in the desired direction, using a coordinated effort between the trunk and the extremities and muscles that control or produce these motions. Any interference that alters this relationship may result in a deviation or disturbance of the normal gait pattern, which, in turn, may result in increased energy expenditure or functional impairment. The physical therapist assistant (PTA) must be able to differentiate between compensated and uncompensated deviations, even though it is the supervising physical therapist (PT) who will be determining the cause. A compensated deviation occurs when the patient intentionally moves in a certain way to decrease pain or to maintain the COG over the BOS, whereas an uncompensated deviation occurs involuntarily. For example, a patient with weak left hip abductors will demonstrate a lateral trunk lean to the right over the right standing leg to keep the COG over the right leg (compensated) but will demonstrate a pelvic drop to the left during the swing of the left leg (positive Trendelenburg).

Perry[21] lists four *priorities* of normal gait:

1. Stability of the WB foot throughout the stance phase
2. Clearance of the non–WB foot during the swing phase
3. Appropriate prepositioning (during the terminal swing) of the foot for the next gait cycle
4. Adequate step length

Gage[23] added a fifth priority, energy conservation. The typical energy expended in normal gait (2.5 kcal/min) is less than twice that spent while sitting or standing (1.5 kcal/min).[23] Two-dimensional kinetic data have revealed that approximately 85% of the energy for normal walking comes from the ankle plantarflexors and 15% from the hip flexors.[47] It has been proposed that the type of gait selected is based on metabolic energy considerations.[48] Current commonly used parameters used to measure walking efficiency include oxygen consumption, heart rate, and comfortable walking speed.[49-51] Economic mobility is a measurement of submaximal oxygen uptake (submax VO_2) for a given speed.[52,53] A decline in functional performance may be evidenced by an increase in submax VO_2 for walking.[54] This change in the economy of mobility may be indicative of an abnormal gait pattern.[54] Some researchers have reported no gender differences for the economy of mobility,[55-57] whereas others suggest that men are more economical or have lower energy costs than women at the same absolute work.[58-60] Age-related declines in economy of mobility also have been reported in the literature, with differing results. Some researchers reported that older adults were less economical than younger adults while walking at various speeds.[52,61,62] Conversely, the economy of mobility appears to be unaffected by aging for individuals who maintain higher levels of physical activity.[63-65]

Some authors have claimed that a limb-length discrepancy leads to mechanical and functional changes in gait[66] and increased energy expenditure.[67] Intervention has been advocated for discrepancies of less than 1 cm to discrepancies greater than 5 cm,[66-68] but the rationale for these recommendations has not been well defined, and the literature contains little substantive information regarding the functional significance of these discrepancies.[69] For example, Gross found no noticeable functional or cosmetic problems in a study of 74 adults who had less than 2 cm of discrepancy and 35 marathon runners who had as much as 2.5 cm of discrepancy.[68]

For gait to be efficient and to conserve energy, the COG must undergo minimal displacement:

▶ Any displacement that moves the COG beyond normal maximum excursion limits wastes energy.

▶ Any abrupt or irregular movement will waste energy even when that movement does not exceed the normal maximum displacement limits of the COG.

To minimize the energy costs of walking, the body uses several biomechanical mechanisms. In 1953, Saunders, Inman, and Eberhart[72] proposed that six kinematic features—the six determinants—can reduce the energetic cost of human walking. The six determinants are[73]:

▶ *Lateral displacement of the pelvis:* to avoid significant muscular and balancing demands, the pelvis shifts side to side (approximately 2.5–5 cm or 1–2 inches) during walking to center the body's weight over the stance leg. If the lower extremities dropped directly vertical from the hip joint, the center of mass would be required to shift 3–4 inches to each side to be positioned effectively over the supporting foot. The combination of femoral varus and anatomical valgum at the knee permits a vertical tibial posture with both tibias close to each other. This narrows the walking base to 5–10 cm (2–4 inches) from heel center to heel center, thereby reducing the lateral shift required of the COG toward either side.

▶ *Pelvic rotation:* the rotation of the pelvis normally occurs about a vertical axis in the transverse plane toward the WB limb. The total pelvic rotation is approximately 4° to each side.[23] Forward rotation of the pelvis on the swing side prevents an excessive drop in the body's COG. The pelvic rotation also results in a relative lengthening of the femur by lessening the angle of the femur with the floor, and thus step length, during the termination of the swing period.[74]

▶ *Vertical displacement of the pelvis:* vertical pelvic shifting keeps the COG from moving superiorly and inferiorly more than 5 cm (2 inches) during normal gait. Because of the shift, the high point occurs during midstance, and the low point occurs during initial contact. The amount of vertical displacement of the pelvis may be accentuated

in the presence of a leg-length discrepancy, a fusion of the knee, or hip abductor weakness, the last of which results in a Trendelenburg sign. The Trendelenburg sign is positive if standing on one leg; the pelvis drops on the side opposite the stance leg. The weakness is present on the side of the stance leg—the gluteus medius cannot maintain the COG on the stance leg's side.

▶ *Knee flexion in midstance:* knee motion is intrinsically associated with foot and ankle motion. At initial contact, before the ankle moves into a plantarflexed position and thus is relatively more elevated, the knee is in relative extension. Responding to a plantarflexed posture at loading response, the knee flexes. Midstance knee flexion prevents an excessive rise in the body's COG during that period of the gait cycle. If not for the midstance knee flexion, the COG's rise during midstance would be larger, as would its total vertical displacement. Passing through midstance as the ankle remains stationary with the foot flat on the floor, the knee again reverses its direction into extension. As the heel comes off the floor in terminal stance, the heel begins to rise as the ankle plantarflexes and the knee flexes. In preswing, as the forefoot rolls over the metatarsal heads, the heel elevates even more as further plantarflexion occurs and flexion of the knee increases.

▶ *Ankle mechanism:* for normal foot function and human ambulation, the amount of ankle joint motion required is approximately 10° of dorsiflexion (to complete midstance and begin terminal stance) and 20° of plantarflexion (for full push-off in pre-swing). At initial contact, the foot is in relative dorsiflexion due to the action of the pretibial muscles and the triceps surae. This muscle action produces a relative lengthening of the leg, resulting in smoothing the COG pathway during the stance phase.

▶ *Foot mechanism:* the controlled lever arm of the forefoot at pre-swing is particularly helpful as it rounds out the sharp downward reversal of the COG. Thus it does not reduce a peak displacement period of the COG, as the earlier determinants did, but instead smooths the pathway. An adaptively shortened gastrocnemius muscle may produce movement impairment by restricting the ankle's normal dorsiflexion from occurring during the midstance-to-heel-raise portion of the gait cycle. This motion is compensated for by increased pronation of the subtalar joint, increased internal rotation of the tibia, and stress to the knee joint complex.

PRE-AMBULATION EXERCISES

The strength and control of several muscle groups are required for gait, and some patients may need a gradual introduction to be upright and weight bear through the lower extremities.

Neurodevelopmental treatment (NDT) techniques, devised by Berta and Karel Bobath, use fundamental postural reflex mechanisms to enhance motor learning while improving strength and balance.[75] Many of these techniques, which place a progressive and increased demand on the patient during functional movements and positions, can be used as pre-ambulation exercises to prepare a patient for gait training. All of the following exercises can be used in isolation to address specific weaknesses or deficits or in combination based on patient need. The exercises are designed to gradually decrease the base of support (BOS) while increasing the height of the patient's center of gravity (COG) and follow the four stages of motor control: mobility → stability → controlled mobility → skill.

Hooklying. The patient is positioned supine with the hips and knees flexed and the feet flat on the bed (Figure 11-2). Depending on the patient's ability, maintaining the lower extremity position may be difficult, so pillows or bolsters can be used. Once this position can be maintained, extra challenges can be added, such as asking the patient to lift one foot a few inches off the bed, holding it raised for a few seconds, and then returning it to the starting position before similarly lifting the other foot. Alternatively, a pillow can be placed between the patient's knees, and the patient is asked to squeeze the pillow.

Bridging. The patient is positioned in the hooklying position. The patient is taught how to do an anterior and posterior pelvic tilt and to hold each of these positions. The patient is then instructed on how to perform bridging (Figure 11-3) and attempts to maintain the position for increasing lengths of time.

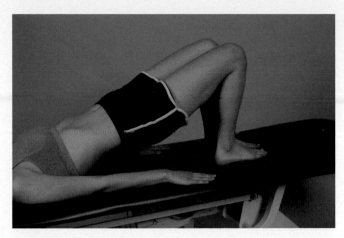

FIGURE 11-3 Bridging.

Rolling. Rolling from supine to prone back to supine is taught to the patient with varying use of the upper extremities and lower extremities to perform both log rolling and segmental rolling (see Chapter 7).

Prone Lying into Prone on Elbows. As with the supine position, the prone position (Figure 11-4) is an extremely stable patient position. As tolerated, the patient is asked to prop themselves up into the prone on elbows position (Figure 11-5). The progression from prone lying to prone on elbows is an excellent way to strengthen the shoulders and upper extremities while gradually increasing lumbar extension. Further strengthening and lumbar extension can be added by asking the patient to perform varying degrees of a prone push-up (Figure 11-6). These exercises help prepare the patient for the erect standing position and use their upper extremities with the prescribed assistive device.

Supine to Long Sitting. Moving from supine to the long sit position requires good upper extremity strength. The patient begins in the hooklying position before raising themselves on their elbows (Figure 11-7). From this position, the patient straightens both legs and then, in a series of side-to-side movements, straightens both arms so that the palms are on the bed and the trunk is elevated into an L position with respect to the lower extremities.

Seated Scooting Forward and Backward. This exercise requires very good strength of the upper extremities but is an excellent exercise to help prepare a patient for using an assistive device. The patient is positioned in the long sitting position and pushes down toward the bed with the upper extremities to raise their buttocks off the bed to move their buttocks either forward or backward. This movement is repeated so that the patient can scoot either up the bed or down the bed.

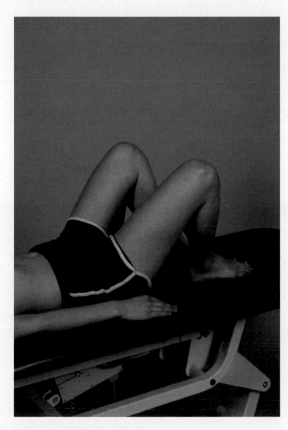

FIGURE 11-2 Hooklying position.

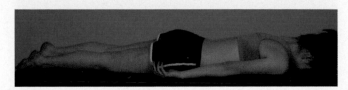

FIGURE 11-4 Prone lying.

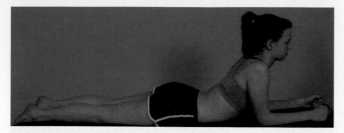

FIGURE 11-5 Prone on elbows.

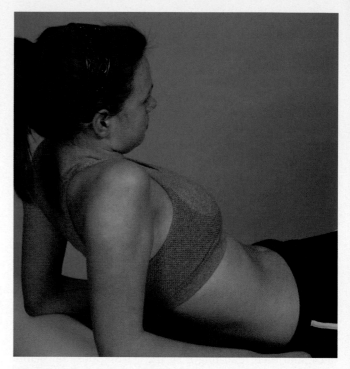

FIGURE 11-7 Supine on elbows.

Quadruped. Despite its relatively large BOS, because the points of contact are small, the quadruped position (Figure 11-8) is much less stable than the previous positions and is a very good position to introduce weight-shifting and more advanced balance activities. For example, once the patient can maintain the quadruped position without assistance, they can be asked to gradually raise one of the lower extremities (Figure 11-9) while attempting to maintain balance. This activity is extremely difficult to perform on a soft surface, so it is usually performed on a mat table or similarly firm surface.

Short Sitting. This task involves the patient moving from the supine position to sitting over the edge of the bed (see Chapter 7) so that the feet are dangling. Sitting in this position significantly reduces the patient's BOS, so the patient may initially require some assistance for balance. This task can be made more challenging by having the patient perform alternating seated knee extensions before progressing to seated hip flexions.

Sitting and Reaching. Various balance exercises can be performed in unsupported sitting. For example, reaching exercises with one upper extremity and then both upper extremities progressively challenge the patient's ability to move the COG out of the BOS.

Seated Toe Raises and Heel Raises. The patient is progressed from sitting on the edge of the bed to sitting in a regular chair so that their feet flat on the floor. In this position, the patient can perform heel slides (Figure 11-10) and toe raises (Figure 11-11). These two exercises will help increase passive dorsiflexion and strengthen the ankle dorsiflexors, respectively, in preparation for gait.

Sitting to Squatting. This task is performed with the patient seated in a chair. Using their arms to push off, the patient moves from a seated position into a half-standing/squatting

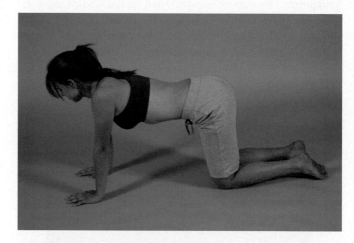

FIGURE 11-8 The quadruped position.

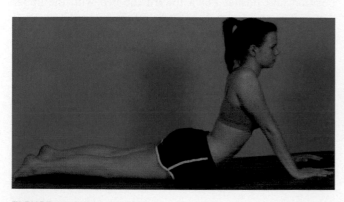

FIGURE 11-6 Prone push up.

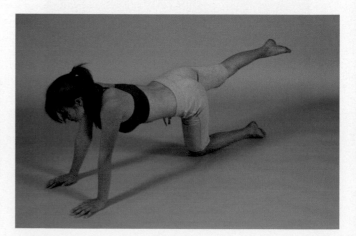

FIGURE 11-9 Hip extension in quadruped.

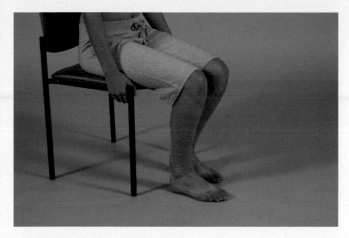

FIGURE 11-10 Heel slides.

position (Figure 11-12), maintains the position briefly, and then returns to the seated position. This is a very challenging exercise, so the patient should be closely monitored.

PRE-AMBULATION EQUIPMENT

Tilt Table

A tilt table, a table designed to move from the horizontal to a vertical position, consists of a padded table with a footplate and restraint straps. The tilt table is used to evaluate how a patient regulates their vital signs in response to simple stresses, including gravity, while being slowly tilted toward a vertical position (approximately 80–90°) or down toward a horizontal position (0°). The tilt table was originally designed to evaluate

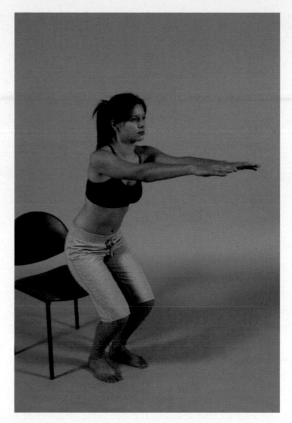

FIGURE 11-12 Sitting to squatting.

patients with fainting spells (syncope), but is now used for a wide variety of patient diagnoses, including orthostatic hypotension, pulmonary ventilation dysfunction, dizziness, and patients with WB restrictions. The tilt table is contraindicated for unstable spinal cord injuries, unstable or erratic blood pressure, or poor cardiac responses to cardiovascular challenges. The speed with which the table is elevated is based on the patient response that the physical therapist monitors, but it is usually elevated in about 15° about every 15–20 minutes. Adverse reactions include excessive blood pressure changes, increased heart rate, low oxygen saturation, complaints of dizziness, nausea, and changes in the level of consciousness. A typical tilt table procedure follows.

▶ The patient is transferred or asked to lie supine on the tilt table with his or her feet flat on the footplate and is then secured by a series of straps or belts around the hips, knees, and trunk (Figure 11-13), based on the level of control that the patient has over the trunk and lower extremities. Also, compression stockings or an abdominal binder may be necessary for the patient's blood pressure to remain stable.

▶ Baseline data are recorded, including resting pulse rate, blood pressure, oxygen saturation, and subjective reports.

▶ The table is raised to a 15–30° angle or according to the physician's orders (Figure 11-14). This position is maintained for about 15–20 minutes while the baseline data are recorded. The table is lowered to a level where the patient stabilizes if there are any negative changes in the patient's condition.

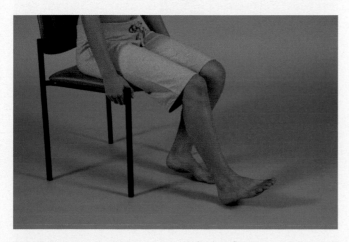

FIGURE 11-11 Toes raises/active ankle dorsiflexion.

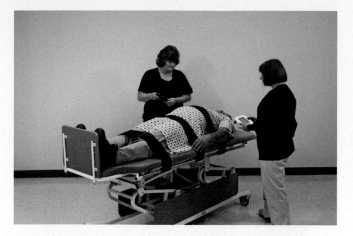

FIGURE 11-13 Tilt table—patient set up.

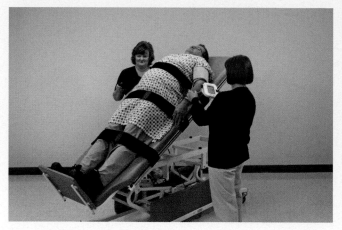

FIGURE 11-15 Tilt table at approximately 60°.

▶ If the patient experienced no adverse effects at 15–30°, the tilt table is raised a further 15–30° (Figure 11-15). The degree of elevation and the time spent at each level depends on the patient's response and treatment goal. If the therapeutic goal is for the patient to ambulate, the table is progressively raised from near-vertical (Figure 11-16) to fully vertical.

At the end of the session, the tilt table is lowered to the horizontal position, the straps are removed, and the patient is transferred from the tilt table. Over time, or a series of sessions, the tilt table is raised farther while monitoring the patient's vital signs and subjective reports. While parallel bars may be necessary for some patients, they have little to no functional carryover other than to increase tolerance for the upright position.

Parallel Bars

Parallel bars can provide maximum stability and security for patients during the beginning stages of ambulation or standing. However, despite the stability provided by the parallel bars, the amount of functional carryover is low. When adjusting the height of the parallel bars, the correct height of the bar should allow for approximately 20–30° of elbow flexion from

the patient while the patient is grasping on the bars approximately 4–6 inches in front of the body.

CLINICAL PEARL

Parallel bars should be set at approximately the level of the greater trochanter, wrist crease, or ulnar styloid process of the standing patient so that when the patient's hands are placed on the bars about 4–6 inches anterior to the hips, the elbows should be flexed to approximately 20–30°.

CLINICAL PEARL

Pre-ambulatory training within the parallel bars can include:

▶ Development of standing balance and tolerance
▶ Weight shifting
▶ Proper stance and foot placement
▶ Proper gait pattern training

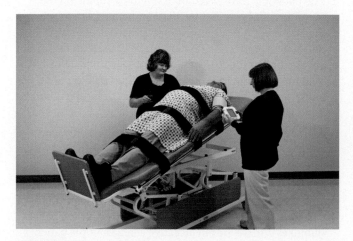

FIGURE 11-14 Tilt table at approximately 30°.

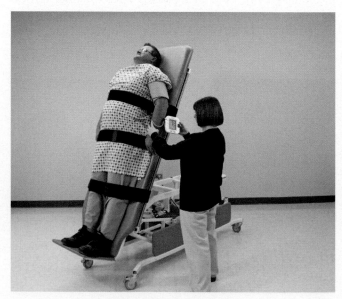

FIGURE 11-16 Tilt table at approximately 80°.

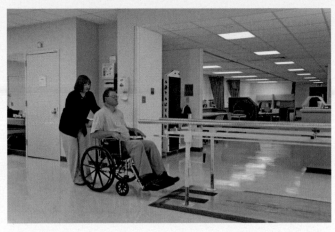

FIGURE 11-17 Wheelchair transport to parallel bars.

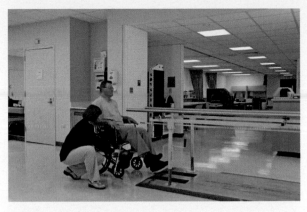

FIGURE 11-19 The leg rests are removed.

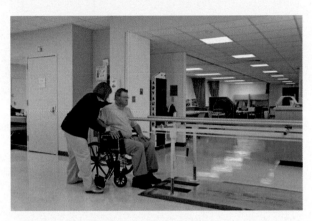

FIGURE 11-20 The patient is asked to place the hands on the armrests and to slide forward in the wheelchair.

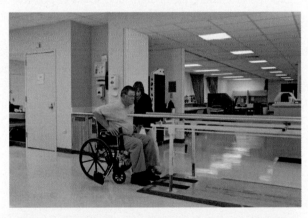

FIGURE 11-21 The patient is asked to lean forward in the chair.

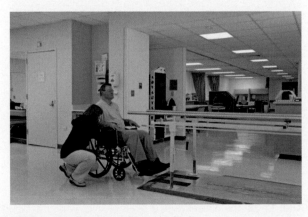

FIGURE 11-18 The wheelchair is locked.

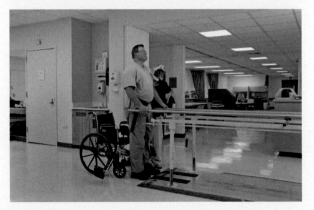

FIGURE 11-22 Once in a standing position, the patient is asked to grasp the parallel bars.

A typical sequence of gait training using the parallel bars follows.

1. The patient is transported in a wheelchair to the end of the parallel bars, and the clinician makes sure that the patient is wearing a gait belt (Figure 11-17).
2. The wheels of the wheelchair are locked (Figure 11-18).
3. The leg rests of the wheelchair are removed (Figure 11-19).
4. The patient is asked to place the hands on the armrests and slide forward in the wheelchair (Figure 11-20).
5. The patient is asked to lean forward in the chair and, when ready to stand, push up from the armrests (Figure 11-21). The patient should be instructed not to pull himself or herself up using the parallel bars.
6. Once in a standing position, the patient is asked to grasp the parallel bars (Figure 11-22), and the clinician asks the patient how he or she feels (weak, dizzy, nauseous, etc) (Figure 11-23) before proceeding. At this point, depending on the patient's status and ability, the clinician may choose to ask the patient to shift his or her body from side to side and forward and backward while maintaining the correct WB status. The clinician may also ask the patient to lift one or both of their hands from the bars to challenge their balance or to step

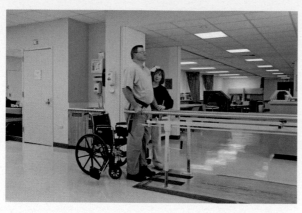

FIGURE 11-23 The clinician asks the patient how he or she feels.

in place, depending on their WB status. Parallel bars enable a patient to practice a particular gait pattern in a safe environment. If necessary, an appropriate assistive device (see Assistive Devices) can also be fitted and used by the patient within the parallel bars.

7. The clinician adjusts his or her position to grasp the gait belt and provide manual cues for the patient (Figure 11-24). Whenever possible, the clinician should remain inside the bars with the patient to enhance control and safety. When the clinician and patient are ready, they are asked to take a step (see Figure 11-24). The choice to stand in front of or behind the patient is based on whether the clinician wants to watch the patient's face and eyes for signs of distress or possible fainting and whether the plan is for the patient to turn within the parallel bars.

8. As the patient continues to take steps within the parallel bars, the clinician follows closely, asking questions about the patient's status (Figures 11-25 through 11-28).

9. If the clinician decides that the patient is to turn within the parallel bars, the patient is asked to stand still and then to turn in the chosen direction (Figures 11-29 through 11-31) until he or she is facing the clinician. Turning within the bars involves asking the patient to turn toward the stronger side.

10. Once the turn is completed, the clinician asks the patient how they feel (Figure 11-32). This is important

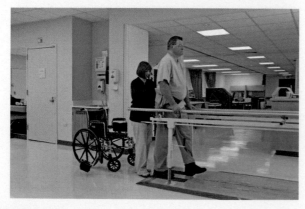

FIGURE 11-24 The clinician adjusts his or her position to be able to grasp the gait belt and to provide manual cues for the patient.

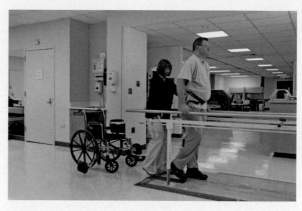

FIGURE 11-25 The patient takes a series of steps while maintaining good posture.

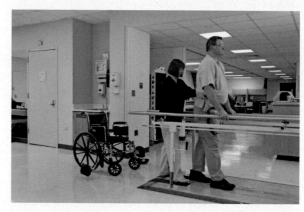

FIGURE 11-26 The patient takes a series of steps while trying to look ahead.

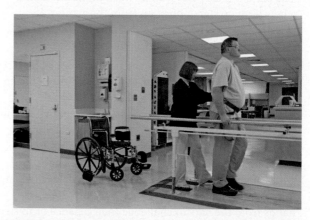

FIGURE 11-27 The patient takes a series of steps using a safe stride length.

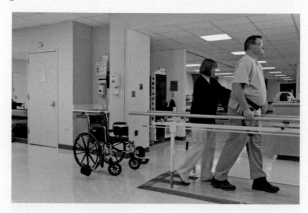

FIGURE 11-28 The patient takes a series of steps while the clinician follows closely.

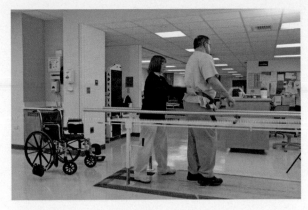

FIGURE 11-29 The patient begins to turn to the left.

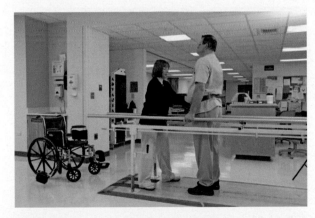

FIGURE 11-30 The patient continues to turn to the left.

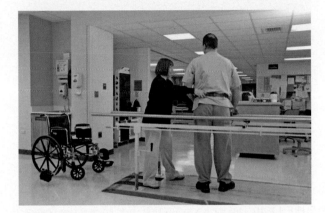

FIGURE 11-31 The patient completes the turn.

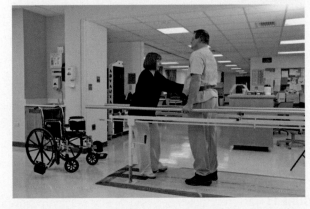

FIGURE 11-32 The clinician asks the patient how he or she feels.

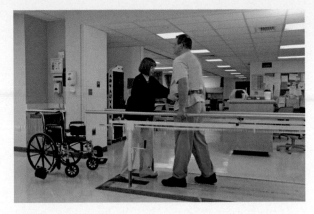

FIGURE 11-33 The patient begins walking toward the clinician.

after any turning activities, as these can provoke dizziness.

11. Once the patient reports having no problems, they are asked to begin walking toward the clinician (Figures 11-33 through 11-36).

12. At the end of the parallel bars (Figure 11-37), the patient is again asked to turn (Figures 11-38 and 11-39), and a wheelchair is positioned appropriately.

13. The patient is asked to shuffle backward until they can feel the seat of the wheelchair against the back of the legs (Figure 11-40). At this point, the patient is asked to reach back for the chair using the hands (Figure 11-41) and then to slowly lower himself or herself into the chair in a controlled manner (Figures 11-42 and 11-43).

Video Description

VIDEO 11-1

There are several points to note in the video demonstrating gait within the parallel bars:

▶ The clinician is constantly aware of patient safety. For example, when the wheelchair is brought to the parallel bars, the clinician makes sure that the wheels are locked and that any obstructions, such as the leg rests, are removed. Also, the patient is wearing a gait belt, and

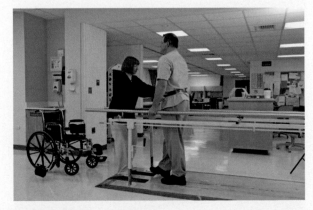

FIGURE 11-34 The patient begins walking toward the clinician while the clinician moves back slowly.

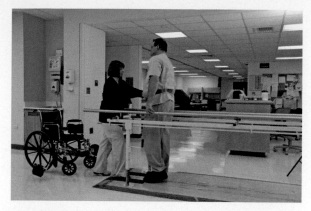

FIGURE 11-35 The patient continues to maintain good posture.

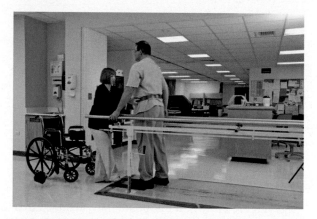

FIGURE 11-36 The patient adjusts his arm positions as he approaches the end of the parallel bars.

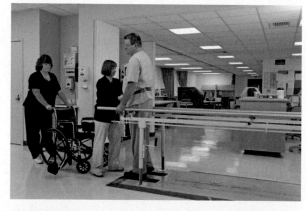

FIGURE 11-37 Patient reaches the end of the parallel bars.

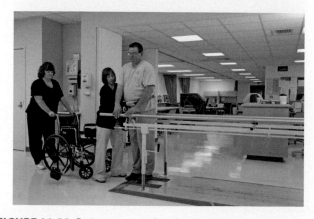

FIGURE 11-38 Patient turns within the parallel bars.

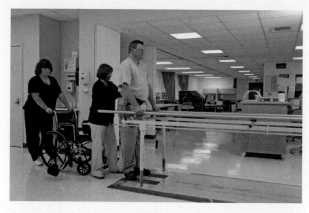

FIGURE 11-39 Patient completes turn within the parallel bars.

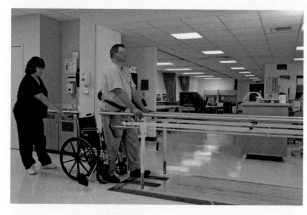

FIGURE 11-40 Patient backs up until he can feel the seat of the wheelchair against the back of his legs.

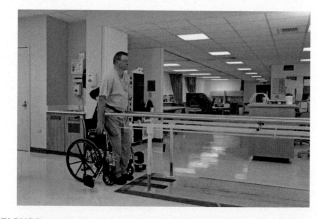

FIGURE 11-41 Patient reaches back with hands.

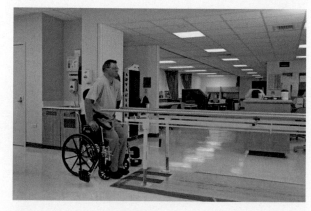

FIGURE 11-42 Patient slowly begins to take his weight through his arms.

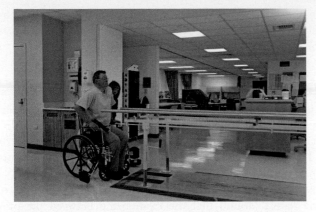

FIGURE 11-43 Patient slowly lowers himself into the chair.

the clinician repetitively asks how the patient is feeling, especially when the patient has changed position or has turned.

▶ The clinician prepares the patient to stand up in the wheelchair by emphasizing the importance of moving forward in the chair, leaning forward, and pushing up with the arms.

▶ When the patient is turning, he always has at least one hand in contact with a bar (**Figures 11-44** through **11-47**).

▶ The clinician asks for assistance in positioning the wheelchair, thus avoiding having to leave the patient unattended.

▶ The patient is instructed to lower himself or herself slowly into the chair, thereby reducing the chance of the chair sliding away or the patient injuring himself or herself.

Although parallel bars are frequently used for weight-shifting exercises and gait training, patients can also perform exercises within them. These can be strengthening exercises, such as performing a push-up using the bars, or balance and

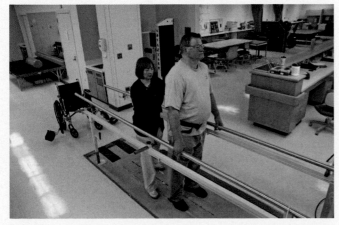

FIGURE 11-44 Detailed view of patient turning to show both hands on the parallel bars.

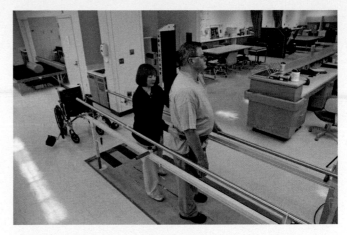

FIGURE 11-45 Detailed view of patient turning to show the release of one hand from the parallel bar.

coordination exercises that reduce the patient's BOS. The goal is to progress the patient out of the bars as quickly as possible to increase overall mobility and decrease dependence on the parallel bars. In consultation with the supervising PT, the time to progress a patient from the parallel bars can be determined by verifying that the patient can transfer from sit to stand, weight shift, and ambulate the bars' length without using the bars for stability.

WEIGHT-BEARING STATUS

The proper gait pattern to instruct the patient depends on the plan of care, which is determined by the PT's assessment of the patient's balance, strength, cardiovascular status, coordination, functional needs, and WB status. One of the major reasons for using an assistive device is that a physician/surgeon has imposed a WB restriction. This restriction is listed in the patient's medical record or, in the case of a patient visiting an outpatient facility, a prescription. Other considerations include the patient's current physical and mental status and where and when to use the assistive device.

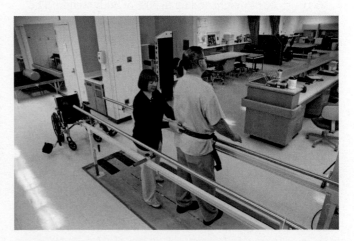

FIGURE 11-46 Detailed view of patient turning to show the one hand moving toward the same parallel bar as the other hand.

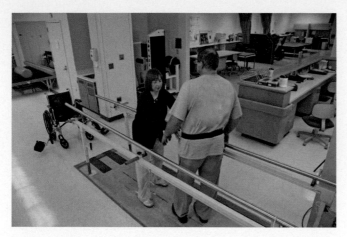

FIGURE 11-47 Detailed view of patient turning to show one hand on the parallel bar with the other hand moving toward the other parallel bar.

CLINICAL PEARL

It is important to remember that changes in WB status occur as the patient progresses but that these changes can only occur with the physician's permission.

Four terms are commonly used to describe the various types of WB restrictions:

▶ *Non–weight bearing (NWB):* The patient is not permitted to bear any weight through the involved limb (VIDEO 11-2). Even though the patient is not bearing weight through the limb, several internal forces are at work. These include stretching of the soft tissues around the joint and joint compression forces. Ironically, it has been reported that forces acting on the hip may be greater during NWB gait than they are during ambulation with touchdown WB.[76]

▶ *Touchdown weight bearing (TDWB)/toe-touch weight bearing (TTWB):* The patient is permitted minimal contact of the injured limb with the ground for balance. Of the four terms, this one causes the most confusion because of the various definitions. For example, the APTA defines it as a contact for balance purposes only, but it is also defined as 10–15 kg of weight and up to 20% of body weight. The most commonly used expression to help the patient understand is, "Imagine as though you are walking on eggshells."

▶ *Partial weight bearing (PWB):* The patient is permitted to bear a portion of their weight through the injured limb. This portion is typically described as a percentage (25%, 50%, etc). However, it is important to remember that 25% of body weight for a person weighing 150 pounds and 25% of body weight for a person who weighs 350 pounds are significantly different.

▶ *Weight bearing as tolerated (WBAT):* The patient is permitted to bear as much weight through the involved limb as can be moderately tolerated.

Despite the preceding definitions, the clinician must consider several variables when determining the actual amount of WB occurring. For example, the amount of force exerted on the joint varies depending on the gait cycle phase as each joint in the lower extremity undergoes different forces throughout the cycle.

Monitoring Weight-Bearing Status

Although the NWB and the WBAT WB restrictions are relatively straightforward to describe to a patient, it is more difficult for the clinician to describe the PWB and the TDWB/TTWB to the patient. It is also difficult for many patients to perceive their WB during ambulation based on verbal instructions or objective measurement of their WB. Indeed, one report[77] found that the relationship between the prescribed WB and the actual weight bearing performed by healthy volunteers or patients with recent lower extremity injury or surgery varied significantly. In fact, another study[78] that used physicians, nurses, physical therapists, and occupational therapists as subjects found that the subjects exceeded the PWB limit by 4–13 kg.

Perhaps the most commonly used clinical method to demonstrate WB to a patient is to use two simple bathroom scales. The patient is asked to place each foot on two separate bathroom scales and then shift the body weight from the involved extremity until the designated amount is reached. This exercise is repeated several times until the patient develops a better sense of what the restriction feels like. However, it is one thing to weight shift in a controlled and static environment; it is another to control their WB during the more dynamic task of ambulation.

Limb load monitors (LLMs), which are relatively inexpensive, have been used to monitor WB status during gait dynamically. The patient wears a lightweight boot over the involved extremity foot, fitted with a strain gauge built into the boot's sole (Figure 11-48).[79-81] During ambulation, the patient is provided with an auditory feedback signal when the WB limits are reached or exceeded.

More recently, computer technology has been used to monitor WB during gait. The computerized air-insole auditory biofeedback system (CAIBS) is a portable system that senses the amount of load and provides auditory feedback in addition to using a wireless receiver connected to a computer. The CAIBS is a valid and reliable system,[82] and has also been shown to increase compliance in subjects with WB restrictions during gait compared to those provided only with verbal instructions.[83]

ASSISTIVE DEVICES

Assistive devices are designed to make ambulation as safe and as painless as possible. In essence, an assistive device is an extension of the upper extremity, used to provide support, balance, and WB that is normally provided by an intact functioning lower extremity.[84] Assistive devices function to reduce ground reaction forces, with the BOS size that they provide proportional to the reduction in these forces. The indications for using an assistive device include[85]:

▶ Decreased ability to bear weight through the lower extremities

▶ Muscle weakness or paralysis of the trunk or lower extremities

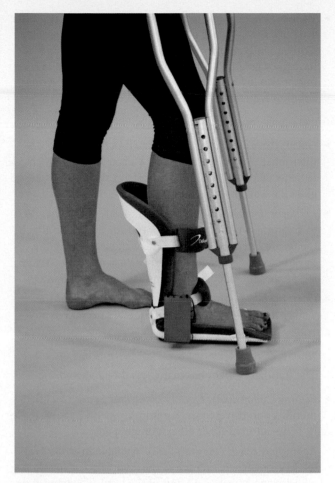

FIGURE 11-48 Limb-load monitor.

- Structural deformity, amputation, injury, or disease resulting in decreased ability to bear weight through a lower extremity
- Decreased balance and proprioception in the upright posture
- Decreased sensation
- Limited passive range of motion
- Joint instability and excessive skeletal loading
- Fatigue or pain
- Fear of falling or history of falling

Choosing a Device

In addition to the WB restriction, the clinician must consider several factors when determining the most suitable assistive device for a patient. These factors include:

- *Amount of support required.* This is a factor of the WB restriction (Table 11-1). The only assistive devices that allow a person to put their full weight through both arms simultaneously are parallel bars, walkers (standard, wheeled, or folding), and bilateral crutches (axillary, or forearm [Lofstrand]), so these devices would be appropriate for a patient with an NWB, TTWB/TDWB, PWB (depending on the percentage allowed), or WBAT

TABLE 11-1	Appropriate Device Based on Weight-Bearing Restriction	
Weight-Bearing Restriction	**Appropriate Device**
Non–weight bearing (NWB)	Parallel bars Walker Bilateral crutches
Partial weight bearing (PWB)	Parallel bars Walker Axillary crutches (one or two) Cane (one or two) Lofstrand crutches

(depending on the level of pain) restriction in one lower extremity. Devices such as hemi-walkers (Figure 11-49) and canes are more suitable for patients with a WBAT restriction.

CLINICAL PEARL

An NWB, TTWB, and PWB restriction limit an assistive device's selection to either a walker or bilateral crutches.

A WBAT restriction allows for any unilateral or bilateral device that provides the necessary support.

- *Amount of stability required.* Generally speaking, the more mobility a device provides, the less stability it provides, and vice versa. Any device with a large BOS, such as a

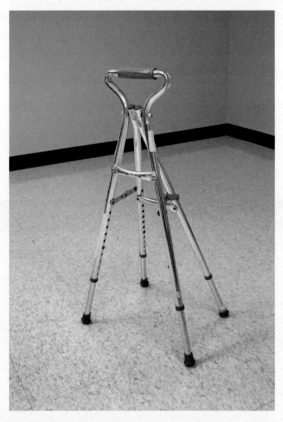

FIGURE 11-49 A hemi-walker.

321

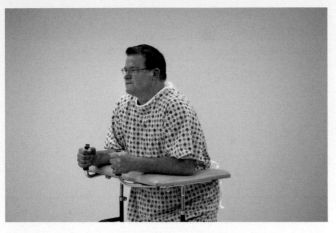

FIGURE 11-50 Modified walker with platform attachment.

standard walker or a platform-style walker (Figure 11-50) with four points of contact will provide the most stability. In order of the stability they provide, assistive devices include parallel bars, platform-style walker, standard walker, bilateral axillary crutches, bilateral forearm crutches, bilateral canes, hemi-walker, quad cane, straight cane, and bent cane.

▶ *Patient strength.* Any assistive devices that use a handgrip require that the patient have good strength in the wrist stabilizers, elbow extensors, and shoulder depressors.

▶ *Patient endurance.* It is worth remembering the energy cost associated with using various assistive devices (Table 11-2).

▶ *Patient coordination.* The list of assistive devices, ordered from those requiring the least coordination by a patient to those requiring the most, is as follows: parallel bars, platform-style walker, one cane, two canes, axillary crutches, forearm (Lofstrand) crutches.

Description of Devices

▶ *Parallel bars.* Parallel bars (see Pre-Ambulation Equipment) provide the greatest stability of any assistive device but the least functional carryover.

TABLE 11-2	Energy Costs Associated with Various Assistive Devices
Assistive Device	**Energy Cost**
Crutches	Energy demand increased 13–80%, in part because of increased demands placed on arms and shoulder-girdle muscles
Standard walker	Oxygen consumption increased >200%
Front-wheeled walker	Lesser impact compared with a standard walker
Cane	No significant energy cost

Reproduced with permission from Placzek JD, Boyce DA: *Orthopaedic Physical Therapy Secrets.* Philadelphia, PA: Hanley & Belfus; 2001.

▶ *Walkers.* Walkers can be used with all WB levels and offer a significant BOS and good anterior and lateral stability. Consequently, walkers are often used with patients who have poor balance and coordination or decreased WB on one or two lower extremities, and they are also the most commonly prescribed assistive device for the elderly.

Attachments include:

▶ *Glides:* these are small, plastic attachments that replace the rubber tips on the bottom of walker legs, which enable patients who cannot lift and advance a standard walker to glide the walker on a smooth surface.

▶ *Platform (forearm) attachments:* these are used when WB through the wrist or hand is contraindicated. The attachments are fitted to the side of the walker, allowing the forearm to rest in a padded trough, held in place with Velcro straps, and include handle grips with a vertical handle.

▶ *Carrying basket:* these are attached to the front of the walker to provide storage for frequently needed items.

▶ *Fold-down seats:* as the name suggests, these attachments allow a patient to sit down using the walker.

The standard walker has many variations, including:

▶ *Folding (collapsible) (Figures 11-51 and 11-52):* facilitate mobility and travel in the community as they are easier to fit in an automobile or other storage space.

▶ *Rolling (wheeled) (Figure 11-53):* available in either two wheels (one wheel on each of the front legs) or four wheels (one wheel on all four of the legs). The latter type requires a hand brake to provide added stability in stopping, which means that the patient must have sufficient grip strength. The rolling walker's advantage is that it requires less energy to use and facilitates walking as a continuous movement sequence. The disadvantage of this type of walker is that it provides less stability.

▶ *Posterior (reverse):* these have the crossbar positioned behind the patient rather than in front of the patient. This type of walker is often used by children who have cerebral palsy to promote a more upright posture.

▶ *Stair climbing:* fitted with two posterior extensions and additional handgrips off the rear legs for use on stairs.

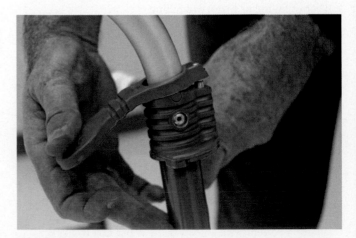

FIGURE 11-51 Folding mechanism on a walker.

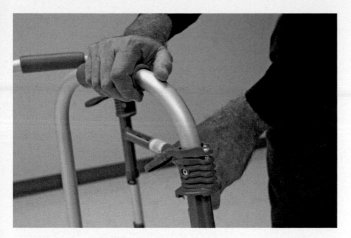

FIGURE 11-52 A folded walker.

▶ *Reciprocal:* fitted with hinges that allow advancement of one side of the walker at a time, thereby facilitating a reciprocal gait pattern.

▶ *Hemi:* this type of walker (see Figure 11-49), sometimes referred to as a walk-cane, is a unilateral assistive device with four legs modified for use with one hand only. It is used when more stability is needed than a single-point or quad cane, but only one upper extremity can be used.

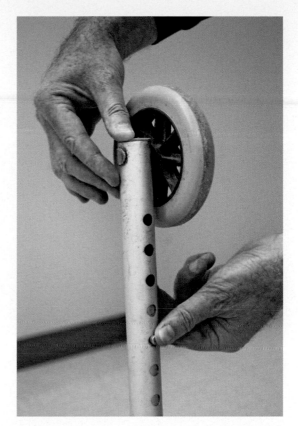

FIGURE 11-53 The wheel of a walker with adjustable height.

CLINICAL PEARL

Common problems to look out for during gait training with a walker include:

▶ The patient ambulates with an excessively flexed posture. This could indicate that either the assistive device is too short or the patient is subconsciously lowering the COG to improve balance.

▶ The patient looks down instead of ahead. This could indicate that the assistive device is too short or the patient is relying too heavily on visual input rather than proprioceptive input.

▶ Subjective complaints of pain and numbness of the hand. This could indicate that the patient is leaning too heavily on the walker.

▶ Excessive gripping. The most common cause for this is a fear of falling.

▶ The patient rocks the walker. This occurs when the patient makes initial contact with only the walker's rear two legs instead of simultaneously placing all four legs down on the floor.

▶ *Axillary crutches.* Axillary crutches (regular or standard), typically used bilaterally, are made from wood or aluminum and are prescribed for patients who need to partially or fully decrease WB on one of the lower extremities. Axillary crutches provide an increased BOS and a moderate degree of lateral stability, and they can be used with all levels of WB. They can also be used for stair climbing. However, crutches are less stable and require more upper extremity strength, some trunk support, and a higher level

of coordination than walkers; are awkward in small areas; and can cause pressure at the radial groove (spiral groove) of the humerus, creating a situation of potential damage to the radial nerve as well as to adjacent vascular structures in the axilla.[86]

CLINICAL PEARL

Crutch palsy, a radial nerve neuropathy, can result from poorly fitted axillary crutches or if the patient rests on the crutch's axillary bars.

▶ *Lofstrand (forearm or Canadian) crutches.* This type of crutch, which is generally constructed of aluminum, can be used at all levels of WB, provide increased ease of movement, and allow the wearer to use the hands because of a forearm cuff without dropping the crutches. Also, the absence of an axillary portion of the crutch allows for more stair-climbing options. However, this type of crutch is slightly more difficult to use than standard crutches, requires good trunk strength, and requires the greatest coordination for proper use.

▶ *Straight canes.* Canes are usually made out of wood, plastic, or aluminum (adjustable with a pushpin lock—Figure 11-54). Using a straight cane to aid walking is perhaps as old as the history of humankind. In ancient times, straight canes were used for support, defense, and the procurement of food.[87] Later, canes became a symbol of power and aristocracy.[88] Currently, straight canes are

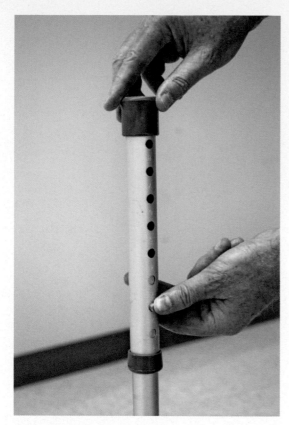

FIGURE 11-54 Adjustable cane.

prescribed for patients with slight weakness of the lower extremity/extremities to provide support and protection, reduce pain in the lower extremities, and improve balance during ambulation.[89] The function of a straight cane is to widen the BOS and improve balance. However, because straight canes provide minimal stability and support for patients during ambulation activities, they are not intended for use with restricted WB gaits.

CLINICAL PEARL

Patients are typically instructed to hold a straight cane in the hand opposite the involved extremity. The cane and involved extremity are advanced together, followed by the uninvolved extremity. The use of a cane in the contralateral hand helps preserve reciprocal motion and a more normal pathway for the COG.[90] Use of a cane in this fashion also helps in reducing forces created by the abductor muscles acting at the hip, as estimated by external kinematics and kinetics.[91-94] Use of a cane can transmit 20–25% of body weight away from the lower extremities.[95,96] Holding the cane in the hand opposite the involved extremity also widens the BOS with less lateral shifting of the COG.

In addition to the straight cane, canes come in a variety of designs:

► *Quad cane:* This type of cane provides a very broad base with four points of floor contact. The legs farther from the patient's body are angled to maintain floor contact and

to improve stability. Walk canes fold flat and are adjustable in height. However, this cane cannot be used on most stairs and requires a slower speed of ambulation.

► *Rolling cane:* provides a wide wheeled base allowing uninterrupted forward progression. A pressure-sensitive brake is built into the handle and can be engaged using pressure from the base of the hand. This cane allows weight to be continuously applied because the need to lift and place the cane forward is eliminated, allowing for a faster progression.

CLINICAL PEARL

Weight limits on standard walkers, canes, and crutches are approximately 300 pounds. Special bariatric gait devices can support 500 pounds or more.

The PTA must appreciate when a patient is ready to progress to a less restrictive device to provide timely feedback for the supervising PT. This decision is based on several factors, including noted objective improvements, whether the current assistive device meets all of the patient's needs, and whether any progression would present safety concerns.

Fitting the Device

Correct fitting of an assistive device is important to ensure patient safety, maintain good posture, and allow for minimal energy expenditure. For the correct fitting, the patient is positioned in a bilateral support stance, wearing the footwear that he or she will typically wear for ambulation, with the toes slightly out, the ankle in neutral, the knee in neutral extension, and the hip in neutral extension. The upper extremity should be positioned so that the elbows and the shoulders are relaxed and level.

CLINICAL PEARL

The bony landmark in the lower extremities used for the correct fitting of an assistive device is the greater trochanter.
The bony landmark in the upper extremities used for the correct fitting of an assistive device is the ulnar styloid.

Once fitted, the patient should be taught the correct walking technique with the device. The fitting depends on the device chosen:

► *Walkers, hemi-walkers, quad canes, and standard canes.* The device handle's height should be adjusted to the greater trochanter level of the patient's hip or the upper extremity's ulnar styloid (Figures 11-55 and 11-56). If measuring for a standard cane, the cane tip should be approximately 3–4 inches anterior to the foot at a 45° angle.

► *Standard crutches.* Several methods can be used for determining the correct crutch length for axillary crutches:

  ■ Ask for a patient's height and then adjust according to the height markings on the crutch.

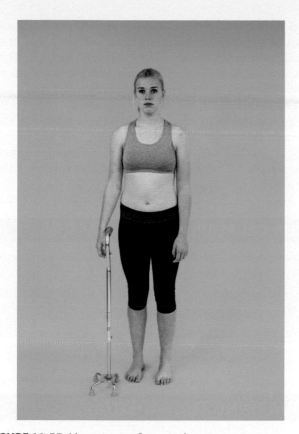

FIGURE 11-55 Measurement for a quad cane.

- Calculate 77% of the patient's height.
- Subtract 16 inches from an adult patient's height.
- Measure from the patient's axillary fold to a point 6–8 inches lateral to the heel's bottom (including footwear).
- Have the patient stand or sit with both arms abducted to 90°. Ask the patient to flex one of the elbows to 90°. The measurement is then taken from the olecranon process of the patient's flexed elbow to the tip of the long finger of the opposite hand (Figure 11-57).
- When the crutches are fitted correctly, there is a 5–8-cm (2–3-inch) gap between the tops of the axillary pads and the patient's axilla (Figure 11-58) when the crutch tip is vertical to the ground and positioned approximately 5 cm (2 inches) lateral to and 15 cm (6 inches) at a 45° angle anterior to the patient's foot. The crutch's handgrips are adjusted to the height of the greater trochanter of the patient's hip or at the ulnar styloid of the upper extremity with the elbow flexed 20–30°.

CLINICAL PEARL

Bauer and colleagues[97] found that the best calculation of ideal crutch length was either 77% of the patient's height or the height minus 40.6 cm (16 inches). The proximal stability of axillary crutches comes from the placement of the axillary bar against the rib cage.

▶ **Forearm/Lofstrand crutches.** The crutch is adjusted so that the handgrip is level with the greater trochanter of the patient's hip and the top of the forearm cuff just distal to the elbow.

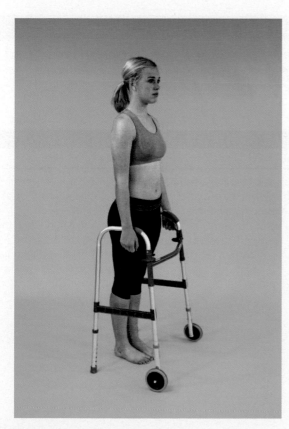

FIGURE 11-56 Measurement for a walker.

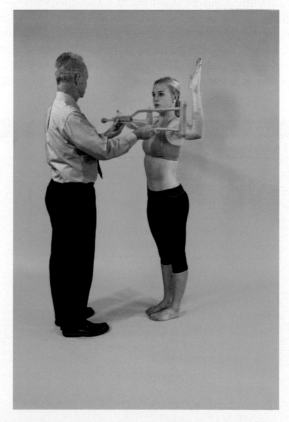

FIGURE 11-57 Measurement for crutches.

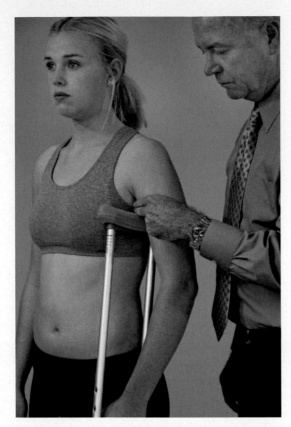

FIGURE 11-58 Ensuring sufficient space in the axilla.

PATIENT INSTRUCTIONS

When providing gait training, it is important that the patient receives verbal and illustrated instructions. Patient instruction should initially be provided in a safe environment free from distraction so that the patient can concentrate. Ideally, the clinician should demonstrate how to use the assistive device before asking the patient to do so. The patient should be encouraged to look ahead rather than down to help with proprioceptive training. The training should be initiated on level surfaces and then advanced to include the negotiation of curbs and stairs, ambulating in busy corridors, and sit-to-stand/stand-to-sit transfers from different surfaces. These instructions should also include any WB precautions pertinent to the patient, the appropriate gait sequence, and a contact number to reach the clinician if questions arise. Finally, the patient should be educated on creating a safe home environment to prevent falls and the device's care and maintenance (replacing rubber tips as needed, tightening any loose fasteners, etc.). The more common methods to prevent falling are outlined in Table 11-3.

CLINICAL PEARL

Patient education and instruction should involve problem-solving. For example:

▶ Getting in and out of a chair that has no armrests

▶ Negotiating stairs that have no railings

Feedback about performance is an extremely important component of skill learning.

GUARDING THE PATIENT

The clinician must always provide adequate physical support and instruction while working with a patient using an assistive gait device. Guarding is the process of protecting a patient from excessive WB, incorrect gait pattern, loss of balance, or falling. Proper guarding requires using a gait belt fitted around the patient's waist to enable the clinician to assist the patient.

CLINICAL PEARL

The most effective way for a clinician to guard a patient is to maintain central control, which involves keeping hand placement close to the patient's COG.

TABLE 11-3	Preventing Falls in the Home		
All Living Spaces		**Bathrooms**	**Outdoors**
_____ Remove throw rugs.		_____ Install grab bars in the bathtub or shower and by the toilet.	_____ Repair cracked sidewalks.
_____ Secure carpet edges.			_____ Install handrails on stairs and steps.
_____ Remove low furniture and objects on the floor.		_____ Use rubber mats in the bathtub or shower.	_____ Trim shrubbery along the pathway to the home.
_____ Reduce clutter.		_____ Take up floor mats when the bathtub or shower is not in use.	_____ Install adequate lighting by doorways and along walkways leading to doors.
_____ Remove cords and wires on the floor.			
_____ Check lighting for adequate illumination at night (especially in the pathway to the bathroom). This can include changing the wattage of a bulb.		_____ Install a raised toilet seat.	
_____ Secure carpet or treads on stairs.			
_____ Install handrail or additional handrail on staircases.			
_____ Eliminate chairs that are too low to sit in and get out of easily.			
_____ Avoid floor wax (or use nonskid wax).			
_____ Ensure that the telephone can be reached from the floor.			
_____ Have medications reviewed by an appropriate healthcare professional.			
_____ Have regular vision examinations by an appropriate healthcare professional.			

When guarding a patient during gait training, the clinician should be positioned with feet astride at a 45° angle slightly to the side and behind the patient. The key is to minimize the distance between the patient's COG and the clinician's COG. Normally, the clinician positions himself or herself slightly posteriorly on the side where the patient will most likely have difficulty. Most frequently, this is the patient's involved side, although in some cases, the patient may tend to fall toward the uninvolved side. If using a gait belt, the clinician should grasp it using a supinated forearm position with the palm facing the ceiling, as this provides a stronger and more reliable grip than using a pronated forearm. A common mistake for the novice clinician is to overguard the patient. This typically includes holding the patient back by pulling too hard on the gait belt or at the patient's shoulder (VIDEO 11-3). This is very frustrating for the patient and can introduce several safety concerns, as it can cause the patient to lose his or her balance.

CLINICAL PEARL

Two types of falls are recognized:
- *Angular:* occurs when the COG moves too far beyond the BOS in any direction for the patient to control.
- *Collapsing:* occurs when there is a loss of support from either the patient's lower extremities or an assistive device.

Whatever side is chosen, if the patient falls forward, backward, or to either side, the aim is to return the combined COG of the patient and the clinician within the BOS of the clinician, with only a shift of the clinician's weight and with no large foot movements by the clinician. Thus, the clinician's BOS must be large enough to support such shifts in the COG should the patient start to fall. The closer the clinician is to the patient, the easier this is to maintain. Although falls typically occur in one direction, the clinician must remember that sometimes the patient's lower extremities can give way, resulting in a collapsing fall. In such instances, the clinician should move closer to the patient and lift on the gait belt to provide time for the patient to regain support.

CLINICAL PEARL

As the COG of most patients is in the lower trunk, the best way to control a patient and thereby prevent a fall is through a gait belt placed around the patient's hip girdle. Because the gait belt is typically fitted when the patient is sitting, the clinician should recheck the belt after the patient stands up to ensure that it still fits snugly.

To prevent any unencumbered weight shifting or foot movement in the event of a fall, the clinician's knee should be slightly bent, and the feet should not be crossed during gait training, nor should they become entangled with the patient's feet or ambulatory equipment. Hand placement is also important. The clinician should try to keep the upper extremity that is holding the gait belt such that the forearm is horizontal to the level of the patient's COG, with the other hand, if necessary, on the superior anterior aspect of the patient's shoulder.

CLINICAL PEARL

If a patient starts to fall, the clinician must decide whether to maintain the patient in an upright position or permit a controlled descent. Either the clinician can adopt a stride stance so that the patient can temporarily rest on the clinician's thigh (VIDEO 11-4), or the clinician can help guide the patient to the floor in a manner that will prevent injury to the patient and the clinician (VIDEO 11-5). The latter option involves keeping the patient's body close to the clinician while maintaining good body mechanics.

FALLING

Although every effort is made to prevent a patient from falling while they are in the clinic, it is not uncommon for a patient to fall outside of the clinic, whether at home or in the community, even if they have been provided with instructions on prevention. Most falls occur when a patient is using axillary crutches. The clinician can help train the patient to fall safely with crutches by practicing on a cushioned surface placed on the floor and slowing down the fall's motion in the initial stages by using a gait belt. The clinician can also help train the patient to get up from the floor following a fall using the crutches.

Falling Safely

As the patient starts to fall, he or she casts the crutches to the side, far enough out of the way to prevent landing on them but near enough for the patient to reach them to rise back to a standing position. The patient attempts to break the fall by landing on the palms with the elbows flexed while simultaneously turning the head to one side to minimize the risk of facial injury.

Getting Up from the Floor

The easiest way for a patient to get up from the floor is to crawl to a nearby chair or another sturdy object and use it to pull up to a sitting or standing position. If no such object is available, the patient collects both crutches and moves into a quadruped position. From there, the patient moves into a tall kneeling position and stands both crutches on the involved side, holding both handgrips with one hand. The patient then moves into a partial kneeling position with the stronger lower extremity forward and then pushes down through the handgrips and the forward leg to achieve a standing position. Once standing, the patient repositions the crutches, with one crutch under each arm.

GAIT TRAINING WITH ASSISTIVE DEVICES

A patient must wear adequate footwear for gait training. At a minimum, the patient should receive gait training to use the assistive gait device on level surfaces and, as appropriate, to negotiate stairs, curbs, ramps, doors, and transfers.

Gait training includes:

► An observation of any abnormality or deviation of a patient's gait noted in the plan of care (POC)

► Teaching the patient how to establish a normal gait pattern

► Gait training in various environments (different surfaces, different lighting, etc)

Gait training with assistive devices can begin in the parallel bars, as they provide maximum stability while requiring the least amount of coordination from the patient. The correct height of the assistive device can also be measured while the patient stands within the bars (see Pre-Ambulation Equipment). However, the need for parallel bars is very much patient-dependent. For example, more active patients with good coordination are unlikely to need parallel bars.

Sit-to-Stand Transfers

When observing a patient moving from a sitting position to a standing position, the clinician should note the biomechanics challenges behind such a move. If the patient remains seated at the back of the wheelchair, the COG remains outside of the BOS created by the feet. If the patient slides forward in the wheelchair, the COG is brought within the BOS. As the patient assumes a standing position, some forces must be overcome:

► Gravity is attempting to force the knees into flexion.

► Gravity is attempting to force the ankles into dorsiflexion.

If the patient does not have sufficient strength, some incorrect compensations can occur (see Clinical Pearl). The correct technique involves asking the patient to lean the trunk over the knees, which ultimately creates an extensor moment at the knee.

Before the patient can begin gait training, they must first learn to transfer from a sitting position to a standing position safely. The following procedure is recommended.

► The bed or wheelchair wheels are locked, and the patient is reminded of any WB restrictions.

► The patient is asked to slide to the front edge of the chair or bed, and the WB foot is placed underneath the body, with the knees flexed to approximately 110° and the

ankles in slight dorsiflexion, so that the COG is closer to the BOS, which will make it easier for the patient to stand. The other lower extremity is positioned appropriately (usually with the knee extended) depending on the WB status and whether a brace has immobilized it.

► The patient is then instructed to lean forward from the hips, which brings the patient's COG over the BOS, and to push up with the hands from the bed or armrests of the wheelchair and extend the elbows while simultaneously extending the legs and standing erect.

► If the patient is being instructed on using a walker, they should grasp the walker's handgrips only after becoming upright (VIDEO 11-6). The patient should not be permitted to pull up to a standing position using the walker (VIDEO 11-7) because this can cause the walker to tip over and increase the potential for falls (VIDEO 11-8).

► If the patient uses crutches, they are instructed to hold both crutches with the hand on the same side as the involved lower extremity (VIDEO 11-9). The patient then presses down on the crutches' handgrips, armrest, bed, and uninvolved lower extremity to stand. Once standing and with adequate balance, the patient moves the crutches into position and begins to ambulate (VIDEO 11-10).

► If the patient uses one or two canes, they are instructed to push up with the hands from the bed or armrests (VIDEO 11-11). Once standing, the patient should grasp the handgrip(s) of the cane(s) with the appropriate hand and begin to ambulate (VIDEO 11-12).

► A hemi-walker can be used similarly to one cane (VIDEO 11-13), but it can also be used for a specific purpose (VIDEO 11-14).

Video Description

Notice how the clinician in Videos 11-10 through 11-14 coaches the patient in the following manner:

► To move forward in the chair

► To place the feet slightly apart and under the chair

► To lean the trunk forward

► To place the hands on the armrests in a manner that allows the patient to push downward

Notice also how the clinician positions herself in the following manner:

► Standing close to the patient to provide sufficient stabilization and assistance

► Flexing the trunk so that she is leaning slightly toward the patient

Note also how the clinician continues to interact with the patient. This includes providing explanations and instructions but also inquiring as to how the patient feels. Repeated cueing is an important component of training—for example, reminding the patient to feel the edge of the seat at the back of both legs before sitting and reminding the patient to lower himself slowly and gently into the chair.

Several compensations can occur as the patient attempts to stand upright. These include:

- Pressing the knees together or bracing the lower legs against the chair to create leverage
- Rocking backward and forward to gain momentum
- Increased use of arm strength to push the body up from the chair

As these are all abnormal movement patterns, the clinician must determine the cause. The most common causes are a weakness of the lower extremities and poor trunk flexion.

Stand-to-Sit Transfer

The stand-to-sit transfer is essentially the reverse of the sit-to-stand transfer. Normally, to return to the chair or bed, the patient has to turn 180°. To enhance safety, the patient should be encouraged to turn using multiple small steps, as these provide increased stability because double contact time is at its highest. Before the patient sits, the clinician must ensure that the bed or wheelchair is locked. To sit down using an assistive device, the patient must first back up against the edge of the bed or chair to touch the back of their legs. Suppose the patient has WB restrictions of the involved lower extremity or cannot flex the knee. In that case, he or she is instructed to advance this lower extremity forward slowly. Once in position:

- The patient using a walker, reaches for the bed or armrest with both hands, flexes the trunk forward, and slowly sits down.
- The patient using crutches, moves both crutches to the hand on the side of the involved lower extremity. With that hand holding onto both handgrips of the crutches, the patient reaches back for the bed or armrest with the other hand and flexes the trunk forward before slowly sitting down.
- The patient, using one or two canes, places the handgrip of the cane(s) against the edge of the chair or bed. Next, the patient reaches back for the bed or armrest and slowly sits down.

Turning

Making changes in direction can prove challenging for many patients. Common findings include hesitancy, decreased speed, multiple steps, and multiple stops during the turn. Generally speaking, it is easier for the patient to turn toward the stronger side than the weaker side. This is also important for patients who have undergone a posterolateral approach to hip arthroplasty to minimize the risk of internal rotation of the involved hip and lower extremity.

Gait Patterns

Several gait patterns are recognized, the most common of which are described here.

Two-Point Pattern

The two-point gait pattern, which closely approximates the normal gait pattern (VIDEO 11-15), requires the use of an assistive gait device (canes or crutches) on each side of the body. This pattern requires the patient to move the assistive gait device and the contralateral lower extremity simultaneously. This pattern requires coordination and balance. The uninvolved lower extremity can be advanced to a point where it is parallel to the involved lower extremity (VIDEO 11-16), or it can be advanced ahead of the uninvolved lower extremity.

Two-Point Modified

The two-point modified pattern is the same as the two-point, except that it requires only one assistive device, positioned on the opposite side of the involved lower extremity. This pattern cannot be used if there are any WB restrictions such as PWB or NWB, but it is appropriate for a patient with unilateral weakness or mild balance deficits. The patient is instructed to move the cane and the involved leg simultaneously, and then the uninvolved leg.

Three-Point Gait Pattern

This pattern is used for non-WB—when the patient is permitted to bear weight through only one lower extremity. The three-point gait pattern, which demands a high degree of energy from the patient, involves using two crutches or a walker (VIDEO 11-17). It cannot be used with a cane or one crutch. The three-point gait pattern requires good upper body strength, good balance, and good cardiovascular endurance. The pattern is initiated with the forward movement of the assistive gait device. Next, the involved lower extremity is advanced. The patient then presses down on the assistive gait device and advances the uninvolved lower extremity. Two methods of advancing the lower extremity can be used:

- *Swing to:* the uninvolved lower extremity is advanced to a point where it is parallel to the involved lower extremity (see VIDEO 11-17).
- *Swing through:* the involved lower extremity is advanced ahead of the uninvolved lower extremity.

Three-Point Modified or 3 Point 1

A modification of the three-point gait pattern requires two crutches or a walker. This pattern is more stable, slower, and requires less strength and energy than the three-point gait pattern. This pattern is used when the patient can bear full weight through one lower extremity, but it only allows PWB through the involved lower extremity. Only part of the patient's weight is allowed to be transferred through the involved lower extremity in partial WB. It must be remembered that most patients have difficulty replicating a prescribed WB restriction and will need constant reinforcement.[103]

The pattern is initiated with the forward movement of one of the assistive gait devices, and then the involved lower extremity is advanced. The patient presses down on the assistive gait device and advances the uninvolved lower extremity, using either a *swing-to* or a *swing-through* pattern described for the three-point pattern.

Four-Point Pattern

The four-point gait pattern, which requires an assistive gait device (canes or crutches) on each side of the body, is used when the patient has compromised balance and stability. This pattern provides a slow gait speed but requires a low amount of energy to perform. The pattern is initiated with the forward movement of one of the assistive gait devices, then the contralateral lower extremity, then the other assistive gait device, and finally the opposite lower extremity (eg, right crutch, then left foot; left crutch, then right foot; VIDEO 11-18).

Four-Point Modified

The four-point modified pattern is the same as the four-point, except that it requires only one assistive device, positioned on the side opposite the involved lower extremity. This pattern cannot be used if there are any WB restrictions such as PWB or NWB, but it is appropriate for a patient with unilateral weakness or mild balance deficits. The patient is instructed to move the cane, then the involved leg, and then the uninvolved leg (VIDEO 11-19).

Stair Negotiation

Stair negotiation brings its own set of challenges. In addition to being more strenuous than walking on a level surface, stair negotiation has more potential risks and requires more coordination and balance by the patient. The three rules to remember for stair negotiation are:

1. "Up with the good and down with the bad." This means that the patient leads with the uninvolved (good) extremity when ascending (VIDEO 11-20) but leads with the involved (bad) extremity when descending (VIDEO 11-21). There appears to be controversy about using value-laden terms such as *good* and *bad* when referring to a patient's injury. Some prefer to use the phrase "good people go to heaven, and bad people go to hell." Whichever phrase is used, it must be easy to remember for the patient.

2. The assistive device remains with the involved extremity. This means that if the assistive device is used to support a weak or unstable lower extremity, it remains with and moves with the involved lower extremity.

3. The clinician always guards the patient from below. This means that the clinician should stand between the patient and the direction toward which the patient is most likely to fall. Thus, the clinician stands behind a patient who is ascending the stairs but in front of a patient descending the stairs. As with gait training on the level, a gait belt should be used, and the clinician should maintain a wide BOS and control the patient's movement centrally through the patient's pelvis and shoulder girdles. Maintaining a wide BOS on the stairs involves the clinician avoiding having both feet on one step simultaneously.

Ascending Stairs

To ascend steps, the patient must first move to the front edge of the step.

- To ascend stairs using a standard walker, the walker will have to be turned toward the opposite side of the handrail or wall. Ascending more than two to three stairs with a standard walker is not recommended. The patient is instructed to grasp the stair handrail with one hand and turn the walker sideways to place the walker's two front legs on the first step. When ready, the patient pushes down on the walker handgrip and the handrail and advances the uninvolved lower extremity onto the first step. The patient then advances the uninvolved lower extremity to the first step and moves the walker's legs to the next step. This process is repeated as the patient moves up the steps.

CLINICAL PEARL

Walkers that are specifically designed for stair negotiation exist but are not common.

- To ascend steps or stairs with crutches, the patient should grasp the stair handrail with one hand and grasp both crutches by the handgrips with the other hand (see VIDEO 11-20). If the patient cannot grasp both crutches with one hand, or if the handrail is not stable or available, then the patient should use both crutches only, although this is not recommended if there are more than two to three steps. When in the correct position at the front edge of the step, the patient pushes down on the crutches and handrail, if applicable, and advances the uninvolved lower extremity to the first step. The patient then advances the involved lower extremity, and finally, the crutches. This process is repeated for the remaining steps.

- To ascend steps or stairs with one or two canes, the patient should use the handrail and the cane(s). If the handrail is not stable or available, the patient should only use the cane(s). The patient pushes down on the cane(s) or handrail, as applicable, and advances the uninvolved lower extremity to the first step. The patient then advances the involved lower extremity. This process is repeated for the remaining steps.

Descending Stairs

To descend steps, the patient must first move to the front edge of the top step.

- To descend stairs using a walker, the walker is turned sideways so that the walker's two front legs are placed on the lower step. Descending more than two to three stairs with a walker is not recommended. One hand is placed on the rear handgrip, and the other hand grasps the stair handrail. When ready, the patient lowers the involved lower extremity down to the first step. Then the patient pushes down on the walker and handrail and advances the uninvolved lower extremity down the first step. This process is repeated as the patient moves down the steps.

- To descend steps or stairs with crutches, the patient should use one hand to grasp the stair handrail and the other to grasp both crutches and handrail (see VIDEO 11-21).

If the patient cannot grasp both crutches with one hand, or if the handrail is not stable, then the patient should use both crutches only, although this is not recommended if there are more than two to three steps. When ready, the patient lowers the involved lower extremity down to the first step. Next, the patient pushes down on the crutches and handrail, if applicable, and advances the uninvolved lower extremity down to the first step. This process is repeated for the remaining steps.

▶ To descend steps or stairs with one or two canes, the patient should use the cane(s) and handrail. If the handrail is not stable, then the patient should use the cane(s) only. When ready, the patient lowers the involved lower extremity down to the first step. Next, the patient pushes down on the cane(s) and handrail, if applicable, and advances the uninvolved lower extremity down to the first step. This process is repeated for the remaining steps.

CLINICAL PEARL

Several studies[104-106] have looked at the required degrees of range of motion for stair negotiation at the various lower extremity joints. These approximate ranges are:

Hip flexion: 7–65° for ascending; 15–40° for descending

Knee flexion: 8–94° for ascending; 10–92° for descending

Ankle dorsiflexion: 11–14° for ascending; 20–34° for descending

Ankle plantarflexion: 20–31° for ascending; 22–40° for descending

Opening Doors

Most doors open in one of two directions—inward or outward.

Door Opens Outward Toward the Patient

The patient is instructed to stand close to the door, turned slightly to face the door opening (VIDEO 11-22). Using the hand closest to the hinges, the patient pulls the door open and then shifts the hand to the inside of the door to give the door a push, opening it wider. The patient then uses his or her prescribed gait pattern to walk through the doorway, being careful to avoid the closing door hitting the assistive device's tip. Alternatively, if the patient is using bilateral axillary crutches, he or she can place the tip of the crutch that is closer to the door in the path of the door so that the door rests against the crutch tip.

Door Opens Inward Away from the Patient

The patient is instructed to stand close to the door, face the door handle, and then open and push the door with the hand nearest the door (see VIDEO 11-22). The patient then walks through the doorway using his or her prescribed gait pattern. Alternatively, suppose the patient is using bilateral axillary crutches. In that case, the patient can turn sideways, facing away from the hinges, and then push against the door with the hip so that when the door opens, the patient positions the crutch tip against the bottom edge of the door to prevent it from closing.

Video Description

Note the differences in techniques between VIDEO 11-22 and VIDEO 11-23. When the door opens toward the patient, there is a high potential for the door to hit the assistive device or obstruct the assistive device if the door is not opened wide enough. When the door opens away from the patient, there is no problem with the door hitting or obstructing the assistive device. However, the problem arises if the patient has to close the door after passing through because the assistive device can obstruct the door from closing. Try to determine some strategies that you would provide to the patient to counteract these problems.

Inclines

Several adaptations need to be made when ambulating up and down on an incline.[107,108] The patient should be instructed to:

▶ Take slightly longer steps when ascending moderate inclines, and take slightly shorter steps when descending inclines

▶ Lean forward when ascending

Different Surfaces

Depending on the treatment environment, sit-to-stand and stand-to-sit transfers can present some challenges. Whereas transferring to and from a relatively hard surface provides a high degree of stability for the patient, transferring to and from a soft surface is more difficult. This difficulty results from the patient being unsure of how the push-off surface is going to react. This is best illustrated by viewing VIDEO 11-24.

Bodyweight-Supported Treadmill

A bodyweight-supported treadmill (BWST) is a device used in various physical therapy practice settings, including schools, outpatient clinics, and inpatient rehabilitation settings. BWSTs, which provide varying levels of support, vary in cost and setup, and run the gamut from manually assisted treadmills to robotically controlled devices that guide the patient's legs while supporting their weight to produce a more normal walking pattern. A BWST works by partially suspending the patient in a harness either from the ceiling or from an apparatus frame. The amount of suspension force can be adjusted according to patient need. The advantage of this type of device is that it allows the clinician to focus on the patient's gait without being concerned about patient safety. It also provides reassurance to a patient who may have a fear of falling. However, the harness's proper fitting is critical to avoid discomfort, particularly with those requiring higher suspension force levels. To date, despite the obvious advantages of safety and support, it remains unclear how beneficial these devices are in improving gait function. It is already known that walking on a treadmill versus the ground alters certain gait parameters, including gait speed and stride length, both of which can be manipulated and controlled by a treadmill.

Also, quite how a BWST device alters spatiotemporal input, and such parameters as the duration of stance and double-limb support remains elusive.

REFERENCES

1. Rose J. Dynamic lower extremity stability. In: Hughes C, ed. *Movement Disorders and Neuromuscular Interventions for the Trunk and Extremities—Independent Study Course 1825*. La Crosse, WI: Orthopaedic Section, APTA, Inc.; 2008:1-34.

2. Lovejoy CO. Evolution of human walking. *Sci Am*. 1988;259:118-125.

3. Korr IM, Wright HM, Thomas PE. Effects of experimental myofascial insults on cutaneous patterns of sympathetic activity in man. *J Neural Transm*. 1962;23:330-355.

4. Simons DG, Travell JG, Simons SL. *Myofascial Pain and Dysfunction—The Trigger Point Manual*, 2nd ed. Philadelphia: Lippincott Williams & Wilkins; 1998.

5. Beal MC. The short leg problem. *JAOA*. 1977;76:745-751.

6. Das P, McCollum G. Invariant structure in locomotion. *Neuroscience*. 1988;25:1023-1034.

7. Mann RA, Hagy JL, White V, Liddell D. The initiation of gait. *J Bone and Joint Surg*. 1979;61A:232-239.

8. Luttgens K, Hamilton N. Locomotion: Solid surface. In: Luttgens K, Hamilton N, eds. *Kinesiology: Scientific Basis of Human Motion*, 9th ed. Dubuque, IA: McGraw-Hill; 1997:519-549.

9. Dobkin BH, Harkema S, Requejo P, Edgerton VR. Modulation of locomotor-like EMG activity in subjects with complete and incomplete spinal cord injury. *J Neurol Rehabil*. 1995;9:183-190.

10. Donatelli R, Wilkes R. Lower kinetic chain and human gait. *J Back Musculoskel Rehabil*. 1992;2:1-11.

11. Levine D, Whittle M. *Gait Analysis: The Lower Extremities*. La Crosse, WI: Orthopaedic Section, APTA, Inc.; 1992.

12. Mann RA, Hagy J. Biomechanics of walking, running, and sprinting. *Am J Sports Med*. 1980;8:345-350.

13. Murray MP. Gait as a total pattern of movement. *Am J Phys Med*. 1967;46:290.

14. Luttgens K, Hamilton N. The center of gravity and stability. In: Luttgens K, Hamilton N, eds. *Kinesiology: Scientific Basis of Human Motion*. 9th ed. Dubuque, IA: McGraw-Hill; 1997:415-442.

15. Epler M. Gait. In: Richardson JK, Iglarsh ZA, eds. *Clinical Orthopaedic Physical Therapy*. Philadelphia: WB Saunders; 1994:602-625.

16. Subotnick SI. Variations in angles of gait in running. *Phys Sportsmed*. 1979;7:110-114.

17. Perry J. Stride Analysis. In: Perry J, ed. *Gait Analysis: Normal and Pathological Function*. Thorofare, NJ: Slack, Inc.; 1992:431-441.

18. Ostrosky KM, Van Sweringen JM, Burdett RG, Gee Z. A comparison of gait characteristics in young and old subjects. *Phys Ther*. 1994;74:637-646.

19. Adelaar RS. The practical biomechanics of running. *Am J Sports Med*. 1986;14:497-500.

20. Basmajian JV. *Therapeutic Exercise*, 3rd ed. Baltimore: Williams & Wilkins; 1979.

21. Perry J. Gait Analysis: *Normal and Pathological Function*. Thorofare, NJ: Slack, Inc.; 1992.

22. Rogers MM. Dynamic foot mechanics. *J Orthop Sports Phys Ther*. 1995;21:306-316.

23. Gage JR, Deluca PA, Renshaw TS. Gait analysis: Principles and applications with emphasis on its use with cerebral palsy. *Inst Course Lect*. 1996;45:491-507.

24. Frey C. Foot health and shoewear for women. *Clin Orthop Relat Res*. 2000;372:32-44.

25. Oberg T, Karsznia A, Oberg K. Basic gait parameters: reference data for normal subjects, 10-79 years of age. *J Rehab Res Dev*. 1993;30:210-223.

26. Molen NH, Rozendal RH, Boon W. Fundamental characteristics of human gait in relation to sex and location. *Proc K Ned Akad Wet C*. 1972;45:215-223.

27. Finley FR, Cody KA. Locomotive characteristics of urban pedestrians. *Arch Phys Med Rehabil*. 1970;51:423-426.

28. Sato H, Ishizu K. Gait patterns of Japanese pedestrians. *J Hum Ergol (Tokyo)*. 1990;19:13-22.

29. Richard R, Weber J, Mejjad O, et al. Spatiotemporal gait parameters measured using the Bessou gait analyzer in 79 healthy subjects: Influence of age, stature, and gender. *Rev Rhum Engl Ed*. 1995;62:105-114.

30. Murray MP, Kory RC, Sepic SB. Walking patterns of normal women. *Arch Phys Med Rehabil*. 1970;51:637-650.

31. Murray MP, Drought AB, Kory RC. Walking patterns of normal men. *J Bone Joint Surg Am*. 1964;46A:335-360.

32. Bhambhani Y, Singh M. Metabolic and cinematographic analysis of walking and running in men and women. *Med Sci Sports Exerc*. 1985;17:131-137.

33. Giannini S, Catani F, Benedetti MG, Leardini A. Terminology, parameterization and normalization in gait analysis. *Gait Analysis: Methodologies and Clinical Applications*. Washington, DC: IOS Press; 1994:65-88.

34. Perry J. The hip. Gait Analysis: Normal and Pathological Function. Thorofare, NJ: Slack, Inc.; 1992:111-129.

35. Reinking MF. Knee anatomy and biomechanics. In: Wadsworth C, ed. *Disorders of the Knee—Home Study Course*. La Crosse, WI: Orthpaedic Section, APTA, Inc.; 2001.

36. Norkin C, Levangie P. *Joint Structure and Function: A Comprehensive Analysis*. Philadelphia: F.A. Davis Company; 1992.

37. Kuster MS, Wood GA, Stachowiak GW, Gachter A. Joint load considerations in total knee replacement. *J Bone and Joint Surg*. 1997;79B:109-113.

38. Andriacchi TP, Ogle JA, Galante JO. Walking speed as a basis for normal and abnormal gait measurements. *J Biomech*. 1977;10:261-268.

39. Corrigan J, Moore D, Stephens M. The effect of heel height on forefoot loading. *Foot Ankle*. 1991;11:418-422.

40. Arsenault AB, Winter DA, Marteniuk RG. Is there a "normal" profile of EMG activity in gait? *Med Biol Eng Comput*. 1986;24:337-343.

41. Berchuck M, Andriacchi TP, Bach BR, Reider B. Gait adaptations by patients who have a deficient anterior cruciate ligament. *J Bone Joint Surg*. 1990;72-A:871-877.

42. Boeing DD. Evaluation of a clinical method of gait analysis. *Phys Ther*. 1977;57:795-798.

43. Dillon P, Updyke W, Allen W. Gait analysis with reference to chondromalacia patellae. *J Orthop Sports Phys Ther*. 1983;5:127-131.

44. Hunt GC, Brocato RS. Gait and foot pathomechanics. In: Hunt GC, ed. *Physical Therapy of the Foot and Ankle*. Edinburgh: Churchill Livingstone; 1988:39-57.

45. Krebs DE, Robbins CE, Lavine L, Mann RW. Hip biomechanics during gait. *J Orthop Sports Phys Ther*. 1998;28:51-59.

46. Luttgens K, Hamilton N. The Standing Posture. In: Luttgens K, Hamilton N, eds. *Kinesiology: Scientific Basis of Human Motion*. 9th ed. Dubuque, IA: McGraw-Hill; 1997:445-459.

47. Winter DA. Biomechanical motor patterns in normal walking. *J Motor Behav*. 1983;15:302-329.

48. Hoyt DF, Taylor CF. Gait and the energetics of locomotion in horses. *Nature*. 1981;292:239-240.

49. Corcoran PJ, Brengelmann G. Oxygen uptake in normal and handicapped subjects in relation to the speed of walking beside a velocity-controlled cart. *Arch Phys Med Rehabil*. 1970;51:78-87.

50. Gonzalez EG, Corcoran PJ, Reyes RL. Energy expenditure in below-knee amputees: correlation with stump length. *Arch Phys Med Rehabil*. 1974;55:111-119.

51. Waters RL, Hislop HJ, Perry J, Antonelli D. Energetics: application to the study and management of locomotor disabilities. *Orthop Clin North Am*. 1978;9:351-377.

52. Martin PE, Rothstein DE, Larish DD. Effects of age and physical activity status on the speed-aerobic demand relationship of walking. *J Appl Physiol*. 1992;73:200-206.

53. Prampero PE. The energy cost of human locomotion on land and in the water. *Int J Sports Med*. 1986;7:55-72.

54. Davies MJ, Dalsky GP. Economy of mobility in older adults. *J Orthop Sports Phys Ther*. 1997;26:69-72.

55. Daniels J, Krahenbuhl G, Foster C, Gilbert J, Daniels S. Aerobic responses of female distance runners to submaximal and maximal exercise. *Ann N Y Acad Sci*. 1977;301:726-733.

56. Pate RR, Barnes CG, Miller CA. A physiological comparison of performance-matched female and male distance runners. *Res Q Exerc Sport*. 1985;56:245-250.

57. Wells CL, Hecht LH, Krahenbuhl GS. Physical characteristics and oxygen utilization of male and female marathon runners. *Res Q Exerc Sport*. 1981;52:281-285.

58. Bransford DR, Howley ET. Oxygen cost of running in trained and untrained men and women. *Med Sci Sports Exerc*. 1977;9:41-44.

59. Daniels J, Daniels N. Running economy of elite male and females runners. *Med Sci Sports Exerc*. 1992;24:483-489.

60. Howley ET, Glover ME. The caloric costs of running and walking one mile for men and women. *Med Sci Sports Exerc*. 1974;6:235-237.

61. Larish DD, Martin PE, Mungiole M. Characteristic patterns of gait in the healthy old. *Ann N Y Acad Sciences*. 1987;515:18-32.

62. Waters RL, Hislop HJ, Perry J, Thomas L, Campbell J. Comparative cost of walking in young and old adults. *J Orthop Res*. 1983;1:73-76.

63. Allen W, Seals DR, Hurley BF, Ehsani AA, Hagberg JM. Lactate threshold and distance running performance in young and older endurance athletes. *J Appl Physiol*. 1985;58:1281-1284.

64. Trappe SW, Costill DL, Vukovich MD, Jones J, Melham T. Aging among elite distance runners: A 22-year longitudinal study. *J Appl Physiol*. 1996;80:285-290.

65. Wells CL, Boorman MA, Riggs DM. Effect of age and menopausal status on cardiorespiratory fitness in masters women runners. *Med Sci Sports Exerc*. 1992;24:1147-1154.

66. Moseley CF. Leg-length discrepancy. In: Morrissy RT, ed. *Lovell and Winter's Pediatric Orthopaedics*, 3rd ed. Philadelphia: J. B. Lippincott; 1990:767-813.

67. Beaty JH. Congenital anomalies of lower extremity. In: Crenshaw AH, ed. *Campbell's Operative Orthopaedics*, 8th ed. St. Louis: Mosby-Year Book; 1992:2126-2158.

68. Gross RH. Leg length discrepancy: How much is too much? *Orthopedics*. 1978;1:307-310.

69. Song KM, Halliday SE, Little DG. The effect of limb-length discrepancy on gait. *J Bone Joint Surg Am*. 1997;79A:1690-1698.

70. Lange GW, Hintermeister RA, Schlegel T, Dillman CJ, Steadman JR. Electromyographic and kinematic analysis of graded treadmill walking and the implications for knee rehabilitation. *J Orthop Sports Phys Ther*. 1996;23:294-301.

71. Croskey MI, Dawson PM, Luessen AC, et al. The height of the center of gravity in man. *Am J Physiol*. 1922;61:171-185.

72. Saunders JBD, Inman VT, Eberhart HD. The major determinants in normal and pathological gait. *J Bone Joint Surg Am*. 1953;35:543-558.

73. Whitehouse PA, Knight LA, Di Nicolantonio F, Mercer SJ, Sharma S, Cree IA. Heterogeneity of chemosensitivity of colorectal adenocarcinoma determined by a modified ex vivo ATP-tumor chemosensitivity assay (ATP-TCA). *Anticancer Drugs*. 2003;14:369-375.

74. Perry J. Gait Cycle. In: Perry J, ed. *Gait Analysis: Normal and Pathological Function*. Thorofare, NJ: Slack Inc; 1992:3-7.

75. Bobath K, Bobath B. The facilitation of normal postural reactions and movements in the treatment of cerebral palsy. *Physiotherapy*. 1964;50:246-262.

76. Givens-Heiss DL, Krebs DE, Riley PO, Strickland EM, Fares M, Hodge WA, et al. In vivo acetabular contact pressures during rehabilitation, Part II: Postacute phase. *Phys Ther*. 1992;72:700-705; discussion 6-10.

77. Dabke HV, Gupta SK, Holt CA, O'Callaghan P, Dent CM. How accurate is partial weightbearing? *Clin Orthop Relat Res*. 2004:282-286.

78. Sutton P, Stedman J, Livesley P. Perception and education of unilateral weightbearing amongst health care professionals. *Injury*. 2007;38:163-164.

79. Miyazaki S, Ishida A, Iwakura H, Takino K, Ohkawa T, Tsubakimoto H, et al. Portable limb-load monitor utilizing a thin capacitive transducer. *J Biomed Eng*. 1986;8:67-71.

80. Gapsis JJ, Grabois M, Borrell RM, Menken SA, Kelly M. Limb load monitor: evaluation of a sensory feedback device for controlled weight bearing. *Arch Phys Med Rehabil*. 1982;63:38-41.

81. Wannstedt G, Craik RL. Clinical evaluation of a sensory feedback device: the limb load monitor. *Bull Prosthet Res*. 1978:8-49.

82. Isakov E. Gait rehabilitation: a new biofeedback device for monitoring and enhancing weight-bearing over the affected lower limb. *Eura Medicophys*. 2007;43:21-26.

83. Hershko E, Tauber C, Carmeli E. Biofeedback versus physiotherapy in patients with partial weight-bearing. *Am J Orthop*. 2008;37:E92-E96.

84. Hoberman M. Crutch and cane exercises and use. In: Basmajian JV, ed. *Therapeutic Exercise*, 3rd ed. Baltimore: Williams & Wilkins; 1979:228-255.

85. Duesterhaus MA, Duesterhaus S. *Patient Care Skills*, 2nd ed. East Norwalk, Connecticut: Appleton and Lange; 1990.

86. Schmitz TJ. Locomotor training. In: O'Sullivan SB, Schmitz TJ, eds. *Physical Rehabilitation*, 5th ed. Philadelphia: FA Davis; 2007:523-560.

87. Lyu SR, Ogata K, Hoshiko I. Effects of a cane on floor reaction force and center of force during gait. *Clin Orthop Relat Res*. 2000;375:313-319.

88. Blount WP. Don't throw away the cane. *J Bone Joint Surg*. 1956;38A:695-708.

89. Joyce BM, Kirby RL. Canes, crutches and walkers. *Am Fam Phys*. 1991;43:535-542.

90. Baxter ML, Allington RO, Koepke GH. Weight-distribution variables in the use of crutches and canes. *Phys Ther*. 1969;49:360-365.

91. Edwards BG. Contralateral and ipsilateral cane usage by patients with total knee or hip replacement. *Arch Phys Med Rehabil*. 1986;67:734-740.

92. Oatis CA. Biomechanics of the hip. In: Echternach J, ed. *Clinics in Physical Therapy: Physical Therapy of the Hip*. New York: Churchill Livingstone; 1990:37-50.

93. Olsson EC, Smidt GL. Assistive devices. In: Smidt G, ed. *Gait in Rehabilitation*. New York: Churchill Livingstone; 1990:141-155.

94. Vargo MM, Robinson LR, Nicholas JJ. Contralateral vs. ipsilateral cane use: Effects on muscles crossing the knee joint. *Am J Phys Med Rehabil*. 1992;71:170-176.

95. Jebsen RH. Use and abuse of ambulation aids. *JAMA*. 1967;199:5-10.

96. Kumar R, Roe MC, Scremin OU. Methods for estimating the proper length of a cane. *Arch Phys Med Rehabil*. 1995;76:1173-1175.

97. Bauer DM, Finch DC, McGough KP, et al. A comparative analysis of several crutch-length-estimation techniques. *Phys Ther*. 1991;71:294-300.

98. Barbur JL, Konstantakopoulou E. Changes in color vision with decreasing light level: Separating the effects of normal aging from disease. *J Opt Soc Am A Opt Image Sci Vis*. 2012;29:A27-A35.

99. Owsley C. Aging and vision. *Vision Res*. 2011;51:1610-1622.

100. Smith SC. Aging and vision. *Insight*. 2008;33:16-20; quiz 1-2.

101. Wood JM. Aging, driving and vision. *Clin Exp Optom*. 2002;85:214-220.

102. Kline DW, Kline TJ, Fozard JL, Kosnik W, Schieber F, Sekuler R. Vision, aging, and driving: The problems of older drivers. *J Gerontol*. 1992;47:P27-P34.

103. Li S, Armstrong CW, Cipriani D. Three-point gait crutch walking: variability in ground reaction force during weight bearing. *Arch Phys Med Rehabil*. 2001:86-92.

104. Reeves ND, Spanjaard M, Mohagheghi AA, Baltzopoulos V, Maganaris CN. The demands of stair descent relative to maximum capacities in elderly and young adults. *J Electromyogr Kinesiol*. 2008;18:218-227.

105. Protopapadaki A, Drechsler WI, Cramp MC, Coutts FJ, Scott OM. Hip, knee, ankle kinematics and kinetics during stair ascent and descent in healthy young individuals. *Clin Biomech*. 2007;22:203-210.

106. Powers CM, Perry J, Hsu A, Hislop HJ. Are patellofemoral pain and quadriceps femoris muscle torque associated with locomotor function? *Phys Ther*. 1997;77:1063-1075; discussion 75-78.

107. Leroux A, Fung J, Barbeau H. Postural adaptation to walking on inclined surfaces: I. Normal strategies. *Gait Posture*. 2002;15:64-74.

108. McIntosh AS, Beatty KT, Dwan LN, Vickers DR. Gait dynamics on an inclined walkway. *J Biomech*. 2006;39:2491-2502.

Putting It All Together

CHAPTER 12

CHAPTER OBJECTIVES

At the completion of this chapter, the reader will be able to:

1. Understand the various components of an initial examination document

2. Be able to recognize the most important information from the medical record

3. Recognize various common abbreviations

4. Use a structured thought process to assimilate information from a typical medical record

5. Appreciate that most patients present with more than one diagnosis

6. Formulate an approach for the first visit with a patient

OVERVIEW

A physical therapist assistant (PTA) must be able to transfer classroom knowledge to the clinic. Part of that ability involves interpreting the supervising physical therapist's documentation and then putting that interpretation into action. The electronic health record (EHR) of a patient with multiple diagnoses is used as an example, as are standard abbreviations (Table 4-1). Various pointers are provided throughout the document to give insight into the thought processes and methods used by a physical therapist (PT) as they complete their initial examination and to emphasize that the PTA should accumulate insights throughout the document review.

The patient used in this example is an 85-year-old female admitted to an acute care hospital with chronic obstructive pulmonary disease (COPD) and congestive heart failure (CHF). It is extremely uncommon in the acute care setting to find a patient with a single diagnosis, and most will have several comorbidities, each of which can impact their treatment.

PATIENT HISTORY			
Name:	Gladys Night	**Precautions:**	Monitor SpO₂ with ADLs
Admission diagnosis:	COPD (J 44.9) CHF (I50.9)	**Weight-bearing Status:**	WBAT
Date of admission:	Mar 16, 2021	**BMI:**	31 (slightly obese)
Date of birth:	Feb 21, 1936	**Living Situation:**	Lives alone in bungalow
Age:	85	**Prior Level of Function:**	IND
Sex:	F	**Assistance Available at Home:**	Very limited, but the neighbor checks in every day. Son and daughter live in different states
Medical Record #:	555-45213	**Physical barriers at home:**	Lives on one level. 2 steps to get into the house
Attending Physician:	Dr. G. Altman	**Assistive Device Used Before Admission:**	FWW
Room #/Bed #:	403/2	**Prior Driving Status:**	Unable to drive
Isolation:	N/AP	**Primary Language:**	English
Medication Allergies:	Penicillin	**Occupation/Life role:**	Home keeper
Food Allergies:	NKA	**Demographics:**	Widow for 20 years. Regular churchgoer. Very social
Diagnostic Test Results:	CXR reveals hyperinflation	**Laboratory Results:**	pH 3.75; PaCO₂ 39 mm Hg; FiO₂ 0.21; BUN 10, creatinine 0.4

Current medications: Albuterol nebulizer (PRN), theophylline (400 mg PO once daily), Lasix (50 mg PO once daily), bisoprolol (5 mg PO once daily)

Pertinent information for the PTA: The PTA needs to focus on any information that is going to impact a physical therapy intervention (weight-bearing status, prior level of function, the assistive device used before admission), and try to determine whether any of the medications, or the laboratory or diagnostic test results could impact any increase in the patient's activity level. In reality, the physician would not have ordered PT if the patient wasn't stable enough, and the nursing staff would be aware of any subsequent change in the patient's status. However, the patient has been prescribed bisoprolol, which is a beta-blocker. Beta-blockers work by lowering the heart rate and blood pressure. It is worth spending some time making a notecard that has all of the normal laboratory values. The diagnostic and laboratory test results are typical for this patient type, but her cardiovascular status indicates that she will need her vital signs and oxygen saturation levels monitored frequently. The patient's weight-bearing status, BMI, prior level of function, and the assistive device (FWW) also provide useful information. So, even at this early stage in the document, the PTA has a fairly good idea of the patient's status.

Pertinent Past Medical History:	Significant for COPD, CHF, bilateral knee replacements (15 years ago), and chronic LB pain. Admitted for increasing SOB and A. fib. Currently prescribed 2 L of supplemental oxygen via nasal cannula. SpO₂ at 86% on admittance. No family history of COPD/CHF. Smoked for 70 years but recently quit.
Observation:	Slightly obese female with evidence of peripheral edema in the lower extremities. Pt ambulates with FWW and waddling gait.
Subjective:	*Chief complaint*: Pt reports increasing levels of fatigue with activity, orthopnea, and nocturnal dyspnea *Pain* Pt reports minor chest discomfort, LB pain, and generalized stiffness of B knees. Pain level for LB assessed with a VAS Resting level/scale: 4/10 Location: Across the LB at the beltline level Characteristic: Dull ache Medication: Ibuprofen 200 mg PRN Post-activity: 6/10 *Patient's Goals* To increase activity level without losing breath To decrease SOB when lying down and when sleeping

(continued)

PATIENT HISTORY (continued)

Pertinent information for the PTA: More information has been added that requires consideration, particularly the impact that activity has on the patient and the fact that the patient does not tolerate lying down very well. The waddling gait pattern suggests a degree of instability, as does the need for a FFW. It should also be clear that the patient is in some degree of pain and that the knees' generalized stiffness may impact function.

SYSTEMS REVIEW

Vision:	20/80 as per chart	**Resting O$_2$ Saturation:**	95% on 2 LPM supp O$_2$
Speech:	Intact	**Blood pressure:**	132/85
Hearing:	Moderately severe as per chart	**Alertness:**	Alert/focussed
Heart Rate at Rest (bpm)	100	**Orientation:**	x4
Respiratory Rate (breaths/min):	25	**Short-term Memory:**	Intact

Changes to vital signs post-activity: Pt amb 30 feet. SpO2 90% on 2 LPM supp O$_2$; HR 115; RR 34; BP 140/90

Pertinent information for the PTA: It should be clear that the patient has a low exercise tolerance. The clinician must also be aware that the prescribed bisoprolol maintains the heart rate within a specific range.

TESTS AND MEASURES

ROM:	WNL for age x̄ b/l knees. Rt—110 flex/-8 ext; Lt—115 flex/-5 ext	**Sitting Balance/Tolerance:**	Balance good at EOB. Altered vital signs initially but stabilized within one minute. Able to sit for 10-minute limit as per test
Strength:	4/5 for major groups	**Standing Balance:**	Fair
Bed Mobility:	IND but slow	**Gait:**	Timed gait: CGA 30 ft c̄ FWW and SOB – 90 secs
Supine to Sit to Supine:	Elevated HOB	**Wheelchair Mobility:**	IND for use in room
Sit to Stand to Sit:	CGA	**Stair negotiation**	Not assessed

Pertinent information for the PTA: Given the previous information, some of the findings in the tests and measures reinforce the patient's poor tolerance for activity and the need for supervision with gait. The elevated HOB should emphasize the precaution of not allowing the patient to lie down flat. The clinician should also note that although the patient can perform bed mobility, she requires more time than normal.

EVALUATION

Diagnosis:	Cardiovascular/pulmonary, pattern C
Prognosis:	Pt IND before admission. Pt remains IND with bed mobility but requires CGA c̄ simple transfers. Sitting balance is G, but standing balance is F, and gait requires CGA. Pt is capable of ambulating short distances but has low energy levels and fluctuating vital signs. Pt has good potential to meet goals but may require short-term SNF placement depending on LOS.

PLAN OF CARE

Discharge Plan:	D/C to home if goals are met. Otherwise SNF placement
Short-term Goals (STG):	At d/c, pt will be able to perform the following: 1. Gait: IND c̄ FWW, 100 ft within 3 mins 2. Transfers: IND with sit-stand-sit 3. Standing balance to be rated at Good

(continued)

PATIENT HISTORY (continued)	
Treatment frequency:	BID
Interventions:	Transfer training Balance training Gait training Therapeutic exercise Therapeutic activities Home program

Pertinent information for the PTA: The physical therapist has listed several functional goals with the interventions to achieve those goals. No specifics are given within the interventions, which will allow the PTA a degree of latitude while remaining within the POC boundaries. Each of the STGs outlines the levels that the patient is expected to reach. For example, the patient's current standing balance is Fair—maintains balance with limited postural sway, no challenges, but with support. The goal is to get the patient to the level of Good—maintains balance with limited postural sway against minimal challenges with no external support. The PTA must try to achieve all of these goals while monitoring the patient carefully for any fluctuations in her vital signs and oxygen saturation levels.

FIRST ENCOUNTER

Having reviewed the patient's medical record and taken notes, the clinician would be well advised to review Table 3-8 and the first two rows of Table 3-9 before meeting the patient for the first time to ensure that all of the necessary information has been gleaned from the medical record and the necessary preparations have occurred. Over time, such a review will not be necessary, as many actions will become second nature as the clinician becomes more confident. Before entering the patient's room, it is well worth taking the time to formulate a plan on the introductions, what to say to the patient about what is planned for the session, and ensuring that all of the necessary equipment is at hand.

As you move through the PTA curriculum, the student will be provided with numerous treatment strategies and techniques to deploy in most clinical situations, and, as experience builds, the correct selection from those strategies and techniques becomes easier. One should always strive to think out of the box and be as creative as possible. For example, although not a documented short-term goal for this patient, the patient expressed a desire to lie down and sleep without shortness of breath. So, would a tilt table help increase the patient's tolerance for supine lying? Unlike the traditional method of using a tilt table where the patient begins the session in the supine position and is slowly raised to a more erect position, perhaps this patient would benefit from beginning in the more erect position and then being slowly lowered while monitoring her vital signs. Although any such intervention would require a discussion with the supervising physical therapist, it should not prevent the PTA from thinking creatively and making suggestions.

After the encounter, the PTA should refer to Table 3-9 for guidance while completing the initial post-visit documentation.

Standards of Ethical Conduct for the Physical Therapist Assistant

APPENDIX A

HOD S06-09-20-18 [Amended HOD S06-00-13-24; HOD 06-91-06-07; Initial HOD 06-82-04-08] [Standard]

PREAMBLE

The *Standards of Ethical Conduct for the Physical Therapist Assistant* (*Standards of Ethical Conduct*) delineate the ethical obligations of all physical therapist assistants as determined by the House of Delegates of the American Physical Therapy Association (APTA). The *Standards of Ethical Conduct* provide a foundation for conduct to which all physical therapist assistants shall adhere. Fundamental to the *Standards of Ethical Conduct* is the special obligation of physical therapist assistants to enable patients/clients to achieve greater independence, health and wellness, and enhanced quality of life.

No document that delineates ethical standards can address every situation. Physical therapist assistants are encouraged to seek additional advice or consultation in instances where the guidance of the *Standards of Ethical Conduct* may not be definitive.

STANDARDS

Standard #1: Physical therapist assistants shall respect the inherent dignity, and rights, of all individuals.

▶ 1A. Physical therapist assistants shall act in a respectful manner toward each person regardless of age, gender, race, nationality, religion, ethnicity, social or economic status, sexual orientation, health condition, or disability.

▶ 1B. Physical therapist assistants shall recognize their personal biases and shall not discriminate against others in the provision of physical therapy services.

Standard #2: Physical therapist assistants shall be trustworthy and compassionate in addressing the rights and needs of patients/clients.

▶ 2A. Physical therapist assistants shall act in the best interests of patients/clients over the interests of the physical therapist assistant.

▶ 2B. Physical therapist assistants shall provide physical therapy interventions with compassionate and caring behaviors that incorporate the individual and cultural differences of patients/clients.

▶ 2C. Physical therapist assistants shall provide patients/clients with information regarding the interventions they provide.

▶ 2D. Physical therapist assistants shall protect confidential patient/client information and, in collaboration with the physical therapist, may disclose confidential information to appropriate authorities only when allowed or as required by law.

Standard #3: Physical therapist assistants shall make sound decisions in collaboration with the physical therapist and within the boundaries established by laws and regulations.

▶ 3A. Physical therapist assistants shall make objective decisions in the patient's/client's best interest in all practice settings.

▶ 3B. Physical therapist assistants shall be guided by information about best practice regarding physical therapy interventions.

▶ 3C. Physical therapist assistants shall make decisions based upon their level of competence and consistent with patient/client values.

▶ 3D. Physical therapist assistants shall not engage in conflicts of interest that interfere with making sound decisions.

▶ 3E. Physical therapist assistants shall provide physical therapy services under the direction and supervision of a physical therapist and shall communicate with the physical therapist when patient/client status requires modifications to the established plan of care.

Standard #4: Physical therapist assistants shall demonstrate integrity in their relationships with patients/clients, families, colleagues, students, other healthcare providers, employers, payers, and the public.

▶ 4A. Physical therapist assistants shall provide truthful, accurate, and relevant information and shall not make misleading representations.

▶ 4B. Physical therapist assistants shall not exploit persons over whom they have supervisory, evaluative, or other authority (eg, patients/clients, students, supervisees, research participants, or employees).

▶ 4C. Physical therapist assistants shall discourage misconduct by health care professionals and report illegal or unethical acts to the relevant authority, when appropriate.

▶ 4D. Physical therapist assistants shall report suspected cases of abuse involving children or vulnerable adults to the supervising physical therapist and the appropriate authority, subject to law.

▶ 4E. Physical therapist assistants shall not engage in any sexual relationship with any of their patients/clients, supervisees, or students.

▶ 4F. Physical therapist assistants shall not harass anyone verbally, physically, emotionally, or sexually.

Standard #5: Physical therapist assistants shall fulfill their legal and ethical obligations.

▶ 5A. Physical therapist assistants shall comply with applicable local, state, and federal laws and regulations.

▶ 5B. Physical therapist assistants shall support the supervisory role of the physical therapist to ensure quality care and promote patient/client safety.

▶ 5C. Physical therapist assistants involved in research shall abide by accepted standards governing protection of research participants.

▶ 5D. Physical therapist assistants shall encourage colleagues with physical, psychological, or substance-related impairments that may adversely impact their professional responsibilities to seek assistance or counsel.

▶ 5E. Physical therapist assistants who have knowledge that a colleague is unable to perform their professional responsibilities with reasonable skill and safety shall report this information to the appropriate authority.

Standard #6: Physical therapist assistants shall enhance their competence through the lifelong acquisition and refinement of knowledge, skills, and abilities.

▶ 6A. Physical therapist assistants shall achieve and maintain clinical competence.

▶ 6B. Physical therapist assistants shall engage in lifelong learning consistent with changes in their roles and responsibilities and advances in the practice of physical therapy.

▶ 6C. Physical therapist assistants shall support practice environments that support career development and life-long learning.

Standard #7: Physical therapist assistants shall support organizational behaviors and business practices that benefit patients/clients and society.

▶ 7A. Physical therapist assistants shall promote work environments that support ethical and accountable decision-making.

▶ 7B. Physical therapist assistants shall not accept gifts or other considerations that influence or give an appearance of influencing their decisions.

▶ 7C. Physical therapist assistants shall fully disclose any financial interest they have in products or services that they recommend to patients/clients.

▶ 7D. Physical therapist assistants shall ensure that documentation for their interventions accurately reflects the nature and extent of the services provided.

▶ 7E. Physical therapist assistants shall refrain from employment arrangements, or other arrangements that prevent physical therapist assistants from fulfilling ethical obligations to patients/clients.

Standard #8: Physical therapist assistants shall participate in efforts to meet the health needs of people locally, nationally, or globally.

▶ 8A. Physical therapist assistants shall support organizations that meet the health needs of people who are economically disadvantaged, uninsured, and underinsured.

▶ 8B. Physical therapist assistants shall advocate for people with impairments, activity limitations, participation restrictions, and disabilities in order to promote their participation in community and society.

▶ 8C. Physical therapist assistants shall be responsible stewards of healthcare resources by collaborating with physical therapists in order to avoid over-utilization or under-utilization of physical therapy services.

▶ 8D. Physical therapist assistants shall educate members of the public about the benefits of physical therapy.

Reprinted from [http://www.apta.org], with permission of the American Physical Therapy Association. © 2021 American Physical Therapy Association. All rights reserved.

DIRECTION AND SUPERVISION OF THE PHYSICAL THERAPIST ASSISTANT HOD P06-18-28-35 [Amended: HOD P06-05-18- 26; HOD 06-00-16-27; HOD 06-99-07-11; HOD 06-96-30-42; HOD 06-95-11-06; HOD 06-93-08-09; HOD 06-85-20-41; Initial: HOD 06-84-16-72/HOD 06-78-22-61/HOD 06-77-19-37] [Position]

Physical therapist practice and the practice of physical therapy are synonymous. Both phrases are inclusive of patient and client management, and direction and supervision. Direction and supervision apply to the physical therapist assistant, who is the only individual who assists a physical therapist in practice. The utilization of other support personnel, whether in the performance of tasks or clerical activities, relates to the efficient operation of the physical therapy service.

Physical therapists are responsible for providing safe, accessible, cost-effective, and evidence-based services. Services are rendered directly by the physical therapist and with responsible utilization of physical therapist assistants. The physical therapist's practice responsibility for patient and client management includes examination, evaluation, diagnosis, prognosis, intervention, and outcomes. Physical therapist assistants may be appropriately utilized in components of intervention and in collection of selected examination and outcomes data.

Direction and supervision are essential in the provision of quality physical therapist services. The degree of direction and supervision necessary for ensuring quality physical therapist services is dependent upon many factors, including the education, experiences, and responsibilities of the parties involved, as well as the organizational structure where physical therapist services are provided.

Regardless of the setting in which the physical therapist service is provided, the following responsibilities must be borne solely by the physical therapist:

1. Interpretation of referrals when available

2. Evaluation, diagnosis, and prognosis

3. Development or modification of a plan of care, which is based on the initial examination or reexamination, and includes the physical therapy goals and outcomes

4. Determination of when the expertise and decision-making capability of the physical therapist requires the physical therapist to personally render services and, when it may be appropriate, to utilize the physical therapist assistant

5. Revision of the plan of care when indicated

6. Conclusion of an episode of care

7. Responsibility for any "hand off" communication

8. Oversight of all documentation for services rendered to each patient or client

Only the physical therapist performs the initial examination and reexamination of the patient and may utilize the physical therapist assistant in collection of selected examination and outcomes data.

The physical therapist is responsible for services provided when the physical therapist's plan of care involves the physical therapist assistant. Regardless of the setting in which the service is provided, the determination to utilize physical therapist assistants requires the education, expertise, and professional judgment of a physical therapist as described by the *Standards of Practice for Physical Therapy*, the *Code of Ethics for the Physical Therapist*, and the *APTA Guide for Professional Conduct*.

In determining the appropriate extent of assistance from the physical therapist assistant, the physical therapist considers:

▶ The physical therapist assistant's education, training, experience, and skill level

▶ Patient or client criticality, acuity, stability, and complexity

▶ The predictability of the consequences

▶ The setting in which the care is being delivered

▶ Federal and state statutes

▶ Liability and risk management concerns

▶ The mission of physical therapist services for the setting

▶ The needed frequency of reexamination

PHYSICAL THERAPIST ASSISTANT

Definition

The physical therapist assistant assists the physical therapist in the provision of physical therapy. The physical therapist assistant is a graduate of a physical therapist assistant program accredited by the Commission on Accreditation in Physical Therapy Education.

Utilization

The physical therapist is directly responsible for the actions of the physical therapist assistant in all practice settings. The physical therapist assistant may provide services under the direction and at least general supervision of the physical therapist. In general supervision, the physical therapist is not required to be on site for direction and supervision but must be available at least by telecommunication. The ability of the physical therapist assistant to provide services shall be assessed on an ongoing basis by the supervising physical therapist.

Services provided by the physical therapist assistant must be consistent with safe and legal physical therapist practice and shall be predicated on the following factors: complexity and acuity of the patient's or client's needs; proximity and accessibility to the physical therapist; supervision available in the event of emergencies or critical events; and type of setting in which the service is provided. The physical therapist assistant makes modifications to elements of the intervention either to progress the patient or client as directed by the physical therapist or to ensure patient or client safety and comfort.

When supervising the physical therapist assistant in any offsite setting, the following requirements must be observed:

1. A physical therapist must be accessible by telecommunication to the physical therapist assistant at all times while the physical therapist assistant is providing services to patients and clients.

2. There must be regularly scheduled and documented conferences with the physical therapist assistant regarding patients and clients, the frequency of which is determined by the needs of the patient or client and the needs of the physical therapist assistant.

3. In situations in which a physical therapist assistant is involved in the care of a patient or client, a supervisory visit by the physical therapist:

   a. Shall be made upon the physical therapist assistant's request for a reexamination, when a change in the plan of care is needed, prior to any planned conclusion of the episode of care, and in response to a change in the patient's or client's medical status

   b. Shall be made at least once a month, or at a higher frequency when established by the physical therapist, in accordance with the needs of the patient or client

   c. Shall include:

      i. An onsite reexamination of the patient or client

      ii. Onsite review of the plan of care with appropriate revision or termination

      iii. Evaluation of need and recommendation for utilization of outside resources

Explanation of Reference Numbers:

HOD P00-00-00-00 stands for House of Delegates/month/year/page/vote in the House of Delegates minutes; the "P" indicates that it is a position (see below). For example, HOD P06-17-05-04 means that this position can be found in the June 2017 House of Delegates minutes on Page 5 and that it was Vote 4.

P: Position | S: Standard | G: Guideline | Y: Policy | R: Procedure

Standards of Practice for Physical Therapy

APPENDIX C

APTA House of Delegates Standard (Last Updated: 10/1/13)

PREAMBLE

The physical therapy profession's commitment to society is to promote optimal health and functioning in individuals by pursuing excellence in practice. The American Physical Therapy Association attests to this commitment by adopting and promoting the following Standards of Practice for Physical Therapy. These Standards are the profession's statement of conditions and performances that are essential for provision of high-quality professional service to society, and provide a foundation for assessment of physical therapist practice.

I. ETHICAL/LEGAL CONSIDERATIONS

A. Ethical Considerations

The physical therapist practices according to the *Code of Ethics* of the American Physical Therapy Association.

The physical therapist assistant complies with the *Standards of Ethical Conduct for the Physical Therapist Assistant* of the American Physical Therapy Association.

B. Legal Considerations

The physical therapist complies with all the legal requirements of jurisdictions regulating the practice of physical therapy.

The physical therapist assistant complies with all the legal requirements of jurisdictions regulating the work of the assistant.

II. ADMINISTRATION OF THE PHYSICAL THERAPY SERVICE

A. Statement of Mission, Purposes, and Goals

The physical therapy service has a statement of mission, purposes, and goals that reflects the needs and interests of the patients/clients served, the physical therapy personnel affiliated with the service, and the community.

B. Organizational Plan

The physical therapy service has a written organizational plan.

C. Policies and Procedures

The physical therapy service has written policies and procedures that reflect the operation, mission, purposes, and goals of the service, and are consistent with the association's standards, policies, positions, guidelines, and *Code of Ethics*.

D. Administration

A physical therapist is responsible for the direction of the physical therapy service.

E. Fiscal Management

The director of the physical therapy service, in consultation with physical therapy staff and appropriate administrative personnel, participates in the planning for and allocation of resources. Fiscal planning and management of the service is based on sound accounting principles.

F. Improvement of Quality of Care and Performance

The physical therapy service has a written plan for continuous improvement of quality of care and performance of services.

G. Staffing

The physical therapy personnel affiliated with the physical therapy service have demonstrated competence and are sufficient to achieve the mission, purposes, and goals of the service.

H. Staff Development

The physical therapy service has a written plan that provides for appropriate and ongoing staff development.

I. Physical Setting

The physical setting is designed to provide a safe and accessible environment that facilitates fulfillment of the mission, purposes, and goals of the physical therapy service.

The equipment is safe and sufficient to achieve the purposes and goals of physical therapy.

J. Collaboration

The physical therapy service collaborates with all disciplines as appropriate.

III. PATIENT/CLIENT MANAGEMENT

A. Physical Therapist of Record

The physical therapist of record is the therapist who assumes responsibility for patient/client management and is accountable for the coordination, continuation, and progression of the plan of care.

B. Patient/Client Collaboration

Within the patient/client management process, the physical therapist and the patient/client establish and maintain an ongoing collaborative process of decision-making that exists throughout the provision of services.

C. Initial Examination/Evaluation/Diagnosis/Prognosis

The physical therapist performs an initial examination and evaluation to establish a diagnosis and prognosis prior to intervention.

D. Plan of Care

The physical therapist establishes a plan of care and manages the needs of the patient/client based on the examination, evaluation, diagnosis, prognosis, goals, and outcomes of the planned interventions for identified impairments, functional limitations, and disabilities.

The physical therapist involves the patient/client and appropriate others in the planning, implementation, and assessment of the plan of care.

E. Intervention

The physical therapist provides or directs and supervises the physical therapy intervention consistent with the results of the examination, evaluation, diagnosis, prognosis, and plan of care. The physical therapy intervention may be provided in an episode of care, or in a single visit/encounter, such as for a wellness and prevention visit/encounter or a specialty consultation or for a follow-up visit/encounter after episodes of care, or may be provided intermittently over longer periods of time in cases of managing chronic conditions.

An *episode of care* is the managed care provided for a specific problem or condition during a set time period and can be given either for a short period or on a continuous basis, or it may consist of a series of intervals marked by one or more brief separations from care.

F. Reexamination

The physical therapist reexamines the patient/client as necessary during an episode of care, during follow-up visits/encounters after an episode of care, or periodically in the case of chronic care management, to evaluate progress or change in patient/client status. The physical therapist modifies the plan of care accordingly or concludes the episode of care.

G. Conclusion of Episode of Care

The physical therapist concludes an episode of care when the anticipated goals or expected outcomes for the patient/client have been achieved, when the patient/client is unable to continue to progress toward goals, or when the physical therapist determines that the patient/client will no longer benefit from physical therapy.

H. Communication/Coordination/Documentation

The physical therapist communicates, coordinates, and documents all aspects of patient/client management, including the results of the initial examination and evaluation, diagnosis, prognosis, plan of care, interventions, responses to interventions, changes in patient/client status relative to the intervention, reexamination, and episode of care summary. The physical therapist of record is responsible for "hand off" communication.

IV. EDUCATION

The physical therapist is responsible for individual professional development. The physical therapist assistant is responsible for individual career development.

The physical therapist and the physical therapist assistant, under the direction and supervision of the physical therapist, participate in the education of students.

The physical therapist educates and provides consultation to consumers and the general public regarding the purposes and benefits of physical therapy.

The physical therapist educates and provides consultation to consumers and the general public regarding the roles of the physical therapist and the physical therapist assistant.

V. RESEARCH

The physical therapist applies research findings to practice and encourages, participates in, and promotes activities that establish the outcomes of patient/client management provided by the physical therapist.

VI. COMMUNITY RESPONSIBILITY

The physical therapist demonstrates community responsibility by participating in community and community agency activities, educating the public, formulating public policy, or providing pro bono physical therapy services.

Criteria for Standards of Practice for Physical Therapy

APPENDIX D

APTA Board of Directors Standard BOD S03-06-16-38

The Standards of Practice for Physical Therapy are promulgated by APTA's House of Delegates; criteria for the standards are promulgated by APTA's Board of Directors. Criteria are italicized beneath the standards to which they apply.

PREAMBLE

The physical therapy profession's commitment to society is to promote optimal health and function in individuals by pursuing excellence in practice. The American Physical Therapy Association attests to this commitment by adopting and promoting the following Standards of Practice for Physical Therapy. These Standards are the profession's statement of conditions and performances that are essential for provision of high-quality professional service to society, and provide a foundation for assessment of physical therapist practice.

I. ETHICAL/LEGAL CONSIDERATIONS

A. Ethical Considerations
The physical therapist practices according to the Code of Ethics of the American Physical Therapy Association.
The physical therapist assistant complies with the *Standards of Ethical Conduct for the Physical Therapist Assistant* of the American Physical Therapy Association.

B. Legal Considerations
The physical therapist complies with all the legal requirements of jurisdictions regulating the practice of physical therapy.
The physical therapist assistant complies with all the legal requirements of jurisdictions regulating the work of the assistant.

II. ADMINISTRATION OF THE PHYSICAL THERAPY SERVICE

A. Statement of Mission, Purposes, and Goals
The physical therapy service has a statement of mission, purposes, and goals that reflects the needs and interests of the patients/clients served, the physical therapy personnel affiliated with the service, and the community.

The statement of mission, purposes, and goals:

▶ *Defines the scope and limitations of the physical therapy service.*

▶ *Identifies the goals and objectives of the service.*

▶ *Is reviewed annually.*

B. Organizational Plan
The physical therapy service has a written organizational plan.

The organizational plan:

▶ *Describes relationships among components within the physical therapy service and, where the service is part of a larger organization, between the service and the other components of that organization.*

▶ *Ensures that the service is directed by a physical therapist.*

▶ *Defines supervisory structures within the service.*

▶ *Reflects current personnel functions.*

C. Policies and Procedures
The physical therapy service has written policies and procedures that reflect the operation, mission, purposes, and goals of the service, and are consistent with the Association's positions, standards, guidelines, policies, procedures, and Code of Ethics.

The written policies and procedures:

▶ *Are reviewed regularly and revised as necessary.*

▶ *Meet the requirements of federal and state law and external agencies.*

▶ *Apply to, but are not limited to:*

  ■ *Care of patients/clients, including guidelines*

  ■ *Clinical education*

  ■ *Clinical research*

  ■ *Collaboration*

  ■ *Collection of patient data*

  ■ *Competency assessment*

  ■ *Criteria for access to care*

  ■ *Criteria for initiation and continuation of care*

- Criteria for referral to other appropriate health care providers
- Criteria for termination of care
- Documentation
- Environmental safety
- Equipment maintenance
- Fiscal management
- Improvement of quality of care and performance of services
- Infection control
- Job/position descriptions
- Medical emergencies
- Personnel-related policies
- Rights of patients/clients
- Staff orientation

D. Administration

A physical therapist is responsible for the direction of the physical therapy service.

The physical therapist responsible for the direction of the physical therapy service:

► *Ensures compliance with local, state, and federal requirements.*

► *Ensures compliance with current APTA documents, including Standards of Practice for Physical Therapy and the Criteria, Guide to Physical Therapist Practice, Code of Ethics, Guide for Professional Conduct, Standards of Ethical Conduct for the Physical Therapist Assistant, and Guide for Conduct of the Physical Therapist Assistant.*

► *Ensures that services are consistent with the mission, purposes, and goals of the physical therapy service.*

► *Ensures that services are provided in accordance with established policies and procedures.*

► *Ensures that the process for assignment and reassignment of physical therapist staff supports individual physical therapist responsibility to their patients and meets the needs of the patients/clients.*

► *Reviews and updates policies and procedures.*

► *Provides for training of physical therapy support personnel that ensures continued competence for their job description.*

► *Provides for continuous in-service training on safety issues and for periodic safety inspection of equipment by qualified individuals.*

E. Fiscal Management

The director of the physical therapy service, in consultation with physical therapy staff and appropriate administrative personnel, participates in planning for, and allocation of, resources. Fiscal planning and management of the service is based on sound accounting principles.

The fiscal management plan:

► *Includes a budget that provides for optimal use of resources.*

► *Ensures accurate recording and reporting of financial information.*

► *Ensures compliance with legal requirements.*

► *Allows for cost-effective utilization of resources.*

► *Uses a fee schedule that is consistent with the cost of physical therapy services and that is within customary norms of fairness and reasonableness.*

► *Considers option of providing pro bono services.*

F. Improvement of Quality of Care and Performance

The physical therapy service has a written plan for continuous improvement of quality of care and performance of services.

The improvement plan:

► *Provides evidence of ongoing review and evaluation of the physical therapy service.*

► *Provides a mechanism for documenting improvement in quality of care and performance.*

► *Is consistent with requirements of external agencies, as applicable.*

G. Staffing

The physical therapy personnel affiliated with the physical therapy service have demonstrated competence and are sufficient to achieve the mission, purposes, and goals of the service.

The physical therapy service:

► *Meets all legal requirements regarding licensure and certification of appropriate personnel.*

► *Ensures that the level of expertise within the service is appropriate to the needs of the patients/clients served.*

► *Provides appropriate professional and support personnel to meet the needs of the patient/client population.*

H. Staff Development

The physical therapy service has a written plan that provides for appropriate and ongoing staff development.

The staff development plan:

► *Includes self-assessment, individual goal setting, and organizational needs in directing continuing education and learning activities.*

► *Includes strategies for lifelong learning and professional and career development.*

► *Includes mechanisms to foster mentorship activities.*

► *Includes knowledge of clinical research methods and analysis.*

I. Physical Setting

The physical setting is designed to provide a safe and accessible environment that facilitates fulfillment of the mission, purposes, and goals of the physical therapy service. The equipment is safe and sufficient to achieve the purposes and goals of physical therapy.

The physical setting:

► *Meets all applicable legal requirements for health and safety.*

► *Meets space needs appropriate for the number and type of patients/clients served.*

The equipment:

- Meets all applicable legal requirements for health and safety.
- Is inspected routinely.

J. Collaboration
The physical therapy service collaborates with all disciplines as appropriate.

The collaboration when appropriate:

- Uses a team approach to the care of patients/clients.
- Provides instruction of patients/clients and families.
- Ensures professional development and continuing education.

III. PATIENT/CLIENT MANAGEMENT

A. Patient/Client Collaboration
Within the patient/client management process, the physical therapist and the patient/client establish and maintain an ongoing collaborative process of decision-making that exists throughout the provision of services.

B. Initial Examination/Evaluation/Diagnosis/Prognosis
The physical therapist performs an initial examination and evaluation to establish a diagnosis and prognosis prior to intervention.

The physical therapist examination:

- Is documented, dated, and appropriately authenticated by the physical therapist who performed it.
- Identifies the physical therapy needs of the patient/client.
- Incorporates appropriate tests and measures to facilitate outcome measurement.
- Produces data that are sufficient to allow evaluation, diagnosis, prognosis, and the establishment of a plan of care.
- May result in recommendations for additional services to meet the needs of the patient/client.

C. Plan of Care
The physical therapist establishes a plan of care and manages the needs of the patient/client based on the examination, evaluation, diagnosis, prognosis, goals, and outcomes of the planned interventions for identified impairments, functional limitations, and disabilities.

The physical therapist involves the patient/client and appropriate others in the planning, implementation, and assessment of the plan of care.

The physical therapist, in consultation with appropriate disciplines, plans for discharge of the patient/client, taking into consideration achievement of anticipated goals and expected outcomes, and provides for appropriate follow-up or referral.

The plan of care:

- Is based on the examination, evaluation, diagnosis, and prognosis.
- Identifies goals and outcomes.

- Describes the proposed intervention, including frequency and duration.
- Includes documentation that is dated and appropriately authenticated by the physical therapist who established the plan of care.

D. Intervention
The physical therapist provides, or directs and supervises, the physical therapy intervention consistent with the results of the examination, evaluation, diagnosis, prognosis, and plan of care.

The intervention:

- Is based on the examination, evaluation, diagnosis, prognosis, and plan of care.
- Is provided under the ongoing direction and supervision of the physical therapist.
- Is provided in such a way that directed and supervised responsibilities are commensurate with the qualifications and the legal limitations of the physical therapist assistant.
- Is altered in accordance with changes in response or status.
- Is provided at a level that is consistent with current physical therapy practice.
- Is interdisciplinary when necessary to meet the needs of the patient/client.
- Documentation of the intervention is consistent with the Guidelines: Physical Therapy Documentation of Patient/Client Management.
- Is dated and appropriately authenticated by the physical therapist or, when permissible by law, by the physical therapist assistant.

E. Reexamination
The physical therapist reexamines the patient/client as necessary during an episode of care to evaluate progress or change in patient/client status and modifies the plan of care accordingly or discontinues physical therapy services.

The physical therapist reexamination:

- Is documented, dated, and appropriately authenticated by the physical therapist who performs it.
- Includes modifications to the plan of care.

F. Discharge/Discontinuation of Intervention
The physical therapist discharges the patient/client from physical therapy services when the anticipated goals or expected outcomes for the patient/client have been achieved.

The physical therapist discontinues intervention when the patient/client is unable to continue to progress toward goals or when the physical therapist determines that the patient/client will no longer benefit from physical therapy.

Discharge documentation:

- Includes the status of the patient/client at discharge and the goals and outcomes attained.
- Is dated and appropriately authenticated by the physical therapist who performed the discharge.

- *Includes, when a patient/client is discharged prior to attainment of goals and outcomes, the status of the patient/client and the rationale for discontinuation.*

G. Communication/Coordination/Documentation

The physical therapist communicates, coordinates, and documents all aspects of patient/client management, including the results of the initial examination and evaluation, diagnosis, prognosis, plan of care, interventions, response to interventions, changes in patient/client status relative to the interventions, reexamination, and discharge/discontinuation of intervention and other patient/client management activities.

Physical therapist documentation:

- *Is dated and appropriately authenticated by the physical therapist who performed the examination and established the plan of care.*

- *Is dated and appropriately authenticated by the physical therapist who performed the intervention or, when allowable by law or regulations, by the physical therapist assistant who performed specific components of the intervention as selected by the supervising physical therapist.*

- *Is dated and appropriately authenticated by the physical therapist who performed the reexamination, and includes modifications to the plan of care.*

- *Is dated and appropriately authenticated by the physical therapist who performed the discharge, and includes the status of the patient/client and the goals and outcomes achieved.*

- *Includes, when a patient/client is discharged prior to achievement of goals and outcomes, the status of the patient/client and the rationale for discontinuation.*

- *As appropriate, records patient data using a method that allows collective analysis.*

IV. EDUCATION

The physical therapist is responsible for individual professional development. The physical therapist assistant is responsible for individual career development.

The physical therapist, and the physical therapist assistant, under the direction and supervision of the physical therapist, participate in the education of students.

The physical therapist educates and provides consultation to consumers and the general public regarding the purposes and benefits of physical therapy.

The physical therapist educates and provides consultation to consumers and the general public regarding the roles of the physical therapist and the physical therapist assistant.

The physical therapist:

- *Educates and provides consultation to consumers and the general public regarding the roles of the physical therapist, the physical therapist assistant, and other support personnel.*

V. RESEARCH

The physical therapist applies research findings to practice and encourages, participates in, and promotes activities that establish the outcomes of patient/client management provided by the physical therapist.

The physical therapist:

- *Ensures that their knowledge of research literature related to practice is current.*

- *Ensures that the rights of research subjects are protected, and the integrity of research is maintained.*

- *Participates in the research process as appropriate to individual education, experience, and expertise.*

- *Educates physical therapists, physical therapist assistants, students, other health professionals, and the general public about the outcomes of physical therapist practice.*

VI. COMMUNITY RESPONSIBILITY

The physical therapist demonstrates community responsibility by participating in community and community agency activities, educating the public, formulating public policy, or providing pro bono physical therapy services.

The physical therapist:

- *Participates in community and community agency activities.*

- *Educates the public, including prevention, education, and health promotion.*

- *Helps formulate public policy.*

- *Provides pro bono physical therapy services.*

Reprinted from [http://www.apta.org], with permission of the American Physical Therapy Association. © 2021 American Physical Therapy Association. All rights reserved.

Code of Ethics

APPENDIX E

CODE OF ETHICS HOD S06-09-07-12 [Amended HOD S06-00-12-23; HOD 06-91-05-05; HOD 06-87-11-17; HOD 06-81-06-18; HOD 06-78-06-08; HOD 06-78-06-07; HOD 06-77-18-30; HOD 06-77-17-27; Initial HOD 06-73-13-24] [Standard]

PREAMBLE

The *Code of Ethics for the Physical Therapist* (*Code of Ethics*) delineates the ethical obligations of all physical therapists as determined by the House of Delegates of the American Physical Therapy Association (APTA). The purposes of this *Code of Ethics* are to:

1. Define the ethical principles that form the foundation of physical therapist practice in patient/client management, consultation, education, research, and administration.

2. Provide standards of behavior and performance that form the basis of professional accountability to the public.

3. Provide guidance for physical therapists facing ethical challenges, regardless of their professional roles and responsibilities.

4. Educate physical therapists, students, other healthcare professionals, regulators, and the public regarding the core values, ethical principles, and standards that guide the professional conduct of the physical therapist.

5. Establish the standards by which the American Physical Therapy Association can determine if a physical therapist has engaged in unethical conduct.

No code of ethics is exhaustive, nor can it address every situation. Physical therapists are encouraged to seek additional advice or consultation in instances where the guidance of the *Code of Ethics* may not be definitive.

This *Code of Ethics* is built upon the five roles of the physical therapist (management of patients/clients, consultation, education, research, and administration), the core values of the profession, and the multiple realms of ethical action (individual, organizational, and societal). Physical therapist practice is guided by a set of seven core values: accountability, altruism, compassion/caring, excellence, integrity, professional duty, and social responsibility. Throughout the document, the primary core values that support specific principles are indicated in parentheses. Unless a specific role is indicated in the principle, the duties and obligations being delineated pertain to the five roles of the physical therapist. Fundamental to the *Code of Ethics* is the special obligation of physical therapists to empower, educate, and enable those with impairments, activity limitations, participation restrictions, and disabilities to facilitate greater independence, health, wellness, and enhanced quality of life.

PRINCIPLES

Principle #1: Physical therapists shall respect the inherent dignity and rights of all individuals.
(Core Values: Compassion, Integrity)

▶ 1A. Physical therapists shall act in a respectful manner toward each person regardless of age, gender, race, nationality, religion, ethnicity, social or economic status, sexual orientation, health condition, or disability.

▶ 1B. Physical therapists shall recognize their personal biases and shall not discriminate against others in physical therapist practice, consultation, education, research, and administration.

Principle #2: Physical therapists shall be trustworthy and compassionate in addressing the rights and needs of patients/clients.
(Core Values: Altruism, Compassion, Professional Duty)

▶ 2A. Physical therapists shall adhere to the core values of the profession and shall act in the best interests of patients/clients over the interests of the physical therapist.

▶ 2B. Physical therapists shall provide physical therapy services with compassionate and caring behaviors that incorporate the individual and cultural differences of patients/clients.

▶ 2C. Physical therapists shall provide the information necessary to allow patients or their surrogates to make informed decisions about physical therapy care or participation in clinical research.

▶ 2D. Physical therapists shall collaborate with patients/clients to empower them in decisions about their healthcare.

2E. Physical therapists shall protect confidential patient/client information and may disclose confidential information to appropriate authorities only when allowed or as required by law.

Principle #3: Physical therapists shall be accountable for making sound professional judgments.
(Core Values: Excellence, Integrity)

▶ 3A. Physical therapists shall demonstrate independent and objective professional judgment in the patient's/client's best interest in all practice settings.

▶ 3B. Physical therapists shall demonstrate professional judgment informed by professional standards, evidence (including current literature and established best practice), practitioner experience, and patient/client values.

▶ 3C. Physical therapists shall make judgments within their scope of practice and level of expertise and shall communicate with, collaborate with, or refer to peers or other healthcare professionals when necessary.

▶ 3D. Physical therapists shall not engage in conflicts of interest that interfere with professional judgment.

▶ 3E. Physical therapists shall provide appropriate direction of and communication with physical therapist assistants and support personnel.

Principle #4: Physical therapists shall demonstrate integrity in their relationships with patients/clients, families, colleagues, students, research participants, other healthcare providers, employers, payers, and the public.
(Core Value: Integrity)

▶ 4A. Physical therapists shall provide truthful, accurate, and relevant information and shall not make misleading representations.

▶ 4B. Physical therapists shall not exploit persons over whom they have supervisory, evaluative, or other authority (eg, patients/clients, students, supervisees, research participants, or employees).

▶ 4C. Physical therapists shall discourage misconduct by healthcare professionals and report illegal or unethical acts to the relevant authority, when appropriate.

▶ 4D. Physical therapists shall report suspected cases of abuse involving children or vulnerable adults to the appropriate authority, subject to law.

▶ 4E. Physical therapists shall not engage in any sexual relationship with any of their patients/clients, supervisees, or students.

▶ 4F. Physical therapists shall not harass anyone verbally, physically, emotionally, or sexually.

Principle #5: Physical therapists shall fulfill their legal and professional obligations.
(Core Values: Professional Duty, Accountability)

▶ 5A. Physical therapists shall comply with applicable local, state, and federal laws and regulations.

▶ 5B. Physical therapists shall have primary responsibility for supervision of physical therapist assistants and support personnel.

▶ 5C. Physical therapists involved in research shall abide by accepted standards governing protection of research participants.

▶ 5D. Physical therapists shall encourage colleagues with physical, psychological, or substance-related impairments that may adversely impact their professional responsibilities to seek assistance or counsel.

▶ 5E. Physical therapists who have knowledge that a colleague is unable to perform their professional responsibilities with reasonable skill and safety shall report this information to the appropriate authority.

▶ 5F. Physical therapists shall provide notice and information about alternatives for obtaining care in the event the physical therapist terminates the provider relationship while the patient/client continues to need physical therapy services.

Principle #6: Physical therapists shall enhance their expertise through the lifelong acquisition and refinement of knowledge, skills, abilities, and professional behaviors.
(Core Value: Excellence)

▶ 6A. Physical therapists shall achieve and maintain professional competence.

▶ 6B. Physical therapists shall take responsibility for their professional development based on critical self-assessment and reflection on changes in physical therapist practice, education, healthcare delivery, and technology.

▶ 6C. Physical therapists shall evaluate the strength of evidence and applicability of content presented during professional development activities before integrating the content or techniques into practice.

▶ 6D. Physical therapists shall cultivate practice environments that support professional development, lifelong learning, and excellence.

Principle #7: Physical therapists shall promote organizational behaviors and business practices that benefit patients/clients and society.
(Core Values: Integrity, Accountability)

▶ 7A. Physical therapists shall promote practice environments that support autonomous and accountable professional judgments.

▶ 7B. Physical therapists shall seek remuneration as is deserved and reasonable for physical therapist services.

▶ 7C. Physical therapists shall not accept gifts or other considerations that influence or give an appearance of influencing their professional judgment.

▶ 7D. Physical therapists shall fully disclose any financial interest they have in products or services that they recommend to patients/clients.

▶ 7E. Physical therapists shall be aware of charges and shall ensure that documentation and coding for physical therapy services accurately reflect the nature and extent of the services provided.

▶ 7F. Physical therapists shall refrain from employment arrangements, or other arrangements, that prevent physical therapists from fulfilling professional obligations to patients/clients.

Principle #8: Physical therapists shall participate in efforts to meet the health needs of people locally, nationally, or globally.
(Core Values: Social Responsibility)

▶ 8A. Physical therapists shall provide pro bono physical therapy services or support organizations that meet the health needs of people who are economically disadvantaged, uninsured, and underinsured.

▶ 8B. Physical therapists shall advocate to reduce health disparities and healthcare inequities, improve access to healthcare services, and address the health, wellness, and preventive healthcare needs of people.

▶ 8C. Physical therapists shall be responsible stewards of healthcare resources and shall avoid overutilization or underutilization of physical therapy services.

▶ 8D. Physical therapists shall educate members of the public about the benefits of physical therapy and the unique role of the physical therapist.

Index

Note: Page numbers followed by *b, f,* and *t* indicate boxes, tables, and figures, respectively.